Primer on the Rheumatic Diseases
Eighth Edition

Library of Congress Cataloging in Publication Data

Main entry under title:

Primer on the rheumatic diseases. Eighth edition.

Includes bibliographical references and index.
1. Rheumatism. I. Rodnan, Gerald P., 1927–
II. Schumacher, H. Ralph. III. Arthritis Foundation.
[DNLM: 1. Rheumatism. 2. Arthritis. WE 344 P953]
RC927.P67 1983   616.7′23   83-7107

Published by the Arthritis Foundation, Atlanta, Georgia. All rights reserved. No part of this book may be reproduced, stored in a retrieval system, or transmitted in any form or by any means, electronic, mechanical, photocopying, recording, or otherwise, without written permission of the publisher. Printed in the United States of America by William Byrd Press, Richmond, Virginia.

Designed by Maureen Stephens

Production staff: Jerelyn Jordan and Maureen Stephens

Printing 10 9 8 7 6 5 4

Arthritis Foundation catalog number 3250. ISBN 0-912423-00-5

Primer on the Rheumatic Diseases

Eighth Edition

Editors: Gerald P. Rodnan, MD and H. Ralph Schumacher, MD
Associate Editor: Nathan J. Zvaifler, MD

Published by the Arthritis Foundation, Atlanta GA

Contributors

The following people contributed to this edition of the Primer on the Rheumatic Diseases by writing sections, reviewing material, or otherwise giving invaluable aid and assistance (credits for illustrations are given in figure captions):

Mrs Henrietta Aladjem
Dr Donato Alarcon-Segovia
Dr Frank Arnett
Dr William J Arnold
Dr Gene V Ball
Dr John Baum
Dr Thomas G Benedek
Dr J Claude Bennett
Dr Rodney Bluestone
Dr Kenneth Brandt
Dr W Watson Buchanan
Dr RB Buckingham
Dr Eric GL Bywaters
Dr John J Calabro
Dr Andrei Calin
Mr Clifford Clarke
Dr Alan S Cohen
Dr JJ Combs, Jr
Dr Joseph Croft
Dr William A D'Angelo
Dr John S Davis IV
Dr John L Decker
Prof Florian Delbarre
Dr Bonnie Dorwart
Dr Richard H Ferguson
Dr Edward C Franklin†
Dr IL Freeman
Dr Osvaldo Garcia-Morteo
Dr Edward Goetzl
Dr Donald L Goldenberg
Dr Duncan A Gordon
Dr Bevra H Hahn
Dr Barry Handwerger
Dr Virgil Hanson
Ms Barbara Hapoienu
Dr Edward D Harris, Jr
Dr Evelyn Hess
Dr Gene G Hunder

Dr Edward C Huskisson
Dr Stephania Jablonska
Dr Hugo E Jasin
Dr Malcolm IV Jayson
Dr Sergio Jimenez
Dr Heljo Julkunen
Dr Warren Katz
Dr William N Kelley
Dr Alan Kirsner
Dr James R Klinenberg
Dr John Klippel
Dr Stephen M Krane
Prof Veikko Laine
Dr Ossi Laitinen
Dr E Carwile LeRoy
Dr Jack Lichtenstein
Dr Peter Lipsky
Dr Robert Lisak
Dr Stephen E Malawista
Dr Henry J Mankin
Dr William Martel
Dr Alfonse T Masi
Dr Daniel J McCarty, Jr
Dr Frederic C McDuffie
Dr Dennis J McShane
Dr Thomas A Medsger, Jr
Dr Ronald P Messner
Dr Roland W Moskowitz
Dr Allen Myers
Prof Valentina Nassonova
Dr David H Neustadt
Dr Desmond J O'Duffy
Dr Carl M Pearson†
Dr Robert H Persellin
Dr Paulding Phelps
Dr Robert S Pinals
Dr Paul H Plotz
Dr Howard F Polley

Dr Mordechai Pras
Dr Eric L Radin
Dr Donald Resnick
Dr Dwight Robinson
Dr RG Robinson
Dr Gerald P Rodnan
Dr Lawrence R Rosenberg
Dr Jaime Rotés-Querol
Dr Naomi Rothfield
Dr Emmanuel Rudd
Dr Shaun Ruddy
Prof Satoshi Sasaki
Dr Jane Schaller
Dr H Ralph Schumacher, Jr
Dr Peter H Schur
Dr James T Scott
Prof Hilton Seda
Dr Gordon C Sharp
Dr Robert P Sheon
Dr Tamotsu Shimizu†
Prof Stefan Sitaj
Dr Clement B Sledge
Dr Hugh A Smythe
Dr Allen C Steere
Dr Alfred Steinberg
Dr Ivan Stojanovic
Dr Robert L Swezey
Dr Norman Talal
Dr George Thompson
Dr Stanley L Wallace
Dr Gerald Weissmann
Dr Ralph Williams
Dr John Winfield
Dr Alan Winkelstein
Dr Verna Wright
Dr Jack Zuckner
Dr Nathan Zvaifler
† Deceased.

Contents

Introduction

This is the eighth edition of the *Primer on the Rheumatic Diseases* (Primer-8). The *Primer* is descended from two publications of the American Committee for the Control of Rheumatism, an early forebear of the American Rheumatism Association (ARA) (1,2). The first of these—*What is Rheumatism?*—was issued in 1928; the second, *Rheumatism Primer: Chronic Arthritis,* was privately distributed in 1932 (1).

The next publication in this line, entitled *Primer on Rheumatism, Chronic Arthritis,* was put forth in 1934 by the American Committee for the Control of Rheumatism, immediate predecessor of the ARA. This work, generally considered the first of the *Primers,* consisted of a brochure that had been prepared for distribution in connection with a scientific exhibit on arthritis at the Annual Convention of the American Medical Association (1). A revision of this abecedarium, identified by its authors as the "Second Primer on Arthritis" appeared in the *Journal of the American Medical Association* in 1942 under the title *Primer on Arthritis* (3). The third through the seventh editions of the *Primer,* also published in the *Journal of the American Medical Association,* appeared in 1949 (3rd), 1953 (4th), 1959 (5th), 1964 (6th), and 1973 (7th) (4–8).

The *Primer* is widely used in teaching programs throughout this country and in a number of countries abroad. More than 250,000 copies of the seventh edition were provided to medical schools and hospitals by the Arthritis Foundation for distribution to students and house officers.

The chief purpose of the present edition of the *Primer* remains the same as that of previous versions—to provide a reasonably thorough yet concise description of the rheumatic diseases, with particular emphasis on clinical manifestations, pathogenesis, diagnosis, and management. The period that has elapsed since the appearance of the seventh edition (1973) has been one of vigorous worldwide research that has yielded a wealth of new information concerning the rheumatic diseases.

The new *Primer* has been completely rewritten. Many sections have been added. Attention is given to a number of newly recognized rheumatic disorders, including eosinophilic fasciitis, mixed connective tissue disease, yersinial arthritis, Lyme disease, apatite deposition disease, and the arthropathy associated with intestinal bypass. Lastly, there are new appendices of criteria dealing with the determination of remission in rheumatoid arthritis and the classification of rheumatic diseases of childhood, systemic lupus erythematosus, progressive systemic sclerosis (scleroderma), gouty arthritis, and finally, the Uniform Database for rheumatic diseases.

In recognition of the worldwide scope of clinical activity and research in rheumatology and in order to enhance the potential usefulness of the *Primer* as an international teaching document, the new edition contains a record high number of contributions from foreign rheumatologists. These individuals are Dr. Stephania Jablonska, Warsaw, Poland; Dr. Satoshi Sasaki, Tokyo, Japan; Dr. Donato Alarcon-Segovia, Mexico City, Mexico; Dr. W Watson Buchanan, Hamilton, Canada; Dr. Verna Wright, Leeds, UK; Dr. Heljo Julkunen and Dr. Ossi Laitinen, Helsinki, Finland; Dr. Eric GL Bywaters, London, UK; Dr. Tamotsu Shimizu, Tokyo, Japan; Dr. Mordechai Pras, Tel Hashomer, Israel; Dr. Stefan Sitaj, Piestany, Czechoslovakia; Dr. Hugh A Smythe, Toronto, Canada; Dr. Malcolm IV Jayson, Salford, UK; Dr. Duncan A Gordon, Toronto, Canada; and Dr. Edward C Huskisson, London, UK.

Furthermore, the editors sought and obtained the generous assistance of a distinguished panel of foreign authorities in reviewing particular sections of *Primer-8.* The individuals who thus served as corresponding editors were Dr. Donato Alarcon-Segovia, Mexico City; Prof. Florian Delbarre, Paris; Dr. Osvaldo Garcia-Morteo, Buenos Aires; Dr. Duncan A Gordon, Toronto; Prof. Veikko Laine, Heinola; Prof. Valentina Nassonova, Moscow; Dr. RG Robinson, Lane Cove, Australia; Dr. Jaime Rotés-Querol, Barcelona; Prof. Satoshi Sasaki, Tokyo; Dr. James T Scott, London; Prof. Hilton Seda, Rio de Janiero; and Dr. Ivan Stojanovic, Belgrade.

1. Stecher RM: The American Rheumatism Association—its origins, development and maturity. Arthritis Rheum 1:4–19, 1958
2. Rodnan GP: Growth and development of rheumatology in the United States: a bicentennial report. Arthritis Rheum 20:1149–1168, 1977
3. Jordan EP, et al: Primer on Arthritis. JAMA 119:1089–1104, 1942
4. McEwen C, et al: Primer on the Rheumatic Diseases. JAMA 139:1068–1076, 1139–1146, 1268–1273, 1949
5. Ragan C, et al: Primer on the Rheumatic Diseases. JAMA 152:323–331, 405–414, 522–531, 1953
6. Crain DC, et al: Primer on the Rheumatic Diseases. JAMA 171:1205–1220, 1345–1356, 1680–1691, 1959
7. Decker JL, et al: Primer on the Rheumatic Diseases. JAMA 190:127–140, 425–444, 509–530, 741–751, 1964
8. Rodnan GP, et al: Primer on the Rheumatic Diseases. JAMA 224:661–812, 1973

1. History of the rheumatic diseases

The term *rheuma* belongs to the humoral theory of disease causation and is first encountered in the portion of the Hippocratic corpus, *On the Locations in the Human Body* (4th century BC). Rheuma literally meant flowing and the ancient Greeks used it interchangeably with the even earlier term catarrhos, flowing down. The source of these humors was believed to be the brain. In the 13th century, an analogous term began to be used to refer to the flowing of gouty humor. This was "gutta" (Latin: a drop) from which gout was derived.

The association of rheumatism with joint ailments originated with the Parisian physician Guillaume Baillou (Ballonius, 1558–1616), who propounded the idea in a posthumously published work, *The Book on Rheumatism and Back Pain* (1642). Baillou's concept of rheumatism remained that of a noxious humor (which he sought to distinguish from catarrh) that was not limited to musculoskeletal symptoms. He wrote picturesquely that "one may designate the condition we are considering inexactly as rheumatism, better as a sort of precipitation like a seasickness of the vessels (which vomit), until better terms offer themselves."

Care must be exercised not to overinterpret the sketchy descriptions of most of the older authors. For centuries "gout" or "gouty diathesis" was used as non-specifically as "arthritis" is used today. Credit for being the first to isolate individual specific diseases from the mix of rheumatic disorders belongs to Thomas Sydenham (1624–1689). Himself a victim of gout, he clearly distinguished an acute febrile polyarthritis,"chiefly attacking the young and vigorous," from gout. Most of the description is compatible with acute rheumatic fever, but it also touches on a chronic phase, perhaps rheumatoid arthritis, in which the patient may become "a cripple to the day of his death and wholly lose the use of his limbs whilst the knuckles of his fingers shall become knotty and protuberant." Beside his description of gout (1683) and acute rheumatism (1685), Sydenham described St. Vitus' dance (Sydenham's chorea, 1686), and in his discussion of *Hysteric Diseases* (1681) may have described fibrositis.

Some authors at the beginning of the 19th century realized how little progress had been made in distinguishing discrete diseases. For example, William Heberden (1710–1801) wrote: "The rheumatism is a common name for many aches and pains, which have yet got no peculiar appellation, though owing to very different causes. It is besides often hard to be distinguished from some, which have a certain name and class assigned them."

Gout. "Gutta" in medieval medicine was a synonym for podagra. It meant a drop resulting from "a defluxion of the humors." The term podagra was employed if the foot was affected, chiragra if the wrist, gonagra if the knee, etc. Despite the venerable history of gout, little of significance was learned between the 4th century BC and the end of the 18th century. Two concepts prevailed throughout the 2 millenia: that the disease occurs predominantly in sexually mature men, as pointed out by Hippocrates and that gustatory and sexual excesses predispose to its acute attacks. A huge folklore derived from these beliefs.

Antonj van Leeuwenhoek (1632–1723) described the microscopic appearance of urate crystals from a tophus (1684, Delft). Nearly a century later in 1776, Carl Wilhelm Scheele (1742–1786) demonstrated that urinary stones were composed of a hitherto unknown organic acid, originally called lithic acid, and renamed acide ourique in 1798. Lithic acid was also found to be a constituent of normal urine.

In 1797 at Cambridge, William H Wollaston (1766–1828) reported that the principal constituent of gouty tophi was a "neutral compound consisting of lithic (i.e., uric) acid and mineral alkali." A half century passed before uric acid was shown to be even more intimately related to gout.

Alfred B Garrod (1819–1909) analyzed the serum of a gouty man by a laborious gravimetric method in which uric acid was identified by its color reaction with ammonium purpurate (Murexide) (1847, London). He found that "1000 grains of serum gave of uric acid 0.050 grain," i.e., 5 mg/dl. Uric acid was barely detectable in the serum of healthy persons, but was found regularly in patients with gout or renal failure. Garrod, who was the first to demonstrate the connection of gout with hyperuricemia, concluded by asking rhetorically, "Might it not, in doubtful cases, be possible to determine the nature of the affliction from an examination of the blood?" Garrod also found urate in tophaceous deposits in subcutaneous tissue and articular cartilage. He hypothesized that gout might result either from a loss of the renal excretory capacity or from increased formation of uric acid, concepts which were proved correct the century after the appearance of Garrod's great monograph on the gout (1859). In 1876 he postulated that acute gout results from the precipitation of sodium urate in a joint or adjacent tissue.

In 1854 Garrod reported that when acidified serum of gouty perons is evaporated, crystals of uric acid precipitate on a thread immersed in the serum. Several other gravimetric methods were devised in efforts to improve the sensitivity of the analysis before Otto Folin and W Denis (1912, Boston) developed the first colorimetric assay for uric acid. Numerous procedures based on colorimetry followed before E Praetorius and H Poulsen (1953, Copenhagen) published a specific enzymatic spectrophotometric technique.

Max Freudweiler (1871–1901), a trainee in the laboratory of Wilheim His, induced acute inflammation experimentally by injecting microcrystalline sodium urate subcutaneously (1899, Leipzig). This forgotten observation was confirmed independently in 1962 with intraarticular injections by Joseph Hollander and Daniel J McCarty, Jr (Phildelphia) and JE Seegmiller (Bethesda) and their respective collaborators.

Rheumatic fever. Although Hippocrates mentioned an acute, migratory arthritis of young people, no definite contributions to the delineation of rheumatic fever were made until the writing of Sydenham (1665), and more than a century passed before further elucidation of "acute rheumatism" began. David Dundas (1808, London) published a good description of heart failure in patients with acute rheumatism and therein appears to have been the first to use the term rheumatic fever. He concluded that "The knowledge that this [heart] disease is always the consequence of, or is connected with, rheumatic affection, points out the necessity of attending to the translation of rheumatism to the chest."

Both Matthew Baillie (1761–1823) and William C Wells (1757–1817) gave credit to David Pitcairn (1749–1809) for first having noted "that persons subject to rheumatism were attacked more frequently than others with symptoms of an organic disease of the heart" (1788, unpublished). Baillie, in his pathology text of 1797 noted "an ossification or thickening of some heart valves" of patients who had suffered from acute rheumatism. Wells (1810, London) confirmed the clinical findings of Dundas and added the description of subcutaneous nodules. Jean-Baptiste Bouillaud (1796–1881) concluded that "In the great majority of cases of acute articular rheumatism with fever, there exists in a variable degree a rheumatism of the serofibrinous tissue of the heart..." (1840, Paris), an observation that became known as the law of coincidence. Ludwig Aschoff (1866–1942) described the myocardial granuloma which came to be considered characteristic of rheumatic carditis (1904, Marburg).

Chorea, from the Greek for dance, was introduced as a medical term by Paracelsus (1493–1541). Sydenham in 1686 unmistakably described, under the designation of St. Vitus' dance, the type of chorea that is now associated with his name. Richard Bright (1789–1858) seems to have been the first to associate this behavior with rheumatic fever (1831, London), a suggestion that George See (1818–1896) substantiated with an epidemiologic study (1850, Paris).

JK Fowler in 1880 reported that tonsillitis is a common precursor of rheumatic fever. He had had this experience himself and had been a patient of AB Garrod who had told him that he had noticed the association. Although Frederick J Poynton (1869–1943) and Alexander Paine isolated a streptococcus from the tonsils of a patient with rheumatic fever in 1900, this was only one of several bacteria implicated as pathogens. HF Swift (1881–1953) et al advanced the theory that the pathogenesis of rheumatic fever can be explained by the development of hypersensitivity to streptococci: "When under suitable circumstances streptococci or products of streptococci are disseminated to the tissues, these tissues over-react and the characteristic picture of the disease results," (1928, New York).

The epidemiologic work of Alvin F Coburn (1899–1976) in the United States and of WR Collis in England (1900—), both published in 1931, led to the final identification of the beta hemolytic streptococcus as the initiator of the process which Swift had suggested.

Rheumatoid arthritis. Credit for the first description of rheumatoid arthritis is usually given to AJ Landré-Beavais (1772–1840) who, in his Paris thesis of 1800 described 9 women who had a disease that he considered to be a variation of gout and therefore called "goute asthenique primitive." He believed that this diease occurred in people with a "primary weakness" and that it was associated with poverty, while true gout occurred in affluent persons who were generally robust. Some have suggested that changes in the hands in several of the oil paintings of Peter Paul Reubens (1577–1640), himself a victim of arthritis, could be evidence that rheumatoid arthritis may have existed long before the account of Landré-Beauvais.

Benjamine C Brodie (1783–1862) described rheumatoid arthritis clearly (1819, London). He pointed out its typically slow progression and that not only joints, but bursae and tendon sheaths may be affected. His most important contribution was the recognition that the disease begins as a synovitis which may secondarily lead to deterioration of articular cartilage.

Jean-Martin Charcot (1825–1893) made excellent clinical distinctions between gout, rheumatic fever, rheumatoid arthritis, and osteoarthritis, but felt that "It is quite impossible to make an actual distinction between the various forms of rheumatism, but on the contrary, it is frequently

possible to show that they all proceed from one and the same cause." He perpetuated Landré-Beauvais' sociologic error, but may have been the first to recognize that rheumatoid arthritis is not a rare disease. He wrote (1867): "While gout is almost unknown in the Salpetriére, chronic rheumatism is, on the contrary, one of the commonest infirmities in this institution; and indeed, this disease prevails among women and among the least-favored classes of society. In this way the proportion of patients admitted to the hospital for this kind of lesion is about one-fifteenth of the total number of inmates."

AB Garrod coined the term rheumatoid arthritis in 1858. He wrote in 1892: "The study of articular affections some thirty years ago led me to the conclusion that the majority of cases then called 'rheumatic gout' were related neither to true gout nor true rheumatism, and that they had an independent pathology of their own; and if such is the case, the term 'rheumatoid gout' was doubly wrong . . . I propose the name of 'rheumatoid arthritis'—a name which does not imply any error, but assumes the disease to be an arthritic or joint disease having some of the external characters of rheumatism . . . Arthritis deformans [Rudolf L.K. Virchow, (1821–1902), 1869] has been applied to the malady, and this again is not an erroneous name, though in the earlier stages of the disease it is by no means a characteristic one. The term 'rheumatic arthritis' is nearly, or at least half, as bad as that of 'rheumatic gout,' as it implies the existence of one error instead of two."

Nosologic conflicts continued even after the British Ministry of Health in 1922 adopted rheumatoid arthritis as the official designation, a step which the American Rheumatism Association did not take until 1941.

The first roentgenogram of joints affected by rheumatoid arthritis was published by GA Bannatyne (1896, London). Joel E Goldthwait (1866–1961) attempted to differentiate rheumatoid arthritis from osteoarthritis (which he designated *atrophic* and *hypertrophic* arthritis, respectively) by roentgenographic criteria (1904, Boston).

The discovery of **rheumatoid factor** ultimately began with the hypothesis of Frank Billings (1854–1932) that rheumatoid arthritis is a response to various chronic focal infections (1912, Chicago). By 1929 from bacteriologic research stimulated by this hypothesis, Russell L Cecil (1881–1965) et al (New York) had concluded that rheumatoid arthritis "is a streptococcal infection, caused in a large proportion of cases by a biologically specific strain of this organism." They believed that they had cultured this streptococcus from the blood or joints of many patients with rheumatoid arthritis and could agglutinate suspensions of the bacteria with sera from

94% of their patients with this disorder. The nonspecificity of this finding was shown by Martin H Dawson (1897–1945) who noted that rheumatoid serum agglutinated other micro-organisms in addition to streptococci (1932, New York).

E Waaler (1940, Oslo), while studying complement fixation, observed that sheep erythrocytes to which rabbit anti-sheep cell serum had been added were agglutinated by some rheumatoid sera. This observation was not pursued and was unknown in the laboratory of Harry Rose (New York), where serologic studies of a Q fever epidemic in New York were being done. Elizabeth Pearce, a technician who had rheumatoid arthritis, used her own serum in a test and found that it agglutinated sheep erythrocytes in high titer. From this observation, Rose and Charles A Ragan (1911–1976) developed in 1948 the sensitized sheep erythrocyte agglutination reaction as a diagnostic procedure. Numerous modifications, including the use of a variety of agglutinating reagents, have been devised to improve the specificity and sensitivity. Jacques M Singer and Charles M Plotz (1956, New York) devised the technique in which a suspension of polystyrene latex particles coated with human gamma globulin is used.

Juvenile chronic polyarthritis. Although the report of George F Still (1868–1941) about "a form of chronic joint disease in children" was antedated by several brief descriptions, his was the first detailed investigation devoted to this subject (1897, London). Still described 12 children who had a polyarthritis which he concluded should be distinguished from rheumatoid arthritis and another 6 children with a disease that was clinically indistinguishable from adult rheumatoid arthritis. The distinctive findings in the first group included generalized lymphadenopathy and splenomegaly, the frequent occurrence of pericarditis, and an unusual predilection for cervical spine involvement. Still also pointed out the febrile component of the disease and the tendency toward growth retardation. Eric GL Bywaters has found that the rash which is characteristic of this disease was recorded on the charts of some of these patients, even though Still neglected to include this finding in his report.

Ankylosing spondylitis. The first clinical report of ankylosing spondylitis (1831) concerned a man from the Isle of Man and the first female patient was described in 1856 in Baltimore. Interest in the disease was stimulated by a series of publications (1893–1899) by Vladimir von Bechterew (1857–1927) in St. Petersburg, Russia. The first patients he described were a woman and 2 of her daughters, and he hypothesized that the principal etiologic factors were a hereditary predisposition and trauma, and that the symptoms result from a myelopathy. Adolf Strümpell (1853–1926;

1897, Erlangen) and Pierre Marie (1853–1940; 1898, Paris) disagreed and considered spondylitis to be a rheumatic disease in which neither trauma nor heredity are of pathogenetic importance.

The earliest roentgenographic examination was published by Valentini in 1899 (Danzig). This study was limited to the lower cervical and upper thoracic region, but syndesmophytes were recognized. Despite numerous publications concerning roentgenographic changes in this disorder, the characteristic obliteration of the sacroiliac joints was not described until 1934 (W Krebs, Aachen).

The occurrence of iritis in patients with ankylosing spondylitis was mentioned by Bechterew (1893) and E Fraenkel (1904, Hamburg). However, the likelihood that this is a manifestation of the disease was first suggested by German opthalmologists (E Kunz and E Kraupa) in 1933.

The first study of heart disease in ankylosing spondylitis included 6 patients with aortic insufficiency, but the findings were attributed to antecedent rheumatic fever (1949, Lilli Bernstein and OJ Broch, Oslo). Attention was serendipitously called to the association between this arthropathy and aortic insufficiency in 1956 when the first 100 patients with aortic insufficiency into whom Charles A Hufnagel (Washington, DC) had inserted a prosthetic aortic valve were reviewed. Five were found to have ankylosing spondylitis, a frequency which was recognized to be far greater than could be attributed to chance. The first adequate pathologic study of the valvular lesion was reported by William S Clark et al (1957, Boston).

The epidemiologic evidence of a heritable predisposition to the development of ankylosing spondylitis led Lee Schlosstein et al (Los Angeles) and Derek Brewerton et al (London) to evaluate the HLA antigens of patients with this disease. In 1973 they reported that 96% and 88% of their subjects, respectively, carried the antigen that is now designated HLA-B27, which occurs in 4–8% of the white population. The finding of such a strong association opened the floodgates on studies of the relationship of histocompatibility antigens to the various rheumatic diseases. The 1963 decision of the American Rheumatism Association to adopt the term ankylosing spondylitis in preference to rheumatoid spondylitis has been supported by the lack of an association between HLA phenotypes of patients with rheumatoid arthritis and spondylitis.

Osteoarthritis. The term osteoarthritis was introduced by JK Spender (1886, Bath) in preference to rheumatoid arthritis and not to designate the disease or diseases to which it is now applied. The modern usage and the clinical differentiation from rheumatoid arthritis were established by Archibald E Garrod (1857–1936; 1907, London). Aside from the older age of onset of osteoarthritis, Garrod was impressed by an even stronger female predominance than that which he had found with rheumatoid arthritis, as well as a heritable tendency. He was unable to make consistent distinctions, however.

With the description of "generalized osteoarthritis" by Jonas H Kellgren (1952, Manchester), similarities to rheumatoid arthritis again have come under consideration. The first differentiation was made by William Heberden (published 1802), who distinguished nodosities on the fingers from tophi. His topographic description clearly identified "Heberden's nodes." In 1805 John Haygarth (1740–1827) described nodosities which occur mainly in women after menopause. It is unclear what he was describing since less than one-fifth of the nodes of his patients were on fingers. In 1884 CJ Bouchard (1837–1915) described nodes adjacent to the proximal interphalangeal joints that are identical to those at the distal interphalangeal joints. AE Garrod related Heberden's nodes to osteoarthritis. Robert M Stecher (1896–1972) demonstrated the strong genetic predisposition and female dominance of the nodes, but questioned their relationship with other varieties of osteoarthritis (1944, Cleveland).

Lupus erythematosus. Ferdinand von Hebra (1816–1880) described an eruption that occurs "mainly on the face, on the cheeks and nose in a distribution not dissimilar to a butterfly" (1845, Vienna). Lupus érythémateux was the designation introduced by Pierre Louis Alphée Cazenave (1795–1877) for a skin disease that was probably discoid lupus erythematosus (1851, Paris). The latter term was used by Moritz Kaposi (1837–1902) to distinguish between different skin manifestations, but not to differentiate these from a visceral disease (1872, Vienna). Many of the visceral features of systemic lupus erythematosus were first described by William Osler (1849–1919) under the name exudative erythema (1895–1904, Baltimore).

Emanual Libman (1872–1946) and Benjamin Sacks (1896—) added nonrheumatic, atypical verrucous endocarditis to the syndrome (1924, New York). George Baehr et al (1887–1978) published a study that included 23 autopsied cases, the largest series to that time, and described the exacerbating effect of solar exposure and the "wire loop" glomerular lesions (1935, New York).

The association of biologic false positive serologic tests for syphilis was pointed out by H Keil (1940, New York) and by AF Coburn and DH Moore (1943, Baltimore). This reaction was studied systematically by J Earle Moore (1892–1957) et al (1940–1957, Baltimore).

The LE cell phenomenon, which was initially demonstrated with bone marrow aspirates, was described by Malcolm M Hargraves et al (1948, Rochester, MN).

This gave great impetus to both case finding and clinical investigations. P Miescher and M Fauconnet (1956, Lausanne) observed that the factor which induces LE cells can be absorbed from serum by exposure to isolated cell nuclei and therefore suggested that the LE cell factor is an antinuclear antibody. The detection of antinuclear antibodies by fluorescent anti-human globulin was described by George Friou (1958, West Haven, CT).

"Diffuse collagen disease" was introduced by Paul Klemperer et al (1887–1964) who applied the term to certain "acute and chronic maladies which are characterized anatomically by generalized alterations of the connective tissue, particularly by abnormalities of its extracellular components," (1942, New York). The idea that the histopathologic changes found in rheumatic fever and rheumatoid arthritis reflected a disturbance in the connective tissue system had first been proposed by F Klinge in his pathology studies of rheumatic fever (1933, Leipzig). The hypothesis of Klemperer et al that certain diseases including systemic lupus erythematosus and progressive systemic sclerosis primarily affect "the connective tissues considered as a colloid system" gained rapid acceptance and the concept of "collagen diseases" (now designated more accurately as connective tissue disorders) did much to call attention to this group of disorders.

Progressive systemic sclerosis. No unequivocal descriptions of scleroderma exist before the reports of WD Chowne (1842, London) and James Startin (1846, London). Several cases were described by French clinicians in 1847 and the term sclérodermie suggested by E Gintrac (1791–1877) of Bordeaux. The term "skleroderma" had been introduced in 1836 by GB Fantonetti (1791–1861), an Italian physician, to describe an uncertain dermatosis. The case reported by Carlo Curzio (1753, Naples) probably was an instance of the self-limited disease, scleredema, which was defined by Abraham Buschke (1868–1943; 1900, Berlin). Heinrich Auspitz (1835–1886) described death due to renal failure with probable hypertension (1863, Vienna). This was not recognized as more than a chance association until 1952 (H Moore and H Sheehan, Liverpool).

Maurice Raynaud (1834–1881) described the phenomenon which bears his name in 1862 (Paris) and commented on the occurrence of this phenomenon in a patient with systemic sclerosis in 1863. It was Jonathan Hutchinson (1828–1913) who pointed out the consistent association of Raynaud's phenomenon with progressive systemic sclerosis (PSS) (1899, London).

Calcinosis was described in 1878 by H Weber, a Swiss physician, and was clearly related to scleroderma by Georges Thibierge and RJ Weissenbach (1910, Paris). Albrecht von Notthafft (1899, Munich) described parenchymatous and vascular pulmonary fibrosis. Salomon Ehrmann (1903, Vienna) suggested that dysphagia was due to the occurrence in the esophagus of the same process as in the skin, and Rudolf Schmidt (1916, Prague) demonstrated the typical roentgenographic changes.

Despite several descriptions of myocardial fibrosis, beginning with that of CF Westphal (1833–1890; 1876, Berlin), this form of heart disease was not established as a manifestation of PSS until the work of Soma Weiss (1899–1942) et al (1943, Boston). In view of the extensive evidence of visceral involvement in this disease, RH Goetz (1945, Capetown) proposed the term progressive systemic sclerosis as more descriptive than scleroderma.

Polymyositis. Ernst L Wagner (1829–1888) first used the term polymyositis (1886, Leipzig). Heinrich Unverricht (1858–1912) in 1891 introduced the title dermatomyositis in a description of a case. The association between dermatomyositis and cancer was first described by Rudolf Bezecny (1935, Prague). The more impressive of 2 patients was a woman who underwent resection of an ovarian carcinoma. Despite peritoneal metastases, her skin began to revert toward normal a few days later, and the myopathy improved during the subsequent roentgen therapy.

Polyarteritides. From the earliest descriptions of polyarteritis to the present, both the etiology and the number of subdivisions that may be valid on clinical or pathologic grounds have remained in dispute. The first certain case was described by Karl Rokitansky (1804–1878) in a general study of arterial aneurysms (1852, Vienna). This case was in part reexamined microscopically by Hans Eppinger (1846–1916); 1887, Graz). Adolf Kussmaul (1822–1902) and Rudolf Maier (1824–1888) published a report of a case with autopsy findings (1866, Freiburg) and called the disease periarteritis nodosa because of the presence of aneurysmal dilatations in most of the medium and smaller arteries. Enrico Ferrari (1903, Trieste) introduced the term polyarteritis nodosa describing a patient with severe arteritis without aneurysms.

Giant cell arteritis was described by Jonathan Hutchinson (1890) and rediscovered by Bayard T Horton (1895—) et al as "arteritis of the temporal vessels," (1934, Rochester, MN). Heinz Klinger (1931, Berlin) reported another restricted form of arteritis, which was described in greater detail by F Wegener (1936–1939, Breslau) and is now called Wegener's granulomatosis. Jacob Churg and Lotte Strauss (1951, New York) described allergic granulomatosis, a variant characterized clinically by bronchospasm and eosinophilia.

Gonococcal arthritis and Reiter's disease. The early history of gonococcal arthritis and of Reiter's disease must be considered together because, prior to the discovery of the gonococcus by Albert Neisser (1855–1914; 1879, Breslau), it would have been impossible to differentiate the 2 diseases. The association between arthritis and urethritis (blenorrhagia) was first described by FX Swediaur (1748–1826; 1784, Paris). By 1883 when LM Petrone (Bologna) demonstrated gonocci in urethral exudates and synovial aspirates of 2 men, the disease was well known. The culture of gonocci from synovial fluid was first accomplished in an infant by Heinrich Höck (1893, Vienna) and in the following year in an adult by Neisser. The unity of gonococcal urethritis and arthritis was proved in 1894 in Vienna (Ernst Finger, published 1896). Cultures made from joint fluid from a patient with gonococcal arthritis were innoculated into the urethra of a man who, then, developed typical gonorrhea.

One criterion that suggests that some of the early descriptions of arthritis with urethritis did not represent gonococcal disease was recurrence of arthritis and/or ocular inflammation with urethritis after totally asymptomatic periods. The first such case was probably that of Thomas Whately (1801, London). Beginning in 1818, Benjamine C Brodie (1783–1862) described several men who had a recurrent syndrome of urethritis, conjunctivitis, and arthritis. One had 9 attacks in 20 years. The first report of a case that began with bacillary dysentery was reported from Germany by Adolf Vossius in 1904.

In 1916 Noël Fiessinger and Edgar Leroy published a report about dysentery among French troops on the Somme front. They incidentally gave a brief description of a "conjunctivo-uretero-synovial syndrome" of which they had seen 4 cases. One week later, Hans Reiter (1881–1969) published his first report on the disease later associated with his name. His one patient developed urethritis, conjunctivitis, and febrile polyarthritis after a bout of dysentery.

Emil Vidal (1825–1893) described a man who had suffered 2 bouts of a heretofore unknown hyperkeratotic eruption in association with what was believed to be recurrent gonorrheal arthritis (1893, Paris). The term keratodermia blennorrhagica was introduced and Anatole Chauffard and Georges Froiu described a case (1896, Paris). Despite little evidence in support of a gonococcal etiology, Wiedmann (1934, Vienna) was the first to suggest that keratodermia blennorrhagica is a manifestation of Reiter's disease, as gradually came to be accepted.

Introduction of corticosteroid therapy. The introduction of corticosteroid therapy resulted from the clinical studies of Philip S Hench (1896–1965) and the biochemical investigations of Edward C Kendall (1886–1972) (both Rochester, MN) and Tadeus Reichstein (1897—) who in 1950 shared the Nobel Prize for medicine for this work. Hench had observed (1929–1934) that the occurrence of nonhemolytic jaundice in patients with rheumatoid arthritis usually ameliorated the inflammation and, subsequently, that treatment with bile pigments or bile acids did not reproduce this effect. The improvement of rheumatoid arthritis during pregnancy was studied during 1931–1938, and Hench concluded that "the agents reponsible for both these phenomena are...perhaps identical." He also commented on the close structural relationships between "some of the sex hormones, cortin adrenocortical extract, and bile acids."

The dramatic initial results reported in 1949 resulted in great optimism and mass production of cortisone, and soon thereafter a number of analogs including hydrocortisone 1949, prednisone and prednisolone 1954, triamcinolone 1956, methylprednisolone 1957, and dexamethasone 1958. Corticotrophin, which had been isolated in 1943, was also introduced clinically by Hench and collaborators in 1949. The intraarticular administration of hydrocortisone was presented by JL Hollander (1951, Philadelphia).

For extensive references, see Rodnan, GP: Bull Rheum Dis 32:59–68, 1982.

2. International organizations

It is noteworthy that an international effort to study and control the rheumatic diseases preceded any nationally organized efforts. In 1928, a Dutch physician, Dr J Van Breeman, brought together concerned physicians from 6 European countries to establish the International League Against Rheumatism (ILAR). Then as now, the aims of the League were the exchange of medical information, the formation of national professional societies, and the stimulation of awareness of the social significance of rheumatic diseases. After 6 international congresses were held in Europe, physicians on other continents formed committees for ILAR in their respective countries. In the United States, such a committee for the study and control of rheumatic diseases was the beginning of the American Rheumatism Association.

Representatives from 25 countries attended a second landmark, the Seventh International Congress of Rheumatology held in 1949 in New York. A new constitution was adopted. Two regional groupings—the European League Against Rheumatism (EULAR) and the Pan American League Against Rheumatism (PANLAR), created during the war years—were formally recognized (1,2).

In subsequent years, there was a rapid growth of national activities to fight rheumatic disease. In 1965 a third regional league, the South East Asia and Pacific region (SEAPAL), was created. A world congress is now convened by ILAR every 4 years, with regional leagues holding congresses in intervening years.

Outstanding clinical achievements and biomedical research have brought rheumatology into the mainstream of medicine. Recognized as an independent specialty in some countries, rheumatology is accepted as a subspecialty of internal medicine in others (3,4). In the past decade, the growth of national professional societies has brought ILAR membership to over 5,000 members in 60 countries. Social and community agencies concerned with rheumatic disease patients in European countries have become full-fledged members of EULAR. Similar arrangements are being made for such agencies, where they exist, in the other 2 regions.

The third landmark in the organized world-wide attack on rheumatic disease occurred in 1974 when ILAR adopted a new structure and became a federation of the 3 regional leagues. A permanent Secretariat of ILAR was established in Basle, Switzerland, assuring continuity of activities in the succession of elected officers coming from various regions.

Six working committees have been created, with corresponding committees of the regional leagues: National and International Agencies, Social and Community Agencies, Education, Training and Accreditation; Epidemiology; Clinical Studies; Publications (5,6).

As a nongovernmental organization with formal relations with the World Health Organization (WHO), ILAR has stimulated interest and concern of public health authorities. The year 1977 was proclaimed World Rheumatism Year by ILAR with the support of WHO. Activities in countries at all stages of economic development brought awareness of rheumatic diseases to community leaders and to the public at large. At the 28th and 29th World Health Assemblies held in 1975 and 1976 (7), WHO urged the Member-States to support national programs concerned with rheumatic disease. The stage is now set for an increasing world-wide effort in the study and control of rheumatic diseases.

1. Ligue International Contre Le Rheumatisme: Yearbooks. ILAR Executive Secretariat. Basle, 1950, 1955, 1961, 1967, 1973, 1977
2. Rudd E: Rheumatology and international health. Arthritis Rheum 14:417–424, 1972
3. World Health Organization: The medical research programme of the WHO: 1958–1963. Geneva, WHO, 1964
4. World Health Organization: Future cooperation in the field of rheumatoid arthritis and related diseases. WHO Bulletin (Geneva) 51:597–607, 1974
5. European League Against Rheumatism: A strategy for conquering rheumatism. EULAR Bulletin (Basle) 4:51, 1975
6. International League Against Rheumatism: Prospectus of the leagues against rheumatism. EULAR Bulletin Supplement (Basle) 1977
7. World Health Organization: World Health Assembly resolutions (WHA 28.59, WHA 29.66). Geneva, WHO, 1975, 1976

3. The Arthritis Foundation

Founded in 1948, the Arthritis Foundation is the only national voluntary health association in the USA seeking the answers to this major health problem.

Its 71 chapters and local divisions 1) support biomedical and clinical research on the many forms of arthritis; 2) finance research training at several levels for scientists working in arthritis and related fields; 3) provide community services to people with arthritis and their families; 4) help provide expert care at low cost to those who cannot afford private care; 5) develop and provide programs for people with arthritis, aimed at improving the quality of their lives and helping them deal successfully with the problems created by having a chronic disease; 6) work closely with governmental agencies at the national and local level to encourage greater funding of research and providing better services for those with arthritis; 7) develop and provide educational programs in arthritis for health professionals (physicians, social workers, nurses, physical and occupational therapists); 8) provide information to the public on important issues related to arthritis, such as economic and social costs of arthritis, identification of quack remedies, and the latest research accomplishments.

Arthritis Foundation chapters. Local chapters engage in fundraising activities and act as information and referral centers concerning arthritis and available community services. They distribute informative literature and sponsor forums and lectures to keep the public, people with arthritis, and health professionals aware of the latest developments in arthritis research and treatment, and the dangers of "quack" remedies. Chapters support a wide variety of community services, from diagnosis to back-to-work programs, including clinics aimed at improving available care.

Professional sections. Two professional organizations are sections within the Foundation. The American Rheumatism Association (the world's largest professional society of physicians and scientists interested in arthritis) provides leadership in the study and control of rheumatic diseases and encourages national and international cooperation in this effort. The Arthritis Health Professions Association represents nurses, physical and occupational therapists, medical social workers, and others with special training and interest in the care of people with arthritis. This Association holds annual scientific meetings and provides educational activities for its members.

American Juvenile Arthritis Association. This organization is a section within the Foundation made up of parents who have children with arthritis and of other interested lay and professional volunteers. It works closely with various departments of the national office and the chapters to promote and review activities related to the problem of juvenile arthritis.

Research programs. Four types of research training fellowships are available from the national office: regular postdoctoral fellowship (2–3 years), Arthritis Investigator award, Senior Investigator award, and arthritis health professions fellowship (for non-physician investigators working in health care fields). Grants are awarded to Arthritis Clinical Research Centers which meet certain tests of excellence. A few grants are available for work in health care research under the national arthritis health professionals research program. Most chapters have research programs that provide support for local research projects, institutions, and training. Information on all these programs can be obtained by writing the Research Department of the national office.

4. The connective tissues: structure, function, and metabolism

Connective tissue

The connective tissue comprises the large mass of the supporting system and integument, as well as the fibers and ground substance which invest individual cells, tissues, and organs throughout the body. Both in the condensed connective tissue of structures such as cartilage and tendons and in the diffuse connective tissue, the connective tissue cells sit within an environment of interstitial fluid containing, in addition to plasma constituents, fibers (collagen, reticulin, and elastin), proteoglycans (also known as mucopolysaccharides), and other extracellular proteins which they have synthesized. Connective tissues are often characterized as relatively inert structural tissues of low metabolism and low cell content, with structural and mechanical rather than biochemical functions, but they are so diverse in structure and so great in regenerative capacity that such generalizations are misleading.

In the rheumatic diseases, critical events take place not only in the synovium, but in interstitial tissue throughout the body. The connective tissue supplies the terrain on which the battles of the rheumatic diseases are fought. The properties of connective tissue may then be crucial in directing the course of inflammation and repair. The connective tissue, however, can also be involved more directly: in Marfan's syndrome and many other hereditary disorders, there are genetically abnormal structural components (1); in lathyrism and scurvy, an environmental agent and a nutritional deficiency cause abnormal synthesis of matrix macromolecules; in relapsing polychondritis (2) and perhaps in rheumatoid arthritis (3), an immune response may be directed against a connective tissue component.

The interaction between components thought of as primarily connective tissue (fibroblasts and their relatives, extracellular fibers, and ground substance) and inflammatory cells (monocytes, lymphocytes, and polymorphonuclear leukocytes) is probably crucial to the pathogenesis and recovery in many rheumatic diseases.

Composition. The principal elements of connective tissue are the cells and the ground substance. The **cells** are principally mesodermal in origin and are responsible for the synthesis of the fibers and proteoglycans of the ground substance. The **fibers** are 1) *collagen*, a helical polymer which is the most abundant protein in the body, 2) *reticulin*, a close relative of collagen which is also widely dispersed, and 3) *elastin*, a polymer whose unusual cross-

linking gives it the elastic properties valuable in some distensible tissues such as arterial wall. The proteoglycans are molecules in which long chains of repeating disaccharide units (called *glycosaminoglycans*) are generally attached along a protein backbone. The structure and properties of these macromolecules are discussed in more detail below.

The cells of connective tissue can be conveniently divided into two categories, extrinsic and intrinsic. The **extrinsic cells**—mast cells, lymphocytes, monocytes, and polymorphonuclear leukocytes—are generally not permanent residents of the tissue in which they are found. The **intrinsic cells,** responsible for the synthesis and maintenance of the extracellular matrix, are fibroblasts (Fig 4–1) or more differentiated relatives of fibroblasts such as chondrocytes and osteoblasts. They are almost entirely of mesodermal origin.

In response to various stimuli, the cells may divide and turn to active synthesis (4). Experiments in tissue culture have shown that even well-differentiated resting cells from apparently inactive tissue can divide in culture and synthesize matrix and macromolecules. Furthermore, the type of macromolecule synthesized (i.e., the type of collagen) is influenced by culture conditions (5,6), by the presence of proteoglycans (7), and by substances derived from the extrinsic cells (8). These

latter molecules, including lymphokines and monokines, may have an important role in the pathogenesis of the connective tissue diseases.

The physical or structural properties of connective tissue depend on the proportions and physical properties of the various cellular and extracellular elements—for example, the proportion of fiber is very high in tendon and skin and very low in mucous connective tissue such as umbilical cord—and on such factors as the geometry of the fibers and the ionic composition of the fluid.

The fibers of connective tissue can influence physical properties by their relative proportions, the degree of *intra*molecular crosslinking, the degree of *inter*molecular crosslinking; aggregation into fibrils, fibril density, fibril diameter, the orientation of fibrils with respect to one another (e.g., the strong alignment of collagen in tendons and cornea as compared with the apparently random alignment in skin or the zones of horizontal, arcuate, and vertical collagen in cartilage), and the interaction of fibers with proteoglycans or other proteins such as osteocalcin and fibronectin.

Proteoglycans, the abundant, large, and perhaps least understood molecules of the connective tissue, also influence bulk properties in many ways. Their composition is determined not only by which individual disaccharide units predominate, but

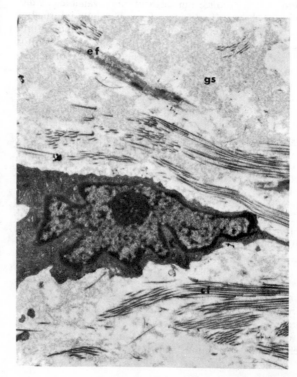

Fig 4–1. Normal human skin (dermis), illustrating composition of loose fibroelastic connective tissue. The cellular component is represented by a portion of a fibrocyte (**fc**), the nucleus of which contains a large nucleolus. Collagen fibrils (**cf**) and an elastic fibril (**ef**) are imbedded in ground substance (**gs**) which appears as an amorphous matrix of precipitated protein (original magnification ×11,200). (Illustration provided by Dr RL Hayes)

also by which modifications have taken place after chain synthesis (9). These factors, in turn, affect their interactions with themselves and with other molecules (for example, the supramolecular aggregation of proteoglycans with hyaluronate and link protein in cartilage) (10). Their interactions with water and with ions are responsible for the powerful osmotic and ionic properties of the proteoglycans (11). In addition, they interact with fibers and with cell surfaces (9). Physical forces can deform proteoglycans and thereby alter their physical and chemical properties. The cells of connective tissue may respond to physical forces, such as compression or stretch, as with synthesis of fibers or proteoglycans.

The **interstitial fluid** is an important solvent with special properties. It is the source of the small molecules involved in connective tissue metabolism such as metabolic substrates, glucose, calcium, phosphate, and uric acid. The distribution of serum proteins and enzymes is determined in part by the gel-filtering properties of the proteoglycans. The proteoglycans and fibers normally allow solvent and small molecules to move freely in the interstices of the matrix, but may exclude some large molecules such as degradative enzymes and can impede the migration of anions such as phosphate. The flow of molecules from the blood to the tissues is determined in part by the properties of the connective tissue in structures such as the vascular wall, the glomerular basement membrane, and the alveolar membrane.

Other proteins of the extracellular matrix include not only the serum proteins but also proteins that may be important in calcification (osteocalcin) or in cell attachment and differentiation (fibronectin).

1. McKusick VA: Heritable Disorders of Connective Tissue. Ed 4. St. Louis, CV Mosby, 1972
2. Foidart J-M, Abe S, Martin GR, Zizic TM, Barnett EV, Lawley TJ, Katz SI: Antibodies to type II collagen in relapsing polychondritis. N Engl J Med 299:1203–1207, 1978
3. Trentham D, Dynesius RA, Rocklin RE, David JR: Cellular sensitivity to collagen in rheumatoid arthritis. N Engl J Med 299:327–332, 1978
4. Sokoloff L: Articular chondrocytes in culture: matrix production and hormonal effects. Arthritis Rheum 19:426–429, 1976
5. Miller EJ: The collagen of joints, The Joints and Synovial Fluid. L Sokoloff, ed. New York, Academic Press, 1978, pp 205–242
6. Nimni M: Molecular structure and function of collagen in normal and diseased tissues, Dynamics of Connective Tissue Macromolecules. PMC Burleigh, AR Poole, eds. New York, Elsevier, 1978, pp 51–76
7. Wiebkin OW, Hardingham TE, Muir H: The interaction of proteoglycans and hyaluronic acid and the effect of hyaluronic acid on proteoglycan synthesis by chondrocytes of adult cartilage. Dynamics of Connective Tissue Macromolecules. PMC Burleigh, AR Poole, eds. New York, Elsevier, 1978, pp 81–98
8. Castor CW, Whitney SL: Connective tissue activation. XIII. Stimulation of sulfated glycosaminoglycan synthesis in human connective tissue cells by peptide mediators from lymphocytes and platelets. J Lab Clin Med 91:811–821, 1978
9. Lindahl U, Höök M: Glycosaminoglycans and their binding to biological macromolecules. Ann Rev Biochem 47:385–417, 1978
10. Hascall VC: Interaction of cartilage proteoglycans with hyaluronic acid. J Supramolec Struct 7:101–120, 1977
11. Comper WD, Laurent TC: Physiological function of connective tissue polysaccharides. Physiol Rev 58:255–315, 1978

Proteoglycans

Proteoglycans are a diverse class of large molecules which permeate the ground substance of connective tissue throughout the body (1). They consist of a **polypeptide core** with multiple **linear polysaccharide side chains.** The basic subunit of the polysaccharide side chains is a **disaccharide,** usually an acid sugar (**hexuronic acid**) attached to an amino sugar (**hexosamine**). The chains are named according to their dominant disaccharide unit (Table 4–1). Often they are not monotonous chains of a repeating disaccharide but have variations along their length imposed after polymerization. Acetylation, sulfation, and epimerization (to produce iduronic acid) all modify individual sugars (2). For example, the dominant disaccharide in chondroitin-4-sulfate is N-acetylgalactosamine, sulfated at position 4, attached to glucuronic acid, but some of the sugars may have the sulfate at position 6 of the N-acetylgalactosamine or no sulfate at all. Only the hyaluronic acid subunit (N-acetylglucosamineglucuronic acid) appears to undergo no modification after synthesis. In some polysaccharides, other sugars (mannose, fucose, N-acetyl neuraminic acid) are found. The reducing end of the chain commonly terminates in the stereotyped sequence glucuronic acid-galactose-galactose-xylose which binds to the hydroxyl group of a peptide-bonded serine. In cartilage keratan sulfate chains and mucins, the termination is galactosamine bound to serine. In corneal keratan sulfate and in most glycoproteins, the linkage is glucosamine bound to asparagine. Considering the possibility for variety in distribution of different subunits within an individual polysaccharide chain and the variety of chains which may be attached to a single protein backbone, the potential for diversity of structure and function is very great.

Compared with our knowledge about the specific sequences of amino acids in proteins and nucleotide bases in nucleic acids, relatively little is known of the fine structure of proteoglycans. Fine structure is certainly responsible for many properties of the polysaccharide chains, such as

Table 4–1. Polysaccharides of connective tissue proteoglycans*

Name	MW range × 10⁻³	Dominant disaccharide	Common modifications	Major locations
Hyaluronate	4,000–8,000	N-acetylglucosamine-glucuronate	None	Skin, cartilage, synovial fluid, vitreous humor, umbilical cord
Chondroitin-4 sulfate	5–50	N-acetylgalactosamine-glucuronate	Sulfate at position 4 of hexosamine	Cartilage, bone, skin, cornea
Chondroitin-6 sulfate	5–50	N-acetylgalactosamine-glucuronate	Sulfate at position 6 of hexosamine	Cartilage, skin, umbilical cord, intervertebral disc, heart valve
Dermatan sulfate	15–40	N-acetylgalactosamine-iduronate and -glucuronate	Sulfate at position 4 and/or 6 of hexosamine and position 2 of iduronate	Skin, tendon, heart valve, intervertebral disc, bone
Keratan sulfate	4–19	Galactose-N-acetylglucosamine	Sulfate at position 6 of either sugar	Cornea, cartilage, nucleus pulposus
Heparin and heparan sulfate	5–50	Iduronate and glucuronate / N-acetylglycosamine and glucosamine-N-sulfate	Sulfate at position 6 of the hexosamine and position 2 of the iduronate and N-sulfate of the hexosamine	Lung, skin, liver

* Compiled from references 1 and 2

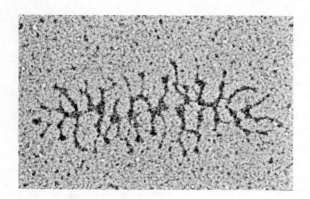

Fig 4–2. Proteoglycan subunit isolated from bovine nasal cartilage. Some side chains of chondroitin sulfate appear to be intertwined with neighboring chains. Other side chains are bridged by short strands that run perpendicularly from the middle of one chain to another (original magnification ×270,000). (Illustration provided by Dr LC Rosenberg—Ref 6)

their binding to and uptake by cells and their degradation. Studies of the interaction of proteoglycans with proteins, with other proteoglycan molecules, and with cell surfaces have clearly established that some properties of the molecules depend critically on fine structure. Conversely, other properties, such as the electrochemical and osmotic potentials of proteoglycans, probably do not.

Because the sugar subunits in most polysaccharide chains bear a net negative charge due to their sulfate and carboxylate groups, they bind a large number of cations. The overall electrical and osmotic properties of a large polyelectrolyte surrounded by abundant obligatory small ions are doubtless of great importance in determining some of the bulk properties of proteoglycans such as resistance to the diffusion of ions and the resilience of cartilage in the face of physical compression when water is expressed from the intertices of the matrix (3). The negative charge over the surface of the chain, the great flexibility of the glycosidic bonds along the chain, and the abundant possibilities for hydrogen bonding between water and the sugar hydroxyls leads to great flexibility of the chains in solution. Consequently, an individual polysaccharide chain, either free or attached to a protein, has no well-defined tertiary structure and occupies a far greater space in solution than does a protein of the same molecular weight.

Protein molecules above a certain size in solution with a proteoglycan can therefore occupy only a fraction of the space they would occupy in a simple solution of the same volume. This molecular sieving not only restricts the passage of large molecules in proteoglycan solutions but also raises the effective concentration of such molecules, which in turn may have significant physiological consequences. For example, it may influence how fibrous proteins, such as collagen, aggregate in connective tissue or when and where amyloid deposits. The distribution and therefore the effective concentration of antigen and antibody may vary strikingly in the presence of proteoglycans. Such a local change in the ratio of antigen to antibody might, under some circum-

stances, lead to the precipitation of immune complexes.

Cartilage proteoglycan. The best studied proteoglycans are those from mammalian cartilage. Most of the proteoglycan in normal cartilage is in the form of supramolecular aggregates (4,5). Each such aggregate contains a single, central, linear backbone consisting of a molecule of hyaluronic acid, often $1–10 \times 10^3$ nm long. Arrayed at intervals of 40–50 nm along this backbone, like bristles on a bottle brush, are individual proteoglycan molecules about 300–400 nm long (Figs 4–2 and 3). Each bristle consists of a protein backbone out of which stick chains of polysaccharides of various lengths. The polysaccharide chains at the end of the protein that attaches to the hyaluronic acid are mostly keratan sulfate; those further out are mostly chondroitin sulfate. At the junction between the proteoglycan subunits and the hyaluronic backbone are special proteins (*link* proteins) which strengthen the attachment. The bonds holding together the hyaluronic acid, the link protein, and the proteoglycan are noncovalent. The molecular weight of the proteoglycan subunits ranges from 1–4 million, of which over 90% is polysaccharide, and each aggregate has many such subunits, leading to an enormous overall size. During extraction the components may be dissociated and allowed to reassemble in vitro for study. In intact cartilage, the proteoglycans exist in a considerably higher concentration than can be reached in vitro (3).

It is not yet understood what factors (possibly the presence of collagen or other glycoproteins) contribute to this ability to exist in high concentration.

The overall composition of cartilage proteoglycan changes with age: the proportion of keratan sulfate rises and that of chondroitin sulfate falls. It is possible, but by no means established, that the changes in the properties of cartilage with age, disease, disuse, and injury are related to changes in its composition which affect the ability of the elements to aggregate with one another or to interact with collagen (7).

Synthesis and metabolism. Individual proteoglycan units are synthesized within a single cell. Synthesis of the protein backbone is under ordinary genetic control as is synthesis of the enzymes which add and modify the sugar moieties. However, the interplay of the synthetic and modifying enzymes responsible for determining the fine structure is still largely obscure. The sugar moieties are added one by one, not as the disaccharide repeating units. An inherited genetically determined template does not determine the sequence of sugars as it does the sequence of amino acids in proteins or of nucleotide bases in nucleic acids, nor does any single gene appear to direct the synthesis of an individual polysaccharide chain.

Post-synthetic modification of the polysaccharide chains takes place within the cell of synthesis, but some degradative modification may take place extracellularly. Since physical forces can alter the configuration of these large molecules and hence their susceptibility to enzymatic degradation, it is possible that the molecules of the extracellular matrix are modified in response to their environment and that these modifications may influence interaction of proteoglycans with surrounding molecules such as collagen.

The synthesis of 2 of the 3 components of cartilage proteoglycan aggregates—proteoglycan and link protein—is probably coordinated, since there does not appear to be a disproportionate amount of either component free in the cartilage matrix. They are synthesized in the same cell but

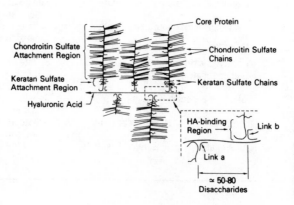

Fig 4–3. A schematic diagram of a whole cartilage proteoglycan molecule. Each bottle brush–like structure is a subunit like the one in Figure 4–2. (Illustration provided by Dr V Hascall (4), with permission of the publisher)

assemble into aggregates only upon leaving.

Although chondrocyte cultures can synthesize both collagen and proteoglycan, it is unknown whether or not they are always synthesized in the same cell at the same time or in what way, if any, their synthesis is coordinated. It is possible to disconnect their synthesis in culture. Under some circumstances, the presence of hyaluronic acid in culture may inhibit proteoglycan synthesis, but it has no such effect under other circumstances. In the early embryo, hyaluronic acid may even repress the synthesis of connective tissue (8).

Turnover of proteoglycan molecules in the extracellular matrix is generally very slow, measured in terms of months or years, although a small fraction may undergo a more rapid metabolism. The combination of modification by incomplete extracellular degradation and very slow turnover of proteoglycan molecules may allow molecular changes in response to injury or disease to persist long after the insult has passed (9). In response to injury, the cells of some connective tissues, which may appear to lie dormant much of the time, can produce large quantities of new matrix, both fiber and proteoglycan. With the stress of injury, cartilage may undergo a repair process in which fibrocartilage rather than hyaline cartilage is made.

It is increasingly apparent that inflammatory and immunologic events can influence both the synthesis and degradation of connective tissue in a number of circumstances in vitro. The histologic picture of inflammatory joint disease—with an advancing edge of proliferating synovium packed with inflammatory and antibody-producing cells creeping along a cartilage surface and destroying it locally—is adequate evidence that there must be powerful interactions between the immune system and connective tissue. For example, lymphokines can cause connective tissue cells to synthesize new proteoglycans or, under other circumstances, they can inhibit synthesis and increase degradation of proteoglycans (10,11). They can also stimulate synthesis of **collagenase,** the collagen-degradative enzyme (12).

Conversely, the components of connective tissue may influence the behavior of the immune system, e.g., serving as chemotactic factors. Some components of connective tissue, such as cartilage collagen and proteoglycan, can be immunogenic and lead not only to antibody formation, but also to active inflammation wherever the component is present (13). To what extent such mechanisms operate as primary events in the pathogenesis of rheumatoid arthritis, in sustaining an injury due to another cause, or in influencing the course of inflammation in connective tissue remains unknown.

Other proteins of connective tissue. The glycoprotein, **fibronectin** (also known as LETS or cold insoluble globulin), is found widely on cell surfaces and in the intercellular matrix as well as in the circulation (14). Fibronectin appears to be related to cell proliferation and differentiation and to the adherence of cells to collagen and to surfaces in tissue culture. Its function in the circulation is unknown.

A major protein (20% of the noncollagenous bone protein) in calcifying tissues is **osteocalcin,** which contains the unusual amino acid, γ-carboxyglutamic acid. This amino acid, which is formed by a vitamin K–dependent post-translational carboxylation of glutamic acid, is also found in the calcium-dependent vitamin K clotting factors. It seems likely that osteocalcin has a role in calcification since it is found in ectopically calcifying tissues as well as in bone (15).

1. Serafini-Fracassini A, Smith JW: The Structure and Biochemistry of Cartilage. Edinburgh, Churchill Livingstone, 1974
2. Lindahl U, Hook M: Glycosaminoglycans and their binding to biological macromolecules. Ann Rev Biochem 47:385–417, 1978
3. Comper WD, Laurent TC: Physiological function of connective tissue polysaccharides. Physiol Rev 58:255–315, 1978
4. Hascall VC: Interaction of cartilage proteoglycans with hyaluronic acid. J Supramolecular Structure 7:101–120, 1977
5. Hascall VC, Hascall GK: Proteoglycans, Cell Biology of Extracellular Matrix. ED Hay, ed. New York, Plenum, 1981, pp 39–63
6. Hamerman D, Rosenberg LC, Schubert M: Diarthrodial joints revisited. J Bone Joint Surg 52A:725–744, 1970
7. Moskowitz RW, Howell DS, Goldberg VM, Muniz O, Pita JC: Cartilage proteoglycan alterations in an experimentally induced model of rabbit osteoarthritis. Arthritis Rheum 22:155–163, 1979
8. Wiebkin OW, Hardingham TE, Muir H: The interaction of proteoglycans and hyaluronic acid and the effect of hyaluronic acid on proteoglycan synthesis by chondrocytes of adult cartilage, Dynamics of Connective Tissue Macromolecules. PMC Burleigh, AR Poole, eds. New York, Elsevier, 1978, pp 81–98
9. Schubert M, Hamerman D: A Primer on Connective Tissue Biochemistry. Philadelphia, Lea & Febiger, 1968
10. Castor W, Whitney SL: Connective tissue activation. XIII. Stimulation of sulfated glycosaminoglycan synthesis in human connective tissue cells by peptide mediators from lymphocytes and platelets. J Lab Clin Med 91:811–821, 1978
11. Herman JH, Musgrave DS, Dennis MV: Phytomitogen-induced, lymphokine-mediated cartilage proteoglycan degradation. Arthritis Rheum 20:922–932, 1977
12. Dayer J-M, Russell RGG, Krane SM: Collagenase production by rheumatoid syniovial cells: stimulation by a human lymphocyte factor. Science 195:181–183, 1977
13. Trentham DE, Townes AS, Kang AH: Autoimmunity to type II collagen: an experimental model of arthritis. J Exp Med 146:857–868, 1977
14. Ruoslahti E. Engvall E, Hayman EG: Fibronectin: current concepts of its structure and function. Coll Res 1:95–128, 1981
15. Gallop P, Lian J, Havscka P. Carboxylated calcium-binding proteins and vitamin K. N Engl J Med 302:1460–1466, 1980

Collagen

The term collagen describes a family of specialized molecules with common structural features that provide an extracellular framework for all multicellular animals. Collagen accounts for more than 20% of total body protein. By subtle control of polypeptide structures (collagen type) and subtle modifications of the newly synthesized chains (fine-tuning), cells can produce diverse support structures like ropes (tendons), woven sheets (skin), transparent lenses (the cornea), a scaffold for mineralization (bone), weight-bearing joints, and basement membranes (1–8).

In addition to structural roles, the collagen family has been implicated in morphogenesis and the various complex regulatory processes which occur during growth and aging, and in wound healing (2). Alterations in the structure and metabolism of collagen are widely believed to be involved, either directly or indirectly in the etiology of many disorders (1,5,7).

Common structural features. The definitive property of all collagen molecules is the **triple helix** (1,2). This unique protein conformation is the result of the winding of the 3 constituent polypeptide chains of the collagen molecule (known as α-chains) around each other at 2 levels of organization. Each chain is coiled into a left-handed helix with about 3 amino acid residues per turn. The 3 chains are then twisted around each other into a right-handed super helix to form a rigid structure similar to a thin segment of rope. This unique 3-dimensional conformation is made possible by a distinctive amino acid sequence in the polypeptide chains. With the exception of short sequences at the ends of the chains, every third amino acid residue in each chain is glycine.

Since the side-chain of this amino acid is an H atom, glycine is the only amino acid residue small enough to occupy the restricted space in which the helical α-chains cluster together in the center of the triple helix. Fully 25% of the total residues consist of proline and hydroxyproline, amino acids with ring structures that impose restrictions on the α-chain conformation and, thereby, strengthen the triple helix and stiffen the collagen molecule. These compositional features make it possible to represent the approximately 1,000-residue helical region of the collagen α-chain of fibrous collagens by the molecular formula $(X-Y-Gly)_{333}$ where X and Y are residues other than glycine. In mammals, about 100 of the X positions are occupied by prolyl residues and about 100 of the Y positions by hydroxyprolyl residues. Hydroxyproline is produced during the biosynthetic process by modification of specific proline residues. Most of the hydroxyproline is present in collagen as the *trans-4-*isomer, but all known collagens contain a very small amount of *trans-*

3-hydroxyproline. In the collagens of basement membranes, relatively large amounts of 3-hydroxyproline are found (2,4).

The precise sequence of amino acid residues that fill the remaining X and Y positions differs from collagen to collagen and may account to some extent for the tissue-specific properties of the fibers of cartilage and skin. One residue that occupies these positions and which is characteristic of the collagens is hydroxylysine. This is produced by a post-translational modification of lysine and is involved in many of the further fine-tuning processes of fiber formation as a precursor of crosslinking compounds and as a site for attachment of carbohydrate. In the latter instance, the hydroxyl group is involved in an O-glycoside linkage to a galactose or to glucosyl galactose (2).

At both ends of the helical region are terminal sequences (**telopeptides**) that do not have glycine as every third residue and are, therefore, nontriple helical. These regions, comprising about 12 residues each, are the persistent remains of the propeptides. These regions appear to be the primary sites of crosslinking where the molecules interact to assemble into a collagen fiber.

Variation of the common triple helical theme in terms of primary structure and post-translational modification enable the collagens to participate in a vast array of structural complexes (2).

Collagen polymorphism. The total genetic potential for collagen production has not yet been determined, but at least 10 distinct α-chains have been described in vertebrate tissues. Each type has a unique amino acid sequence and has been firmly identified as a distinct gene product (2,4).

The different collagen types can be classified according to their locations and functions (Table 4–2). The **fibrillar interstitial collagens,** forming the extracellular fabric of the major connective tissues, are the most familiar class. A second class is the **nonfibrous collagens** of the basement lamina of epithelial cell layers. The third class comprises the poorly defined **collagenous molecules** that appear to be located in the immediate pericellular environment, perhaps as part of the external skeleton of the cell.

In addition to these classes, 2 quite

unrelated proteins contain collagen-like sequences. It is presumed that the collagen-like sequences of these molecules enable them to perform their specialized biological functions. For example, the collagenous sequences in the C1q subcomponent of the blood complement system are thought to provide the molecules with a rigid segment that enables them to self-aggregate. The collagenous sequences in acetylcholinesterase serve to anchor the enzyme to basement membranes (2).

The discovery of new chain types and the identification of families of molecules already necessitates a reevaluation of current chain nomenclature. Presumably, this will occur when further molecular and genetic information is available for each collagen chain. To avoid this confusion, we will examine the different collagens according to location and function.

Fibrillar collagens. The major fibrillar collagens are known as types I, II, and III. In electron micrographs these collagens exhibit the same characteristic 64–67 nm periodicity (1).

The characteristic periodicity of the collagen fibril is generated by the packing of the collagen molecules in a precise axial register that is usually described as a near-quarter-stagger with overlap. This axial stagger has been precisely defined at 234 ± 1 residues for type I collagen. No lateral substructure is obvious by electron microscopy, and it is not yet clear whether the side-to-side aggregation of molecules, ultimately responsible for the fiber diameter, is due to accretion of the molecules as microfibrillar sub-units or whether the lateral organization is amorphous like a type A smectic liquid crystal. What is clear, however, is the fact that the primary structure of the chains contains all the information needed to fold the precursor molecules into native molecules, to pack these molecules into fibers, and then to determine the type and number of intermolecular crosslinks that will eventually be formed. Primary structure of the chains also appears to dictate the nature of the interaction of the collagen with the other connective tissue components, namely glycoproteins and proteoglycans.

Type I collagen consists of two identical α1(I) chains and a genetically distinct α2 chain in the molecular form $\alpha1(I)_{2\alpha2}$. This species accounts for about 90% of the

collagen in the body and is the major collagenous component of cornea, conjunctiva, skin, sclera, synovium (9), bone, and tendon. Recent genetic and biochemical studies appear to indicate that the type I collagens are not identical from tissue to tissue, but represent closely related products of a family of type I collagen genes.

Type II collagen fibers appear much thinner than those of type I in electron micrographs. Type II collagen is composed of 3 identical α-chains and designated $\alpha1(II)_3$. This molecular species is found in cartilage and vitreous. However, 2 structurally different chains designated α1(II) Major and α1(II) Minor have recently been identified in cartilage. Also, several properties of the α1(II) chains of vitreous humor differ from those of the α1(II) chains of cartilage. These differences strongly suggest that $\alpha1(II)_3$ molecules are not a homogenous population, but like those in type I collagen represent a family of closely related molecules. To add further to the current confusion in classification and nomenclature, 3 other α-chains, not identical to classic type II collagen, have recently been described in human hyaline cartilage.

Type III collagen is encountered with type I in skin, synovium, and blood vessel wall tissue. This form of collagen also contains 3 identical chains that are readily distinguishable from the previously described fibrillar types. The type III molecule is therefore designated $\alpha1(III)_3$. Because of its presence in substantial quantities in fetal tissue, this molecular species was first thought to be fetal type collagen. Although α1(III) chains have not been sufficiently characterized at the biochemical level to state with any certainty that a family of closely related molecules exists, molecular heterogeneity is strongly suggested by evidence from the genetic mapping of "embryonic" type III collagen to a different chromosome from that of "adult" type III collagen.

The physiologic significance of the various genetic types is not yet known. However, the fact that type III collagen forms fibrils of smaller diameter and of different fibrillar organization than type I collagens suggests that the expression of separate collagen genes is an important step in establishing and maintaining the individual characteristics of a particular connective tissue. For example, the relative proportions of type I and type III were found to change drastically in studies of healing skin wounds. Similar notable changes in collagen gene expression have also been found during embryonic development. However, it should be noted that physiologic correlations with the relative ratios of collagen types are complicated by the effects of post-translational modifications of the collagen molecules and interaction of these molecules with other components of the connective tissues (1,2,7).

A molecule apparently composed of

Table 4–2. Classification of collagen

Type	Chain structure	Comments
I	$\alpha1(I)_{2\alpha2}$	Collagen vulgaris: major type in many tissues including cornea, tissue differences due mainly to post-translational modifications
II	$\alpha1(II)_3$	Major collagen type of cartilage, may be more than one species
III	$\alpha1(III)_3$	Major type of blood vessels
IV	$\alpha(IV)_3$	Classical basement membrane collagen
V	$\alpha A(\alpha B)_2$	Placenta, normal corneal stroma, posterior elastic lamina of the cornea, and other membranes
VI	$\alpha1(I)_3$	Embryonic tissue; certain cell lines in culture, corneal scar α1(I) chain may not be identical with α1(I) of type I

$\alpha1(I)_3$ has been found in low concentrations in cornea, skin, embryonic bones and tendons, and rat dentin. This molecular species has also been identified as a product of various cell cultures and tumors. The α-chain of this molecular species appeared to be identical, by peptide mapping, to the $\alpha1(I)$ chain of type I collagen and gave rise to the nomenclature collagen type I trimer. Recent work has indicated that the chains are non-identical but are closely related genetic variants. Although its functional role is not understood, type I trimer appears in higher concentrations in healing wounds and embryonic tissues.

Basement membrane collagens. Basement membranes contain collagenous components that are probably responsible for the structural integrity of the membranes and act as anchors for other membrane components. Unlike those collagens discussed above, basement membrane collagens are not fibrillar when seen in the electron microscope. A discrete collagen α-chain with a distinctive amino acid composition has been isolated from glomerular basement membrane and lens capsule and posterior elastic lamina of the cornea. For the past several years, this α-chain has been considered to be derived from a distinct basal lamina collagen, termed collagen **type IV** to distinguish it from the fibrillar types I–III.

The structural role of this molecular species has been a controversial matter, however, since later work has identified several collagenous polypeptides differing in molecular size and composition from classic $\alpha1(IV)$ chains. One explanation for the presence of several small collagenous segments is the recently identified susceptibility of the basement membrane collagens to proteolytic attack. Resolution of the exact number of basement membrane collagens will probably be obtained by biosynthetic studies. In fact, results of several recent experiments indicate that the assembly of basement membrane collagens occurs from only 1 or 2 procollagen chains. However, unlike the interstitial collagens, the basement membrane precursor molecules appear to be inserted directly into the membrane structure without prior clipping of the pro-peptide extensions.

Pericellular collagens. Type V collagen surrounds fibroblasts and other mesenchymal cells. This type of collagen contains distinct chains known as αA and αB that are minor components in pepsin digests of placenta, cornea, skin, and blood vessels and have been identified in surface-associated materials of cells in culture. These chains are gene products independent of the previously known collagen types.

The biosynthetic process. Attempts have been made to localize the collagen genome using the techniques of somatic cell hybridization. Genes for skin type I collagen have been traced to chromosome 17 by one group of researchers and to chromosome 7 by another. Corneal type I collagen has also localized to chromosome 7. However, it is still unclear whether the codes for 1 type of collagen will be found on more than 1 chromosome (2,3).

Studies of the translation of messenger RNA (mRNA) for procollagen type I in cell-free systems indicate that the molecule is synthesized on the ribosomes as **pre-procollagen** and each chain contains a short (approximately 20 residue) leader sequence at the extreme amino terminus. This hydrophobic leader sequence is thought to channel the nascent polypeptide through the membrane into the cisternae of the rough endoplasmic reticulum where it is immediately cleaved off by a protease to yield **procollagen.**

Thus far, only a few procollagens have been studied in detail. Chicken type I procollagen is composed of 2 pro $\alpha1$ and 1 pro $\alpha2$ chains which have estimated molecular weights of about 150,000 daltons compared with 95,000 daltons for the corresponding chains of the processed molecule. Each of the pro α chains contains 2 polypeptide extensions, 1 at the amino terminal end and 1 at the carboxy terminal end of the triple-helical region. The amino and carboxy-terminal extensions are estimated to be 20,000 daltons and 35,000 daltons, respectively (1,8).

These extensions, or **propeptides,** appear to prevent the unwanted formation of collagen fibrils before the molecules reach the desired cell export site. They may also be involved in directing the assembly of the collagen molecules from their constituent chains and in regulating triple-helix formation. Recent evidence has further suggested a role for the propeptides in feedback inhibition of collagen biosynthesis and an ability to direct extracellular fibrillogenesis.

During the biosynthetic process, the polypeptide chains of procollagen are subject to at least 6 different enzyme-mediated modifications prior to secretion. Further post-translational modifications involving crosslink formation occur extracellularly. These enzyme-mediated modifications are not usually found in the biosynthetic pathways of other proteins and each offers a unique control point for the synthetic pathway. Intracellular post-translational modifications include hydroxylation of proline and of lysine, addition of galactose to certain hydroxylysines and of glucose to certain galactose-hydroxylysines, and finally extrusion from the cell coupled with proteolytic cleavage of the extension peptides from the amino and carboxy termini of the molecule.

It should be appreciated that the post-translational microheterogeneity resulting from these enzyme-mediated modifications probably represents the fine-tuning which adapts the collagen molecule for its ultimate biological function. The molecule is only secreted after hydroxylation, glycosylation, and triple-helix formation is complete. Secretion appears to be a stepwise process, first requiring packing into a Golgi vacuole before exocytosis.

Although almost all the procollagens of most tissues are converted to collagen molecules, some unprocessed procollagen molecules may be retained at the cell surface to interact specifically with various structural components of the interfibrillar matrix. Basement membrane procollagens appear to be incorporated into the membrane structure without prior processing.

Processed molecules destined to form fibrils self-assemble into 3-dimensional fibrillar complexes which are then stabilized by a series of covalent inter- and intra-chain crosslinks. Most of these bonds originate from lysine or hydroxylysine and from modified forms of amino acid residues derived by oxidative deamination. Control of the extent of polymerization and of crosslinking is poorly understood, but has far ranging effects on mechanical properties of collagen fiber (1–3).

Collagen degradation. The native tissue contains collagen in the form of insoluble paracrystalline aggregates in close association with many other tissue components. Degradation is thus extremely complex (5,6). The rate of degradation seems to depend, at any one moment, both on the amount of active specific degradative enzymes present and on the degree of substrate susceptibility. Much current knowledge of mammalian collagenases refers to the enzyme responsible for the cleavage of the native molecule at a single specific site within the triple-helical region that produces 2 pieces: 1 (the TC$_A$ peptide) accounts for 75% of the length of the molecule, the other (the TC$_B$ peptide) for 25% of the length of the molecule. These peptides are unstable at physiologic temperatures and after denaturation become susceptible to the hydrolytic action of nonspecific tissue proteases.

Several investigators have evidence that collagenases are secreted as inactive precursor molecules, while others suggest that these latent enzymes are in reality enzyme-inhibitor complexes. In fact, both mechanisms may be operating within a connective tissue depending on the prevailing set of circumstances. Additionally, hormones and other factors may play as yet undefined operational roles (5).

Collagen and collagenases in disease. The basic lesions in 3 recessive types and 1 sex-linked type of Ehlers-Danlos syndrome have been traced to specific abnormalities in collagen (3,10). Three of the lesions affect enzymes responsible for post-translational events, the fourth is a failure of the synthesis of type III collagen and is therefore analogous to the thalassemia syndromes of hemoglobin pathology. A defect in the synthesis of type I collagen is suspected in certain types of osteogenesis imperfecta.

In addition to the heritable disorders, there are many acquired diseases that appear to be associated with secondary abnormalities in collagen metabolism. For example, changes in the synthetic patterns of cartilage collagen may be a causative factor in osteoarthritis.

A knowledge of collagenase has special significance for understanding chronic inflammatory diseases such as rheumatoid arthritis and other pathologic processes in which excessive collagen degradation occurs.

1. Prockop DJ, Kivirikko KI, Tuderman L, Guzman NA: The biosynthesis of collagen and its disorders. N Engl J Med 301:13–23, 77–85, 1979
2. Eyre DR: Collagen: molecular diversity in the body's protein scaffold. Science 207:1315–1322, 1980
3. Bornstein P, Byers PH: Disorders of collagen metabolism, Metabolic Control and Disease. 8th ed. PK Bondy, L Rosenberg, eds. Philadelphia, WB Saunders, 1980, pp 1089–1153
4. Rojkind M: Chemistry and biosynthesis of collagen. Bull Rheum Dis 30:1006–1010, 1979
5. Perez-Tamayo R: The degradation of collagen. Bull Rheum Dis 30:1012–1015, 1979
6. Barrett AJ, Saklatvala J: Proteinases in joint disease, Textbook of Rheumatology. WN Kelley, ED Harris Jr, S Ruddy, C Sledge, eds. Philadelphia, WB Saunders, 1981, pp 195–209
7. Gay S, Miller EJ: Collagen in the Physiology and Pathology of Connective Tissue. Stuttgart, Gustav Fischer Verlag, 1978
8. Fessler JH, Fessler LI: Biosynthesis of procollagens. Ann Rev Biochem 47:129–162, 1978
9. Gay S, Ray RE, Miller EJ: The collagens of the joint. Arthritis Rheum 23:937–941, 1980
10. Jimenez SA, Lally EV: Disorders of collagen structure and metabolism. Bull Rheum Dis 30:1016–1022, 1979

Elastin

Elastin fibers are easily identified by their characteristic tinctorial properties (e.g., with acid-orcein stain) and their ability to stretch when wet. These widely distributed fibers stretch and return to their original length after initiation and removal of a deforming force. Elastic fibers are the most prominent component of the ligaments (70–80% of the dry weight of ligamentum nuchae) and they contribute their unique properties to the walls of the larger blood vessels (aorta contains 30–60% elastin). Elastic fibers constitute 2–5% of the dry weight of dermis (1,2).

Main structural features. Electron microscopic examination reveals that elastic fibers consist of 2 distinct components. The major component has an amorphous appearance and demonstrates no distinct periodicity. This component, the protein elastin, forms 5 nm diameter ropes which are aligned in parallel to form a 5–6 μm diameter core in the elastic fiber. This core is surrounded by a sheath of microfibrillar structures that measure 10–12 μm in diameter (3,4).

Biochemical characterization of the microfibrillar protein is not yet complete. However, it has been shown that this component is totally distinct in composition from the elastin core. It contains smaller amounts of the amino acids glycine, alanine, and valine than elastin, and it does not contain hydroxyproline. It is relatively rich in those amino acids that are entirely lacking in elastin or are only present in small amounts: cystine, methionine, and histidine. In fact, the content of cystine in microfibrillar protein is particularly high (70–80 residues per 1,000 amino acid residues). The microfibrils also contain a large number of hexose and hexosamine sugar residues revealing the glycoprotein nature of this component (4).

The fibrous elastin core is a polymer of **tropoelastin** sub-units. Each tropoelastin monomer contains 850 amino acids and has a molecular weight of about 72,000 daltons. Four amino acids—glycine, alanine, proline, and valine—constitute 80% of all the amino acids of tropoelastin. Hydroxyproline is present in the molecule, but it is much less plentiful than in collagen. The protein lacks tryptophan, crystine, and methionine. This unusual composition leads to a unique primary structure containing repeating peptide sequences. For example, the pentapeptide (Val-Pro-Gly-Val-Gly) appears to be a dominant feature since it is repeated more than 6 times in a single sequence and occurs elsewhere in the chain (1–4).

When tropoelastin molecules associate to form a fiber, they do so in a way that favors juxtaposition of a limited number of the 38 lysine residues present in the polypeptide chain. This alignment process is probably brought about by pairing of like amino acid sequences and interlocking of particular chain segments. The lysine residues occur in alanine-rich sequences with 2 or 3 alanine residues between the 2 lysine residues that serve as crosslink precursors. Crosslinking involves 2 lysine residues from each of 2 chains. Thus the major crosslinks, **desmosine** and **isodesmosine**, derive from the side chain of 4 lysine residues. These crosslinks appear to be unique to elastin (2–4).

The resultant polymeric insoluble fibrous matrix is a twisted-rope structure held together by hydrophobic ridges stacked at 65A intervals that run at angles to the axis. Three well-defined regions can be recognized in the stabilized structure: a dynamic β-spiral region largely responsible for the elastometric properties, an interlocked β-spiral region, and the essentially α-helical crosslinking region which convalently binds the tropoelastin sub-units into the fibrous network (4).

Biosynthesis. Elastin biosynthesis follows the same basic principles as that of collagen and other proteins destined for export from the cell. Translation of the messenger RNA for the monomer sub-units takes place in the rough endoplasmic reticulum of connective tissue cells. After translation, the newly synthesized polypeptides are fed through the cisternae, packaged, and discharged into the extracellular space where they undergo chemical modifications in preparation for incorporation into polymeric elastin.

The first step in the formation of the crosslinks, desmosine and isodesmosine, is the oxidative deamination of 3 lysine residues to form aldehydes. The fourth lysine is incorporated into the crosslink without modification.

Thus, the generation of activated crosslink precursors in elastin is similar to that which occurs with collagen. The oxidative deamination reaction is catalyzed by lysyl oxidase. In diseases in which there is a genetic deficiency or a reduced level of activity of this enzyme, abnormal crosslinking of elastin appears to be partly responsible for the clinical manifestations. Deficient lysyl oxidase activities have been encountered, for example, in an inbred strain of mice demonstrating aortic aneurysms, a reduced tensil strength of the skin, and bone abnormalities. Ehlers-Danlos syndrome type V may represent an analogous situation in humans (3,5).

Degradation. Although the metabolic turnover of elastin in adult animals is relatively slow, there is normally a continuous degradation of small amounts of the protein. A specific family of enzymes, the **elastases,** degrade elastin at neutral pH. They are serine proteases that appear to be inactivated by serum inhibitors such α1-antitrypsin and α2-macroglobulin. Analysis of the digestion products of the elastases has shown that these enzymes preferentially cleave the peptide bonds adjacent to the smallest amino acids found in nature, namely, glycine, alanine, and valine (3,4).

Although the first specific elastase was isolated from pancreatic tissue, elastolytic enzymes have been found in other tissues and in macrophages, leukocytes, and platelets. The leukocyte elastase is particularly interesting because release of this enzyme together with other lysosomal proteolytic enzymes, probably contributes to the damage of blood vessels in diseases such as leukocytoclastic vasculitis. The elastases may play a role in other disease processes, such as arteriosclerosis, pulmonary emphysema, and the invasion of various tumors into adjacent connective tissues. Furthermore, a specific elastolytic activity in aortic tissue has been shown to increase with advancing age, suggesting that aging and degenerative changes of the cardiovascular system might be partly explained by an increased rate of degradation of elastic fibers (2,3).

1. Franzblau C: Elastin, Comprehensive Biochemistry. Vol 26. M Florkin, EN Stotz, eds. Amsterdam, Elsevier, 1971, pp 659–712
2. Sandberg LB, Gray WR, Franzblau C, eds: Elastin and Elastic Tissue. New York, Plenum, 1977
3. Sandberg LB: Elastin structure in health and disease. Int Rev Connect Tissue Res 7:159–210, 1976
4. Urry DW: Molecular perspective of vascular wall structure and disease: the elastic component. Prospective Biol Med 21:265–295, 1978
5. Uitto J: Biochemistry of the elastic fibers in normal connective tissues and its alterations in diseases. J Invest Dermatol 72:1–10, 1979

5. Biology of the joints

Nearly all the articulations of the extremities are synovial or diarthrodial joints. These possess a joint cavity and are, therefore, freely movable. In diarthroses, the articular cartilage and the articulation are enveloped by a joint capsule and held together by ligaments. The outer stratum of the joint capsule (**fibrosum**) is made up of dense fibrous tissue. The inner layer (**synoviale**) consists of loose highly vascularized connective tissue and synovium (1–3). The radiocarpal, sternoclavicular, and knee joints contain intraarticular fibrocartilaginous menisci which act as washers and help maintain the stability of these joints in rotation (3,4). These menisci are attached at their periphery to the fibrous capsule. Fascia and other periarticular connective tissues blend with the joint capsule, adjacent ligaments, and the musculotendinous structures that pass over the joints, as well as invest the nerves and blood vessels entering the joint. Increased fibrosis of the periarticular tissues and edema, particularly after periods of relative inactivity, are probably responsible in great measure for the limitation of motion and "morning stiffness" that characterize patients with inflammatory arthritis (5).

The joints of the spine and pelvis are of several types. True diarthrodial joints exist in the intervertebral facet joints and in the joints of Luschka (uncovertebral joints) in the cervical spine. The joints between the vertebral bodies are amphiarthrodial (slightly movable) and contain an intervertebral disc. The pubic symphysis is also an amphiarthrodial joint. The sacroiliac joint, in the adult, has elements of both a di- and amphiarthrodial joint (Table 5–1).

Synovium. The synovium or joint lining represents a condensation of connective tissue that covers the inner surface of the fibrous capsule and forms a sac enclosing the synovial cavity (1,2). The synovium also invests tendons that pass through the joint as well as the free margins of the intraarticular structures such as ligaments and menisci. The synovium is thrown into folds that surround the margin of the articular cartilage, but it does not cover the loadbearing surface of the cartilage. Normally the synovial cavity contains a small amount of highly viscous fluid that lubricates the joint surfaces (cartilage on cartilage, cartilage on synovium, and synovium on synovium). The folds of the synovium permit this tissue to be stretched with joint motion without tissue damage. The lining of the bursae resembles a rudimentary synovium.

The innermost or intimal portion of the synovium consists of a layer of specialized cells, known as synoviocytes or synovial lining cells. Beneath this coat, which is normally 1–3 cells deep, there is a loose meshwork of vascular areolar or fibrous connective tissue (Fig 5–1). The deeper or subintimal portion of the synovium differs in thickness and appearance from place to place within the joints, being more or less fibrous or fatty. This layer merges with the periosteum. There is no periosteum on bone within the joint capsule. At the margin of the articular cartilage, the conjoined tissue becomes continuous with cartilage by means of a transitional zone of fibrocartilage.

Synoviocytes. The cells lining the synovial cavity resemble other connective tissue cells but differ from ordinary fibroblasts in their ultrastructural features and metabolic activities. They possess long cytoplasmic processes that overlap and intertwine. Although these cells do not form a fully continuous lining, grossly the synovium presents a relatively smooth surface with a variable number of villi, folds, and fat pads projecting into the joint cavity.

Scanning electron microscopy (EM) has demonstrated that the individual synoviocytes appear relatively uniform in size and exhibit evidence of surface activity with knobby and foldlike processes (Fig 5–2) (6). There are striking changes in these

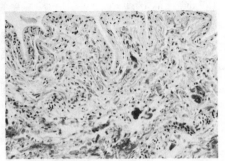

Fig 5–1. Normal human synovium obtained from knee joint. Note small villi covered by layer of specialized synovial lining cells (*synoviocytes*), 1–3 cells in depth. The more superficial portion of the lining (*stratum synoviale*) consists of loosely textured fibrous connective tissue containing numerous capillary vessels, whereas the deeper portion approaching the capsule (*stratum fibrosum* or *subsynovialis*) is made up of more densely compact fibrous tissue.

features in pathologic states such as rheumatoid arthritis, which may explain abnormalities in diffusion and resulting changes in synovial fluid contents.

Transmission EM studies reveal 2 main types of surface lining cells (2,7). Type A cells, which are somewhat more numerous, are characterized by the presence of a rich collection of cytoplasmic organelles, including numerous lysosomes, smooth walled vacuoles, and micropinocytotic vesicles, and by scanty endoplasmic reticulum (Fig 5–3). These cells are active in phagocytosis and secretion. Type B cells possess abundant endoplasmic reticulum and relatively few vacuoles and vesicles (Fig 5–4). The B cells are thought to synthesize the hyaluronate of synovial fluid. In addition, there is an intermediate or type C cell that combines features of both A and B, suggesting that A and B cells represent different functional phases of the same basic cell. Some intermediate or phagocytic type cells also appear to be of monocytic origin (8,9).

The synovium is further distinguished by a rich network of capillaries and venules adjacent to the joint cavity. This tissue is also supplied with lymphatic and sympathetic nerve fibers. The underlying subsynovialis contains fibroblasts, mast cells, and variable amounts of collagen fibers and fatty tissue.

Synovia. The liquid found in all synovial joints was given the name synovia by Paracelsus (1493–1541) who credited the origin of the word to the early wound surgeons who compared the consistency of the sticky gelatinous fluid to that of egg whites (10). Synovia (synovial fluid) is a highly viscous liquor that assists in the lubrication of joints and serves as a source of nutriment for the articular cartilage. Normal synovia is clear, colorless or pale yellow and does not clot. Its characteristic

Table 5–1. Classification of the joints

1. Fibrous joints—synarthroses, or immovable joints
   a. Suture, e.g., skull
   b. Syndesmoses, e.g., tibiofibular attachment
   c. Gomphoses, e.g., tooth sockets
2. Cartilaginous joints—including amphiarthroses, or slightly movable joints
   a. Hyaline cartilaginous joints or synchondroses, e.g., epiphyseal plate in growing bone
   b. Fibrocartilaginous joints or symphyses, e.g., the intervertebral discs, pubic symphysis
3. Synovial joints—diarthroses, or freely movable joints*
   a. Plane or gliding joint, e.g., the carpal and tarsal joints
   b. Hinge joint or ginglymus, e.g., the interphalangeal joints
   c. Condylar joint, e.g., the knee
   d. Spheroidal or ball-and-socket joint, or enarthrosis, e.g., the shoulder and the hip
   e. Ellipsoidal joint, e.g., radiocarpal joint
   f. Pivot or trochoid joint, e.g., the proximal radioulnar joint
   f. Saddle or sellar joint, e.g., the carpometacarpal joint of the thumb

* Subclassified according to axes of movement

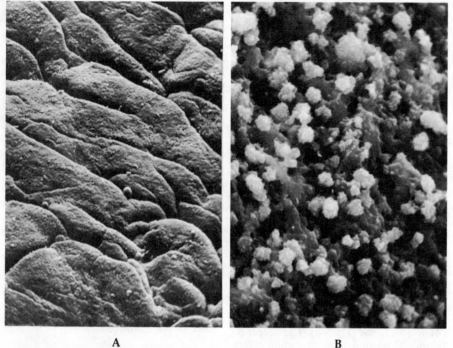

A   B

Fig 5–2. Near normal human synovium (scanning electron microscopy). **A**, At low magnification the surface topography is arranged in a series of shallow folds which provide the capability for expansion during joint movement (original magnification ×95). **B**, At higher magnification individual synoviocytes are seen randomly distributed over the synovial surface. They are separated by wide areas, appear to be partially embedded within the intercellular matrix, and their surface exhibits folds and projections—the morphologic expression of pinocytotic activity (original magnification ×2,500). (Illustration provided by Dr JM Riddle and Dr GB Bluhm)

the synovial fluid which bathes its surface. In the immature animal, diffusion of substances from blood coursing through the vessels in the subchondral area also contributes (13). The matrix of articular cartilage is hyperhydrated; the water content varies from 65–80% of total weight. This water plays an important role in joint lubrication and wear resistance.

The solid matter of the matrix consists chiefly of collagen (type II) and proteoglycan, synthesized locally by the chondrocytes. Collagen fibers form over half the dry weight and play a major role in maintaining the integrity of the tissue. The remainder of the solids are made up largely of proteoglycans, a family of molecules consisting of a protein core to which are attached long chains of negatively charged repeating units of sulfated disaccharide. Most of the units in the cartilage are chondroitin-4 sulfate, in which the component sugars are N-acetyl galactosamine and glucuronic acid. The sulfate is linked to the galactosamine. Chondroitin-6-sulfate, an isomer differing in that the sulfate is attached to the sixth position of the N-acetyl galactosamine, is also present. In addition there are quantities of keratan sulfate, in which the repeating disaccharide consists of sulfated N-acetyl glucosamine and galactose. The relative concentration of these glycosaminoglycans varies markedly with age.

In immature cartilage, there is a preponderance of chondroitin-4-sulfate and little keratan sulfate. With advancing age, there is an appreciable increase in keratan sulfate content and a corresponding fall in chondroitin-4-sulfate. The proteoglycan is highly viscous and strongly hydrophilic, properties which are of key importance in the resiliency of the articular cartilage and lubrication of its bearing surfaces under compressive loads.

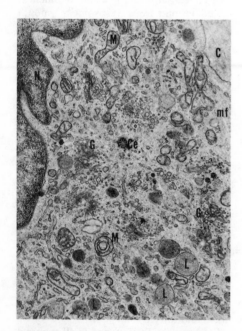

Fig 5–3. Human synovium, type A cell. Cytoplasm of a type A synoviocyte demonstrating nucleus (**N**), mitochondria (**M**), a small centriole cut in a cross section (**Ce**), and several lysosomes (**L**). The Golgi apparatus is extensive (**G**) and consists of lamellae and vesicles occurring in groups. Interspersed between the cytoplasmic organelles are fine microfilaments (**mf**) and outside this cell lie a few collagen fibrils (**C**) (original magnification ×18,000). (Illustration provided by Dr CR Wynne-Roberts)

high viscosity is related to the presence of a complex macromolecule hyaluronate which is synthesized by synovial lining cells (2,11,12). Hyaluronate is a high molecular weight glycosaminoglycan composed of regularly alternating units of glucosamine and glucuronic acid.

Synovial fluid is thought to be a transudate of plasma to which hyaluronate is added by the type B cells in the synovial lining (2). Certain larger proteins, such as fibrinogen, are normally absent or present in very small quantity compared to plasma. Molecular charge and shape as well as molecular weight appear to be important in determining the permeability of synovium to different plasma proteins. Synovial fluid normally contains less than 200 cells/mm^3. These consist chiefly of mononuclear cells believed to be derived from the lining tissue. Inflammation and other pathologic processes affecting the synovium alter the composition, cellular content, and physical characteristics of the synovia. Examination of this fluid plays an important role in the diagnosis of joint diseases (see Section 90).

Articular cartilage. Articular cartilage is the weight-bearing surface of the joint and is distinguished by a relatively low concentration of cells and preponderance of intercellular materials. In the adult blood vessels, lymphatic channels and nerves are lacking. Nourishment is derived from

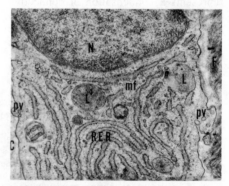

Fig 5–4. Human synovium, type B cell. Part of a type B (synthetic) synoviocyte showing nucleus (**N**), well-developed lamellae of rough endoplasmic reticulum (**RER**), lysosomes (**L**), a few pinocytotic vesicles at the edge of the cell (**pv**), and a small group of microfilaments (**mf**). Some fibrin (**F**) and a small amount of collagen (**C**) lie outside the cell (original magnification ×24,000). (Illustration provided by Dr CR Wynne-Roberts)

Articular cartilage is highly active metabolically, chiefly in the synthesis of proteoglycan (PG). Although the half-life of adult human articular cartilage PG may exceed 800 days (14), the turnover of at least a portion of the PG is so rapid (8 days) (15) as to suggest the existence of an internal remodeling system. Proteoglycan synthesis dramatically increases in damaged articular cartilage (16,17). Clinical and experimental evidence for cartilage healing has been reported (15) but it appears that the material synthesized is mainly fibrocartilaginous and may not be an adequate replacement for hyaline cartilage as a bearing surface, particularly over long periods of time (18). The variables controlling cartilage healing and the transition of fibrocartilage to hyaline cartilage are yet to be completely understood.

Blood and nerve supply. The blood supply of the joint arises from vessels that enter the subchrondral bone at or near the line of capsular attachment and form an arterial circle around the joint. These vessels subdivide into a rich capillary network that is specially prominent in the portions of synovium immediately adjacent to the joint cavity. Constitutents of plasma diffuse rapidly between these vessels and the joint cavity. Colloidal and fine particulate suspensions injected into the joint enter the subsynovialis, but these substances, as well as proteins, are removed mainly via lymphatic channels.

The articular nerves carry fibers derived from several spinal segments and vary in number and course. As a rule, joints are innervated by all peripheral nerves that cross the articulation. This may help explain the "referral" of pain from one joint to the next. For example, hip pain may be perceived as pain in the knee, or lumbar pain as pain in the hip, posterior thigh, and calf. Joints are richly innervated and the nerves to them carry autonomic as well as sensory fibers. The larger sensory fibers form proprioceptive endings in the ligaments and capsule and are sensitive to position and movement, in particular stretching and twisting. Under normal circumstances, we are aware of the position of our back and limbs without regard to visual confirmation. The superficial synovium is innervated only by autonomic fibers which control blood flow; thus the synovium itself is relatively insensitive to painful stimuli. When the joint is swollen, there is significant pressure on the pain sensitive capsule. Pain arising from the capsule tends to be diffused or poorly localized.

The proprioceptive responses accompanying joint motion are extremely important in maintaining proper muscular balance around the joint. Joint stability is dependent to a great extent on such reflexural muscle activity. Shock absorption is largely the result of joint motion and the controlled stretching of partially contract-

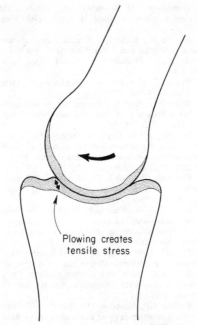

Fig 5–5. Cartilage compression associated with simultaneous oscillation can create tensile stresses within cartilage.

ed muscle (19). Thus loss of proprioception and abolition of this reflexural activity lead to progressive destructive change in the joint (see Section 37).

Joint lubrication. The diarthrodial joints possess lubrication mechanisms that permit free motion with a minimum of friction (20). This lubrication is more effective than in most mechanical bearings and relies primarily on a combination of hydro-

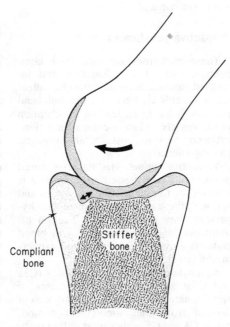

Fig 5–6. The relative stiffness of the underlying bone determines the amount of deformation to which the overlying cartilage will be subjected. Regions of cartilage that overlie gradients in the stiffness of the underlying bone will be subjected to significant tensile stresses.

static and boundary lubrication mechanisms. Pressures applied to articular cartilage cause its interstitial fluid to "weep" out. The greater the load on the cartilage, the greater the hydrostatic pressure on the fluid and the more tendency it will have to weep. Most of this fluid emerges from the cartilage peripheral to the zone of impending contact. When opposing surfaces of cartilage rub together, the bulk of the load can be borne by the interstitial fluid which is reimbibed when the pressure on the cartilage is reduced. The cartilage also appears to be lubricated by a boundary surface phenomenon, wherein a specific glycoprotein lubricating fraction, found in synovial fluid, preferentially binds to the articular cartilage surfaces and keeps them apart (21). Thus animal joints operate within a mixed film region of lubrication throughout the range of load and motion, the boundary phenomenon predominating at low loads and low speeds and the hydrostatic (weeping) mechanism predominating at high loads and high speeds.

Articular cartilage possesses excellent elastic properties and the fluid flow that accompanies cartilage deformation under load contributes to the fluid film which maintains separation between the joint surfaces. Thus joints cannot be made to wear out by rubbing them, even under severe conditions, as long as a fluid film is present (19,22).

Articular cartilage has an extremely low frictional resistance to movement even when simply lubricated by physiologic saline. The major friction created by joint motion is from the soft tissues rubbing on themselves or on the articular cartilage. Soft tissue lubrication depends on the hyaluronate in the synovial fluid. This is extremely sensitive to the molecular weight and concentration of the hyaluronate (12) and appears to be a boundary lubrication phenomenon. The large hyaluronate molecules give synovial fluid its viscosity. Synovial fluid, without hyaluronate, will not lubricate the synovium but as long as it contains the glycoprotein lubricating fraction, it will still lubricate articular cartilage. The glycoprotein lubricating fraction seems to have no effect on soft tissue (synovial) lubrication within the joint. Since the hyaluronate is responsible for the high viscosity of synovial fluid, cartilage on cartilage lubrication, which is independent of hyaluronate, is also not dependent on the viscosity of the lubricant (20).

Natural mechanisms protecting the joint from wear. The friction of joints is so low that articular cartilage is normally never subjected to significant shear stresses. But when cartilage is highly compressed, simultaneous oscillation can provoke tensile stresses within the cartilaginous tissue (Fig 5–5). The major factor limiting the compressive loads on joints is the neuromuscular shock-absorbing reflex (4). The wide potential contact area of the bearing surface also helps to spread out the load. The cartilage sits on a bed of cancellous bone which can deform to decrease local concentrations of stress. Cartilage deformation occurring over areas of significant gradients in stiffness of the underlying subchondral bone, such as the margins of habitually loaded and nonloaded areas of the joint, will create potentially deleterious tensile stresses in cartilage. Over time, this can cause fatigue failure of the cartilage (Fig 5–6) (4). It is not unusual to find surface fragmentation of the articular cartilage (fibrillation) in these areas in the normal joints of adults (22). The integrity of normal adult articular cartilage depends on the proper action of the natural shock-absorbing mechanisms—neuromuscular and bony. Alterations in the quality of either can have significant effects on the joint.

1. Barnett HCH, Davies DV, MacConaill RA: Synovial Joints: Their Structure and Mechanics, Springfield IL, Charles C Thomas, 1961

2. Hammerman D, Rosenberg LC, Schubert M: Diarthroidal joints revisited. J Bone Joint Surg 52A:725–744, 1970
3. Mankin HJ, Radin EL: Structure and function of joints , Arthritis and Allied Conditions. Ed 9. DJ McCarty, Jr., ed. Philadelphia, Lea & Febiger, 1979, pp 151–166
4. Radin EL: Biomechanics of the knee joint. Orth Clin N Am 4:539–546, 1973
5. Radin EL, Paul IL, Swann DA, Schottstaedt ES: The lubrication of synovial membrane. Ann Rheum Dis 30:322–325, 1971
6. Woodward DH, Gryfe A, Gardner DL: Comparative study by scanning electron microscopy of synovial surfaces of four mammalian species. Experientia 25:1301–1303, 1969
7. Ghadially FN, Roy S: Ultrastructure of Synovial Joints in Health and Disease. New York, Appleton-Century Crofts, 1969
8. Edwards JCW, Willoughby DA: Demonstration of bone marrow derived cells in synovial lining by means of giant intracellular granules as genetic markers. Ann Rheum Dis 41:177–182, 1982
9. Edwards JCW, Sedgwick AD, Willoughby DA: Membrane properties and esterase activity of synovial fluid of synovial lining cells: further evidence for a mononuclear phagocyte population. Ann Rheum Dis 41:282–286, 1982
10. Rodnan GP, Benedek TG, Panetta WC: The early history of synovia (joint fluid). Ann Intern Med 65:821–842, 1966
11. Schubert M, Hamerman D: A Primer on Connective Tissue Biochemistry. Philadelphia, Lea & Febiger, 1968
12. Swann DA, Radin EL, Nazimiec M, Weisser PA, Curran N, Lewinneck G: Role of hyaluronic acid in joint lubrication. Ann Rheum Dis 33:318–326, 1974
13. McKibbin B: Nutrition in Adult Articular Cargilage. MAR Freeman, ed. New York, Grune and Stratton, 1973, pp 277–286
14. Maroudas A: Glycosaminoglycan turnover in articular cartilage. Phil Trans Res Soc Lond B271:293–313, 1973
15. Mankin HJ: The structure, chemistry, and metabolism of articular cartilage. Bull Rheum Dis 17:447–451, 1967
16. Radin EL, Ehrlich MM, Weiss CA, Parker GH: Osteoarthrosis as a state of altered physiology, Recent Advances in Rheumatology, Part I. WW Buchanan, WC Dick, eds. New York, Churchill Livingstone, 1976, pp 1–18
17. Cheung HS, Cottrell WH, Stephenson K, Nimni M: In vitro collagen biosynthesis in healing and normal rabbit articular cartilage. J Bone Joint Surg 60A:1076–1081, 1978
18. Akeson W, Coletti J, Woo S: A comparison of the physical behavior of normal articular cartilage and the arthroplasty surface. J Bone Joint Surg 54A:147–159, 1972
19. Radin EL: Mechanical aspects of osteoarthrosis. Bull Rheum Dis 26:862–865, 1976
20. Radin EL, Paul IL: A consolidated concept of joint lubrication. J Bone Joint Surg 54A:607–616, 1972
21. Swann DA: Macromolecules of synovial fluid, The Joints and Synovial Fluid. Vol 1. L. Sokoloff, ed. New York, Academic Press, 1978, pp 407–435
22. Radin EL: Mechanics of joint degeneration, Practical Biomechanics for the Orthopedic Surgeon. EL Radin, SR Simon, RM Rose, IL Paul, eds. New York, John Wiley and Sons, 1979

6. The inflammatory process

Inflammation protects the host from foreign invaders by isolating and destroying bacteria, viruses, and other agents. It is a highly complex process involving many types of cells, a number of enzymes, and many physiologically active materials that alter local blood flow and cell behavior. In many of the rheumatic diseases, the offending agent causing inflammation is unknown (e.g., rheumatoid arthritis); in others the inciting agent is recognized (e.g., sodium urate monohydrate crystals in gouty arthritis). In both of these cases, the inflammatory reaction becomes deleterious to the host, causing pain and limitation of function of joints and leads to the destruction of skeletal and extraskeletal tissues. The therapy of the rheumatic diseases is based primarily on drugs that suppress inflammation.

Inflammation may occur in different forms, involving different mechanisms. Although the detailed mechanism of the inflammatory reaction is not fully understood, these reactions are almost certainly dependent on a number of chemical signals or mediators which will be subject of this Section. For convenience we may consider factors primarily active in 3 areas, although some overlap occurs between these: vasoactive substances, chemotactic factors, and agents leading to cell and tissue damage.

Vasoactive substances

These mediators are vasoactive compounds, causing vasodilatation and increased vascular permeability. They affect the contractile elements in endothelial and periendothelial cells, leading to dilatation of the vessels and to opening of junctions between cells in postcapillary venules, causing edema.

Vasoactive amines. Histamine is stored in basophils and tissue mast cells and is released by the interaction of antigen and IgE with these cells during immediate hypersensitivity reactions (see Section 8). Serotonin released from stores in blood platelets may also contribute to vasopermeability (1).

Anaphylatoxins. These substances (C3a and C5a) are polypeptide fragments of approximately 10,000 molecular weight derived from the complement components, C3 and C5, either by standard pathways of complement activation or through action of other proteolytic enzymes, such as plasmin (see Section 7). These components are potent mediators of vascular permeability, acting either directly on vessels or through the release of histamine from mast cells (1).

Kinins. Bradykinin is the most important kinin, an oligopeptide composed of 9 amino acids with potent activity as a vasodilator and promoter of vascular permeability (1). Bradykinin arises as a result of a complex cascade of proteolytic reactions outlined in Fig 6–1.

Hageman factor (coagulation factor XII) activation begins the sequence leading to the production of bradykinin by binding to negatively charged surfaces, such as monosodium urate or calcium pyrophosphate crystals, probably undergoing proteolytic cleavage. Active Hageman factor in turn activates prekallikrein to kallikrein. Kallikrein then cleaves bradykinin from precursor kininogens in plasma (Fig 6–1).

Kallikrein also activates plasminogen to plasmin, and the protein plasminogen activator appears to be a modified form of kallikrein. In addition to its own effects on vasopermeability, bradykinin has the ability to stimulate histamine release from mast cells and to stimulate prostaglandin synthesis in a variety of tissues (1).

Prostaglandins. The prostaglandins (PGs) are a group of compounds derived from polyunsaturated fatty acids (Fig 6–

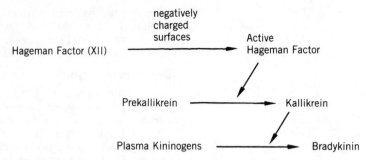

Fig 6–1. Schematic sequences of reactions leading to bradykinin formation.

2). The most important are PGs of the 2-series, which are all derived from arachidonic acid, a component of the phospholipid present in all cell membranes. These molecules have 2 double bonds in their side chains and are therefore designated by a subscript 2, e.g., PGE$_2$. The PGs possess characteristic 5-membered ring structures which are the basis for designation by letters such as E and F. Thromboxane A$_2$ is closely related to prostaglandins but possesses a 6-membered ring structure (2).

Another group of compounds closely related to PGs are the products of lipoxygenase catalyzed reactions (Fig 6–3) (3). These compounds are also products of reactions of molecular oxygen with arachidonic acid. One of them, leukotriene D, has been shown to be a slow-reacting substance released from mast cells and other sources during immediate hypersensitivity reactions, causing bronchoconstriction and vascular permeability (4,5).

The PGs and lipoxygenase products are not stored in cells but are synthesized by almost all cells in response to a variety of stimuli. The fatty acid precursors of PGs are stored in cell membrane lipids, primarily phospholipids, and are released by the action of phospholipases. The enzyme cyclooxygenase converts free arachidonic acid into PGH$_2$ by reactions with molecular oxygen and molecular rearrangements. Isomerases then convert this endoperoxide intermediate into PGs and thromboxane A$_2$.

The distribution of isomerases in tissues determines the types of PGs to be synthesized. For example, blood platelets make primarily thromboxane A$_2$ (2); endothelial cells, PGI$_2$ or prostacyclin (6); and rheumatoid synovial tissue, PGE$_2$ (7). The so-called classic prostaglandins—PGE$_2$ and PGF$_{2\alpha}$—are relatively stable although they are rapidly inactivated in the pulmonary circulation (8). Thromboxane A$_2$ and prostacyclin are chemically labile under physiologic conditions, with half-lives of approximately 30 seconds and 2 minutes, respectively (2,6).

The prostaglandins have potent physiologic effects on many cells and tissues, but the effects of one PG often differ widely from those of another. For example, PGE$_2$

and PGI$_2$, are vasodilators, whereas thromboxane A$_2$ and PGF$_{2\alpha}$ are vasoconstrictors. The PGs are active in tissues containing smooth muscle and their widespread effects on blood vessels and on smooth muscle of the gastrointestinal tract, tracheobroncheal tree, uterus, and many other organs have led to much interest in the PGs.

Many of the effects of PGs may be mediated through cyclic nucleotides. In particular, some PGs, such as PGE$_2$ and PGI$_2$, activate adenylate cyclase, leading to elevated levels of 3′,5′-cyclic AMP in tissues. Other PGs may inhibit adenylate cyclase activation (thromboxane A$_2$) or produce antagonism of cAMP by stimulating guanylate cyclase (PGF$_{2\alpha}$) (7).

There are several lines of evidence that PGs, primarily PGE$_2$ and PGI$_2$, may act as mediators of inflammation (9,10):

1. They cause vasodilatation, potentiate edema induced by other agents, and sensitize tissues to painful stimuli.

2. They are present in elevated concentrations in inflammatory exudates.

3. They act synergistically with other mediators such as bradykinin and histamine.

4. The synthesis of PGs is inhibited by antiinflammatory drugs.

5. Certain lipoxygenase-derived products, substances closely related to PGs, are vasoactive and have chemotactic activity (3–5).

In addition, the synthesis of both prostaglandins and lipoxygenase-derived products generates active oxygen free radicals, including superoxide anion (O$_2^-$) and hydroxyl radical (OH·), reactive species which may cause tissue injury during inflammatory reactions (11). Products of lipoxygenase reactions, although not PGs, may themselves be important in inflammation. Some of these compounds, especially leukotriene B, are chemotactic for leukocytes (3). At least 1 of these compounds (leukotriene D) has been associated with potent slow-reacting substance (SRS) of anaphylaxis activity, leading to histamine release, bronchoconstriction, and increased vasopermeability (4,5).

Although PGs generally act as mediators of inflammation, their effects may be more complex. Certain model systems indicate that PGE may actually inhibit some immune reactions, probably through stimulation of adenylate cyclase and elevations of cyclic AMP levels in tissues. The significance of these findings remains uncertain, but it is possible that under some conditions PGs may suppress some forms of inflammation (7).

Prostaglandins and the mechanism of action of antiinflammatory drugs. It is now generally accepted that a major pharmacologic effect of the nonsteroidal antiinflam-

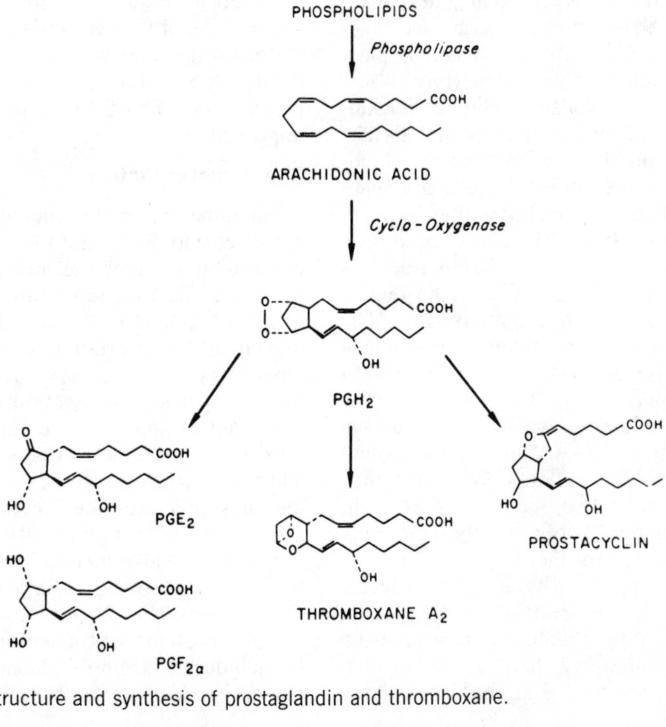

PHOSPHOLIPIDS

Phospholipase

ARACHIDONIC ACID

Cyclo-Oxygenase

PGH$_2$

PGE$_2$

PGF$_{2\alpha}$

THROMBOXANE A$_2$

PROSTACYCLIN

Fig 6–2. Structure and synthesis of prostaglandin and thromboxane.

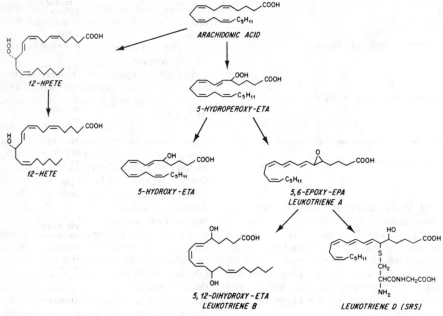

Fig 6–3. Formation of leukotrienes and other oxygenated derivations of arachidonic acid derivatives via action of lipoxygenase.

matory drugs may be accounted for by their ability to inhibit PG synthesis (12). These drugs include aspirin, indomethacin, phenylalkanoic acid derivatives, and others. They interact directly with the enzyme, cyclooxygenase, and inhibit the synthesis of all PGs. Aspirin irreversibly inhibits cyclooxygenase by acetylating the enzyme (13). This action accounts for the anti-platelet effects of aspirin, since platelets are incapable of synthesizing new cyclooxygenase as other cells apparently do. The mechanism of action of other drugs of this class is less clear, but they do directly inhibit the cyclooxygenase reaction at concentrations comparable to plasma levels achieved during therapy (14).

Corticosteroids also inhibit prostaglandin synthesis by intact cells and tissues (15). The inhibition is specific for glucocorticoids since other steroids are inactive. Furthermore, the potency of PG synthesis inhibition by glucocorticoids parallels the relative antiinflammatory potency of these drugs (dexamethasone > prednisolone > hydrocortisone). The mechanism of action of glucocorticoids on PG synthesis is not fully understood, but some evidence suggests that they may inhibit the release of arachidonic acid from phospholipids (16). Although the potent antiinflammatory effects of glucocorticoids are probably based on several mechanisms, inhibition of PG synthesis is likely to be an important factor.

Certain drugs that have a more specific antiinflammatory action than the nonsteroidal drugs or glucocorticoids have no important inhibitory effects on PG synthesis. These include gold-containing compounds, penicillamine, anti-malarials, and colchicine (15).

Effects of PGs on bone. The destruction of juxtaarticular bone is an important aspect of the tissue damage in inflammatory joint disease, especially in rheumatoid arthritis. Rheumatoid synovial tissue produces large quantities of PGE_2, which is known to stimulate osteoclastic bone resorption. It has been suggested that PGE_2 produced by the rheumatoid synovial pannus may mediate osteoclastic resorption in subchondral bone (17) and thus contribute to osseous erosions. It follows that the suppression of PG synthesis by antiinflammatory drugs may be expected to retard the development of such erosions, but this possible benefit of these drugs remains unproved.

Chemotactic factors

Inflammatory cells, including neutrophils, eosinophils, and monocytes, migrate to sites under the influence of chemotactic factors, substances causing increased cell motility and directed cell movement (18). Certain fragments of complement components have active chemotactic properties (see Section 7). The most important of these are the anaphylatoxin, C3a, and the soluble complex, C5, 6, 7. In addition, neutral proteases such as plasmin may generate other chemotactic peptide fragments from C3 and C5. The C5a fragment may also increase neutrophil adhesiveness, allowing margination and escape of these cells from blood vessels (1).

Other proteins with chemotactic activity include kallikrein or plasminogen activator, peptides derived from fibrin and collagen, and bacterial products. Prostaglandins have no important chemotactic activity but several lipoxygenase products are active chemotactic factors (3).

Degradative enzymes

In addition to vasoactive and chemotactic factors, a large number of enzymes are released in inflammatory exudates that catalyze the hydrolysis of tissue components, including proteins, carbohydrates, and lipids. Inflammatory cells contain large quantities of these hydrolases, primarily in granules or lysosomes. The function of these enzymes may be primarily bacteriocidal, since lysosomes fuse with phagosomes containing internalized particles. Other components, such as immune complexes, may be destroyed in this manner.

Many of the hydrolytic enzymes are active at acid pH, apparently in the phagolysosome. However, these enzymes are released in part from leukocytes during phagocytosis and may exert their effects on host tissues. Although enzymes with activities limited to acid pH values may be of little consequence at the pH of the extracellular environment, some enzymes, primarily proteases, are active at neutral pH, and so may attack and destroy host tissues (19).

Collagenase is one of the most important extracellular degradative enzymes. Collagenase is a metalloenzyme, a specific neutral protease, acting on native collagens by cleaving the triple helical structure into 2 fragments, 1 containing the amino-terminal three-fourths and the other the carboxy-terminal one-fourth of the molecules (20). Collagenase is active on all types of collagen investigated, although it degrades type II collagen of articular cartilage less rapidly than types I and III, found in skin, bone, and blood vessels. Collagenases appear to act on extracellular collagen and once cleaved, the 2 collagen fragments are readily denatured at 37°C and become susceptible to degradation by several nonspecific proteases.

Collagenases are produced by several tissues including rheumatoid synovial tissue and by polymorphonuclear leukocytes and macrophages. Proteolytic enzymes may be required for activation of collagenase by either of 2 mechanisms. In the first, macromolecular inhibitors which form inactive complexes with collagenases are present in tissues and serum. Proteolytic enzymes may digest the inhibitors, releasing active collagenase. In the second mechanism, a precursor, procollagenase, may require proteolytic cleavage for activation (21). Since collagens are a major constituent of structural tissues, collagenase activity is likely to mediate the destruction of articular cartilage, tendons, joint capsules, bone, and other tissues in arthritis and other inflammatory processes.

Other neutral proteases. Two neutral proteases are produced by polymorphonuclear leukocytes and macrophages which account for much of the extracellular proteolytic activity in rheumatoid arthritis and other inflammatory states. The first is elastase, a serine protease of broad substrate specificity, which is capable of digesting a wide variety of proteins. Elastase degrades proteoglycans by cleaving the core protein of proteoglycan subunits into several fragments. Elastase is also capable of degrading elastin of blood vessels and many other proteins (19,21).

The second important extracellular protease is cathepsin G, a chymotrypsin-like enzyme active at neutral pH on proteoglycans and other proteins. Other cathepsins, such as cathepsin D, are inactive near neutral pH and therefore are probably insignificant in extracellular locations. Cathepsin D may be important in the intracellular degradation of proteoglycans in phagolysosomes at acid pH. Many other lysosomal enzymes degrade carbohydrates and proteins but appear to be active only at the acid pH of the phagolysosome (19,21).

Proteolytic enzymes may also participate in inflammation by releasing mediators from complement components and from plasma kininogens. The neutral protease, plasmin, is generated by the action of plasminogen activator on the zymogen, plasminogen. Plasmin acts on several substrates, including fibrinogen and fibrin, releasing biologically active peptide fragments. It may also lead to activation of Hageman factor, activation of collagenase from its latent forms, and activation of C1 and C3, by proteolytic cleavage reactions (19,21).

1. Fearon DT, Austen FK: Acute inflammatory response, Arthritis and Allied Conditions. Ed 9, DJ McCarty, Jr, ed. Philadelphia, Lea & Febiger, 1979, pp 214–228
2. Hamberg M, Svensson J, Samuelsson B: Thromboxanes: a new group of biologically active compounds derived from prostaendoperoxides. Proc Natl Acad Sci 72:2994–2998, 1975
3. Goetzl EJ, Sun FF: Generation of unique monohydroxy-eisatetraenoic acids from arachidonic acid by human neutrophils. J Exp Med 150:406–411, 1979
4. Orning L, Hammarstrom S, Samuelsson B: Leukotriene D: a slow reacting substance from rat basophilic leukemia cells. Proc Natl Acad Sci 77:2014–2017, 1980
5. Morris HR, Taylor GW, Piper PJ: Structure of slow-reacting substance of anaphylaxis from guinea-pig lung. Nature 285:104–108, 1980
6. Baenziger NL, Dillender MJ, Majerus PW: Cultured human skin fibroblasts and arterial cells produce a labile platelet-inhibitory prostaglandin. Biochem Biophys Res Commun 78:294–301, 1977
7. Robinson DR, Dayer J-M, Krane SM: Prostaglandins: their regulation in rheumatoid arthritis. Ann NY Acad Sci 332:279–294, 1979
8. Samuelsson B, Granstrom E, Green K: Metabolism of prostaglandins. Ann NY Acad Sci 180:138–163, 1971
9. Vane JR: Prostaglandins as mediators of inflammation, Advances in Prostaglandin and Thromboxane Research. Vol 2. B Samuelsson, R Paoletti, eds. New York, Raven Press, 1976, pp 791–801
10. Trang LE: Prostaglandins and inflammation. Semin Arthritis Rheum 9:153–190, 1980
11. Salin JL, McCord JL: Free radicals and inflammation. J Clin Invest 56:1319–1323, 1975
12. Flower RJ: Drugs which inhibit prostaglandin biosynthesis. Pharm Rev 26:33–65, 1974
13. Roth GJ, Majerus PW: The mechanism of the effect of aspirin on human platelets. J Clin Invest 56:624–632, 1975
14. Robinson DR, McGuire MB, Bastian D: The effects of anti-inflammatory drugs on prostaglandin production by rheumatoid synovial tissue. Prostaglandins Med 1:461–477, 1978
15. Kantrowitz F, Robinson DR, McGuire MB: Corticosteroids inhibit prostaglandin production by rheumatoid synovia. Nature 258:737–739, 1975
16. Blackwell GJ, Flower RJ, Nijkamp FP: Phospholipase A$_2$ activity of guinea-pig isolated perfused lungs: stimulation, and inhibition by anti-inflammatory steroids. Br J Pharmacol 62:79–89, 1978
17. Robinson DR, Tashjian AH Jr, Levine L: Prostaglandin-stimulated bone resorption by rheumatoid synovia. J Clin Invest 56:1181–1188, 1975
18. Snyderman R, Goetzl EJ: Molecular and cellular mechanisms of leukocyte chemotaxis. Science 213:830–837, 1981
19. Smolen JE, Weissmann G: Polymorphonuclear leukocytes, Arthritis and Allied Conditions. Ed 9. DJ McCarty, Jr, ed. Philadelphia, Lea & Febiger, 1979, pp 282–295
20. Harris ED Jr, Krane SM: Collagenases. N Engl J Med 291:557, 605, 652, 1974
21. Krane SM: Mechanisms of tissue destruction in rheumatoid arthritis, Arthritis and Allied Conditions. Ed 9. DJ McCarty, Jr, ed. Philadelphia, Lea & Febiger, 1979, pp 449–456

7. The complement system

Blood plasma contains at least 4 protein systems that affect and amplify inflammation. These are the complement, coagulation, fibrinolytic, and bradykinin-forming systems. The first of these systems to be studied extensively was "complement," recognized in the late 19th century as the heat-labile nonspecific substance in human serum required to "complete" the killing of bacteria coated with specific antibody.

Today it is known that the complement system consists of a group of approximately 20 plasma proteins that interact sequentially to mediate a large number of inflammatory effects, including bacterial killing (1). Virtually all of these proteins have been purified to chemical homogeneity and to a large extent their functions are understood.

Their actions can be divided broadly into 2 categories: those involved in triggering activation of the system, for which there are 2 major pathways, and those involved in effecting a response, for which there is a single final common pathway.

Two pathways for activation: classical and alternative. Although the "classical" pathway is so named because it was discovered first, the "alternative" pathway actually seems to be the older and more primitive as judged by phylogenetic and ontogenetic studies.

The **classical pathway** requires IgG or IgM antibodies combining with their antigens in immune complexes for activation (Fig 7–1): adaptive immunity and specific IgG or IgM antibody are found relatively late in evolution or embryologic development.

In contrast, the **alternative pathway** may be activated without involving antibody;

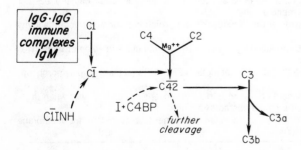

Fig 7–1. The classical activation pathway. Immune complexes containing either **IgG** or **IgM** convert the first component (**C1**) from its precursor form to an active protease. This cleaves the fourth (**C4**) and second (**C2**) components, forming from them the complex enzyme, **C42**, a new protease which in turn is capable of cleaving the third (**C3**) component into **C3a** and **C3b**. C1 Inhibitor blocks the effect of C1. In the presence of the C4 binding protein (**C4BP**), Factor I (**I**) inactivates the C4b produced by C1 by further cleaving it to C4bi. (Illustration provided by Dr Shaun Ruddy)

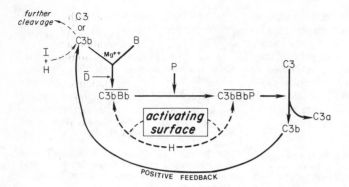

Fig 7–2. The alternative pathway. Either **C3b** or native **C3**, that has been altered by hydrolysis of an internal thioester bond, interacts with Factor B (**B**) which is subsequently cleaved by Factor D (**D**) forming **C3bBb**. The stability of C3bBb is enhanced by combination with properdin (**P**) to form **C3bBbP**. **C3b**, the major fragment of **C3**, interacts with additional Factor B generating additional complex enzyme **C3bBb**, creating a positive feedback loop. Two control proteins oppose this feedback: 1) Factor I (**I**) further degrades C3b to C3bi and 2) Factor H (**H**) interacts with C3b both to block its participation in the loop and to enhance the rate at which the complex enzymes C3bBb and C3bBbP decay. Surfaces that activate the alternative pathway provide a microenvironment inimical to the action of Factor H. (Illustration provided by Dr Shaun Ruddy)

repeating polysaccharides or other polymeric structures may trigger this pathway in blood from animals incapable of mounting an adaptive immune response.

Activation of either pathway involves the conversion of zymogens to proteolytic enzymes and subsequent limited proteolysis of other components. In the classical pathway, precursor C1 undergoes internal proteolysis to the active enzyme C1, which then cleaves its 2 natural substrates C4 and C2. The action of C1 on C4 and C2 is opposed by the C1 inhibitor and alpha-2 globulin which binds tightly to the active site on C1 (2). An additional control mechanism involves the action of Factor I, an endoprotease which, in the presence of the C4 binding protein, degrades the major fragment of C4 into inactive fragments. Major fragments of C4 and C2 combine in the presence of Mg^{++} to form a bimolecular complex (C42) with new enzymatic activity, "C3 convertase," which cleaves C3 and continues the complement sequence (Fig 7–1).

Events in the activation of the alternative pathway parallel those of the classical in that a bimolecular magnesium-dependent C3-cleaving complex is formed from the union of 2 fragments, C3b and Bb (3). Fragment Bb is the major product of the action of Factor D, a C1-like protease, on Factor B, which is homologous to C2. The C3bBb enzyme is stabilized by properdin (P), although both C3bBb and C3bBbP are subject to dissociation by the control protein, Factor H (beta-1-H globulin) (Fig 7–2).

The actions of C42 and C3bBb are identical. Cleavage of C3 occurs at precisely the same site, the 77th residue, an arginine from the amino terminal end of the alpha chain, yielding the cleavage peptide C3a and the major fragment C3b. This proteolytic reaction results in an internal rearrangement of the C3 molecule leading to disruption of an internal thioester bond in the C3 molecule. The active carbonyl group thus formed permits C3b to bind covalently to surfaces via ester or amide linkages.

By interacting with proteins of the alternative pathway, C3b leads into the positive feedback or amplification cycle, in which the product, C3b, generates additional enzyme (C3bBb), which in turn generates more C3b. This positive feedback loop is damped by 2 control proteins: Factor I (C3b inactivator), an endoprotease which further degrades C3b into C3bi, and Factor H (beta-1-H globulin), which combines physically with C3b, preventing its interaction with other proteins and, as mentioned, enhances the dissociation of Bb already bound to C3b. Surfaces that activate the alternative pathway do so by furnishing a microenvironment in which C3b is protected from the controlling effects of Factor H, thereby allowing amplification via the positive feedback loop (4).

The terminal sequence: biologic activities. Either of the endopeptidases (C42 or C3bBb) give rise to the same inflammatory events. The reaction products and the effects they mediate are listed in Table 7–1. The amino acid sequence of human C3a, which causes secretion from histamine-containing mast cells and basophils, is known, and peptide analogs that mimic the inflammatory effects of this fragment have been synthesized. C3a is also a potent suppressor of the humoral immune response, although this effect, like that of histamine release, is abrogated by scission of the terminal arginine from the molecule by carboxypeptidase B, an enzyme normally present in serum.

The biologic activity of C3b varies with the type of cell that bears the receptor to which it binds. Judging from the frequency of sepsis with pyogenic organisms in individuals who are homozygous for C3 deficiency, enhancement of phagocytosis by polymorphonuclear and mononuclear leukocytes is clearly of prime importance. Certain of these reactions can also be promoted by C3bi, the form of C3 produced by the action of Factor I on C3b.

Evidence for the functioning of C3b or other complement proteins in the facilitation of cell-cell interactions required for the processing of antigen, for the initiation of an immune response, or for the maintenance of an effective response has been presented, but precise mechanisms by which these effects are mediated are as yet unclear. The significance of binding sites for C3d, a further cleavage fragment of C3bi, on a small proportion of lymphocytes is even less well understood.

Cleavage of C5 by endopeptidases arising from either the classical or alternative pathways produces C5a, a peptide with chemotactic activity for leukocytes and secretory activity for mast cells and basophils containing histamine. The evolution of C5b, the major fragment of C5, leads to the formation of a trimolecular complex, C5b67, which also has chemotactic activity. Assembly of the membrane attack

Table 7–1. Biologically active products of the complement system

Product	Function
C3a	An "anaphylatoxin"—liberates histamine from mast cells and basophils, suppresses humoral immune response
C3b(bi)	Major fragment of initial C3 cleavage (or of further cleavage by Factor I)—binds to receptors on lymphocytes, monocytes, macrophages, and polymorphonuclear leukocytes, enhancing phagocytosis. Triggers formation of additional C3-cleaving enzyme via the "feedback" or "amplification" loop (Fig 7–2)
C3d	Smaller fragment of C3bi produced by Factor I or other proteases—binds to receptor sites on certain lymphoid cells
C3bBb	Unstable active enzyme of the "feedback" loop which has chemoattractant activity for leukocytes
Bb	Major fragment of B produced by cleavage by D—induces spreading of monocytes and macrophages
C5a	An anaphylatoxin (like C3a). Also chemotactic for mononuclear and polymorphonuclear leukocytes
C5b67	Complex of 3 components that can initiate "innocent bystander" lysis when in its active form, or can promote chemotaxis
C5b6789	Membrane attack complex of terminal components responsible for membrane damage and cell lysis

complex, which involves union of C5b, C6, C7, C8, and C9 by nonenzymatic processes, completes the reaction sequence.

The interaction of the C5b–9 complex with membranes impairs the osmotic integrity of these membranes. It matters little what the source of the membrane is: many bacteria, tumor cells, protozoa, viruses, "innocent bystander" erythrocytes, and platelets are susceptible to complement-induced lysis. In each case, the initial impairment of regulation of small ions and water is followed by osmotic lysis of the cell (5).

Complement deficiencies. Inherited deficiencies of all 11 classical pathway proteins and 3 of the control proteins have been described. A single instance of properdin deficiency has also been described, but none has yet been found for the other alternative pathway components (B and D). With the exception of C1 inhibitor deficiency, which gives rise to the clinical syndrome of hereditary angioedema, all of the others are inherited as autosomal codominant traits. Heterozygotes have half-

normal levels and homozygotes lack the active protein. The genes controlling synthesis of C4, C2, and Factor B are located in the major histocompatibility complex on the sixth autosomal chromosome. Although clinical manifestations associated with complement deficiency are many and varied, certain general patterns have emerged:

1. Rheumatic diseases including systemic lupus erythematosus–like syndromes, vasculitis, glomerulonephritis, and polymyositis occur most frequently with deficiencies of the classical pathway components. C2 deficiency is by far the most common; its gene frequency in the normal population is about 1%. Impaired processing of immune complexes in deficient individuals may be the pathogenetic mechanism common to the association of complement deficiencies with rheumatic diseases (6).

2. Recurrent infections with pyogenic organisms are almost always observed with C3 deficiency or with Factor I or H deficiencies that lead to secondary depressions in C3 levels because of uncontrolled

cycling of the alternative pathway. Decreased phagocytosis of these organisms due to failure of opsonization appears to be responsible for the infections.

3. Recurrent sepsis with *Neisseria* species is common among patients with deficiencies of the terminal components including C5, C6, C7, C8, and C9. Failure of bacteriolysis of the *Neisseria* is presumably the explanation for this association.

1. Atkinson JP, Frank MM: Complement, Clinical Immunology. CW Parker, ed. Philadelphia, WB Saunders Co, 1980, pp 219–271
2. Cooper NR: Activation and regulation of the first complement component. Fed Proc (in press)
3. Fearon DT, Austen KF: The alternative pathway of complement: a system of host resistance to microbial infection. N Engl J Med 303:259–263, 1980
4. Muller-Eberhard HJ: Chemistry and function of the complement system. Hosp Pract 12:33–43, 1977
5. Ruddy S: Plasma protein effectors of inflammation: complement, Textbook of Rheumatology, WN Kelley, ED Harris Jr, S Ruddy, CB Sledge, eds. Philadelphia, WB Saunders Company, 1981, pp 83–96
6. Ruddy S: Complement, rheumatic diseases and the major histocompatibility complex. Clin Rheum Dis 3:215–237, 1977

8. Role of immunologic mechanisms in the pathogenesis of rheumatic disease

In a broad sense, the immune system can be subdivided into 2 distinct components—humoral immunity and cell-mediated immunity. Although the existence of both elements is well established, it is evident that a complex and intricate network of interaction occurs between them. These interactions can result in both amplification and suppression of immune reactivity.

Humoral immunity

Antibodies/immunoglobulins. In the early 1900s it was realized that immunity to a variety of bacterial agents was mediated by serum factors—humoral substances. These factors were subsequently shown to be specific anti-bacterial antibodies (1–8). In serum protein electrophoresis, antibody is found in the β to γ-globulin region. Based on chemical structure and antigenic properties, 5 classes of human immunoglobulins (Ig) have been defined (1,2). These have been designated IgG, IgA, IgM, IgE, and IgD.

Composition of immunoglobulins. The IgG class has 4 subclasses, IgG1 to IgG4, with differing as well as common structural, antigenic, and biological properties. There are 2 subclasses of human IgA and IgM. Fig 8–1 illustrates the basic structure of IgG. It consists of 2 identical γ heavy

(H) chains (MW 50,000) and 2 identical light (L) chains (MW 23,000) which are either kappa or lambda in type. X-ray crystallographic and amino acid sequence studies have demonstrated that IgG molecules are composed of several distinct globular domains, each containing approximately 110 amino acid residues.

The H chains of IgG and IgA have 3 constant region (C_H) domains and 1 variable region (V_H) domain. IgM and IgE heavy chains contain 4 C_H domains and 1 V_H domain. All L chains contain 2 domains, 1 each V_L and C_L domain.

There is a significant, albeit variable, degree of amino acid sequence homology between domains on the same polypeptide chain and on different chains of the same or different Ig molecules. The amino acid sequence of V_H and V_L regions contains areas where the amino acid sequences are hypervariable, interspread between relatively stable framework regions. The hypervariable regions contain the antigen-combining sites and idiotypic determinants of the Ig molecules.

By chemical and enzymatic techniques, Ig molecules can be fractionated into Fab fragments, consisting of a light chain linked to the CH_1 and V_H domains, containing the antigen-combining site, and Fc fragments, containing CH_2 and CH_3 domains and the sites important in com-

plement binding, placental transport, and immune adherence to lymphocytes, monocyte/macrophages, polymorphonuclear leukocytes (PMNs), eosinophils, basophils, and mast cells.

IgM is composed of 5 identical subunits, each consisting of 2 μ heavy chains (MW 70,000) and 2 light chains. The 5 subunits are joined by a junctional polypeptide or J chain (MW 15,000) (9).

IgA exists in serum either as a monomer composed of 2 α heavy chains (MW 55,000) and 2 light chains or as a dimer composed of 2 IgA monomers joined by a J chain. In secretions, IgA exists as a dimer to which secretory component, a 70,000 dalton molecular weight glycoprotein, is added.

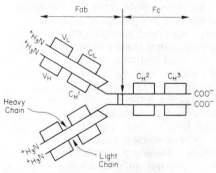

Fig 8–1. The basic structure of IgG

Table 8–1. Properties of human immunoglobulins

Property	IgG	IgA	IgM	IgD	IgE
Normal serum concentration (mg/ml)	8–16	1.4–4	0.5–2	0–0.4	17–450
% of total serum immunoglobulin	70–80	10–15	5–10	0.2–1	0.002
Electrophoretic mobility	γ–α_2 globulin	γ–β globulin	γ–β globulin	γ–β globulin	γ–β globulin
Sedimentation coefficient	7S	7S (85%) (9,11,13S)	19S	7S	8S
Molecular weight	150,000	160,000–385,000*	900,000	180,000	200,000
Number of basic 4-peptide units	1	1,2	5	1	1
Heavy chains	γ	α	μ	δ	ε
Carbohydrate content (%)	2.6	5–6.2	10.5		10.7
Primary distribution	Extracellular fluid	External secretion	Intravascular	Intravascular	Extracellular fluid
Total circulating pool (mg/kg)	494	95	37	1.1	0.02
Biologic half-life (days)	23	5.8	5.1	2.8	2.3
Fractional catabolic rate (% of intravascular pool catabolized per day)	6.7	25	18	37	89
Synthetic rate (mg/kg/day)	33	24	6.7	0.4	0.02
Complement fixation (C1q)	+	–	+	?	–
Cross placenta	+	–	–	–	–
Fix to mast cells (in homologous skin) and basophils	–	–	–	–	+
Cytophilic binding to macrophages	+	–	–	–	–
Major Ig class in secretions	–	+	–	–	–
First antibody formed in response to antigen	–	–	+	–	–
Major Ig on mature B lymphocytes	–	–	+	+	–
Combination with staphylococcal A protein	+	–	–	–	–

* Monomeric MW = 160,000; secretory MW = 400,000.

IgD and **IgE** are monomeric immunoglobulins containing 2 δ or ε heavy chains (MW 62,000 and 70,000, respectively) and 2 light chains.

The physicochemical, metabolic, and biological properties of the 5 classes of immunoglobulins are shown in Table 8–1 (4–7). The properties of 4 subclasses of IgG are listed in Table 8–2.

Roles of immunoglobulins. IgG is the immunoglobulin present in the highest concentration in serum, and most circulating antibodies are of this class. IgG1, IgG3, and to a lesser extent, IgG2 molecules are capable of fixing C1q and activating the classical pathway of complement (see Section 7). In contrast, IgG4 molecules are unable to fix C1q but can activate the alternative pathway of complement. IgG antibodies can participate in antibody-dependent cell-mediated cytotoxic reactions (ADCC) (10,11). IgG1, IgG3, and IgG4 can cross the placenta.

Although IgA exists in serum in a relatively high concentration, its major immunologic role is related to its presence in external secretions (4). IgA predominates in lacrimal, nasopharyngeal, salivary, and respiratory and gastrointestinal tract fluids. The immunoglobulin portion of secretory IgA is synthesized by submucosal plasma cells; the glycoprotein secretory component is produced by epithelial cells. IgA does not fix C1q and, thus, cannot activate the classical complement pathway. IgA, however, can activate the alternative complement pathway (4).

IgM is the first class of antibody formed after primary antigenic challenge; pentameric IgM is extremely effective in fixing the first component of complement (1–3). IgM, in some systems, may mediate antibody-dependent cell-mediated cytotoxicity (10). IgM is largely confined to the intravascular space. The isohemagglutinins, many of the "naturally occurring" antibodies to microorganisms, antibodies to typhoid O antigen, the WR antibodies in syphilis, rheumatoid factors, and antibodies to T helper-independent antigens, are usually of the IgM class. Monomeric IgM and IgD are the major Ig classes present in the plasma membranes of B lymphocytes (5,6).

Little is known about the physiologic role of serum IgD; only a few reports unequivocally demonstrate antibody activity in IgD (5).

IgE, which is found in very low concentrations in serum, plays a predominant role in many allergic reactions (7). The physiologic role of IgE is unknown, but its serum concentration has been noted to increase markedly during the course of systemic infection with certain parasites, especially helminths.

Cellular immunity

A variety of cells are involved in immune reactions. These include polymorphonuclear leukocytes (PMNs), eosinophils, basophils, mast cells, monocytes/macrophages, lymphocytes, and plasma cells.

Polymorphonuclear leukocytes. The mature neutrophil or PMN normally comprises about 60% of the circulating white blood cells in humans. Mature PMNs are end-stage cells, which circulate with a half-life of 6–20 hours when released from bone marrow. The total neutrophil pool is composed of approximately equal numbers of circulating and marginated PMN.

Table 8–2. Properties of human IgG subclasses

	IgG1	IgG2	IgG3	IgG4
Serum concentration (mg/ml)	5–12	2–6	0.5–1	0.2–1
% of total IgG in normal serum	65	23	8	4
Electrophoretic mobility	Slow	Slow	Slow	Fast
Half-life (days)	23	23	16	23
Combination with staphylococcal A protein	+	+	–	+
Cross placenta	+	±	+	+
Complement fixation (C1q)	++	+	+++	–
Binding to:				
neutrophils	+	+	+	+
monocyte/macrophages	++	+/–	++	+/–
lymphocytes	++	+/–	++	+/–
platelets	+	+	+	+
Blocking of IgE binding	–	–	–	+

The PMN is a phagocytic cell containing 2 distinct types of granules—primary or azurophilic granules containing myeloperoxidase, lysozyme, elastase, acid hydrolases, antibacterial cationic proteins, and secondary or specific granules containing lactoferrin and some lysozyme (12–14).

PMNs play a central role in the host defense against most bacteria and are the primary immunologic cell present at sites of acute inflammation. PMNs are capable of chemotaxis, i.e., when exposed to a chemotactic factor, they will migrate toward the highest concentration of that factor (15,16).

Chemotactic factors that have been identified for neutrophils include bacterial products, tissue protease, complement components (C3a, C5a, C567), N-formylmethionyl peptides, and products of sensitized lymphocytes (15). Chemotactic factors attract PMNs to sites of acute inflammation.

Once localized at the inflammatory site, PMNs bind and phagocytose appropriately opsonized materials. Opsonization can occur by: 1) binding of specific IgG antibody to a particle, such as a microorganism or erythrocyte, with subsequent attachment of that antibody–antigen complex to Fc(IgG) receptors on the surface of the PMN; 2) binding of specific antibody and complement to a particle with subsequent attachment of the antibody–antigen–complement complex to C3 receptors on the surface of the PMN; and 3) through heat labile, "nonspecific" opsonins which promote the fixation of activated C3 to a particle through the activation of the alternative pathway of complement.

During and after phagocytosis, a complex series of morphologic and biochemical events occurs within the PMN (16). The morphologic events include the ingestion of the phagocytosed particle, formation of a phagosome, fusion of granules with the phagosome, and degranulation.

As these events occur, there is a burst of oxygen consumption and marked stimulation of the hexose-monophosphate shunt. PMNs kill phagocytosed microorganisms by nonoxidative mechanisms mediated by cationic proteins, lysozyme, lactoferrin, elastase, and low pH and by oxidative mechanisms mediated by hydrogen peroxide and free radicals including superoxide anion and possibly singlet oxygen and hydroxyl radicals (12–14). For a more detailed discussion of the role of PMN in inflammation see Section 6.

Basophils, mast cells, eosinophils. Basophils, mast cells, and eosinophils are involved in anaphylactic and allergic reactions. Mast cells are found in the connective tissue of the skin, the submucosa of the small intestines, the sheaths of peripheral nerves and the meninges, and the reticuloendothelial system. Basophils and mast cells contain a variety of biologically active compounds including heparin, hyaluronic acid, histamine, serotonin, kinins, prostaglandins, slow reacting substance of anaphylaxis (SRS-A), eosinophil chemotactic factor of anaphylaxis (ECF-A), and platelet aggregating factor (PAF). These cells are the targets for IgE in anaphylactic and allergic reactions (9).

Eosinophils, which normally comprise 1–5% of peripheral blood leukocytes, have phagocytic potential and are capable of ingesting antibody–antigen complexes. Peripheral eosinophilia occurs commonly during allergic reactions and is frequently seen during systemic parasitic infections. The exact role of the eosinophil in these diseases, however, has not been totally elucidated (17).

Mononuclear phagocytes. Mononuclear phagocytes originate from precursor monoblasts and promonocytes present in the bone marrow. They circulate in peripheral blood as monocytes, with a half-life in blood of approximately 8-1/2 hours. Monocytes leave the peripheral blood and mature into macrophages in tissues. Tissue macrophages are present in liver (Kupffer cells), lung (pulmonary alveolar macrophages), connective tissue (histiocytes), spleen, lymph node, bone marrow, serous cavities (pleural and peritoneal macrophages), bone (osteoclasts), and nervous, system (microglial cells) (18,19).

Monocyte–macrophage system. Monocytes/macrophages possess plasma membrane receptors for the Fc portion of IgG (IgG1 and IgG3), activated C3, macrophage chemotactic factors, lymphokines such as MIF, and several hormones including insulin, glucagon, calcitonin, and parathyroid hormone (20). Macrophages express cell surface HLA–D and HLA–DR antigens in humans and Ia determinants in the mouse (20,21).

The macrophage plays a crucial role in both the afferent and effector limbs of immunity. Macrophages are required in the generation of an antibody response to T-dependent antigens and for induction of most T lymphocyte–mediated immune responses, including the in vitro generation of cytotoxic cells, the in vitro production of certain lymphokines, and the in vitro blastogenic response to soluble antigens, allogeneic cells, and mitogens such as phytohemagglutinin and concanavalin A (22).

During the induction of antigen-specific T cell and B cell responses, macrophages are thought to play a central role in antigen processing and in presentation of antigen to lymphocytes. A different cell, the dendritic cell, has recently been identified that may also be important as an accessory cell (23). The dendritic cell is Ia positive but nonphagocytic and negative for Fc receptors.

In in vitro systems, macrophages appear to provide nutritional factors important to lymphocytes and to secrete factors capable of enhancing the activation of both T and B cells (22). In several systems, macrophages can also actively suppress immune reactivity (24,25). In some instances this suppression is mediated by macrophage secreted prostaglandins (26).

Macrophages are important effector cells in a variety of immunologic reactions. Macrophages are phagocytic cells and can phagocytose by both nonimmunologic mechanisms as well as those mediated by the Fc and C3 receptor. After phagocytosis, macrophages can kill cells that have been ingested and deposited into phagolysosomes (18,19). Macrophages can also mediate nonphagocytic cytolysis or cytostasis of antibody-coated target cells by a mechanism known as antibody-dependent cell-mediated cytotoxicity (ADCC) (27).

Nonantibody-dependent nonphagocytic cytolysis of tumor cells and erythrocytes by activated macrophages has also been documented (18,19). This form of macrophage-mediated cytolysis may be immunologically specific or nonspecific depending on the mechanism of macrophage activation.

Recently, it has become apparent that macrophages secrete a variety of biologically active products capable of influencing and modulating immunologic reactions (22,23). Table 8–3 lists some of the known macrophage secretory products.

Lymphocytes and plasma cells. There are 2 major classes of lymphocytes—thymus-processed or derived T lymphocytes and bone marrow–derived B lymphocytes. The differentiation of T and B cells is shown in Fig 8–2.

T lymphocytes. Lymphocyte stem cells are initally located in the yolk sac and later in liver and then bone marrow. During T cell differentiation the stem cell migrates to the thymus gland where, under the influence of the thymic epithelium, the cell differentiates into a large, rapidly dividing cortisone-sensitive immature thymocyte found in the thymic cortex (28). In most assays of T cell function, the immature thymocyte is immunoincompetent; in some immunologic assays, however, immature thymocytes have been shown to have suppressor cell activity (29).

In the mouse the immature thymocyte expresses H-2, Thy 1, and TL antigens. Some immature thymocytes differentiate into functionally mature, small, cortisone-resistant thymocytes located in the medulla of the thymus. Mature thymocytes comprise only 5–10% of thymic lymphocytes. In the mouse these cells no longer express the TL antigen and express more cell surface H-2 and less Thy 1 antigen than do immature, cortical thymocytes. Mature thymocytes exit from the thymus gland and differentiate in the periphery into peripheral T cells which populate the spleen, lymph nodes, tonsils, peripheral blood, and the lymphatic system. Like mature

Table 8–3. Secretory products of lymphocytes and macrophages

Lymphocytes

Migration inhibitory factor (MIF)
Macrophage aggregating factor
Macrophage activating factor
Macrophage chemotactic factor
Leukocyte inhibitory factor
Neutrophil chemotactic factor
Chemotactic factor(s) for eosinophils
Lymphotoxin (LT)
Cloning inhibitory factor
Proliferation inhibitory factor (PIF)
Blastogenic factors (BF)
Skin reactive factors (SRF)
Interferon

Lymph node permeability factor (LNPF)
Soluble immune response suppressor (SIRS)
Antigen-specific T helper-factor(s)
Antigen-specific T suppressor factor(s)
Allogeneic effect factor (AEF)
T cell replacing factor(s) (TRF)
Procoagulant factor activity
Platelet slowing factor (PSF)
Platelet aggregating factor
Inducer of plasminogen activator secretion (IPA)
Osteoclast activating factor (OAF)
Proteoglycan degradation factor

Macrophages

Colony stimulating activity
Factors influencing fibroblast growth and activity
Lysozyme
Acid hydrolases (cathepsins, glycosidases, acid phosphatases, aryl sulfatases, and others)
Neutral proteinases (collagenase, elastase, plasminogen activator)
Interferon
Bactericidal factors
Thymocyte-differentiating factor (TDF)

Genetically restricted factor
Thymocyte mitogenic protein (TMF)
Lymphocyte activating factor (LAF)
T cell activating factor (TAF)
B cell activating factor (BAF)
Complement components (C1q, C2, C3, C4, C5, C6, Factor B)
Endogenous pyrogen
Polymorphonuclear leukocyte chemotactic factor
Cyclic nucleotides
Prostaglandins
Macrophage cytotoxic factors

thymocytes, peripheral T cells in the mouse express the Thy 1 antigen but not the TL antigen (30).

B lymphocytes. During B cell differentiation, the lymphocyte stem cell migrates to the bursa of Fabricius in avian species and presumably to bone marrow in humans. There it differentiates into an immature B cell, which possesses surface membrane immunoglobulin but is unable to secrete immunoglobulin into its environment. This cell further differentiates into a mature immunoglobulin-secreting B cell which, in turn, terminally differentiates into an immunoglobulin-secreting plasma cell (30,31).

Null cells. The existence in mice and humans of a third type of lymphocyte, a "null" cell which lacks definitive T and B cell markers, is now well documented. The exact relationship of these null lymphocytes, which are undoubtedly a heterogenous group of cells, to the T and B cell lines of differentiation is controversial and has not as yet been firmly established (32,33).

Table 8–4 lists the approximate percentages of T cells, B cells, and null cells in various lymphoid tissues.

Lymphocyte markers. T, B, and null lymphocytes generally cannot be distinguished from one another morphologically. However, they can be identified and quantitated, by use of cell surface markers (30–34) (Table 8–5).

The definitive marker for B lymphocytes in both mice and humans is the presence of surface membrane immunoglobulin. All mature murine and human B lymphocytes possess readily detectable surface immunoglobulin, while T and null cells do not. Monomeric IgM and IgD are the major immunoglobulin classes present in the plasma membranes of mature B cells (5,6). Human and murine B cells also possess cell surface receptors for the Fc portion of IgG (35) and for activated C3 (36) and express HLA–D and HLA–DR determinants in humans and H2, I-region (Ia) determinants in mice (21–30). Some human B cell subsets also appear to express Fc receptors for IgM (37) and IgE (38).

All murine T cells express the Thy 1 determinant (30); all human T cells have a plasma membrane receptor for sheep erythrocytes (SRBC) and under appropriate in vitro conditions will form rosettes when incubated with SRBC (33). B lymphocytes and null cells do not express the Thy 1 determinant or form SRBC rosettes, but brain cells do express Thy 1 or Thy 1-like determinants. Rabbit antisera raised against mouse or human brain and appropriately absorbed cross react with T lymphocytes (39).

Subpopulations of human and murine T cells have been defined which differentially express cell surface receptors for the Fc portion of IgG or the Fc portion of IgM (40). In addition, subpopulations of murine T cells have been defined by their differential expression of the Lyt* 1, 2, 3 series of surface antigens (30,41) and the presence of specific membrane I-region determinants (30,42). Certain I-region determinants appear to be preferentially expressed on subpopulation of T cells but not on B cells or macrophages, others are on B cells and macrophages but not T cells, and yet others may be expressed on all 3 cell types (30,42–44).

Human T cell subpopulations have also been defined by their differential reactivity with antilymphocyte antibodies present in the sera of patients with systemic lupus erythematosus (45,46) or juvenile arthritis (47,48) and by their reactivity with certain heterologous anti–T cell antisera (32) or hybridoma anti–T cell antibodies (49). Some activated human T cell populations may also express HLA–DR determinants (21).

Lymphocyte function. The principal functional properties of B, null, and T cells are listed in Table 8–6. B cells, as described earlier, differentiate into antibody-secreting plasma cells (31). Null lymphocytes function as cytotoxic effector cells in both antibody-dependent cell-mediated cytotoxicity (10,11) and spontaneous cell-mediated cytotoxic or natural killer assay systems (50).

T lymphocytes can be divided into 4 functional subpopulations:

1. **Helper T (T_H) cells** are important in the induction of antibody responses to most antigens and in generation of cytotoxic T cells after allogeneic stimulation. In murine systems T_H cells are phenotypically Lyt 1+ (30,41). In humans helper T cells bear an Fc receptor for IgM (40) and react with certain monoclonal antibodies such as OK-T4 (49) but do not react with antilymphocyte antibodies present in the sera of patients with active juvenile chronic arthritis (47).

2. **Cytotoxic T (T_C) cells** are capable of directly lysing cells that bear target antigens to which they have been sensitized. Phenotypically, murine alloreactive T_c cells are Lyt 2, 3+ (41). In humans cytotoxic T cells react with monoclonal antibodies such as OK-T5 and 8 (49).

3. **Suppressor T (T_S) cells** regulate or suppress a variety of immunologic reactions (29,51). Defects in suppressor T cell

---

* Sometimes referred to as Ly but more properly Lyt when applied to T cells.

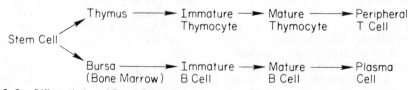

Fig 8–2. Differentiation of T and B lymphocytes

Table 8–4. Approximate percentages of T and B cells and null cells in various lymphoid organs

Organ	% T cells	% B cells	% null cells
Peripheral blood	75	15	5–10
Lymph	95	<5	—
Spleen	35	50	—
Lymph node	75	20	—
Tonsil	50	50	—
Thymus	100	0	—
Bone marrow	<25	>75	—

activity have been demonstrated in several murine models of systemic lupus erythematosus (SLE) (52–57) as well as in patients with this disease (58–60) and juvenile chronic polyarthritis (48).

Suppressor T cells in the mouse, usually Lyt 2, 3+ (40), bear I-J region determinants on their cell surfaces (30,42). In a few systems Lyt 1, 2, 3+ Ts cells have been described (30). In humans Ts cells possess an Fc receptor for IgG (40) and react with antilymphocyte antibodies present in the sera of patients with active juvenile chronic polyarthritis (47,48), SLE (46), and monoclonal antibodies such as OK-T5 (47). In a few immunologic systems, the existence of suppressor macrophages and suppressor B cells has been documented (24,25,61,62).

4. **Delayed hypersensitivity T (T_{DH}) cells** play a critical role in delayed hypersensitivity reactions which are important in host defense in diseases such as tuberculosis, syphilis, and leprosy. Activated T_{DH} cells secrete factors called lymphokines which are important in cell-mediated immune reactions (63,64) (Table 8–3). A few lymphokines such as migration inhibition factor (MIF) are also secreted by B lymphocytes (65). T_{DH} cells are Lyt 1+ (30); in some systems, Lyt 2, 3+ cells may also participate in the production of some lymphokines (66).

The cells that respond by blast transformation after in vitro antigenic stimulation with either soluble antigens or in mixed lymphocyte cultures (MLC) are T lymphocytes (Lyt 1+ in mice, OKT-4+ in humans). Recent evidence suggests that like null cells and macrophages, human T lymphocytes can mediate both antibody-dependent (10,67) and spontaneous cell-mediated cytotoxicity (68).

During the past 15 years, a variety of mitogenic substances have been utilized for the evaluation of T and B cell activation and immunocompetence. Mitogens are naturally occurring or synthetic substances which "nonspecifically" activate lymphocytes from all normal individuals. Activation does not require prior immunologic sensitization to the mitogenic substance. As illustrated in Table 8–7, in the standard 3-day assay system in both mice and humans, phytohemagglutinin and con-

canavalin A are mitogenic for T but not B cells (69,70), while pokeweed mitogen is mitogenic for both T and B lymphocytes (69). Lipopolysaccharide is a B cell–specific mitogen in the mouse (70), but does not consistently stimulate human B cells. Anti-β_2-microglobulin has been reported to be mitogenic for both murine and human B cells (71).

Immunopathologic mechanisms of tissue injury

The idea that many rheumatic diseases are caused, at least in part, by tissue damage by host immune systems has had a strong influence on the approach to research and therapy in the past 30 years. Immune injury can be classified into 4 basic types (72). These types are not mutually exclusive and may occur together in some patients, but separating them conceptually provides a framework for understanding the pathogenesis of immunologic disease.

Anaphylactic type I reactions. This mechanism is responsible for the immediate hypersensitivity reactions that occur in many allergic diseases and for the phenomenon of generalized anaphylactic shock. The principal components of this system are antibodies of the IgE class and basophils or mast cells. Basophils and mast cells contain a variety of vasoactive substances in their granules and possess high affinity surface receptors for the Fc portion of IgE (73).

They circulate with IgE bound to their surface. Binding of monomeric IgE molecules alone to mast cells has no effect on cell function. If, however, an antigen attaches to adjacent cell-associated IgE molecules and crosslinks them, a series of events is triggered within the cell that results in release of vasoactive substances from the cell (Fig 8–3). These substances—histamine, slow-reacting substance of anaphylaxis (SRS-A), serotonin, heparin, kinins, prostaglandins, and an eosinophil chemotactic factor—are responsible for the pathologic manifestations that occur in allergic and anaphylactic reactions, including vasodilation,

edema, bronchospasm, and collection of eosinophils (9).

Experimentally, release of these substances can be obtained with the use of aggregated IgE as well as IgE immune complexes. The optimal ratio of antigen to antibody for release of mast cell granules by IgE complexes is slight to moderate antigen excess. Plasma cells synthesizing IgE are found primarily adjacent to endothelial surfaces, the bronchi, the gastrointestinal tract, and the bladder. They are rare in the liver, spleen, or lymph nodes (74). The development of an IgE response is under genetic control, dependent on helper T cells, and regulated by suppressor T cells (8).

Anaphylactic reactions can be divided into local and generalized types, but this distinction is probably quantitative rather than qualitative. The local reaction is typified by the immediate skin test in which a small amount of antigen, given intradermally, combines with antibody locally fixed to tissue mast cells to give a wheal and flare. The antibody can be of host origin or given passively as in the classic Prausnitz-Küstner reaction.

Passively administered antibody is capable of mediating an immediate hypersensitivity (type I) reaction within 6 hours after injection; however, its maximum effectiveness is not attained for 48–72 hours. It may remain locally fixed for as long as 6 weeks. The immediate-type hypersensitivity reaction obtained when an antigen challenge is given occurs within 20 minutes. Type I reactions may be organ-specific, as in asthma or atopic dermatitis.

Generalized anaphylaxis occurs when the antigen is widely distributed in a sensitized host and is manifest by marked vasodilatation, increased vascular permeability, and shock.

Antibody-mediated type II reactions. Reactions of this type are characterized by combination of antibodies with either intrinsic cell surface antigens or antigens adsorbed to the cell surface. Fig 8–4 illustrates several types of events that may take place after antibody attachment:

1. Complement may be activated, resulting in lysis of the cell.

Table 8–5. Major lymphocyte cell surface determinants in humans and mice

Cell type	Marker	
	Humans	Mice
B	SIg (IgD, IgM) Fc(IgG) receptor C'3 receptor	SIg (IgD, IgM) Fc(IgG) receptor C'3 receptor
T	SRBC receptor Reactivity with anti-T cell antibodies Fc (IgG and IgM) receptors	Thy 1 Lyt 1,2,3
Null	Fc(IgG) receptor C'3 receptor Lacks SIg and SRBC receptor	Fc(IgG) receptor C'3 receptor Lacks SIg and Thy 1

Table 8–6. Primary functions of T lymphocytes, B lymphocytes, null lymphocytes

B lymphocytes
Differentiate into plasma cells, secrete antibody
Can secrete some lymphokines (MIF, LIF)

Null lymphocytes
Effector cell function in antibody-dependent, cell-mediated cytotoxicity
Effector cell function in spontaneous cell-mediated (natural killer) cytotoxicity

T lymphocytes
Helper cell function in antibody formation and in T cell–mediated immune responses
Cytotoxic effector cell function; important in:
   transplantation immunity
   tumor immunity
   graft-versus-host disease
   anti-viral immunity
Suppressor cell function
Delayed-hypersensitivity reactions: important in host defense against fungi, tuberculosis, leprosy, syphilis
Lymphokine secretion
Blastogenic response on antigenic stimulation in vitro
Effector cell function in antibody-dependent cell-mediated cytotoxicity
Effector cell function in spontaneous cell-mediated (natural killer) cytotoxicity

2. The cell may be destroyed through enhanced phagocytosis or opsonization with or without the aid of complement.

3. The cell may be destroyed by a mononuclear cell (K cell, T cell, or macrophage) or PMN via the mechanism of antibody-dependent cellular cytotoxicity.

4. Cell function may be altered through nonlytic events. Antibody bound to surface receptors may a) serve as a positive stimulus and initiate cellular proliferation (71,75) or induce the release of a specific cellular product such as a hormone (76); or b) play a negative role and render the cell unresponsive to an unrelated stimulus by blocking the specific cell surface receptors for that stimulus (77,78).

5. The cell may be protected from damage by "masking" of its antigens (79).

The exact end result of the combination of antibody with a membrane antigen depends to a large extent on the type of antibody involved. For example, complement-mediated lysis occurring via activation of the classical complement pathway is facilitated by antibodies of the IgG or IgM but not IgA or IgE class (3). Opsonization and phagocytosis are enhanced by IgG antibodies but not antibodies of other classes, except IgM antibodies that have fixed complement (12,13,18,19). IgG and, in a few systems, IgM antibodies effectively mediate antibody-dependent cell-mediated cytotoxicity reactions while those of other classes do not (10,11).

Another important variable is the density of cell surface antigen. Fixation of C1 by IgG requires 2 closely spaced antibody molecules, and if the antigens are widely spaced, these conditions may not be met.

Autoimmune hemolytic anemia and thrombocytopenia of systemic lupus erythematosus are examples of antibody-mediated immune damage. Recent evidence suggests that antilymphocyte antibodies through a type II immune reaction may be responsible for the decrease in T cell suppressor function that occurs in patients with systemic lupus erythematosus (46).

Goodpasture's syndrome, in which damage of renal and pulmonary basement membrane occurs secondary to attachment of an autoantibody directed against specific basement membrane antigens, is probably another clinical example of a type II reaction (80). The role of antibody-dependent cellular cytotoxicity in human diseases has not been clearly defined, but evidence now suggests that cellular damage to thyroid acinar cells in autoimmune thyroiditis may be, in part, due to antibodies cooperating with K cells (81,82).

Graves' disease provides an example of autoimmune stimulation. Patients with this disease have antibodies directed against the thyroid-stimulating hormone (TSH) receptor site. These antibodies mimic the action of TSH on thyroid cells (76).

In contrast, in myasthenia gravis, anti-acetylcholine receptor antibodies cause loss of receptors, resulting in muscular weakness (77). In some diabetic patients, insulin resistance appears to result from blocking of insulin receptors by anti-insulin receptor antibodies (78).

Long-term survival of renal allografts in patients who have circulating cytotoxic lymphocytes capable of destroying their graft may be caused by the presence of blocking antibodies in their serum. This phenomenon, called immunologic enhancement, may also be important in the growth of some neoplasms (79). Experimental evidence in animals suggests that blocking or masking of antigens by antibody may be only one of several mechanisms operating in these situations. Others may involve immune complexes or free antigens that are capable of "blinding" the cytotoxic cells.

Immune complex type III reactions. In this type of reaction, damage occurs as a result of localization of immune complexes on the surface of cells or tissues. The classic examples of this mechanism are the Arthus reaction and serum sickness (83,84).

Arthus reaction. In the Arthus reaction, local immune complex disease is induced by intradermal injection of antigen into an active or passively immunized host. Swelling and erythema occur in 1–2 hours, reach a maximum at about 5 hours, and disappear by 12 hours. Vasculitis is seen in the small blood vessels in the area secondary to deposition of complexes of the injected antigen and circulating antibody. Complement is fixed in the vessel walls, followed by an influx of polymorphonuclear neutrophils and later by mononuclear cells.

Local immune complex disease. By use of a similar technique, local immune complex disease can be produced in several organs including the lung, pleura, and thyroid. Repeated intraarticular injection of antigen into immune rabbits or of preformed complexes into nonimmune rabbits causes synovitis.

Clinically, hypersensitivity pneumonitis is thought to represent an example of local immune complex disease. This acute illness characterized by chills, fever, cough, and dyspnea occurs from binding of inhaled antigens to preformed antibody in the lung. Antigens of fungal, insect, and avian origin have been implicated in this syndrome (85).

Serum sickness. The classic clinical pattern of serum sickness was defined when heterologous antisera were used in the treatment of several bacterial infections (see Section 23). Fever, an urticarial or erythematous rash, arthralgia, malaise, and lymphadenopathy occur within 3 weeks of injection of foreign serum and last 1–2 weeks.

Serum sickness can be induced experimentally by injecting bovine serum albumin (BSA) intravenously into nonimmunized rabbits (83). Initially, serum levels of antigen decline rapidly due to equilibration between the intra- and extravascular spaces; the concentration then falls slowly as a result of catabolism of the BSA (Fig 8–5). This phase is followed by rapid immune clearance as the animal begins to produce anti-BSA antibodies. Those rabbits that produce the most vigorous response develop vasculitis with arthritis.

Table 8–7. Mitogens: T cell–B cell specificity*

	Humans		Mice	
	T	B	T	B
Phytohemagglutinin	+	−	+	−
Concanavalin A	+	−	+	−
Pokeweed mitogen	+	+	+	+
Lipopolysaccharide	−	+/−	−	+
Anti-β₂-microglobulin	−	+	−	+

* In standard 3-day assay systems.

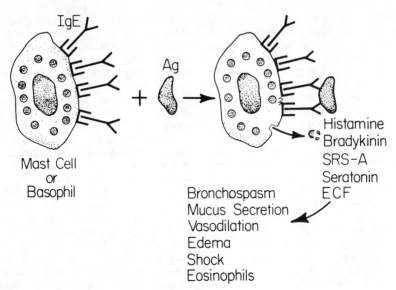

Fig 8–3. Anaphylactic type I reactions

serositis, and glomerulonephritis that begin during the phase of rapid immune clearance. The symptoms peak shortly after clearance of antigen and then subside.

A chronic form of experimental serum sickness can be induced by daily injection of antigen. If a fixed amount of antigen is given, the development of immune complex disease depends on the antibody response of the animal. Those that develop very little or large amounts of antibody remain normal, while those that produce intermediate levels develop glomerulonephritis. If the antigen dose is titrated to maintain the animal in slight antigen excess, all rabbits that mount an immune response develop nephritis. These differences primarily reflect differences in the composition of the immune complexes formed.

The structure of complexes depends on several factors: the ratio of antigen to antibody, the valence of antigen and antibodies, the avidity of the antibodies, and the participation of other serum components such as complement. Changes in any one of these factors may alter the composition of a complex and affect its ability to induce immune damage.

In experimental serum sickness, soluble complexes containing more than 2 antibody molecules and having molecular weights between 500,000 and 700,000 are most likely to cause vasculitis.

Systemic immune complex disease. The sequence of events in systemic immune complex injury is similar to that noted in localized immune complex disease. Deposition of circulating complexes in vessel walls appears to require an increase in vascular permeability (86) (Fig 8–6). This may be accomplished in part through release of vasoactive amines from platelets or from basophils activated by IgE antibodies.

Once complexes are lodged in the vessel, complement is activated, chemotactic factors released, and PMNs infiltrate the area. Lysosomal enzymes are then released from the PMNs, damage vessel walls, and lead to hemorrhage, occlusion, and ischemic changes in the tissue. The initiating complexes may be detectable throughout the process, but failure to distinguish them does not rule out their role in the lesion. It has been demonstrated in animals that complexes may be undetectable as early as 24 hours after initiation of tissue reaction.

Deposition of complexes in vessel walls is enhanced by increased hydrostatic forces and turbulence of flow. The nature of the antigen may also influence complex deposition. For example, DNA has an affinity for glomerular basement membrane; this may be one factor in localization of DNA–anti-DNA complexes in the kidney in systemic lupus erythematosus. In addition to inducing vasculitis, immune complexes may inhibit ADCC-mediated

tissue damage by blocking the Fc receptor on effector cells.

Most types of systemic vasculitis, including systemic lupus erythematosus, periarteritis nodosa, and hypersensitivity and granulomatous vasculitis, involve type III damage (86). Poststreptococcal and idiopathic glomerulonephritis are also clinical examples of this process, as are cryoglobulinemia and vasculitis associated with infectious agents and neoplasms.

In systemic lupus erythematosus, DNA–anti-DNA complexes correlate well with disease activity. A variety of complexes, including those involving other nuclear as well as cytoplasmic antigens, are also found in this disease. Hepatitis B antigen–antibody complexes have been implicated in the pathogenesis of some cases of periarteritis nodosa and mixed cryoglobulinemia, while antigens of the infecting organism have been found in immune complexes in patients with vasculitis and malaria (86).

Cell-mediated type IV reactions. Cell-mediated type IV reactions occur as a direct result of contact between sensitized T lymphocytes and specific antigens. Antibodies and complement are not necessary. The characteristic lesion is the delayed cutaneous inflammatory response or tuberculin reaction that occurs when antigen is injected intradermally into a sensitized individual. Exposure of sensitized T lymphocytes to antigen results in proliferation of these cells and release of soluble mediators, lymphokines, or interleukins (63,64) (Table 8–3).

Macrophage chemotactic factors, macrophage activation factor, and migration inhibition factor (MIF) attract, activate, and contain macrophages in the area of the stimulated lymphocyte. Macrophages release lysosomal enzymes capable of damaging the surrounding tissue. Sensitized T cells also secrete lymphotoxins, which can kill adjacent cells, and blastogenic factors, which can induce other lymphocytes to transform and broaden the response to

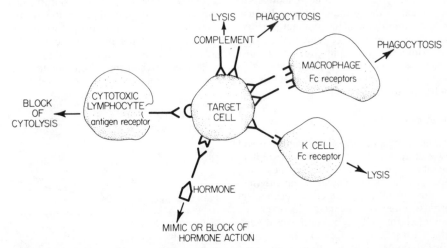

Fig 8–4. Antibody-mediated type II reactions

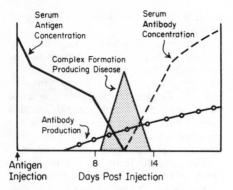

Fig 8–5. One shot serum sickness (Illustration provided by Dr Frank J Dixon)

include proliferation of cells with specifications toward antigens other than that which originated the reaction (Fig 8–7).

The erythema and induration of the delayed cutaneous inflammatory response are first noted at 6 hours, reach a maximum at 24–48 hours, and then subside. Histologically, the lesion consists of a mononuclear infiltrate of small to medium sized lymphocytes and monocytes. About half the cells in the infiltrate are monocytes that enter from the circulation. Lymphocytes specifically sensitized to the inciting antigen make up only a small percentage of the cells (87).

A second mechanism of cell-mediated immunity involves direct cell cytotoxicity. T lymphocytes as well as activated macrophages can kill cells directly. Once a sensitized cytotoxic T cell has been produced, it need not proliferate to exert its killer effect. In vitro tests demonstrate that direct cytotoxicity is rapid, with lysis of the target cell in minutes. Direct cell-to-cell contact is required and the reaction is strongly influenced by the target to killer cell ratio. Generation of this response in a mixed lymphocyte culture leads to the induction of cytotoxic T cells specific for the histocompatibility antigens of the sensitizing cells (86).

In addition to delayed hypersensitivity reactions, type IV immune reactions are important in the granulomatous response to some microorganisms, contact sensitivity, allograft and tumor rejection, lysis of virus-infected cells, and graft-versus-host reactions. Type IV reactions may also play a role in granulomatous vasculitis and polymyositis.

Autoimmunity

The concepts of self-recognition and autoimmunity have undergone radical changes throughout the history of immunology. The immune system was originally conceived as a defense mechanism against infectious agents. However, its potential for self-destruction was recognized early. At the turn of the century, Ehrlich coined the term "horror autotoxi-

cus" to describe what was then the almost unthinkable idea that the body might rebel against itself. He postulated the existence of strict "internal regulating contrivances" to prevent this type of rebellion.

The reality of the self-destructiveness of the immune system became apparent with the description of autoimmune hemolytic anemia and experiments from a number of laboratories demonstrating that proper immunization could induce animals to form autoantibodies. It was postulated that these autoantibodies were products of "forbidden clones" that had somehow escaped destruction. However, as clinical and experimental examples of autoantibodies and autoimmune phenomena became more common, it became obvious that autoreactive cells were normally present in animals and humans.

Immunoregulation. Recently, the concept of self-recognition has been greatly expanded in the network theory which proposes that immunologic control is mediated by a complex network of anti-idiotype antibodies (88). These antibodies are directed against the unique antigens (idiotypes) created by the individual combining sites of antibodies. Idiotypic antigens are present not only on secreted antibodies but also on antigen recognition molecules on the surface of B and T cells. Experimentally, anti-idiotype antibodies can either stimulate or suppress cells bearing the appropriate idiotype antigen.

It has also been shown that recognition of antigens of the major histocompatibility complex (MHC) is important in cooperation between lymphocytes or lymphocytes and macrophages (89). Also, killing of virus-infected cells by cytotoxic T lymphocytes requires recognition not only of the foreign viral antigens but also of self antigens of the major histocompatibility complex (90).

Thus, the concept of self-recognition and autoimmunity has evolved from "never" to "always with control." The immune system appears to be constantly adjusting through negative and positive feedback mechanisms to non-self and self antigens. Increasing appreciation of the complexity of immunoregulation has brought with it a new awareness of the potential for defects in this system.

Possible mechanisms. Autoimmune diseases are probably diseases of defective

immunoregulation. One widely accepted theory is based on the premise that self-reactive B cells which are always present remain dormant because helper T cells capable of recognizing autoantigens are absent or inactive. This control may be bypassed if a foreign antigen and a self antigen are linked together so that a T cell recognizing the foreign portion of a complex antigen can provide help to a B cell capable of recognizing the self portion of that antigen (91). This process may occur when a foreign antigen such as a drug adheres to a cell or when virus antigens appear on the surface of a virus-infected cell. The result is production of antibody to self antigens on the surface of that cell.

Another possibility is the formation of antibodies (rheumatoid factors) against other antibodies that are linked to foreign antigens in an immune complex. The helper T lymphocyte gap can also be bypassed by nonspecific stimulation of B cells by adjuvants.

Other postulated mechanims of deregulation include a viral infection or genetic defect specific for helper or suppressor T cells that would decrease the effectiveness of that cell and tip the balance in favor of its antagonist. Imbalance could also occur from a genetic defect that renders a B cell unable to produce antibody once given the proper signal. This might lead to overreaction in another part of the system as well as a failure of the effector function of the specific antibody involved.

Genetic factors. The genetics of autoimmunity may be quite complicated. Study of autoimmune disease in New Zealand mice suggests that several genes may be involved. One mutant gene may foster autoimmune phenomena through an effect on the regulating system, another is antigen specific and predisposes to production of antinuclear antibody, and a third may exert modifying effects on those at the first locus (92).

In humans certain genes encoded within the major histocompatibility complex are associated with ankylosing spondylitis and the other seronegative spondylarthropathies (B27), rheumatoid arthritis (DR4), SLE (DR2 and DR3), and Sjögren's syndrome (DR3) (93–96). See Section 9 for a more detailed discussion of the immunogenetics of the rheumatic diseases.

Other regulatory systems may also be

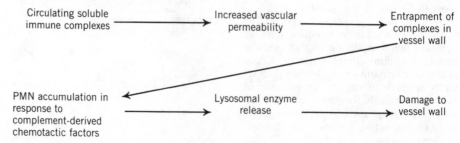

Fig 8–6. Immune complex type III reactions

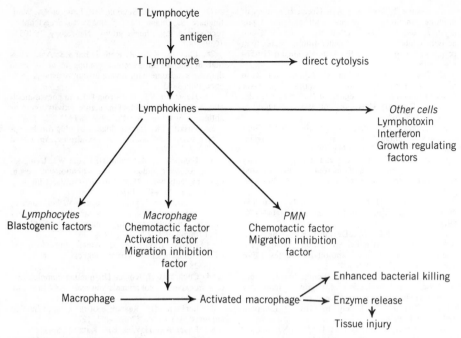

Fig 8–7. Cell-mediated type IV reactions

important in autoimmunity. In NZB/NZW mice female hormones appear to enhance and male hormones diminish autoimmune disease (97). In addition, prostaglandins exert a negative control over lymphocytes (62). An increase in prostaglandin production has been implicated in the defect in cellular immunity seen in Hodgkin's disease and systemic lupus erythematosus (26).

Autoimmunity as a factor in diseases. Many of these concepts have been applied to explain the pathogenesis of systemic lupus erythematosus. A defect has been postulated in suppressor T cells resulting in excessive B cell activity, the production of autoantibodies, and subsequent immune complex disease (52–58). Recent evidence that suppressor T cell function is defective in patients with SLE (52–60) and juvenile chronic polyarthritis (44) and in the NZB and (NZB/NZW) F₁ animal models of SLE (52–57) support this idea as do data showing that a soluble suppressor substance produced by T cells can suppress the disease in animals (55).

The increased occurrence of autoimmune disease in patients with immune deficiency may be another example of immunologic imbalance. Failure of one aspect of the immune response may lead to persistence of endogenous or exogenous antigens and initiate an excessive, self-destructive response in another part of the system.

Thus, some of the diseases now grouped as autoimmune may be the result of a purely endogenous regulatory defect that allows the self-destructive potential of the system to be realized. Others may be autoimmune in the sense that an ineffective or inappropriate response to an exter-

nal challenge leads to immune damage. In both instances treatments that can tune the response by enhancing or diminishing specific aspects such as antibody production or cellular cytotoxicity might be of great value. Defining the external agents and those individuals at risk may also offer a means of prevention of disease.

In either case one of the major challenges for research in rheumatology in the next decade is the understanding of the details of immune regulation and how it relates to the pathogenesis of rheumatic disease.

1. Franklin EC, Frangione B: Immunoglobulins. Ann Rev Med 20:155–174, 1969
2. Cohen S, Milstein C: Structure and biological properties of immunoglobulins. Adv Immunol 7:1–89, 1967
3. Spiegelberg HL: Biological activities of immunoglobulins of different classes and subclasses. Adv Immunol 19:259–294, 1974
4. Tomasi TB, Grey HM: Structure and function of immunoglobulin A. Prog Allergy 16:81–213, 1972
5. Leslie GA, Martin LN: Structure and function of serum and membrane immunoglobulin D (IgD). Curr Top Mol Immunol 7:1–49, 1978
6. Moller G, ed: Immunoglobulin D: structure, synthesis, membrane representation and function. Immunol Rev 37:1–219, 1977
7. Ishizaka T, Ishizaka K: Biology of immunoglobulin E: molecular basis of reaginic hypersensitivity. Prog Allergy 19:61–121, 1975
8. Tada T: Regulation of reaginic antibody formation in animals. Prog Allergy 19:122–194, 1977
9. Pearson GR: In vitro and in vivo investigations on antibody-dependent cellular cytotoxicity. Curr Top Microbiol Immunol 80:65–90, 1978
10. Lovchik JC, Hong R: Antibody-dependent cell-mediated cytolysis (ADCC): analysis and projections. Prog Allergy 22:1–44, 1977
11. Goodfriend L, Sehen AH, Orange RP, eds: Mechanisms in Allergy: Reagin-mediated Hypersensitivity. New York, Marcel Dekker, 1973
12. Bellanti JA, Dayton DH, eds: The Phagocyte Cell in Host Defense. New York, Raven Press, 1975
13. Cline MJ: The White Cell. Cambridge, Mass, Harvard University Press, 1975
14. Stossel TP: Phagocytosis: recognition and ingestion. Semin Hematol 12:83–116, 1975
15. Wilkinson PC: Chemotaxis and Inflammation. Edinburgh, Chruchill Livingston, 1974
16. Snyderman R, Goetzl EJ: Molecular and cellular mechanisms of leukocyte chemotaxis. Science 213:830–837, 1981
17. Weller RF, Goetzl EJ: The regulatory and effector roles of eosinophils. Adv Immunol 27:339–371, 1979
18. VanFurth R, ed: Mononuclear Phagocytes in Immunity, Infection and Pathology. Conference on Mononuclear Phagocytes. Oxford, Blackwell, 1975
19. Nelson DS, ed: Immunobiology of the Macrophage. New York, Academic Press, 1976
20. Zuckerman SA, Douglas SD: Dynamics of the macrophage plasma membrane. Annu Rev Microbiol 33:267–307, 1979
21. Ferrone S, Allison JP, Pellegrino MA: Human DR (Ia-like) antigens: biological and molecular profile. Contemp Top Mol Immunol 7:239–281, 1978
22. Moller G, ed: Role of macrophages in the immune response, Immunological Reviews. Vol 40. Copenhagen, Munksgaard, 1978, pp 1–254
23. Klinkert WEF, LaBadie JH, Bowers WE: Accessory and stimulating properties of dendritic cells and macrophages from various rat tissues. J Exp Med 156:1–19, 1982
24. Kirchner H, Chused TM, Herberman RB, Holden HT, Lavrin DH: Evidence of suppressor cell activity in spleens of mice bearing primary tumors induced by Maloney Sarcoma virus. J Exp Med 139:1473–1487, 1974
25. Broder S, Humphrey R, Durm M, Blockman M, Meade B, Goldman C, Strober W, Waldmann T: Impaired synthesis of polyclonal (nonparaprotein) immunoglobulins by circulating lymphocytes from patients with multiple myeloma: role of suppressor cells. N Engl J Med 293:887–892, 1975
26. Goodwin JS, Messner RP, Bankhurst AD, Peake GT, Saiki IH, Williams RC: Prostaglandin-producing suppressor cells in Hodgkin's disease. N Engl J Med 297:963–968, 1977
27. Handwerger BS, Koren HS: The nature of the effector cell in antibody-dependent, cell-mediated cytolysis (ADCC): the cytotoxic activity of murine tumor cells and peritoneal macrophages. Clin Immunol Immunopathol 5:272–281, 1976
28. Cantor H, Weissman I: Development and function of subpopulations of thymocytes and thymphocytes. Prog Allergy 20:1–64, 1976
29. Gershon RK: T cell control of antibody production. Contemp Top Immunobiol 3:1–40, 1974
30. McKenzie IFC, Potter T: Murine lymphocyte surface antigens. Adv Immunol 27:179–338, 1979
31. Greaves MD, Owen JJT, Raff MC: T and B lymphocytes: origins, properties and roles in immune responses. New York, American Elsevier, 1973
32. Chess L, Schlossman SF: Human lymphocyte subpopulations. Adv Immunol 25:213–241, 1977
33. Jondal M, Wigzell H, Aiuti F: Human lymphocyte subpopulations: classification according to surface markers and/or functional characteristics. Transplant Rev 16:163–195, 1973
34. Winchester RJ, Fu SM, Hoffman T, Kunkel HG: IgG on lymphocyte surfaces: technical problems and the significance of a third cell population. J Immunol 159:1210–1212, 1975
35. Dicker HB: Lymphocyte receptors for immunoglobulin. Adv Immunol 21:167–214, 1976
36. Bianco C, Nussenzweig V: Complement receptors. Curr Top Mol Immunol 6:145–176, 1977
37. Ferrarini M, Hoffman T, Fu SM, Winchester R, Kunkel HG: Receptors for IgM on certain human B lymphocytes. J Immunol 119:1525–1529, 1977
38. Ganzalez-Molina A, Spiegelberg HC: A subpopulation of normal human peripheral B lymphocytes that bind IgE. J Clin Invest 59:616–624, 1977
39. Golub ES: Brain-associated antigen: reactivity of rabbit anti-mouse brain with mouse lymphoid cells. Cell Immunol 2:353–361, 1971
40. Moretta L, Ferrarini M, Cooper M: Characterization of human T-cell subpopulations by specific receptors for immunoglobulins. Curr Top Immunobiol 8:19–53, 1978

41. Cantor H, Boyse EA: Regulation of cellular and humoral immune responses by T cell subsets. Cold Spring Harbor Symp Quant Biol 41:23–32, 1977

42. Murphy DB, Herzenberg LA, Okumura K, Kerzenberg LA, McDevitt HO: A new I subregion (I-J) marked by a locus (Ia-4) controlling surface determinants on suppressor T lymphocytes. J Exp Med 144:699–712, 1976

43. Shreffler DC, David CS: The H-2 complex and the I immune response region: genetic variation, function and organization. Adv Immunol 20:125–195, 1975

44. Nieberhuber JE, Frelingor JA: Expression of Ia antigens on T and B cells and their relationship to immune-response functions. Transplant Rev 30:101–121, 1976

45. Lies RB, Messner RP, Williams RC Jr: Relative T-cell specificity of lymphocytotoxins from patients with systemic lupus erythematosus. Arthritis Rheum 16:369–375, 1973

46. Koike T, Kobayashi S, Yoshiki T, Stoh T, Shirai T: Differential sensitivity of functional subsets of T cells to the cytotoxicity of natural T-lymphocytic autoantibody of systemic lupus erythematous. Arthritis Rheum 22:123–129, 1979

47. Strelkauskas AJ, Schauf V, Wilson BS, Chess L, Schlossman SF: Isolation and characterization of naturally occurring subclasses of human peripheral blood T cells with regulatory functions. J Immunol 120:1278–1282, 1978

48. Strelkauskas AJ, Callery RT, McDowell J, Borel Y, Schlossman SF: Direct evidence for loss of human suppressor cells during active autoimmune disease. Proc Natl Acad Sci (USA) 75:5150–5154, 1978

49. Reinherz EL, Schlossman SF: Regulation of the immune response-inducer and suppressor T-lymphocyte subsets in human beings. N Engl J Med 303:370–373, 1980

50. Kiesling R, Wigzell H: An analysis of the murine NK cell as to structure, function and biological relevance. Immunol Rev 44:165–208, 1979

51. Moller G, ed: Suppressor T lymphocytes, Transplantation Reviews, Vol 26. Copenhagen, Munksgaard, 1975, pp 1–205.

52. Barthold DF, Kysela S, Steinberg AD: Decline in suppressor T-cell function with age in female NZB mice. J Immunol 112:9–16, 1974

53. Gerber, NL, Hardin JA, Chused TM, Steinberg AD: Loss with age in NZB/W mice of thymic suppressor cells in the graft-versus-host reaction. J Immunol 113:1618–1625, 1974

54. Krakauer RS, Waldmann TA, Strober W: Loss of suppressor cells in adult NZB/NZW mice. J Exp Med 144:662–673, 1976

55. Krakauer RS, Strober W, Pippeon D, et al: Prevention of autoimmunity in experimental lupus erythematosus by soluble immune response suppressor. Science 196:56–59, 1977

56. Talal N, Steinberg AD: The pathogenesis of autoimmunity in New Zealand black mice. Curr Top Microbiol Immunol 64:79–103, 1974

57. Talal N: Disordered immunologic regulation and autoimmunity. Transplant Rev 31:240–263, 1976

58. Abdou NI, Sagawa A, Pascual E, Herbert J, Sadeghee S: Suppressor T-cell abnormality in idiopathic systemic lupus erythematosus. Clin Immunol Immunopathol 6:192–199, 1976

59. Breshnihan B, Jasin HE: Suppressor function of peripheral blood mononuclear cells in normal individuals and in patients with systemic lupus erythematosus. J Clin Invest 59:106–116, 1977

60. Sakane T, Steinberg AD, Green I: Studies of immune functions of patients with systemic lupus erythematosus. I. Dysfunction of suppressor T-cell activity related to impaired generation of rather than response to suppressor cells. Arthritis Rheum 21:657–664, 1978

61. Gorcznski RM, Norbury C: Suppressor cells in murine sarcoma virus induced tumors, Suppressor Cells In Immunity. SK Singhal, MRStC Sinclair, eds. London, Ontario, University of Western Ontario, 1975, pp 148–162

62. Goodwin JS, Bankhurst AD, Messner RP: Suppression of human T-cell mitogenesis by prostaglandin. J Exp Med 146:1719–1734, 1977

63. David JR, David RR: Cellular hypersensitivity and immunity: inhibition of macrophage migration and the lymphocyte mediators. Prog Allergy 16:300–449, 1972

64. Waksman BH, Namby Y: On soluble mediators of immunologic regulation. Cell Immunol 21:161–176, 1976

65. Rocklin RE, MacDermott RP, Chess L, Schlossman SF, David JR: Studies on mediator production by highly purified T and B lymphocytes. J Exp Med 140:1303–1316, 1974

66. Newman W, Gordon S, Hammerling U, Senik A, Bloom BR: Production of migration inhibitory factor (MIF) and an inducer of plasminogen activator (IPA) by subsets of T cells in MLC. J Immunol 120:927–931, 1978

67. Handwerger BS, Giroux D, Kay NE, Goodspeed B, Hatfield S, Schmidtke JR: Human T lymphocyte-mediated antibody-dependent cytotoxicity, The Molecular Basis of Immune Cell Function. JG Kaplan, ed. Proceedings of the 13th International Leucocyte Culture Conference, Amsterdam, Elsevier/North Holland, 1979, pp 568–571

68. Herberman RB, Djeu JY, Kay HD, Ortaldo JR, Riccardi B Bonnard GD, Holden HT, Fagnani R, Santoni A, Puccetti P: Natural killer cells: characteristics and regulation of activity. Immunol Rev 44:43–70, 1979

69. Greaves M, Janossy G: Elicitation of selective T and B responses by cell surface binding ligands. Transplant Rev 11:87–130, 1972

70. Andersson J, Sjoberg V, Moller G: Mitogens as probes from immunocyte activation and cellular cooperation. Transplant Rev 11:131–177, 1972

71. Ringden O, Moller E: B-cell mitogenic effects on human lymphocytes of rabbit anti-human beta-2-microglobulin. Scand J Immunol 4:171–179, 1975

72. Coombs RA, Gell PG: Classification of allergic reactions responsible for clinical hypersensitivity and disease, Clinical Aspects of Immunology. PGH Gell, ed. Oxford, Blackwell, 1968, pp 575–596

73. Ishizaka T, Soto CS, Ishizaka K: Mechanisms of passive sensitization: number of IgE molecules and their receptor sites in human basophil granulocytes. J Immunol 111:500–511, 1973

74. Tada T, Ishizaka K: Distribution of IgE forming cells in lymphoid tissues of human and monkey. J Immunol 104:377–387, 1970

75. Sell S, Gell PGH: Studies on rabbit lymphocytes in vitro. I. Stimulation of blast transformation with anti-allotype serum. J Exp Med 122:423–439, 1965

76. Doniach D, Marshall NJ: Autoantibodies to the thyrotropin (TSH) receptors on thyroid epthelium and other tissues, Autoimmunity. N Talal, ed. New York, Academic Press, 1977, pp 621–642

77. Lindstrom JM, Seybold ME, Lennon VA, Whittingham S, Duane DD: Antibody to acetylcholine receptor in myasthenia gravis. Neurology 26:1054–1059, 1967

78. Flier JS, Kahn R, Roth J, Bar RS: Antibodies that impair insulin receptor binding in an unusual diabetic syndrome with severe insulin resistance. Science 190:63–65, 1975

79. Hellstrom KE, Hellstrom I: Lymphocyte-mediated cytotoxicity and blocking serum activity to tumor antigens. Adv Immunol 18:209–277, 1973

80. Poskitt TR: Immunologic and electron microscopic studies in Goodpasture's syndrome. Am J Med 49:250–257, 1970

81. Calder EA, McLeman D, Irvine WJ: Lymphocyte cytotoxicity induced by preincubation with serum from patients with Hasimoto thyroiditis. Clin Exp Immunol 15:467–470, 1974

82. Wasserman J, von Stedingk L-V, Perlmann P, Jonsson J: Antibody-induced in vitro lymphocyte cytotoxicity in Hashimoto thyroiditis. Int Arch Allergy Appl Immunol 47:473–482, 1974

83. Dixon FJ, Vasquez JJ, Weigle WO, Cochrane CG: Pathogenesis of serum sickness. Arch Pathol 64:18–28, 1958

84. Cochran CG, Koffler D: Immune complex disease in experimental animals and man. Adv Immunol 16:185–264, 1973

85. Schlueter DP: Response of the lung to inhaled antigens. Am J Med 57:476–492, 1974

86. Fauci AS, Haynes BF, Katz P: Spectrum of vasculitis: clinical, pathologic, immunologic and therapeutic considerations. Ann Intern Med 89:660–676, 1978

87. Cerottini JC, Brunner KT: Cell-mediated cytotoxicity, allograft rejection and tumor immunity. Adv Immunol 18:67–132, 1974

88. Jerne NK: Towards a network theory of the immune system. Ann Immunol 125C:373–389, 1974

89. Benacerraf B, Germain RN: The immune response genes of the major histocompatibility complex. Immunol Rev 38:70–119, 1977

90. Zinkernagel RM, Doherty PC: MHC-restricted cytotoxic T-cells: studies on the biological role of polymorphic major transplantation antigens determining T-cell restriction-specificity, function and responsiveness. Adv Immunol 27:51–177, 1979

91. Allison AC: Autoimmune diseases: concepts of pathogenesis and control, Autoimmunity. N Talal, ed. New York, Academic Press, 1977, pp 91–139

92. Warner NL: Genetics of autoimmune disease in animals, Autoimmunity. N Talal, ed. New York, Academic Press, 1977, pp. 33–62

93. Brewton DA, Albert E: Rheumatology in HLA and Disease

94. Stasny P: Association of B cell alloantigen DRW4 with rheumatoid arthritis. N Engl J Med 298:869–871, 1978

95. Reinertsen J, Klippel JH, Johnson AH, Steinberg AD, Decker JL, Mann DL: B lymphocyte alloantigens associated with systemic lupus erythematosus. N Engl J Med 299:515–518, 1978

96. Moutsopoulos H, Chused TM, Johnson AH, Knudsen B, Mann DL: B lymphocyte antigens in sicca syndrome. Science 199:1441–1442, 1978

97. Roubiniaen JR, Papovian R, Talal N: Androgenic hormones modulate auto-antibody responses and improved survival in murine lupus. J Clin Invest 59:1066–1070, 1977

9. Immunogenetic aspects of the rheumatic diseases

Recent developments in the field of immunogenetics and the study of HLA antigens and associated diseases have added to our understanding of pathogenetic mechanisms and suggested new classifications of the rheumatic diseases.

HLA antigens are cell surface components of two structural types. HLA–A, B, and C (class I antigens) are present on all nucleated mammalian cells and consist of 2 closely associated polypeptide chains. One chain (the alpha chain) is a glycopeptide encoded by HLA with a molecular weight (MW) of approximately 30,000 and possessing the alloantigen specificity (1,2). The other chain (beta) is a smaller unit (12,000 molecular weight) identical to β2 microglobulin encoded by genes on chromosome 15 (3).

HLA–D antigens. HLA–D related (DR) (class II) antigens show more limited expression on B lymphocytes, macrophages, certain activated T lymphocytes, and other specialized cells (4). These alloantigens are also composed of alpha (34,000 MW) and beta (28,000 MW) polypeptide chains, but both chains are believed to be encoded by genes within the HLA–D region (4).

Recently, several additional class II antigen systems determined by D region genes have been identified. These include the MB and MT specificities (5,6) as well as even newer SB (7) and DS antigens (8). Whether MB and MT antigens are products of distinct D region genes or are "supertypic" specificities physically located on DR molecules is not yet resolved. Nevertheless, certain MB and MT types almost invariably accompany certain DR types, for example MB1 and MT1 with DR 1, 2, and 6; MB2 with DR3 and 7, MT2 with DR3, 5, 6, and 8; and MB3 with DR4 and 5.

It appears that the HLA antigens are not transfixed on the lymphocyte surface but are highly mobile within the fluid-like plane of the membrane. Although the implications of this mobility are not understood, it is clear that a 2-dimensional flexibility would facilitate interactions with various memory determinants as well as with extrinsic antigens (9).

Major histocompatibility complex. The area on chromosome 6 which codes for the HLA antigens is referred to as the major histocompatibility complex (MHC) (2,4). In addition to the genes coding for the serologically detectable HLA antigens (at the A, B, C, and DR loci), there are a number of other immunologic determinants under the genetic control of this chromosomal region (Fig 9–1). The HLA–D region also codes for a discrete set of determinants on the surface of lymphocytes and is functionally recognized by the mixed leukocyte culture (MLC) reaction (10).

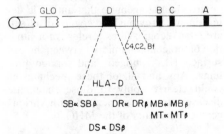

Fig 9–1. Schematic representation of the major histocompatibility complex (MHC) in humans (HLA) located on the short arm of chromosome 6. The circle on the left represents the centromere. The HLA–A, B, and C loci code of glycoprotein antigens are on all nucleated body cells. The HLA–D region codes for DR, MB, MT, and DS alloantigens, selectively expressed on B lymphocytes, macrophages, and activated T cells and for Dw specificities which are defined by mixed lymphoctye culture. Structural genes for complement components C2, C4, and factor B map between HLA–D and HLA–B. (Illustration provided by Dr Frank Arnett)

Other components of the MHC include several genes governing complement production including those coding for C2, C4, and properdin factor B (11,12). Interestingly, some hereditary deficiencies of complement components have been shown to be in linkage disequilibrium with certain HLA genes, including C2 with A10 (25), B18, Dw2, DR2 (12,13).

HLA typing. The most widely recognized alleles coding for the major HLA antigens segregate at the 4 separate loci on the 6th chromosome (A, B, C, and D). These loci have been shown to possess extreme polymorphism within the human species. The HLA antigens coded for the A, B, and C loci are recognized by humoral antibodies and are detected by reacting patients' lymphocytes with complement and exposing them to a large panel of human sera with known anti–HLA specificities (14). Cells rendered nonviable by a specific antiserum can then be recognized by dye uptake.

Typing of B lymphocytes for DR, MB, and MT antigens is performed in a similar manner using a panel of sera containing antibodies to these antigens from which A, B, and C antibodies have been removed. MLC typing for specific D locus (Dw) antigens is much more laborious, usually incorporating a 1-way MLC reaction using a panel of Dw homozygous typing cells (HTC) as stimulators (or not) of the lymphocytes of unknown Dw type (15).

The standard procedure of tissue typing reveals that each locus on chromosome 6 carries 2 codominant alleles—one each at the A, B, C, Dw, and DR loci. Since each individual has 2 of these chromosomes, everyone has 2A, 2B, 2C, 2D, and 2DR antigens—referred to as the HLA **phenotype.** Therefore, each offspring will have in common A, B, C, and D alleles of 1 chromosome with each of his or her parents. By studying HLA phenotypes in families, it is possible to determine which A, B, C, and D alleles segregate with each other on the same chromosome—referred to as the **haplotype.**

Linkage. Thus far about 35 different alleles have been accepted for the A locus, over 40 for the B locus, 12 for the C locus, 12 for D, and 10 for DR. The frequency of any individual HLA antigen within a population is determined largely by ethnic origin. Through family studies it is possible to determine which other genetic loci lie close by or within the HLA region of chromosome 6. If other genetic traits consistently segregate with the A, B, C, or D locus antigens, these traits are said to be "linked" to the HLA region of the chromosome (16,17). Linkage thereby implies a geographic closeness representable as genetic map units between loci on a given chromosome. Moreover, within any population an individual allele will occur at an intrinsic frequency unrelated to the appearance of any other specific linked allele. This is termed **linkage equilibrium.**

However, when 2 alleles at linked loci occur together with a greater or lesser frequency than would be expected from this intrinsic frequency, they are said to be in **linkage disequilibrium.** Examples of such linkage disequilibrium include an excessively high association of A1, B8, and Dw3–DR3, and A3, B7, and Dw2–DR2.

Immune response genes. Interest in the genetic material of the MHC as a key regulatory factor of the immune response has grown from the indisputable evidence generated during the past 2 decades that immune response genes (Ir genes) are located within the analogous chromosomal complex in every nonhuman species thus far studied (18–22). Similar evidence in humans has recently been presented for both immune response (23) and immune suppressor genes (24) linked to HLA.

The fact that some pathogenic Ir genes in animals appear to reside within the MHC and are frequently in linkage disequilibrium with genes coding for major histocompatibility antigens raises the possibility that a similar situation could exist in humans and be responsible for some autoimmune diseases. Thus, the hypothesis has been developed that if pathogenetically significant Ir genes were present in or near the MHC of the 6th chromosome, they too might be linked to certain genes coding for the A,B,C, or D locus antigens. Their presence might, therefore, be revealed by the detection of linkage between some well-characterized autoimmune diseases and a specific HLA allele within an ethnically defined population.

HLA and pathogenesis. This hypothesis has lead to a large number of reports describing HLA-disease associations which appear to support this concept. There are now over 50 diseases, including many autoimmune conditions, clearly associated with a particular HLA antigen or haplotype (2,25–29). Many of these associations with diseases of keen interest to rheumatologists are shown in Table 9–1.

Most of the diseases in the table are characterized by an osteoarticular tissue reaction compatible with an immune-mediated inflammatory response. Some of the HLA-linked metabolic arthropathies are clearly not immunologic diseases but appear to be governed by genes controlling abnormal metabolism which happen to reside within or near the MHC and therefore may be linked to an HLA gene. Some of the strongest HLA human disease associations thus far uncovered have been with the B cell alloantigens, including associations with rheumatoid arthritis and systemic lupus erythematosus.

It should be noted that many of the rheumatic diseases associated with MHC genes are autoimmune. This fact supports the initial hypothesis motivating such a search—that there might indeed be pathogenetically significant human Ir genes within the MHC that exist in linkage disequilibrium with HLA genes. These Ir

Table 9–1. Rheumatic diseases associated with HLA

	Diseases	HLA Association
Seronegative spondylarthropathies	Ankylosing spondylitis	B27
	Reiter's disease	B27
	Post-yersinia and salmonella arthritis	B27
	Juvenile ankylosing spondylitis	B27
	Psoriasis:	
	without arthritis	B13, B17, B37, CW6, DR7
	with axial disease	B27
	with peripheral arthritis	Bw38, Bw39, DR4 (?)*
	Inflammatory bowel disease	
	with spondylitis	B27
	Acute anterior uveitis	B27
	Juvenile arthritis†	DR4, DR5, DRw8, Dw8, TMo, Bw35 (?)*
Autoimmune diseases	Rheumatoid arthritis	Dw4, DR4
	Primary Sjögren's syndrome	B8, Dw3, DR3, MT2
	Systemic lupus erythematosus	DR3, DR2, MB1
	Polymyositis	DR3, DRw6
Metabolic diseases	Hemochromatosis	A3, B14
Complement deficiencies		
C2	SLE-like	A10 (25), B18, Dw2-DR2
C4	SLE-like	‡
Other	Takayasu's arteritis	B5 (Bw52)
	Behcet's syndrome	B5 (Bw51)

* ? = possible association.
† Clinical subgroups of this heterogeneous disease are associated with different HLA antigens, including DR4 with rheumatoid factor–positive polyarticular disease, DR5 with ANA-positive patients who have chronic iridocyclitis, DR and Dw8 and TMo with pauciarticular arthritis, and possibly Bw35 with the acute febrile type (Still's disease).
‡ Associations with specific HLA antigens not clearly defined.

genes may in some way be responsible for generating this type of chronic inflammatory disease. On the other hand, it is also possible that HLA antigens themselves may play a role in pathogenesis.

HLA–B27 and ankylosing spondylitis. The strikingly high association between the gene coding for HLA–B27 and ankylosing spondylitis (AS) has been widely confirmed (30,31). HLA–B27 is present in more than 90% of white patients and in about 50% of American blacks with the disease, compared to control frequencies of about 6–8% and 4%, respectively. Conversely, approximately 20% of B27 positive individuals have evidence of spondylitis (32). This association has served to focus and clarify many aspects of this chronic rheumatic disorder. The apparent familial transmission of ankylosing spondylitis can now be attributed to at least one specific genetic determinant identical to the B27 gene or coexistent with it in marked linkage disequilibrium. Family studies suggest that approximately 20% of family members inheriting the B27 containing haplotype will themselves acquire ankylosing spondylitis or a related disease (33–35).

Clearly other genetic and/or environmental factors are required to promote disease expression. An excess of HLA–B27 cross-reactive antigens (B7, Bw22, B40, Bw42) and the psoriatic arthritis antigen, Bw16 (now Bw38 and Bw39) has been described in B27-negative patients with ankylosing spondylitis (36–39). The association of AS with HLA–B27 has permitted a reconsideration of the epidemiology of this disease and has promoted a similar exploration of many other rheumatic diseases. The various "members" of the seronegative spondylarthropathies probably include idiopathic ankylosing spondylitis, AS seen in association with chronic inflammatory bowel disease, juvenile AS, Reiter's disease, some forms of psoriatic arthritis, and the various types of "reactive" arthropathies following systemic gastrointestinal bacterial infections, notably by yersinia, shigella, and salmonella (33).

The realization that all of these clinical syndromes are often associated with the B27 gene has clarified the long-noted anecdotal observations that any of these clinical syndromes may be recognized among families suffering from a higher than expected incidence of rheumatic disease. Additionally, many puzzling rheumatic syndromes that appear to be "formes frustes" of the seronegative spondylarthropathies are now better recognized.

HLA association with other diseases. Rheumatoid arthritis is associated with increased percentages of HLA–Dw4 and DR4 in whites (40). The DR4 association is maintained across ethnic groups including blacks, Japanese, and Chippewa Indians; however, the Dw4 correlation disassociates from the disease in these populations (40,41). DR4 is not increased in "seronegative rheumatoid arthritis" (40). Primary Sjögren's syndrome shows a striking excess of B8, Dw3, DR3, and MT2, but the sicca complex occurring with rheumatoid arthritis is associated with the rheumatoid antigen, DR4. MT2 may be increased in such patients (42). Systemic lupus erythematosus (SLE) shows weak correlations with DR3, DR2, and MB1 (43,44). Certain autoantibodies (anti–Ro or SS-A, and anti–DNA) in SLE patients, however, may show stronger associations with DR2 and DR3 (44,45). Interestingly, susceptibility to hydralazine-induced lupus has been linked to DR4 rather than DR2 or DR3 (46). In fact, genetic predisposition to several adverse drug reactions has been associated with HLA antigens, including gold-induced nephropathy (47), immune thrombocytopenia (48), and D-penicillamine–induced proteinuria (47).

From the evidence available in animals and humans, it seems likely that the MHC of the human 6th chromosome encompasses genes whose products almost certainly determine how the organism may respond to a variety of antigens within its environment. Such genes may, therefore, play a role in disease susceptibility. The disease susceptibility genes may be those coding for the classic transplantation antigens—such as HLA–B27—or they may be genes within the MHC and in close vicinity to the genes coding for the transplantation antigens and therefore in linkage disequilibrium with them.

Some possible mechanisms for the operation of human HLA–linked disease susceptibility genes have been suggested (49,50). These include an aberrant antibody response, abnormal immune cell interaction, the MHC serving as a receptor for virus, alteration of the MHC by an environmental agent so that antigenic determinants previously recognized as self are later recognized as foreign, or a situation of molecular mimicry between the cell surface HLA antigens and foreign proteins. Any and all of these mechanisms could clearly apply to those rheumatic diseases strongly associated with various gene components of the MHC.

1. Crumptom MJ, Snary D: Isolation and structure of human histocompatibility (HLA) antigen, Contemp Top Mol Immunol 6:52–82, 1977
2. McMichael AJ, McDevitt HO: The association between the HLA system and disease. Prog Med Genet 2:39–95, 1977
3. Goodfellow PN, Jones EA, van Heyningen V, Solomon E, Bobrow M, Miggiano V, Bodmer WF:

The B$_2$-microglobulin gene is on chromosome 15 and not in the HLA region. Nature 254:267–269, 1975

4. Winchester RJ, Kunkel HG: The human Ia system. Adv Immunol 28:221–292, 1979

5. Duquesnoy RJ, Marrari MM, Annen K: Identification of an HLA–DR associated system of B-cell alloantigens. Transplant Proc 11:1757–1760, 1979

6. Duquesnoy RJ, Marrari MM, Vieira J: Definition of MB and MT antigens by 8th International Histocompatibility Workshop B-cell alloantiserum clusters. Histocompatibility Testing 1980. PI Terasaki, ed. UCLA Los Angeles, UCLA Tissue Typing Laboratory Press, 1980, pp 861–863

7. Shaw S, Johnson AH, Shearer GM: Evidence for a new segregant series of B-cell antigens that are encoded in the HLA-D region and that stimulate secondary allogeneic proliferative and cytotoxic responses. J Exp Med 152:565–579, 1980

8. Goyert SM, Silver J: Isolation of I-A subregion–like molecules from subhuman primates and man. Nature (London) 294:266–268, 1981

9. Raff MC: Cell surface immunology. Sci Am 234:30–39, 1976

10. Walford RL, Gossett T, Troup GM, Gatti RA, Mittal KK, Robins A, Ferrara GB, Zeller E: The Merritt alloantigenic system of human B-lymphocytes: evidence for 13 possible factors including one 6-member segregant series. J Immunol 116:1704–1710, 1976

11. Weitkamp LR, Lamm LU: Report of the committee on the genetic constitution of chromosome 6. Cytogenet Cell Genet 32:130–142, 1982

12. Rittner C, Bertrams J: On the significance of C2, C4 and factor B polymorphisms in disease. Human Genet 56:235–247, 1981

13. Ruddy S: Complement, rheumatic diseases, and the major histocompatibility complex. Clin Rheum Dis 3:215–237, 1977

14. Terasaki P, Bernoco D, Park MS, Ozturk G, Iwaki Y: Microdroplet testing for HLA, -B, -C, and -D antigens. Am J Clin Pathol 69:103–120, 1978

15. Dupont B, Hansen JA, Yunis E: Human mixed-lymphocyte culture reaction: genetics, specificity, and biological implications. Adv Immunol 23:107–202, 1976

16. Albert E, Amos DB, Kissmeyer-Nielsen F, Bodmer WF, Mayr W, Trnka Z, Ceppellini R, Payne R, Dausset J, VanRood JJ, Terasaki PI, Walford RL: Nomenclature for factors of the HLA system—1977. Transplantation 25:272–275, 1978

17. Grumet FC: HLA and disease associations. Transplant Proc 9:1839–1844, 1977

18. Shreffler DC, Meo T, David CS: Genetic resolution of the products and functions of I and S region genes of the mouse H-2 complex, The Role of Products of the Histocompatibility Gene Complex in Immune Responses. DH Katz, B Benacerraf, eds. New York, Academic Press, 1976, pp 3–27

19. Katz DH, Armerding D, Eshhar Z: Histocompatibility gene products as mediators of lymphocyte interactions, The Role of Products of the Histocompatibility Gene Complex in Immune Responses. DH Katz, B Benacerraf, eds. New York, Academic Press, 1976, pp 541–552

20. McDevitt HO, Benacerraf B: Genetic control of specific immune responses. Adv Immunol 11:31–74, 1969

21. McDevitt HO, Oldstone MBA, Pincus T: Histocompatibility-linked genetic control of specific immune responses to viral infection. Transplant Rev 19:209–225, 1974

22. Dorf ME, Balner H, Benacerraf B: Mapping of linked immune response genes in the major histocompatibility complex of the Rhesus monkey. J Exp Med 142:673–693, 1975

23. Hsu SH, Chan MM, Bias WB: Genetic control of major histocompatibility complex-linked immune responses to synthetic polypeptides in man. Proc Natl Acad Sci USA 78:440–444, 1981

24. Sasazuki T, Kaneoka H, Nishimura Y, Kaneoka R, Hayama M, Ohkuni H: An HLA-linked immune suppression gene in man. J Exp Med 152:297s–313s, 1980

25. Kemple K, Bluestone R: The major histocompatibility complex and rheumatic diseases. Pathobiol Annual 7:305–326, 1977

26. Dausset J, Svejgaard A, eds: HLA and disease: predisposition to disease and clinical implications. Abstract of Paris symposium. INSERM, Paris, 1976

27. Ryder LP, Svejgaard A: Report from the HLA and diseases registry of Copenhagen. Published by the authors, 1976

28. Bluestone R: Histocompatibility antigens and rheumatic diseases. Current Concepts (in press)

29. Mann DL, Murray C: HLA alloantigens: disease association and biologic implications. Semin Hematol 16:293–308, 1979

30. Schlosstein L, Terasaki PI, Bluestone R, Pearson CM: High association of the HLA antigen W27 with ankylosing spondylitis. N Engl J Med 288:704–706, 1973

31. Brewerton DA, Hart FD, Nicholls A, Caffrey M, James DCO, Sturrock RD: Ankylosing spondylitis and HLA 27. Lancet 1:904–907, 1973

32. Calin A, Fries JF: Striking prevalence of ankylosing spondylitis in "healthy" W27 positive males and females. N Engl J Med 293:835–839, 1975

33. Woodrow JC: Genetics of B27-associated diseases. Ann Rheum Dis 38 (suppl):135–141, 1979

34. Hochberg MC, Bias WB, Arnett FC: Family studies in HLA-B27 associated arthritis. Medicine 57:463–475, 1978

35. Calin A, Barnett M, Marder A, Marks S: The nature and prevalence of spondyloarthropathies among relatives of probands with ankylosing spondylitis and Reiter's syndrome (abstract). Arthritis Rheum 24 (suppl):S78, 1981

36. Arnett FC, Hochberg MC, Bias WB: HLA-27 cross-reactive antigens in B27-negative Reiter's syndrome and sacroiliitis. Johns Hop Med J 141:193–197, 1977

37. Khan MA, Kusher I, Braun WE: A subgroup of ankylosing spondylitis associated with HLA-B7 in American blacks. Arthritis Rheum 21:528–530, 1978

38. Schwartz B, Luehrman LK, Rodey GE: A public antigenic determinant on a family of HLA-B molecules—a basis for cross-reactivity and possible link with disease predisposition. J Clin Invest 64:938–947, 1978

39. Khan MA, Kushner I, Braun WE: Genetic heterogeneity in primary ankylosing spondylitis. J Rheumatol 7:383–386, 1980

40. Stastny P: Joint report on rheumatoid arthritis. Histocompatibility Testing 1980. PI Terasaki, ed. Los Angeles, UCLA Tissue Typing Laboratory Press, 1980, pp 681–686

41. Harvey J, Arnett FC, Bias WB, Hsu SH, Stevens MB: Heterogeneity of HLA-DR4 in the rheumatoid arthritis of a Chippewa band. J Rheumatol 8:797–803, 1981

42. Moutsopoulos HM, Mann DL, Johnson AH, Chused TM: Genetic differences between primary and secondary sicca syndrome. N Engl J Med 301:761–763, 1979

43. Reinertsen JL, Klippel JH, Johnson AH, Steinberg AD, Decker JL, Mann DL: B-lymphocyte alloantigens associated with systemic lupus erythematosus. N Engl J Med 299:515–518, 1978

44. Ahearn JM, Provost TT, Dorsch CA, Stevens MB, Bias WB, Arnett FC: Interrelationships of HLA-DR, MB, and MT phenotypes, autoantibody expression and clinical features in systemic lupus erythematosus. Arthritis Rheum 25:1031–1040, 1982

45. Bell DA, Maddison PJ: Serologic subsets in systemic lupus erythematosus: an examination of autoantibodies in relationship to clinical features of disease and HLA antigens. Arthritis Rheum 23:1268–1273, 1980

46. Batchelor JR, Welsh KI, Tinoco RM, Dollery CT, Hughes GRV, Bernstein R, Ryan P, Naish PF, Aber GM, Bind RF, Russell GI: Hydralazine-induced systemic lupus erythematosus: influence of HLA-DR and sex on susceptibility. Lancet 1:1107–1109, 1980

47. Wooley PH, Griffin J, Panayi GS, Batchelor JR, Welsh KI, Gibson TJ: HLA-DR antigens and toxic reactions to sodium aurothiomalate and D-penicillamine in patients with rheumatoid arthritis. N Engl J Med 303:300–302, 1980

48. Coblyn JS, Weinblatt M, Holdsworth D, Glass D: Gold-induced thrombocytopenia: a clinical and immunogenetic study of twenty-three patients. Ann Intern Med 95:178–181, 1981

49. Dietz MH, Bluestone R: The major histocompatibility complex and disease. J Chron Dis 31:307–311, 1978

50. McDevitt HO, Bodmer WF: HL-A, immune response genes and disease. Lancet 1:1269–1275, 1974

10. Epidemiology of the rheumatic diseases

Most acquired chronic disorders, such as the rheumatic diseases, are believed to result from the interaction of multiple factors relating to the host, environment and, at times, infectious agents. Primary disease mechanisms are often obscured by complex interactions of such factors. Epidemiology, defined as the study of the frequency and distribution of disease in populations and of those factors determining or associated with disease occurrence, may assist in clarifying such interrelationships.

Rheumatoid arthritis and the connective tissue diseases. Rheumatoid arthritis and related connective tissue diseases have now been the subjects of numerous epidemiologic studies (1,2). Some of these findings are summarized in Table 10–1. Similarities in the patterns of occurrence are more striking than the discrepancies. By and large, these are disorders of women, with onset most often during the childbearing ages, and with a tendency to affect blacks more frequently than whites.

Such findings suggest constitutional predisposition and hormonal modulation of disease expression. These influences are more apparent in the spontaneous lupus-like illness of NZB-NZW hybrid mice, one of the few animal models available for the study of these diseases. Immune mechanisms also appear to play an important role in pathogenesis, a concept strengthened by the frequent finding of antinuclear and other autoantibodies in the serum of these individuals (see Section 4).

Estimates of the prevalence of rheumatoid arthritis (RA) have been derived from population surveys which indicate that approximately 1% of the adult population

Table 10–1. Epidemiologic characteristics of connective tissue diseases

	Rheumatoid arthritis	Systemic lupus erythematosus	Progressive systemic sclerosis	Polymyositis/ dermatomyositis
Annual incidence (per million)	750	75	10	10
Sex ratio, all ages (female: male)	2.5:1	5:1	2.5:1	2:1
Race ratio, both sexes (black:white)	1:1	4:1	2:1	3:1
Childhood diagnosis (%)	5–10	10	1	20
Incidence pattern	Increases with age, especially in females; F:M sex ratio of 6:1 in seropositive patients 15–45 years of age and 1:1 in first and oldest decades	Highest in women 20–40 years of age; F:M sex ratio of 8:1 in patients 20–40 years of age and 2:1 in first and oldest decades	Increases with age, especially in women; uncommon in children and men under age 35	Childhood and adult peaks
5-year survival (%)	95+	90+	60	60

is affected with definite RA (see Section 12). The few studies of incidence yield estimates of 0.75/1000 or 750 new cases per million population at risk annually.

Although the overall sex ratio is almost 3 women to 1 man, this relationship seems to vary by age periods. Among adults under age 60, women predominate over men by a ratio of 5:1, whereas from age 60 and older, the sex ratio approximates equality. Sex-related host factors seem to play a role in determining both the onset and severity of rheumatoid arthritis. This concept is consistent with the recognized pregnancy-induced remission of rheumatoid arthritis and the postpartum development of exacerbations or new onsets of disease.

Population surveys of persons with rheumatoid arthritis of all degrees of severity have not revealed impressive evidence of familial aggregation. However, in seropositive erosive rheumatoid arthritis, a 6-fold increase in prevalence has been found among siblings and dizygotic twins of rheumatoid arthritis probands versus controls, and a 30 times expected frequency is reported among monozygotic twins. These studies are buttressed by the observation that a lymphocyte defined histocompatibility antigen (HLA–Dw4) is significantly increased in frequency in a subset of rheumatoid arthritis patients with seropositive erosive disease (see Section 9).

Systemic lupus erythematosus. Population studies of systemic lupus erythematosus (SLE) became feasible after the discovery of the LE cell phenomenon (see Section 13). In New York City the estimated SLE incidence increased steadily from 5–10 new patients per million population per year in the early 1950s to over 30 per million per year by 1965, and since then higher figures (up to 75 per million annually) have been reported in several community studies. It is not known whether this increasing incidence reflects mainly greater physician awareness of lupus or represents a true increase in disease frequency. The female to male ratio is

highest (about 10:1) during the childbearing years (ages 15–45), and is significantly lower both in childhood and among the elderly (2–3:1).

A role for endocrine factors in the pathogenesis and expression of SLE is also suggested by its reported association with Klinefelter's syndrome; metabolic studies have suggested prolonged estrogenic stimulation in such cases. Of note is the frequent exacerbation or new onset of SLE in the postpartum period and the finding that spontaneous lupus in NZB-NZW hybrid mice is accelerated in female animals and worsened after castration of male mice.

An excess of black versus white women of 3–4:1 has now been confirmed in a number of studies. Reports of familial SLE and occurrence of the disease in monozygotic twins (60% concordance) have been frequent. However, in population studies, such familial aggregation appears to operate at a relatively low level, whether genetic, environmental, or infectious agent factors might be contributing. Studies of the histocompatibility antigens in SLE have produced conflicting results (see Section 9).

Progressive systemic sclerosis (PSS, scleroderma; Section 14) and polymyositis-dermatomyositis (Section 16) are less common, with an estimated incidence of approximately 10 new cases diagnosed per million population per year. PSS is characterized by a female to male ratio of 3–4:1 and an incidence that steadily increases with age. The disorder is unusual in childhood and among men less than 35 years of age. There is little, if any, racial predilection in males, but black women seem to be at higher risk than white women. Several occupations have been cited as possibly predisposing to PSS, including stone mason work and underground gold, coal, and uranium mining. An increasing number of familial cases has been described recently, but convincing associations with HLA antigens have not been identified.

Polymyositis has a bimodal age distribution, with incidence peaks in childhood

and between ages 45 and 64; it is uncommon for the disease to commence in late adolescence or young adulthood. Females predominate by 2:1, and black women are at significantly greater risk than white females (4:1). Under age 10 and again after age 60, the female to male ratio is nearly 1, while during the intervening years and especially in the second decade, a significant female excess is noted (8:1). Thus, as in the other connective tissue diseases, female preponderance tends to increase during the childbearing years, reinforcing the concept that factors related to sexual maturation are important in modulating these disorders.

Polyarteritis nodosa and the family of conditions considered under the umbrella of vasculitis offer a particularly difficult challenge in definition and classification (see Section 18). There are few or no pathognomonic clinical or laboratory findings, and nomenclature varies widely, depending on the frame of reference, i.e., clinical, histologic, or immunologic. No systematic epidemiologic studies have been reported. Vasculitis syndromes appear to be less frequent than the connective tissue disorders discussed and show less concentration among young or middle-aged black women, suggesting a somewhat different set of pathogenetic mechanisms.

Ankylosing spondylitis and the seronegative spondylarthropathies. A major contribution of clinical epidemiology during the past decade has been the description of the patterns of occurrence of ankylosing spondylitis and related disorders (seronegative spondylarthropathies) (see Sections 27–30). Even before the discovery of HLA–B27 as an hereditary marker of these disorders, the familial nature and overlapping clinical features of ankylosing spondylitis, Reiter's disease, and the arthropathies associated with psoriasis and chronic inflammatory bowel disease were described.

The frequency of ankylosing spondylitis (AS) reported in population surveys depends not only on the frequency of HLA–

B27 in the group studied, but also on the detection methods used. The prevalence varies from a virtual absence in black Africans to fully 5% in adult Haida Indian men of the Pacific Northwest. When clinical criteria alone were employed, the prevalence of probable and definite ankylosing spondylitis was estimated to be 4/1000 in adult white men. Among HLA–B27 positive individuals, however, and including roentgenographic exmaination of the sacroiliac joints, the reported frequency of sacroiliitis and/or other manifestations of AS approaches 20% in several investigations.

This disorder is typically diagnosed in young adult men with the usual age of onset between 15 and 35 years. Females tend to have milder disease, resulting in underdetection. Ankylosing spondylitis does occur in individuals who lack HLA–B27, more frequently so (up to 50%) in blacks. In these circumstances, several other histocompatibility antigens have been associated with the disease, some closely related to B27, including B7, Bw22, Bw42, Cw1, and Cw2.

Reiter's syndrome bears a close clinical relationship to ankylosing spondylitis, with nearly half the patients eventually developing spinal involvement. Although once considered rare, this condition is perhaps the leading cause of arthritis among young adult males. Its recognition in women is unusual.

Reiter's syndrome is reported in epidemic occurrences, such as after bacillary dysentry and as an endemic or sporadic event after venereal urethritis. In an epidemic aboard an American naval vessel in 1962, 10 (1.5%) of 602 men developed Reiter's syndrome several weeks after shigella dysentery. Recent followup has revealed that 4 of 5 sailors located were positive for HLA–B27 and the fifth had the related B7 antigen. Gastroenteritis due to other Gram-negative organisms (*Yersinia enterocolitica* and *Salmonella*) also appears to precipitate Reiter's syndrome in HLA–B27 positive individuals.

Family studies suggest a wider spectrum of the disease than originally considered, including a number of ''incomplete'' cases. Some of these patients have only a seronegative, asymmetrical, oligo- or polyarthritis. Considering the epidemiologic evidence that Reiter's syndrome follows exposure to an infectious agent, it appears that development of the disease is triggered by the encounter of a genetically susceptible (HLA–B27 positive) host with some triggering environmental inciting event or insult (possibly an infectious agent).

Lymphocytes of Reiter's syndrome patients with onset after venereal infection or urethritis had greater ^{3}H-thymidine uptake responses to ureaplasmal or chlamydial than to enteric bacterial antigens, whereas the reverse was true in those who developed Reiter's after enteric infection. This observation suggests a host-agent cell-mediated immunologic component in the disease (3).

Sacroiliitis and spondylitis. Two other B27 associated spondylarthropathies have been recognized—sacroiliitis or spondylitis—in association with psoriasis and chronic inflammatory bowel disease (both ulcerative colitis and Crohn's disease). A smaller proportion of individuals with these disorders develop a peripheral arthritis and B27 is only minimally more frequent overall than in control populations. Another striking revelation is that acute anterior uveitis (AAU) is reported in as many as 20% of these seronegative spondylarthropathy patients and the frequency of B27 in all patients with AAU is approximately 50%.

Gout and hyperuricemia. The risk of developing hyperuricemia and primary gout depends on a complex interaction of multiple factors including heredity, age, sex, diet, and drugs (see Section 46). In the United States the normal mean serum uric acid level for males is approximately 5 mg/dl for whites, blacks, Indians, orientals, and other groups, whereas surveys in the South Pacific have shown native populations with mean levels ranging as high as 7 mg/dl or greater, with correspondingly high frequency of gouty arthritis.

The average serum urate level is higher in men than women; this discrepancy, which commences at age 15 and reaches a maximum of almost 1.5 mg/dl by age 20–24, is apparently related to the uricosuric influence of estrogenic hormone. The mean value gradually increases in women after age 40, rising *after* menopause to within 0.5 mg/dl of the average level in men.

The frequency of gouty arthritis increases steadily with age in men, but gout is exceedingly rare in premenopausal women, except in those persons with strong hereditary factors. The overall male to female ratio is 7:1 in most large clinical series of gout patients but may be less in population interview studies.

A number of inborn errors of uric acid metabolism have now been described which may be associated with gout, e.g., the Lesch-Nyhan syndrome, a rare complete deficiency of the enzyme hypoxanthine-guanine phosphoribosyltransferase. Hyperuricemia and gout are associated statistically with a number of other metabolic disorders including obesity, hypertension, diabetes mellitus, arterial hypertension, and atherosclerotic heart disease, but the pathogenetic relationships between these conditions is still incompletely defined.

Osteoarthritis. Population studies have indicated that osteoarthritis (degenerative joint disease, osteoarthrosis) is a ubiquitous condition. Its frequency increases steadily with age (see Section 36), especially as observed in roentgenographic surveys, in which articular alterations are found in many asymptomatic individuals.

It has been estimated that approximately 30% of persons with radiographic evidence of osteoarthritis complain of pain in affected sites. Epidemiologic studies suggest that both host (heredity, obesity) and environmental factors (excessive joint use, trauma) contribute to increased susceptibility to osteoarthritis.

1. Lawrence JS: Rheumatism in Populations. London, William Heinemann Medical Books Ltd, 1977
2. Masi AT, Medsger TA Jr: Epidemiology of the rheumatic diseases, Arthritis and Allied Conditions, Ed 9. DJ McCarty Jr, ed. Philadelphia, Lea & Febiger, 1979, 11–30
3. Ford DK, daRoza DM, Schulzer M: The specificity of synovial mononuclear cell responses to microbiological antigens in Reiter's syndrome. J Rheumatol 9:S61–S67, 1982

11. Classification of the rheumatic diseases

With the discovery of a variety of new pathophysiologic mechanisms to explain old observations, the classification of arthritis and rheumatism has undergone rapid changes in recent years. A variety of newly identified patient subsets have been added to the family of rheumatic diseases, and previously recognized entities have been regrouped based on current knowledge.

The most noteworthy achievement in this regard is the grouping of ankylosing spondylitis and closely related conditions having spondylitis in greater than expected frequency (Reiter's syndrome, psoriasis, and chronic inflammatory bowel disease). Progress in this area was dramatically accelerated by the discovery of their association with the histocompatibility antigen HLA–B27, a marker for the susceptible host. Another area of intense interest has been the separation of juvenile arthritis into more meaningful clinical-pathophysiologic subsets. Progress has also been evident in the classification of biochemical and endocrine disorders and nonarticular rheumatism.

Classification is a dynamic process which requires periodic review and revision of existing nomenclature. Change is to be expected, and even applauded, since it nearly always reflects important new information and concepts concerning pathophysiologic mechanisms of disease. Only by such efforts can we make the all-important advances in therapy we seek for our patients.

As evidence of the acquisition of new knowledge, this *Primer on the Rheumatic Diseases* contains 19 sections not covered in the last edition. Table 11–1 represents a revision and updating of the 1963 effort by the Nomenclature and Classification Committee of the American Rheumatism Association and the 1973 *Primer* refinement of that original document. It is the preliminary proposal of the Glossary Committee of the American Rheumatism Association.

Table 11–1. Classification of the rheumatic diseases

I. Diffuse connective tissue diseases
  A. Rheumatoid arthritis
  B. Juvenile arthritis
    1. Systemic onset
    2. Polyarticular onset
    3. Oligarticular onset
  C. Systemic lupus erythematosus
  D. Progressive systemic sclerosis
  E. Polymyositis/dermatomyositis
  F. Necrotizing vasculitis and other vasculopathies
    1. Polyarteritis nodosa group (includes hepatitis B associated arteritis and Churg-Strauss allergic granulomatosis)
    2. Hypersensitivity vasculitis (includes Schönlein-Henoch purpura and others)
    3. Wegener's granulomatosis
    4. Giant cell arteritis
      a. Temporal arteritis
      b. Takayasu's arteritis
    5. Mucocutaneous lymph node syndrome (Kawasaki's disease)
    6. Behcet's disease
  G. Sjögren's syndrome
  H. Overlap syndromes (includes mixed connective tissue disease)
  I. Others (includes polymyalgia rheumatica, panniculitis (Weber-Christian disease), erythema nodosum, relapsing polychondritis, and others)

II. Arthritis associated with spondylitis
  A. Ankylosing spondylitis
  B. Reiter's syndrome
  C. Psoriatic arthritis
  D. Arthritis associated with chronic inflammatory bowel disease

III. Degenerative joint disease (osteoarthritis, osteoarthrosis)
  A. Primary (includes erosive osteoarthritis)
  B. Secondary

IV. Arthritis, tenosynovitis, and bursitis associated with infectious agents
  A. Direct
    1. Bacterial
      a. Gram-positive cocci (staphylococcus and others)
      b. Gram-negative cocci (gonococcus and others)
      c. Gram-positive rods
      d. Mycobacteria
      e. Treponemes
      f. Others
    2. Viral
    3. Fungal
    4. Parasitic
    5. Unknown, suspected (Whipple's disease)
  B. Indirect (reactive)
    1. Bacterial (includes acute rheumatic fever, intestinal bypass, postdysenteric—shigella, yersinia, and others)
    2. Viral (hepatitis B)

V. Metabolic and endocrine diseases associated with rheumatic states
  A. Crystal-induced conditions
    1. Monosodium urate (gout)
    2. Calcium pyrophosphate dihydrate (pseudogout, chondrocalcinosis)
    3. Hydroxyapatite
  B. Biochemical abnormalities
    1. Amyloidosis
    2. Vitamin C deficiency (scurvy)
    3. Specific enzyme deficiency states (includes Fabry's, Farber's, alkaptonuria, Lesch-Nyhan, and others)
    4. Hyperlipidemias (types II, IIa, IV)
    5. Mucopolysaccharides
    6. Hemoglobinopathies (SS disease and others)
    7. True connective tissue disorders (Ehlers-Danlos, Marfan's, pseudoxanthoma elasticum, and others)
    8. Others
  C. Endocrine diseases
    1. Diabetes mellitus
    2. Acromegaly
    3. Hyperparathyroidism
    4. Thyroid disease (hyperthyroidism, hypothyroidism)

      D. Immunodeficiency diseases
      E. Other hereditary disorders
         1. Arthrogryposis multiplex congenita
         2. Hypermobility syndromes
         3. Myositis ossificans progressiva
VI. Neoplasms
      A. Primary (e.g. synovioma, synoviosarcoma)
      B. Metastatic
VII. Neuropathic disorders
      A. Charcot joints
      B. Compression neuropathies
         1. Peripheral entrapment (carpal tunnel syndrome and others)
         2. Radiculopathy
         3. Spinal stenosis
      C. Reflex sympathetic dystrophy
      D. Others
VIII. Bone and cartilage disorders associated with articular manifestations
      A. Osteoporosis
         1. Generalized
         2. Localized (regional)
      B. Osteomalacia
      C. Hypertrophic osteoarthropathy
      D. Diffuse idiopathic skeletal hyperostosis (includes ankylosing vertebral hyperostosis—
           Forestier's disease)
      E. Osteitis
         1. Generalized (osteitis deformans—Paget's disease of bone)
         2. Localized (osteitis condensans ilii; osteitis pubis)
      F. Avascular necrosis
      G. Osteochondritis (osteochondritis dissecans)
      H. Congenital dysplasia of the hip
      I. Slipped capital femoral epiphysis
      J. Costochondritis (includes Tietze's syndrome)
      K. Osteolysis and chondrolysis
IX. Nonarticular rheumatism
      A. Myofascial pain syndromes
         1. Generalized (fibrositis, fibromyalgia)
         2. Regional
      B. Low back pain and intervertebral disc disorders
      C. Tendinitis (tenosynovitis) and/or bursitis
         1. Subacromial/subdeltoid bursitis
         2. Bicipital tendinitis, tenosynovitis
         3. Olecranon bursitis
         4. Epicondylitis, medial or lateral humeral
         5. DeQuervain's tenosynovitis
         6. Adhesive capsulitis of the shoulder (frozen shoulder)
         7. Trigger finger
      D. Ganglion cysts
      E. Fasciitis
      F. Chronic ligament and muscle strain
      G. Vasomotor disorders
         1. Erythromelalgia
         2. Raynaud's disease or phenomenon
      H. Miscellaneous pain syndromes (includes weather sensitivity, psychogenic rheumatism)
X. Miscellaneous disorders
      A. Disorders frequently associated with arthritis
         1. Trauma (the result of direct trauma)
         2. Lyme arthritis
         3. Pancreatic disease
         4. Sarcoidosis
         5. Palindromic rheumatism
         6. Intermittent hydrarthrosis
         7. Villonodular synovitis
         8. Hemophilia
      B. Other conditions
         1. Internal derangement of joints (includes chondromalacia patella, loose bodies)
         2. Familial Mediterranean fever
         3. Eosinophilic fasciitis
         4. Chronic active hepatitis
         5. Other drug-induced rheumatic syndromes

12. Rheumatoid arthritis

Rheumatoid arthritis is a chronic, systemic inflammatory disorder of unknown etiology characterized by the manner in which it involves joints (1). Articular inflammation is sometimes remitting, but if continued usually results in progressive joint destruction and deformity, leading ultimately to variable degrees of incapacitation. Extraarticular features such as rheumatoid nodules, arteritis, neuropathy, scleritis, pericarditis, lymphadenopathy, and splenomegaly occur with considerable frequency. Once thought to be complications of rheumatoid arthritis, they are now recognized as integral parts of the disease and serve to emphasize its systemic nature.

Rheumatoid arthritis has a worldwide distribution and involves all racial and ethnic groups. Women are affected 2–3 times more often than men, although this female preponderance disappears when only patients with positive serologic tests for rheumatoid factor and erosive change on x-ray are considered (2,3). The disease occurs at all ages and generally increases in incidence with advancing age. In women, the peak incidence is between the fourth and sixth decades.

This discussion will be limited to the adult form of the disease. Juvenile arthritis is presented in Section 34.

Etiology

Despite many years of intensive investigative effort, the etiology of rheumatoid arthritis remains obscure. Endocrine, metabolic, and nutritional factors as well as geographic, occupational, and psychosocial variables have all been studied. Although possibly influencing the course of the disease, they clearly cannot be implicated in its causation. Conventional family and genetic studies have provided inconclusive and often conflicting results. The recent finding of an association with certain alleles of the major histocompatibility complex suggests that genetic factors can influence the expression of the disease, perhaps by their effect on the immunologic phenomena that play an important role in its pathogenesis (4).

The occurrence of polyarthritis during many human bacterial and viral diseases and the resemblance of rheumatoid arthritis to certain illnesses in animals caused by microorganisms (such as mycoplasmal disease in rodents and erysipelothrix infections in swine) make infection an attractive hypothesis, but to date no direct evidence of infection has been discovered.

Rheumatoid factors

Tests. Rheumatoid factors are antibodies with specificity for antigenic determinants on the Fc portion of human or animal IgG. The usual clinical tests for rheumatoid factor are agglutination procedures that use sheep red blood cells sensitized with rabbit anti-sheep cell antibodies or inert particles (latex or bentonite) with human IgG adsorbed onto their surface. The sensitized sheep cell test is more specific for rheumatoid arthritis, but is infrequently used in clinical practice because it is more laborious than the latex agglutination or bentonite flocculation tests. These systems detect primarily 19S IgM rheumatoid factors; more recently developed methods can demonstrate anti-gamma globulins (rheumatoid factors) in IgG and IgA in a large percentage of rheumatoid sera, occasionally in the absence of IgM rheumatoid factor (5,6).

Standard flocculation tests detect IgM rheumatoid factors in the sera of approximately 70% of adult patients with rheumatoid arthritis. A positive test is by no means diagnostic of this disorder, since rheumatoid factors are also found in 1–5% of normal subjects, the incidence increasing with advancing age, and in a variety of disease states. Conversely, its absence does not exclude rheumatoid arthritis. Rheumatoid patients usually have more rheumatoid factor than normal individuals or those with other diseases. High titers of rheumatoid factor are generally associated with more severe and active joint disease, the presence of nodules, greater frequency of systemic complications of rheumatoid arthritis, and a poorer outcome (3,6–8).

Reactivity with IgG. The antibody nature of rheumatoid factors is demonstrated by specificity for both genetic (e.g., gamma) and nongenetic (structural) determinants on the IgG molecule, most commonly located in the amino terminal portion of the Fc fragments from IgG1, IgG2, and IgG4 molecules. This reactivity may be to autologous (patient's own), isologous (other human), or heterologous (other species) IgG in either the native or denatured state. Individual sera in general contain an array of anti–gamma globulins with different specificities. The majority lack specificity for genetic determinants and react preferentially with aggregated IgG or antigen–antibody complexes.

Reactivity with native and autologous IgG can be demonstrated for some rheumatoid factors; this presumably accounts for the occurrence of circulating complexes made of IgM rheumatoid factor and IgG in the serum of some patients with rheumatoid arthritis. Intermediate sized complexes, containing only 7S IgG, part having rheumatoid factor activity, can also be detected in some sera. Some rheumatoid factors react with both heterologous and isologous IgG, reflecting shared antigenic determinants. A minority are limited to heterologous IgG (6,9).

Rheumatoid factor. Currently, the most popular notion is that rheumatoid factors arise as antibodies to "altered" autologous IgG. Alteration is thought to occur when a native IgG antibody molecule combines with its specific antigen. This antigen-antibody interaction changes the configuration of the IgG molecule revealing new or previously hidden antigenic determinants, thereby rendering it an autoimmunogen. Support for this hypothesis comes from animal experiments in which chronic, intense immunization with bacteria or bacterial cell wall antigens results in the production of anti–gamma globulin factors and from the finding of rheumatoid

Table 12–1. Occurrence of rheumatoid factor in various diseases

IgM rheumatoid factor frequently present	Rheumatoid factor usually absent
Rheumatic diseases	
Rheumatoid arthritis	Osteoarthritis
Sjögren's syndrome (with or without arthritis)	Ankylosing spondylitis
Systemic lupus erythematosus	Gout
Progressive systemic sclerosis	Chondrocalcinosis
Polymyositis/dermatomyositis	
Infectious diseases	
Bacterial endocarditis	Suppurative arthritis
Tuberculosis	Psoriatic arthritis
Syphilis	Enteropathic arthritis
Infectious hepatitis	Reiter's syndrome
Leprosy	
Kala-azar	
Schistosomiasis	
Noninfectious diseases	
Normal individuals, especially aged	
Diffuse interstitial pulmonary fibrosis	
Cirrhosis of liver, chronic active hepatitis	
Sarcoidosis	
Waldenstrom's macroglobulinemia	

factors in bacterial endocarditis and other human diseases that have chronic antigenic stimulation as a common denominator (Table 12–1).

An alternative explanation derives from the observation that cultured peripheral blood B lymphocytes make immunoglobulins and antibodies when stimulated with pokeweed mitogen or Epstein-Barr virus (polyclonal B cell activation). B cells from normal subjects and rheumatoid patients produce rheumatoid factor; the latter make larger amounts. Thus, it had been proposed that increased serum concentrations of rheumatoid factor reflect polyclonal B cell activation by an as yet unidentified pathogen or defective T cell regulation of rheumatoid B lymphocytes.

The exact biological role of rheumatoid factors is unknown. Antiviral properties have been ascribed to them, and under certain circumstances, they can affect the inflammatory response by enhancing complement fixation, by altering the properties (e.g., size or solubility) of immune complexes, or by rendering them more susceptible to ingestion by phagocytic cells. These latter characteristics are probably especially important in synovial tissues and fluids (10).

Pathogenesis

Etiologic factors. Although difficult to document, the earliest events in rheumatoid arthritis appear to be microvascular injury, edema of subsynovial tissues, and mild synovial lining cell proliferation (11,12). Polymorphonuclear leukocytes, when present, are in the superficial synovium; plasma cells are rare. Small blood vessels may be obliterated by inflammatory cells and organized thrombi.

Electron microscopic examination discloses gaps between vascular endothelial cells and endothelial cell injury. Phagocytosis is prominent in proliferating synoviocytes and in large mononuclear cells. In contrast to established rheumatoid arthritis, the synovial fluids from patients with recent onset usually show more mononuclear cells than polymorphonuclear leukocytes. These early findings suggest that the responsible etiologic factor is carried to the joint by the circulation.

Cellular pathology. In established rheumatoid arthritis, the synovium appears grossly edematous and protrudes into the joint cavity as slender villous projections (Fig 12–1). Light and electron microscopic examination discloses hyperplasia and hypertrophy of the synovial lining cells which may reach a depth of 6–10 cells; normally there are only 1–3 cell layers. Hyperplasia of synoviocytes results from an increase in both A (reticuloendothelial-like) and B type cells. The former show large accumulations of residual bodies and altered lysosomes. Focal or segmental vascular changes are a regular feature. Venous distention, capillary obstruction,

infiltration of the arterial walls by neutrophils, and areas of thrombosis and perivascular hemorrhage are commonly seen.

The normally acellular subsynovial stroma is packed with mononuclear cells, some collected into aggregates or follicles, particularly around small blood vessels. True germinal centers are rare. Lymphocytes predominate in these follicles with a mantle of plasma cells around their periphery. Transitional areas show an intermingling of macrophages, lymphocytes, and plasma cells. Blast cells constitute less than 5% of the cells in either the lymphocyte rich or plasma cell rich zones, but in the transitional areas, two-thirds of the cells are blast cells, suggesting that antibodies and the products of activated lymphocytes and macrophages are generated there (13).

The majority of the lymphocytes in the rheumatoid synovium are T cells, but immunofluorescence shows large numbers of immunoglobulin-producing cells. The plasma cells in the subsynovium contain predominantly IgG but few have anti-Ig activity when tested with fluorescein-labeled aggregated IgG. After pepsin treatment of tissue sections, the number of plasma cells staining for rheumatoid factor increases significantly. This suggests local production of an IgG rheumatoid factor which combines in the plasma cell cytoplasm with similar IgG molecules ("self-associating IgG")(14).

Pathogenic hypotheses. Based on these histologic observations, 2 pathogenetic mechanisms have been advanced to explain rheumatoid arthritis.

The first—the **extravascular immune complex hypothesis**—proposes an interaction of antigens and antibodies in synovial tissues, cartilage, and fluid (15). In general, the antibodies are presumed to be locally produced, especially the self-associating dimers and higher multiples of the IgG anti-IgG complex. Other potentially important immune complexes are those in which the antigens are constituents of articular tissues or byproducts of the inflammatory process, such as collagen, cartilage, fibrinogen or fibrin, partially digested IgG, DNA, and soluble nucleoproteins.

The reaction of antigen with antibody in the joint tissues engages the complement sequence, causing reduced complement levels in synovial fluid, increased vascular permeability, and an accumulation of cellular blood elements. Polymorphonuclear leukocytes, attracted by complement-derived chemotactic factors, ingest the complexes with a subsequent release of large quantities of hydrolytic enzymes, oxygen radicals, and arachidonic acid metabolites that are directly responsible for much of the inflammation and some tissue damage (16).

There is an alternative hypothesis, namely that rheumatoid joint disease results from **cellular hypersensitivity**. The accumulation of activated T lymphocytes in the rheumatoid synovium, the demonstration of soluble factors derived from T cells (lymphokines) in synovial effusions, the dramatic improvement in some patients treated by thoracic duct drainage, and the observation of a rheumatoid-like arthritis in some agammaglobulinemic children are cited as evidence for an important role of cellular immune reaction in rheumatoid synovitis (17).

Destructive processes. Chronic rheuma-

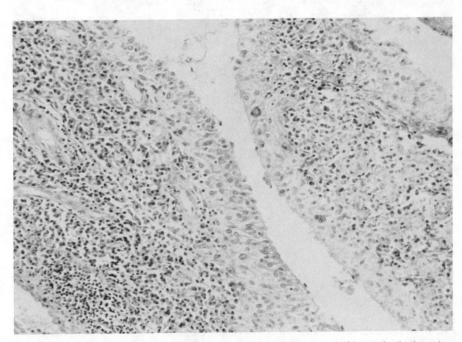

Fig 12–1. Knee synovitis. The multilayered synovial lining is composed of hyperplastic, hypertrophic synoviocytes with occasional multinucleated giant cells. The enlarged villi are diffusely infiltrated by lymphocytes and plasma cells. Moderate capillary proliferation is seen. (From the Revised Clinical Slide Collection on the Rheumatic Diseases)

toid arthritis is characterized by destruction of articular cartilage, ligaments, tendons, and bone. The damage results from a dual attack—from without by digestants in the synovial fluid and from above and below by granulation tissue.

Proteoglycan depletion (loss of metachromatic staining) in normal appearing cartilage at sites distant from the advancing margin of the proliferating synovial membrane is caused by neutral and acid proteases in the fluid that continually bathes the cartilage surfaces. They are insufficient to produce irreversible damage, however, because the structural skeleton of cartilage is provided by collagen. When in its triple helical configuration, collagen resists degradation by nonspecific proteases. But specific collagenases derived from polymorphonuclear leukocytes and rheumatoid synovial cells can cleave the collagen polypeptide chains into 2 fragments, exposing them to further proteolytic digestions (18).

Pannus. The most important destructive element is rheumatoid pannus, a vascular granulation tissue composed of proliferating fibroblasts, numerous small blood vessels, and various numbers of inflammatory cells. Collagen and proteoglycan seem to be dissolved in the region immediately surrounding nests of mononuclear cells at the cartilage-pannus junction (Fig 12–2). Occasionally collagen fibers are seen within phagolysosomes of cells at the leading edge of the pannus (19,20).

Collagenase. Cultured explants of rheumatoid synovial tissue produce large quantities of collagenase and prostaglan-dins. The responsible cells, presumably synoviocytes, are large, with abundant cytoplasm, a big nucleus, and dendritic processes. They lack the conventional surface markers of macrophages. Collagenase production is markedly increased by exposing them to factors derived from blood mononuclear cells (interleukin-1) (21). The collagenase released from isolated synovial cells is an inactive or latent form. Activation is accomplished by proteolytic enzymes. Plasmin is potentially important in vivo because plasminogen activator is also produced by cultured rheumatoid synovial cells. Although latent, the collagenase can bind to collagen fibrils, and thus is near its substrate when activated (22).

The following scheme of collagenolysis has been proposed. The lymphocytes and macrophages in the rheumatoid synovium, individually or in consort, are stimulated to release soluble products that cause inflammation, increased blood vessel permeability, and the production of latent collagenase by synovial cells. Synovial cells also produce a plasminogen activator. Plasminogen from the circulation enters the inflamed joint and is converted to plasmin which activates the latent collagenase bound to collagen fibrils. This leads to a rapid destruction of collagen-containing tissues.

Alternatively, the latent collagenase could be released, but escape activation and remain bound to fibrils. At some later time plasminogen activators produced by the endothelial cells of small blood vessels in the pannus would initiate the collageno-lytic process. It is quite likely that these mechanisms are not unique to rheumatoid arthritis and operate in other forms of chronic synovitis.

Pathologic changes. The end result of the pathologic changes is unpredictable since the disease may arrest at any stage. In chronic long-standing disease the granulation tissue forms adhesions and undergoes cicatrization. Opposing articular surfaces become adherent and organize, causing fibrous ankylosis if large parts of the joint surfaces are involved. Metaplasia of the pluripotential granulation tissue can result in cartilaginous or bone ankylosis. Capsular scarring and shrinkage impair joint mobility. Adhesions between periarticular structures and weakening of the capsular and supporting ligaments alter joint structure and function. Tendon contracture and rupture can occur.

The sum of these pathologic changes, in conjunction with the mechanical forces of weight bearing and muscle pull, produces the characteristic deformities of rheumatoid arthritis.

Clinical features

The clinical course of rheumatoid arthritis is highly inconsistent, ranging from a mild pauciarticular illness of brief duration to a relentlessly progressive, destructive polyarthritis associated with a systemic vasculitis. The extent of articular involvement does not correlate well with the presence or severity of constitutional symptoms or extraarticular manifestations, but destructive arthritis and extraarticular features are more common in patients whose serum contains high titers of rheumatoid factors.

Joint disease. The onset of rheumatoid arthritis is frequently heralded by prodromal symptoms such as fatigue, anorexia, weight loss, weakness, and generalized aching and stiffness. Joint symptoms usually appear gradually and insidiously over weeks to months. Occasionally, there are brief remittent episodes of articular involvement prior to the development of more persistent arthritis.

Approximately 20% of patients have an abrupt onset of polyarthritis, often accompanied by fever, prostration, and constitutional symptoms (1). The mode of onset is not clearly related to the subsequent course or prognosis of the disease, although in one study an acute onset was associated with a high probability of subsequent remission (23).

Articular involvement is manifested clinically by pain, stiffness, limitation of motion, and the signs of inflammation. Pain need not be proportional to the degree of inflammation and is usually most pronounced on movement of the afflicted joint.

Morning stiffness lasting more than 30 minutes (and frequently several hours) is

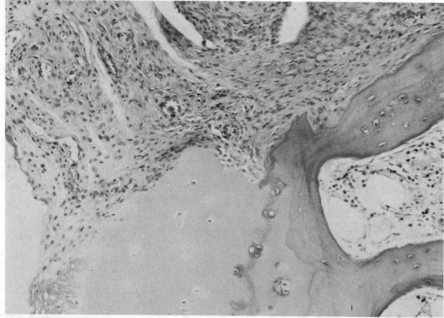

Fig 12–2. Ankle pannus. This microscopic photograph reveals typical pannus formation. Fibrovascular tissue protrudes from the inflamed synovium into the articular cartilage. A portion of the fibrous tissue extends over the surface of the cartilage, which shows death of chondrocytes and loss of basophilia of the matrix. Note the inflammatory exudate in the subchondral bone (H&E, medium power). (From the Revised Clinical Slide Collection on the Rheumatic Diseases)

characteristic of rheumatoid arthritis and is thought to result from congestion in the synovium, joint capsule thickening, and, frequently, from an increase in the volume of synovial fluid (effusion). Early in the disease, joint motion is usually limited by pain but later may be limited by capsular fibrosis, muscle contracture and/or rupture, laxity or shortening of tendons and ligaments, or bony or fibrous ankylosis.

Rheumatoid arthritis can affect any diarthrodial joint; those most commonly involved initially are the small joints of the hands, the wrists, knees, and feet. At the outset there may be any pattern of joint disease, but usually it is bilateral, symmetrical, and polyarticular. In a small percentage of patients the disease remains unilateral or monarticular (usually the knees) for months to years. As the disease becomes established, the arthritis spreads to the elbows, shoulders, sternoclavicular joints, hips, ankles, and subtalar joints. Less commonly the temporomandibular and cricoarytenoid joints are affected. Clinically significant spinal involvement is usually limited to the upper cervical articulations, although radiographic evidence of other spinal disease can occur.

Hands. Joint examination generally reveals a number of characteristic abnormalities, especially in the hands. Early in the disease, swelling of the proximal interphalangeal (PIP) joints produces a fusiform or spindle-shaped appearance of the fingers. Bilateral and symmetrical swelling of the metacarpophalangeal (MCP) joints, particularly the second and third, is very common and remains long after PIP joint inflammation has subsided. The distal interphalangeal (DIP) joints can be involved but are more often spared.

As the disease progresses, laxity of soft tissues increases and under the pressure of regular use, typical hand deformities develop (Fig 12–3). Ulnar deviation of the fingers is particularly common, often accompanied by palmar subluxation of the proximal phalanges. Hyperextension of the PIP joints in conjunction with flexion

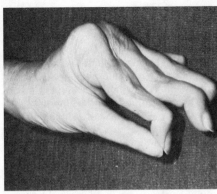

Fig 12–4. "Swan-neck" deformities are present in the second and third fingers of this patient with rheumatoid arthritis. This deformity results from contracture of the interosseous and flexor muscles and tendons, resulting in a flexion contracture of the metacarpophalangeal joint, hyperextension of the proximal interphalangeal joint, and flexion of the distal interphalangeal joint. (From the Revised Clinical Slide Collection on the Rheumatic Diseases)

at the DIP joint constitutes the **swan-neck** deformity (Fig 12–4). The **boutonniere** deformity is a flexion deformity of the PIP joints and extension of the DIP joints.

Rheumatoid involvement of the thumbs causes hyperextension of the interphalangeal joints and flexion at the MCP joints with a resultant loss of pinch. A sudden loss of ability to extend the fingers—especially the third, fourth, and fifth digits—follows rupture of the extensor tendons or their dislocation into the intermetacarpal space. Only prompt surgical repair ensures good results for tendon rupture. The insidious development of weakness of finger extensors suggests dislocation of the metacarpophalangeal joints or entrapment of the posterior interosseous nerve as it traverses the supinator muscle in front of the elbow joint.

Wrists. Wrist disease is an almost invariable accompaniment of rheumatoid arthritis. Active synovitis can be observed at the dorsum of the wrist as a boggy, soft tissue swelling. Synovial hypertrophy and tenosynovitis on the volar aspect may compress the median nerve beneath the transverse carpal ligament, producing a **carpal tunnel syndrome** with paresthesia

and dysesthesia of the thumb, second, third, and radial aspect of the fourth digits (Fig 12–5). The thenar eminence may atrophy and percussion over the flexor retinaculum elicits pain in the median nerve distribution (**Tinel's sign**). Later in the disease, wrist immobility develops, resulting from fibrous or very occasionally, bony ankylosis of the radiocarpal, intercarpal, and/or carpometacarpal joints. Commonly, pronation and supination are severely limited due to involvement of the inferior radioulnar joint.

Elbows. Flexion contractures of the elbow are frequent, even at an early stage of the disease. The paraolecranon grooves are often obliterated by hypertrophied synovium. Shoulder involvement is common, with the glenohumeral, acromioclavicular, and thoracoscapular articulations all being susceptible. Examination generally reveals limitation of motion and tenderness just below and lateral to the corocoid process. Swelling is rarely observed. Frequently, the joint capsule ruptures and subluxation of the humerus occurs.

Hips. Rheumatoid arthritis of the hip joints is a less common, later development. A frequent complaint is discomfort in the groin; less often the pain is referred to the buttocks or lower back. Swelling and tenderness are difficult to note and hip disease may be recognized only because of gait abnormalities or limitation of joint motion.

Knees. The knee is among the most frequently affected joints and is responsible for much disability. Synovial hypertrophy and chronic effusion can be pronounced. When less conspicuous, joint effusions can be detected by ballotting the patella or by the demonstration of a "bulge" alongside the patella when fluid is milked into the suprapatellar pouch and then expressed back into the joint. A regular accompaniment of knee involvement is quadriceps atrophy, often of great severity.

Flexion contractions, valgus deformity, and all degress of ligamentous instability are later complications. Pathologic enlargement of the normal gastrocnemius—semimembranous bursa (**Baker's cyst**)—can be palpated in the popliteal space. Although usually asymptomatic, these

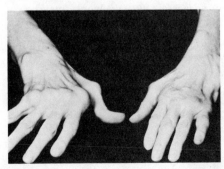

Fig 12–3. Ulnar deviation and subluxation of metacarpophalangeal joints have occurred in the patient's right hand. These joints also appear swollen. Muscle atrophy has developed in the dorsal musculature of both hands. (From the Revised Clinical Slide Collection on the Rheumatic Diseases)

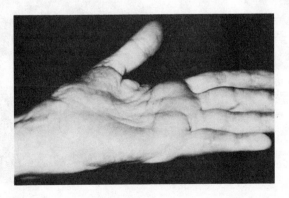

Fig 12–5. In this patient with rheumatoid arthritis, thenar atrophy has occurred due to damage of the median nerve caused by pressure from swollen inflammatory tissue. (From the Revised Clinical Slide Collection on the Rheumatic Diseases)

cysts can cause discomfort by compressing structures behind the knee. Occasionally, they enlarge rapidly or rupture and give rise to symptoms and signs mimicking acute thrombophlebitis.

Arthrography usually confirms the diagnosis (Fig 12–6) and should be performed in any patient with rheumatoid arthritis who develops acute tenderness, warmth, or edema of the lower leg.

Feet and ankles. Arthritis in the feet and ankles creates a number of vexing problems. Pain and limitation of flexion and extension of the foot result from disease of the mortis joint of the ankle, while subtalar involvement gives symptoms with eversion and inversion. Pain on walking may result from inflammation on the un-

dersurface of the heel or the bursa just beneath the insertion of the achilles tendon into the calcaneus.

In the foot proper, synovitis of the metatarsophalangeal joints is particularly common, whereas interphalangeal joint involvement is distinctly unusual. Characteristic deformities that develop with progression of the disease are subluxation of the metatarsal heads, hallux valgus, and lateral deviation and clawing of the toes.

Neck. Symptoms of intermittent neck pain and stiffness are frequent; neurologic complications occur, but are rare. The spinal cord may be compromised by anterior dislocation of the first cervical vertebrae (Fig 12–7) or by vertical subluxation of the odontoid process of the second vertebra into the foramen magnum. Subluxation can also induce torsion and compression of the vertebral arteries with symptoms of vertebrobasilar insufficiency and syncope on downward gaze. Headache, a frequent complaint, is most commonly occipital, but occasionally radiates over the top of the cranium, settling behind one or the other eye. Neck examination discloses localized tenderness, muscle spasm, and limitation of rotary motion. Flexion and extension of the cervical spine are less affected.

Extraarticular manifestations. Although characteristically a joint disease, rheumatoid arthritis can involve a number of other tissues (24,26). These extraarticular manifestations probably occur frequently but are usually occult and of limited clinical significance. Occasionally, however, they dominate the clinical picture. Terms like "rheumatoid disease" and "malignant rheumatoid arthritis" describe this form of the disease. Extraarticular features occur, more often, in patients whose serum contains rheumatoid factor and, in general, correlate with the severity but not the duration of the joint disease. Men develop certain manifestations such as vasculitis, pulmonary disease, and pericarditis more frequently than would be predicted from the disease incidence alone.

Rheumatoid nodules. Subcutaneous nodules, perhaps the commonest extraar-

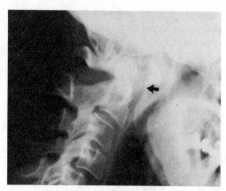

Fig 12–7. Atlantoaxial subluxation of the cervical spine. A lateral view of the upper cervical region reveals posterior displacement of the odontoid process. The preodontoid space measures approximately 8 mm (**arrow**). Normally this measurement should not exceed 2.5–3 mm in the adult, although in the child 4–5 mm may be within normal limits. The measurement is made at the base of the anterior aspect of the dens with the neck held in flexion. (From the Revised Clinical Slide Collection on the Rheumatic Diseases)

ticular feature of rheumatoid arthritis, appear at some time in approximately 20–25% of patients (Fig 12–8). They are almost invariably associated with seropositive (rheumatoid factor) disease and perhaps with a more severe and destructive arthritis. Nodules are firm, rounded, or oval masses in the subcutaneous or deeper connective tissues, varying from less than 0.5 cm to several centimeters in diameter.

Periarticular structures and areas subjected to mechanical pressure are common sites—especially the olecranon bursae, extensor surface of the forearms, and the achilles tendon. Visceral involvement will be discussed in more detail later. Unusual locations include the pleura, meninges, ears, and the bridge of the nose.

Subcutaneous nodules seldom cause symptoms, but occasionally they break down or become infected. Typically, they develop insidiously and once present can persist indefinitely or regress at any time. Nodules have been mistaken for gouty tophi, basal cell carcinoma, xanthomata, or sebaceous cysts; a biopsy may be required to establish the diagnosis.

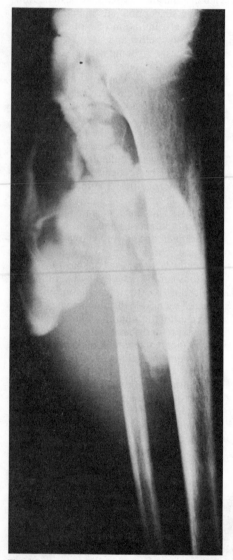

Fig 12–6. This is the lateral projection of an arthrogram of the left knee of a patient with a popliteal cyst. There is good filling of the suprapatellar bursa and knee joint proper. The contrast medium extends posteriorly into the distended gastrocnemio-semimembranosus bursa with extension and/or rupture distally into the calf. (From the Revised Clinical Slide Collection on the Rheumatic Diseases)

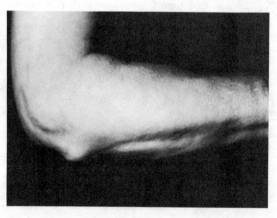

Fig 12–8. A large subcutaneous nodule is located on the extensor surface of the forearm near the elbow. (From the Revised Clinical Slide Collection on the Rheumatic Diseases)

Histologically, the rheumatoid nodule is composed of an irregular central zone of fibrinoid necrosis surrounded by a palisade of elongated connective tissue cells arranged radially in a corona around the necrotic zone. This core is enveloped by an outer zone of granulation tissue containing chronic inflammatory cells, chiefly lymphocytes and plasma cells (Fig 12–9).

Vasculitis. A spectrum of vascular lesions accompanies rheumatoid arthritis. The majority are silent and only discovered at postmortem examination. They take many forms: capillaritis and venulitis, considered important in the development of rheumatoid nodules and synovitis; a bland intimal proliferation commonly affecting digital and mesenteric vessels; subacute lesions of arterioles and venules in scattered locations; and finally, a widespread necrotizing arteritis of small and medium sized arteries that may be indistinguishable from polyarteritis nodosa.

Onset of this "rheumatoid arteritis" can occur in an explosive fashion and characteristically produces a sensorimotor neuropathy, skin necrosis and ulcceration, digital gangrene, and visceral infarction (7). Death may ensue after a few weeks or months. Fortunately, this fullblown picture is rare, and any one of these manifestations can appear insidiously, posing little threat to life.

Ischemic skin lesions appear in crops as small brown spots, usually in the nailfolds and digital pulp. Larger ischemic ulcerations may develop in the lower extremities, particularly over the malleoli. Fatal intestinal and myocardial infarctions have been reported.

Patients with the acute form of rheumatoid arteritis often are febrile, sometimes to 104°F or more, and have polymorphonuclear leukocytosis. Many will have concomitant episcleritis, scleromalacia, pleuritis, myocarditis, and/or pericarditis. The appearance of vasculitis does not necessarily correlate with the activity of the articular disease. The prognosis in the fulminant form of vasculitis is poor and the terminal condition is usually complicated by the superimposition of malnutrition, infection, congestive heart failure, or gastrointestinal bleeding (7,27).

The pathogenesis of rheumatoid vasculitis is uncertain; indirect evidence suggests the participation of immune complexes. Most patients have serum rheumatoid factor, usually in high titer. As a rule, rheumatoid patients have normal or elevated serum complement values, but in those with arteritis, complement levels tend to be lower and may be very low. Materials with the properties of antigen–antibody complexes have been detected in the circulation by a variety of techniques (28). Sural nerve biopsies from subjects with rheumatoid neuropathy show deposition of IgG, IgM, and C3 in the walls of acutely inflamed blood vessels (29).

Neuropathy. Rheumatoid arthritis tends to spare the central nervous system, but causes a number of abnormalities in peripheral nerves. Foot or wrist drop and a patchy sensory loss in one or more extremities (mononeuritis multiplex) are frequent manifestations of vasculitis (30). Patients with rheumatoid arthritis also get a mild, symmetrical distal sensory neuropathy. This is usually more marked in the lower extremities, is not related to vasculitis, and does not carry an unfavorable prognosis (31). Elderly patients are most often affected.

Neurologic complaints in patients with rheumatoid arthritis can result from cervical cord compression or entrapment neuropathy. Median neuropathy is most common (**carpal tunnel syndrome**), but symptoms can result from ulnar nerve involvement at the elbow or wrist or from compression of the radial or posterior interosseous nerves of the elbow. In the lower legs, an anterior tibial nerve palsy causing foot drop and the so-called tarsal tunnel syndrome, with pain and paresthesia in the heel and medial aspect of the foot, may occur.

Cardiac manifestations. A variety of cardiac lesions are demonstrable at postmortem examination, but clinically detectable heart disease attributable solely to the rheumatoid process is unusual (32). Pericarditis, the most frequent histopathologic abnormality, occurs in about 40% of autopsied patients. Less common are granulomatous lesions, similar to rheumatoid nodules, involving the epicardium, myo-

cardium and valves; focal interstitial myocarditis; and arteritis of coronary vessels. Occasionally valvular insufficiency or conduction abnormalities are recognized during life and rarely, myocardial infarction complicates coronary arteritis (33).

The most common symptomatic lesion is acute pericarditis. It appears most often in males with seropositive disease and is unrelated to the duration of arthritis. An associated pleural effusion is often found. Characteristics of the pericardial fluid include a low glucose concentration, increased lactic dehydrogenase (LDH) LDH and IgG levels, and low complement activity. The course of the pericarditis is irregular, ranging from a mild, self-limited process to cardiac tamponade and death. Corticosteroid therapy is usually effective, but chronic effusion or constriction may ensue and necessitate pericardiectomy. Recurrences may be experienced (34–36).

Pleuropulmonary manifestations. Respiratory symptoms encountered in rheumatoid patients usually result from more common disorders, but some findings are intimately related to the rheumatoid process: 1) pleurisy with or without effusions, 2) nonpneumoconiotic intrapulmonary rheumatoid nodules, 3) rheumatoid pneumoconiosis (Caplan's syndrome), 4) diffuse interstitial fibrosis and pneumonitis, and 5) involvement of the intima of small pulmonary arteries and arterioles leading to pulmonary hypertension. Considerable overlap exists among these syndromes.

Rheumatoid pleural disease is most commonly asymptomatic. Pleurisy may appear before or simultaneously with the onset of arthritis. Effusions tend to be chronic and occasionally are of sufficient size to cause respiratory obstruction.

The pleural fluid is typically exudative. White blood cell counts vary greatly, but are usually less than 5,000/mm³. Either mononuclear or polymorphonuclear leukocytes may dominate. LDH enzyme is usually high and glucose values tend to be low, frequently less than 25 mg%. Normal glucose levels do not exclude the diagnosis. Total hemolytic complement, C3, and C4 are significantly lower in the rheumatoid pleural fluid compared to simultaneous serum samples and to nonrheumatoid inflammatory effusions (24,37). Pleural biopsy findings are usually nonspecific.

Solitary or multiple densities are occasionally seen in chest roentgenograms of patients with rheumatoid arthritis, especially those with subcutaneous nodules. Although usually asymptomatic, they may cavitate, become infected, or rupture into the pleural space with the production of pneumothorax or pyopneumothorax. On histologic examination, they are identical to rheumatoid nodules from any other location (38,39).

The presence of numerous rheumatoid nodules in the lungs of patients with a

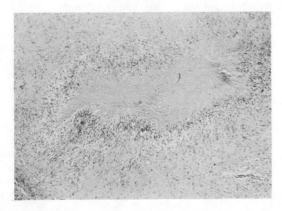

Fig 12–9. Subcutaneous nodule (H&E, medium power). See text for description. (From the Revised Clinical Slide Collection on the Rheumatic Diseases)

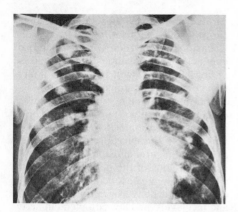

Fig 12–10. Caplan's syndrome. Chest of a 54-year-old coal miner showing characteristic multiple round opacities 1–2 cm in diameter. There was no clinical evidence of rheumatoid arthritis at the time of this roentgenogram, although sheep cell agglutination reaction was positive in a dilution of 1:2,048. Histologic examination of a pulmonary nodule revealed a rheumatoid granuloma. (Illustration provided by Dr Anthony Caplan)

history of rheumatoid arthritis and a pneumoniotic exposure is referred to as **rheumatoid pneumoconiosis** or **Caplan's syndrome** (Fig 12–10) (40). Principally described in Welsh soft coal miners, the same phenomenon has since been observed in asbestos and ceramic workers, gold and chalk miners, and others with arthritis and a particular industrial exposure (26). Chest roentgenograms usually reveal multiple well-defined nodular opacities of 0.5–5 cm in diameter, widely distributed throughout the lungs, but particularly abundant at the periphery. Alternatively, large numbers of smaller nodules present a "snowstorm" appearance or nodules may coalesce into large conglomerate masses. Cavitation has been observed.

Patients with rheumatoid arthritis develop a **diffuse interstitial fibrosis** indistinguishable from the idiopathic variety. Early radiographic findings are diffuse, patchy infiltrates or fine reticulonodular densities most pronounced at the lung bases. Later, a diffuse mottling and interstitial fibrosis develops that progresses to an endstage honeycomb appearance with bronchiolar ectasia. Such a condition may evolve rapidly, or more commonly, over 5–10 years.

Progressive dyspnea and a cough productive of scanty sputum are associated with auscultatory findings of dry crackling rales. Clubbing is common. Pulmonary function tests show a diminished compliance and a restrictive ventilatory pattern. Histologically, there is thickening of alveolar walls, lymphoreticular hyperplasia, and interstitial infiltration with chronic inflammatory cells (38).

Obstructive airway disease has also re-

cently been found in some nonsmokers with RA. This is often associated with Sjögren's syndrome. Peribronchiolar inflammation is found on biopsy (41).

Ocular manifestations. The most common ocular abnormalities are the corneal and conjunctival lesions associated with Sjögren's syndrome (Section 20). Rheumatoid patients also develop inflammatory lesions of the episclera and sclera. **Episcleritis** is a self limited, relatively benign condition that causes mild pain and discomfort in the eyes, but does not interfere with vision. It usually begins abruptly as a raised, cream colored to violaceous lesion surrounded by intense hyperemia which clears in a few weeks (42).

Scleritis is usually an indolent, slowly progressing process. It is a more serious condition that episcleritis and can be accompanied by severe pain and occasionally, visual impairment or blindness. Lesions are most commonly found in the superior sclerae and tend to be bilateral. They appear as raised yellow nodules surrounded by hyperemia of the deep scleral vessels. After a period of time, the sclera at the involved site thins, allowing the dark blue of the choroid beneath to show through (**scleromalacia perforans**). Inflammation may spread to the episclera, choroid, ciliary body, and retina. The histology of both episcleritis and scleritis is that of a rheumatoid nodule (42,43).

Ocular complaints in a rheumatoid patient can result from the drugs used to treat this condition. Gold deposits in the cornea, posterior subcapsular cataracts caused by prolonged corticosteroid ingestion, and corneal or retinal abnormalities related to chloroquine therapy are most important.

Lymphadenopathy, splenomegaly, and Felty's syndrome. Lymph node enlargement is common in rheumatoid arthritis. Nodes proximal to inflamed joints are most likely to be enlarged, but lymphadenopathy may be present in areas remote from articular inflammation. Palpable splenomegaly occurs in up to 10% of patients with rheumatoid arthritis.

A symptom complex of chronic rheumatoid arthritis associated with splenomegaly and leukopenia is called **Felty's syndrome**. Additional features include skin hyperpigmentation, leg ulcers, lymphadenopathy, anemia, and thrombocytopenia. The leukopenia is, in fact, a selective neutropenia and may be profound. Marrow examination usually reveals moderate hypercellularity with a paucity of mature neutrophils. Hypersplenism has been proposed as one cause of the leukopenia, but splenectomy fails to correct the abnormality in some patients. Recurrent Gram positive infections are common and frequently respond poorly to antibiotics. The incidence of infection can decline after splenectomy, even when the neutropenia remains unaltered (26,44–46).

Laboratory findings

Standard tests. A normocytic, normo- or hypochromic anemia of moderate degree associated with low serum iron and a normal or low iron binding capacity is common in rheumatoid arthritis (47). It is generally recalcitrant to iron therapy. The white blood cell count is usually normal. Eosinophilia may be associated with systemic rheumatoid disease (48). The erythrocyte sedimentation rate (ESR) is diversely elevated in most patients and roughly parallels disease activity. Thus, it is a useful parameter for assessing response to therapy.

Serum protein analysis commonly shows an elevation in the alpha$_2$ fraction, a polyclonal increase in gamma globulin, and a diminution in serum albumin. Liver and renal function tests usually show normal results as does the urinary sediment. Persistent proteinuria may indicate complicating amyloidosis.

Serologic findings. A number of serologic abnormalities are encountered in rheumatoid patients. Five to 10% have false positive tests for syphilis; LE cell tests can be positive, and approximately 25% have serum antinuclear antibodies with a diffuse pattern of nuclear immunofluorescence. Antibodies to native double-stranded DNA (characteristic of lupus erythematosus) are rarely, if ever found. As noted, rheumatoid factor can be demonstrated in approximately 70% of adults with rheumatoid arthritis, but is not specific for this disease.

Synovial fluid. Synovial analysis can be of value in establishing the diagnosis of rheumatoid arthritis, although no one finding is specific. Characteristically, the fluid is an exudate. The increased cellular and proteinacious elements render the normally clear yellow synovial fluid turbid in appearance. Depolymerization or dilution of joint fluid hyaluronate reduces its viscosity and probably accounts for the formation of a loose, friable clot on the addition of dilute acetic acid (**the mucin clot test**). The protein content, normally less than 2 gm %, often exceeds 3.5 gm %. Fibrin, absent from normal synovial fluid, is present and may cause the fluid to clot.

Hemolytic complement levels are reduced to less than one-third of the serum values in the vast majority of patients with seropositive disease; C4 and C2 levels are most profoundly depressed. Seronegative fluids tend to have complement reduction of a lesser magnitude. Glucose levels may be low or normal (49).

White blood cell counts usually range from 5,000 to 20,000 mm^3, although values in excess of 50,000 mm^3 are encountered. About two-thirds of the cells are polymorphonuclear in most cases, although mononuclear cells can predominate, especially early in the disease. Unstained wet preparations frequently reveal leukocytes with small intracytoplasmic granules, the so-called RA cells that are characteristic of but not specific for rheumatoid arthritis.

Synovial biopsy. Rheumatoid arthritis appears histologically as a hyperplastic inflammatory synovitis with a constellation of abnormalities that are characteristic, but not pathognomonic for the disease. These include edema and congestion, mononuclear cell infiltration, lining cell proliferation, fibrin deposition, and necrosis. Individual specimens vary greatly depending on the phase of the disease and the site within the articular cavity from which they are obtained.

Radiology

The roentgenographic features of rheumatoid arthritis are detailed in Section 85. None are diagnostic, but the finding of symmetry in well-established disease and the predilection for joint erosions in certain anatomic sites, notably the MCP and PIP joints of the hands, the wrists, and MTP joints of the feet (Fig 12–11), help to differentiate rheumatoid arthritis from degenerative joint disease and other inflammatory arthritides. So, too, is the relative lack of bone formation in the presence of advanced joint destruction.

Course and prognosis

The course that rheumatoid arthritis will follow in a given patient cannot be predicted at the disease onset. Some patients show an unrelenting progression to deformities and occasionally, even death. Alternatively, brief episodes of acute arthritis may be interspersed with longer periods of low grade activity or complete

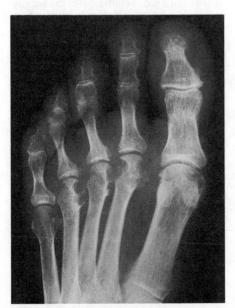

Fig 12–11. Roentgenogram of left foot of a 55-year-old woman with rheumatoid arthritis of 6 months' duration. Note erosion of heads of second, third, and fourth metatarsal bones.

remission. Most commonly, the disease is intermittent at first and becomes more sustained with the passage of time. In any longitudinal study more patients are found to be doing poorly as time goes by, regardless of therapy (1,23,50,51).

Classification. The functional capacity of rheumatoid patients can be roughly divided as follows: remission or ability to perform normal activities (Class I); moderate restriction, adequate for normal activities (Class II); marked restriction, inability to perform most duties of usual occupation or self care (Class III); incapacitation, or confinement to bed or a wheelchair (Class IV).

Studies of the natural history of the disease reveal that after 10–15 years few patients will be in remission, but the majority will be functional (1,23). A good approximation would be Class I—15%, Class II—40%, Class III—30%, and Class IV—15%. Spontaneous remission, when it occurs, usually comes in the first 2 years. Appreciation of this fact is important for determining therapy and evaluating claims of benefits for early treatment of rheumatoid arthritis.

Sustained disease, a long duration of active disease before the initial examination, and the presence of nodules are all unfavorable indices. Men may do slightly better than women, and an abrupt onset with weight loss and fever may portend a better outcome. The amount of rheumatoid factor in the serum is also a significant factor (23,50–53).

Patients rarely die of rheumatoid arthritis, although systemic vasculitis and atlantoaxial subluxation can be responsible. Rheumatoid patients usually succumb to the same diseases as their cohorts, but with a greater frequency (54,55).

Diagnosis

Like most diseases, rheumatoid arthritis is easily diagnosed in its advanced and characteristic form. Early in the course the diagnosis is often obscured, especially when articular manifestations are preceded only by constitutional symptoms such as fatigue, neurasthenia, low grade fever, and morning stiffness. Considerable diagnostic confusion also results when the initial joint disease is spotty or monarticular.

As time passes, the disease assumes its typical form as a bilateral, symmetrical polyarthritis of small and large joints in both the upper and lower extremities. The axial skelton with the exception of the cervical spine is usually spared. The demonstration of subcutaneous or subperiosteal nodules is important confirmatory evidence.

Additional findings that substantiate the diagnosis include positive tests for rheumatoid factor, exudative synovial fluid showing polymorphonuclear leukocytosis

and depressed complement values, and radiographic findings of bone demineralization and erosions around the affected joints. In the majority of patients, the disease has assumed its more characteristic clinical features by the end of 1–2 years. The persistence of articular symptoms without the presence of radiologic joint abnormalties is unusual after this time.

The American Rheumatism Association criteria for the diagnosis of rheumatoid arthritis are outlined in Appendix 2. Any combination of 7 or more of this group of symptoms, signs, and laboratory findings in a patient whose disease has been continuous for at least 6 weeks is designated as classic rheumatoid arthritis. A diagnosis of definite rheumatoid arthritis requires 5 of the criteria.

It should be understood, however, that these criteria were not developed for the bedside diagnosis of rheumatoid arthritis but rather to classify large groups of patients for inclusion in epidemiologic surveys, drug trials, and studies of the natural history of the disease. Therefore, failure to meet an arbitrary set of criteria need not preclude the diagnosis of rheumatoid arthritis, especially in its early stages.

1. Short CL, Bauer W, Reynolds WS: Rheumatoid Arthritis. Cambridge, Harvard University Press, 1957
2. O'Sullivan JB, Cathcart ES: The prevalence of rheumatoid arthritis. Ann Intern Med 76:573–577, 1972
3. Kellgren HJ: Epidemiology of rheumatoid arthritis, Rheumatic Diseases. JJR Dutker, WRM Alexander, eds. Baltimore, Williams & Wilkins, 1968
4. Stastny P: Immunogenetic factors in rheumatoid arthritis. Clin Rheum Dis 3:315–332, 1977
5. Torrigiani G, Roitt IM: Antiglobulin factors in sera from patients with rheumatoid arthritis and normal subjects. Ann Rheum Dis 26:334–340, 1967
6. Stage DE, Mannik M: Rheumatoid factors in rheumatoid arthritis. Bull Rheum Dis 23:720–725, 1973
7. Schmid FR, et al: Arteritis in rheumatoid arthritis. Am J Med 30:56–83, 1961
8. Hart FD: Rheumatoid arthritis: extraarticular manifestations. Br Med J 3:131–136, 1969
9. Kunkel HG, Tan EM: Autoantibodies and disease. Adv Immunol 4:351–395, 1964
10. Greenberg PD, Zvaifler NJ: Rheumatoid arthritis, Mechanisms of Immunopathology. S Cohen, R McCluskey, P Ward, eds. New York, John Wiley & Sons, 1979
11. Kulka JP, Bocking D, Ropes MW, et al: Early joint lesions of rheumatoid arthritis. Arch Pathol 59:129–150, 1955
12. Schumacher HR: Synovial membrane and fluid morphologic alterations in early rheumatoid arthritis: microvascular injury and virus-like particles. Ann NY Acad Sci 256:39–64, 1975
13. Ishikawa H, Ziff M: Electron microscopic observations of immunoreactive cells in the rheumatoid synovial membrane. Arthritis Rheum 19:1–14, 1976
14. Natvig JB, Munthe E: Self-associating IgG rheumatoid factor represents a major response of plasma cells in rheumatoid inflammatory tissue. Ann NY Acad Sci 256:88–95, 1975
15. Zvaifler NJ: Immunopathology of joint inflammation in rheumatoid arthritis. Adv Immunol 16:265–336, 1973
16. Weissman G: Lysosomal mechanisms of tissue injury in arthritis. N Engl J Med 286:141–147, 1972
17. Pearson CM, Paulus HE, Machleder HI: The role of the lymphocyte and its products in the propagation of joint disease. Ann NY Acad Sci 256:150–168, 1975

18. Harris ED Jr, et al: Effects of proteolytic enzymes on structural and mechanical properties of cartilage. Arthritis Rheum 15:497–503, 1972

19. Kobayashi I, Ziff M: Electron microscopic studies of the cartilage-pannus junction in rheumatoid arthritis. Arthritis Rheum 18:475–483, 1975

20. Harris ED, Glauert AM, Merrley AH: Intracellular collagen fibers at the pannus-cartilage junction in rheumatoid arthritis. Arthritis Rheum 20:657–665, 1977

21. Krane SM: Aspects of the cell biology of the rheumatoid synovial lesion. Ann Rheum Dis 40:433–448, 1981

22. Werb Z, et al: Endogenous activation of latent collagenase by rheumatoid synovial cells: evidence for a role of plasminogen activator. N Engl J Med 296:1017–1023, 1977

23. Duthie JJR, et al: Course and prognosis in rheumatoid arthritis. Ann Rheum Dis 23:193–204, 1964

24. Hollingsworth JW: Local and Systemic Complications of Rheumatoid Arthritis. Philadelphia, WB Saunders, 1968

25. Gordon DA, Stein JL, Broder I: The extraarticular features of rheumatoid arthritis: a systematic analysis of 127 cases. Am J Med 54:445–452, 1973

26. Hurd ER: Extraarticular manifestations of rheumatoid arthritis. Semin Arthritis Rheum 8:151–176, 1979

27. Mongan EL, et al: A study of the relation of seronegative and seropositive rheumatoid arthritis to each other and to necrotizing vasculitis. Am J Med 47:23–35, 1969

28. Lambert PH, Casali P: Immune complexes and the rheumatic diseases. Clin Rheum Dis 4:617–642, 1978

29. Conn DL, McDuffie FC, Dyck PJ: Immunopathology of sural nerves in rheumatoid arthritis. Arthritis Rheum 15:135–143, 1972

30. Pallis CA, Scott JT: Peripheral neuropathy in rheumatoid arthritis. Br Med J 1:1141–1147, 1965

31. Chamberlain MA, Bruckner FE: Rheumatoid neuropathy: clinical and electrophysiological features. Ann Rheum Dis 29:609–616, 1970

32. MacDonald WJ, et al: Echocardiographic assessment of cardiac structure and function in patients with rheumatoid arthritis. Am J Med 63:890–896, 1977

33. Weintraub AM, Zvaifer: NJ: The occurrence of valvular and myocardial disease in patients with rheumatoid arthritis. Am J Med 35:145–162, 1963

34. Franco AE, Levine HD, Hall AP: Rheumatoid pericarditis. Ann Intern Med 77:837–844, 1972

35. Kirk J, Cosh J: The pericarditis of rheumatoid arthritis. Q J Med 38:397–423, 1969

36. Thadani W, Iveson JMI, Wright V: Cardiac tamponade, constructive pericarditis and pericardial resection in rheumatoid arthritis. Medicine 54:261–270, 1975

37. Hunder GG, McDuffie FC, Hepper NGG: Pleural fluid complement in systemic lupus erythematosus and rheumatoid arthritis. Ann Intern Med 76:357–363, 1972

38. Walker WC, Wright V: Pulmonary lesions and rheumatoid arthritis. Medicine 47:501–520, 1968

39. Martel W, et al: Pulmonary and pleural lesions in rheumatoid disease. Radiology 90:641–653, 1968

40. Caplan A: Certain unusual radiological appearances in the chest of coal miners suffering from rheumatoid arthritis. Thorax 8:29–37, 1953

41. Bégin, Massé S, Cantin A, et al: Airway disease in a subset of nonsmoking rheumatoid patients. Am J Med 72:743–750, 1982

42. University of California, San Francisco, Medical Staff Conference: Ocular complications of rheumatic diseases. Calif J Med 118:17–22, May, 1973

43. Jayson MIV, Jones DEP: Scleritis and rheumatoid arthritis. Ann Rheum Dis 30:343–347, 1971

44. Barnes CG, Turnbull AL, Vernon-Roberts B: Felty's syndrome: a clinical and pathological survey of 21 patients and their response to treatment. Ann Rheum Dis 30:359–374, 1971

45. Spivak JL: Felty's syndrome: an analytic review. Johns Hopkins Med J 141:156–162, 1977

46. Moore RA, et al: Felty's syndrome: long term followup after splenectomy. Ann Intern Med 75:381–385, 1971

47. Mowat AG: Hematologic abnormalities. Semin Arthritis Rheum 1:195–219, 1971

48. Panush RS, Franco AE, Schur PH: Rheumatoid arthritis associated with eosinophilia. Ann Intern Med 75:199–205, 1971

49. Cohen AJ, Brandt KD, Krey PB: Synovial fluid, Laboratory Diagnostic Procedures in the Rheumatic Diseases. Ed 2. AS Cohen, ed. Boston, Little, Brown, 1975

50. Ragan C, Farrington E: The clinical features of rheumatoid arthritis. JAMA 181:664–667, 1962

51. Sharp JT, et al: Observations on the clinical, chemical and serologic manifestations of rheumatoid arthritis, based on the course of 154 cases. Medicine 43:41–58, 1964

52. Fleming A, Crown JM, Corbett M: Prognostic value of early features in rheumatoid disease. Br Med J 1:1243–1245, 1976

53. Masi AT, et al: Prospective study of the early course of rheumatoid arthritis in young adults: comparison of patients with and without rheumatoid factor positivity at entry and identification of variables correlating with outcome. Semin Arthritis Rheum 5:299–326, 1976

54. Monson RR, Hall AP: Mortality among arthritics. J Chron Dis 29:459–467, 1976

55. Isomaki HA, Mutree O, Koota K: Death rate and cause of death in patients with rheumatoid arthritis. Scand J Rheumatol 4:205–208, 1975

Treatment

A wide range of drugs and procedures are available for the treatment of rheumatoid arthritis and by utilizing these and the facilities now available to help the person with arthritis, deformity can be minimized and the majority of patients can continue a comfortable, productive life.

General approach. The physician must recognize that RA is a systemic disease with irregular onset, course, and outcome. It is particularly important to remember the various courses that the disease may manifest. Physicians and allied health professionals are responsible as soon as the diagnosis has been confirmed for educating the patient and family and providing hope and motivation for their participation in the management of the disease.

The main objectives of management are 1) relief of pain, 2) reduction or suppression of inflammation, 3) minimizing undesirable side effects, 4) preservation of muscle and joint function, 5) return to a desirable and productive life, if possible.

The physician, knowing the divergent courses of the disease, must also make an assessment of the disease status and the patient's functional classification. This can be achieved by using the American Rheumatism Association classification of progression and functional capacity (see Appendix 3). It is also helpful to use criteria of disease activity such as those by the Cooperating Clinics Committee of the American Rheumatism Association (Table 12–2). The patient's own assessment can also be used as a guide, particularly as the physician gets to know the patient better.

It must be stressed that rheumatoid arthritis requires a management plan for all aspects of a patient's life. Using the suggested guidelines to characterize the patient's disease, assimilating the information on the patient's home and work environment, incorporating the patient's goals, the physician then chooses a management plan tailored to the patient.

The so-called pyramid approach provides a helpful guide for the management plan (Table 12–3). A hopeful environment, the utilization of the basic principles of systemic and local rest, good nutrition, family counseling including sex and marital help, availability of social services, incorporation of physical and occupational therapy, and judicious orthopedic consultation are the essentials for any management program. The physician selects appropriate drugs to help control the disease. The ARA Uniform Database and its many modules can provide an easy way to follow the many faceted long-term course of the RA patient (See Appendix 10).

Drug therapy. There is general agreement that every new rheumatoid arthritis patient is started on **aspirin** unless contraindicated. This is still the most tried, effective, and cheapest drug available. It is essential that sufficient drug be given to achieve a clinical response. A serum salicylate level of 23–30 mg/dl is sought. To achieve this, between 3–6 gm per day is usually required. Smaller doses are mainly analgesic and have lesser antiinflammatory effect. Adult patients can be started on three 0.3 gm aspirin tablets 4 times per day. Aspirin dosage can be increased every 5 days to a level producing tinnitus and then reduced a few tablets below this level.

Care must be exercised, particularly in elderly patients who may have preexisting hearing loss (1). Frequent clinical monitor-

Table 12–2. Criteria of disease activity*

	Least disease activity	Median disease activity	Most disease activity
No. of hours of morning stiffness	0	1.5	>5
No. of painful joints	<2	12	>34
No. of swollen joints	0	7	>23
Grip strength			
male—mm Hg	>250	140	>55
female—mm Hg	>180	100	<45
No. of seconds to walk 50 feet	<9	13	>27
Erythrocyte sedimentation rate	<11	41	>92

* Based on a study of 499 patients.

Table 12–3. Treatment pyramid for rheumatoid arthritis

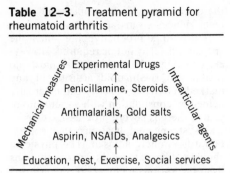

ing, constant "selling" of the drug to the patient, and occasional measurement of plasma salicylate concentrations with appropriate dose adjustments may be necessary to obtain a nontoxic therapeutic level.

Gastrointestinal upsets may occur but can be overcome by taking the aspirin with meals and/or a mild antacid. Buffered as well as enteric coated aspirin are available, though the latter are sometimes not fully absorbed. Other salicylate preparations are available that may have fewer gastrointestinal effects but also may not be as effective as aspirin (2). Some nonacetyl salicylates have been shown to be effective taken only twice a day (3).

Gastrointestinal bleeding, usually occult, is common with aspirin treatment, possibly from mucosal injury or effects on hemostasis or both (4). Usually the amount of blood loss is not related to dyspepsia, previous hemorrhage, or peptic ulcer. Overt gastrointestinal tract hemorrhage is rare.

Intrinsic defects in platelets or other plasma factors involved in platelet aggregation may occur when a person is taking aspirin (5). There may be liver function abnormalities, first reflected by elevated transaminase level along with abnormalities of alkaline phosphatase, bilirubin, and prothrombin (6). These changes are more common in systemic lupus erythematosus and juvenile arthritis (7). The vast majority of patients, given appropriate support, should be able to take therapeutic doses. When aspirin cannot be given or an adequate trial does not provide therapeutic benefit, the physician moves to the next step on the pyramid.

Until recently, only 2 other nonsteroidal antiinflammatory drugs were available, indomethacin and phenylbutazone. **Indomethacin** is an effective analgesic, antipyretic, and antiinflammatory drug and can be a useful drug for some patients. The side effects include gastrointestinal problems and central nervous system symptoms with headache, vertigo, dizziness, and mild confusion occurring very early. Such symptoms usually subside after a few days. The patient must be cautioned about these. The drug is frequently used for long periods in osteoarthritis and can also, when effective, be so used in RA.

Phenylbutazone is used more often today for short-term management of acute episodes, acute bursitis, and other soft tissue symptoms. Its potential side effects usually preclude long-term therapy.

There are now 9 **nonsteroidal antiinflammatory drugs** (NSAIDs) available in the United States and a number of others in Europe and other parts of the world. They include derivatives of phenylacetic acids (*ibuprofen, fenoprofen*), napthalene-acetic acids (*naproxen*), pyrrolealkanoic acid (*tolmetin*), indoleacetic acids (*sulindac*), and a halogenated anthranilic acid (*meclofenamate sodium*). The most recent NSAIDs are *piroxicam, zomepirac,* and *diflunisal*. Piroxicam is a member of the oxicams class which have extended plasma half-lives. The structural formulas of these drugs are given in Appendix 9.

The NSAIDs are beneficial in many patients with RA. Generally, experience has shown that they are no more effective than aspirin in most patients but may be better tolerated. Some patients respond better to one of these drugs than to aspirin.

Most physicians caring for rheumatoid patients realize that a single drug does not help all patients. There is a wide range of individual variation and some who have little response to one drug may respond very well to another. This holds for both the effectiveness and side effects of these drugs. The incidence of gastrointestinal effects is relatively low with ibuprofen; however, bleeding ulcers have been reported. Fenoprofen, naproxen, and tolmetin probably cause fewer gastrointestinal tract and platelet abnormalities than aspirin, though all have an effect on platelet function to some degree (8).

Experience with the recently released NSAIDs is not yet extensive enough to draw conclusions. However, renal effects may occur with all the NSAIDs and the drugs should be given with caution in those with compromised renal function and in the elderly.

There is no proof that the NSAIDs' effect is additive when given together or with aspirin (9). The many drug interactions involving anti-rheumatic agents should be taken into account when prescribing for rheumatoid arthritis patients (10). These agents should be given for a minimum of 3 weeks and dosage levels cautiously increased before effectiveness is ascertained. Unfortunately, bioassays are not yet available to determine effective drug levels. If 1 NSAID fails, it is appropriate to try 1 or 2 more in sequence.

If these agents fail to control the disease, one should consider the slow acting drugs which include gold, antimalarials, and penicillamine. These are given in addition to aspirin or an NSAID. Although the **antimalarials** are used infrequently today, they may benefit some RA patients. The drug usually given is *hydroxychloroquine*

200 mg once to twice daily. This drug and chloroquine may cause retinal lesions with loss of vision, and patients should therefore have baseline and six monthly opthalmologic examinations. If benefit is not noted within 3-4 months, the drug is discontinued.

Gold salts are widely used because they can suppress joint inflammation and have been reported to favorably alter the natural history of rheumatoid arthritis (11). Disadvantages include the necessity for injections, with urine and blood checks and an office visit resulting in considerable cost. Advantages include the knowledge the patient is getting the appropriate therapy and the use of the clinic or office visit for continued education and assessment of the patient. Gold appears to work best in those who have reasonably early, active disease and who are seropositive and male.

The standard treatment schedule consists of 10 mg injection the first week, 25 mg the second week, and then 50 mg weekly. Before each injection side effects are checked for and complete blood count and urinalysis, at least for protein, obtained. At about 1 gm total or earlier if response is dramatic, the dose can be reduced to alternate weeks, and subsequently to every third or fourth week. There is no specific time limit to a gold therapy course and a large number of patients have been and are now on gold therapy for prolonged time periods.

Side effects are fairly common with gold; probably about 30% of patients have treatment discontinued because of troublesome side effects. The commonest are the various pruritic skin rashes. Others include rather painful mouth ulcers, transient leukopenia, and eosinophilia. Injections should be stopped, at least temporarily, if these reactions occur. With minor skin rashes, the drug can be restarted after a period of discontinuation but at a lower dose and with careful observation; very often the rash will not recur. Continuation of the drug while a rash exists could lead to an exfoliative dermatitis.

Hematologic changes also include thrombocytopenia, pancytopenia, granulocytosis, and aplastic anemia. Fortunately, these are very rare but may occur without warning, sometimes with pharyngitis and fever. Should agranulocytosis occur, the drug is stopped and steroids are commenced. If there is not a prompt response, a gold chelating agent such as dimercaprol should be considered. Aplastic anemia is an extremely rare complication that may occur any time or even after treatment has been discontinued.

Transient proteinuria is a fairly common problem (3–10%). Nephrotic syndrome is very uncommon; its prognosis is favorable since the majority of patients recover. Renal biopsies have shown that the predominant lesion is a membranous glomerulonephritis with deposition of IgG, IgM, and complement (12). Steroid treatment may be needed. Minor degrees of proteinuria and hematuria, which may be noted early in the course of treatment, require only interruption of therapy until the urine is again normal.

Oral gold agents have been extensively studied in Europe, but experience is more limited in the United States. They appear to be effective and could prove to be a major therapeutic help.

Penicillamine is now available throughout the world for the treatment of rheumatoid arthritis (13). It should be used in those with serious active disease which has proved refractory to conventional anti-rheumatic therapy. Whether penicillamine, gold, or other drugs of this class may eventually be the first choice is not yet clear. Usage in Europe suggests that penicillamine may be an alternative to gold, particularly if there are medical or economic contraindications to that drug.

Another third-line drug in the management of rheumatoid arthritis is **corticosteroid**. Extensive experience over the years has reduced the role of steroids in this disease since they are not curative and do not prevent progressive joint destruction. There certainly are initial beneficial effects, mostly relief of symptoms, but these are usually not maintained. If used in management for occasional socioeconomic reasons or because of failure of the first and second line drugs, the initial dose should be low, usually 10 mg or less daily of a prednisone equivalent. A once daily morning dose may be effective if therapy is started in this fashion. Experience has shown that alternate day dosage is not well tolerated in RA.

The side effects of corticosteroids are too well known to repeat here. Their incidence has not diminished over the years and the physician should be fully aware of the long-term problems when deciding to start treatment with these agents.

Corticosteroids may be necessary in the treatment of severe unremitting disease with fever, anemia, weight loss, neuropathy, vasculitis, pericarditis, pleuritis, scleritis, and Felty's syndrome. Intraarticular steroids are very useful adjuncts to both basic and advanced therapy programs when only a few joints are affected and temporary relief of pain and inflammation is desired. There are a number of both short and long acting synthetic steroids available for intraarticular injection and all appear to be effective (14). It is a wise procedure always to aspirate fluid from a joint to make certain that the "flare" is not an infection that can occur in rheumatoid arthritis (15).

Other drugs that may be disease modifiers include azathioprine, cyclophosphamide, chlorambucil, methotrexate, and levamisole. Of these, only **azathioprine** has been given FDA approval for the treatment of rheumatoid arthritis. In practice, it provides an antiinflammatory effect and modest control of symptoms. Published studies on these drugs suggest they may help in the management of individual problem patients. It is recommended that patients be given complete information about these drugs and enter into the treatment choice with their physician. See also Section 92.

There are also a number of experimental procedures for the treatment of the severe or drug resistant patient. These include plasmapheresis, leukapheresis, lymphapheresis, thoracic duct drainage, and total body irradiation (16,17). These procedures require special facilities or hospitalization in special centers and their long-term effects are unknown at this time.

Physical measures. Appropriate and skilled therapy can provide notable benefit for the RA patient (see Section 95). As soon as the active, painful phase has been controlled, a muscle evaluation, muscle building, and joint protection program should be started.

Advantage should be taken of hospitalizations to obtain the therapist's aid. Frequently, the patient and family can be taught the various physical therapy modalities and subsequently only supervisory evaluations will be required.

During visits, the physician should include an assessment of joint and muscle function as part of the examination. The encouragement of use of appropriate appliances such as canes and walkers is also the physician's responsibility. Other modalities such as a Hubbard tank, if available, may also be helpful. Swimming in a warm pool for limited time periods is an excellent overall exercise for arthritis patients and they should be encouraged to do their exercise program in this setting.

Orthopedic surgery can be preventative or reparative. The physician should be on the lookout for soft tissue damage and refer a patient for orthopedic evaluation as soon as possible. Corrective surgery has much to offer and deformities require orthopedic evaluation (see Section 94).

Consultation. In many communities, the physician has available knowledgable rheumatologists, orthopedists trained in arthritis surgery, physiatrists with rehabilitation skills, physical and occupational therapists, arthritis nurse specialists, and many other health professionals experienced in arthritis care. If a correct diagnosis of rheumatoid arthritis has been made,

the disease stage is favorable, and treatment induces a satisfactory response with a return to a productive life, then the special skills may not be required. However, experience has shown that most patients with rheumatoid arthritis of any marked activity or severity can be greatly helped by consultation with a rheumatologist. If there is severe progressive disease with systemic complications, such consultation is strongly advised. The physician should not hesitate to obtain consultations from the various members of the arthritis care team. The Arthritis Foundation through its local chapters can provide information about facilities available for the care of the arthritis patient and can provide helpful literature for physician and patient. Education clubs for patients and their families can be a valuable adjunct to therapy.

1. Morgan E, Kelly P, Nies K, et al: Tinnitus as an indication of therapeutic salicylate levels. JAMA 226:142, 1973

2. Smyth CJ, Bravo JF: Antirheumatic drugs. Drugs 10:394–425, 1975

3. Giuliano V, Scharff EV: Clinical comparison of two salicylates in rheumatoid arthritis patients on maintenance gold therapy. Current Therap Res 28:61–71, 1980

4. Davenport HW: Salicylate damage to the gastric mucosal barrier. N Engl J Med 276:1307–1312, 1967

5. Mills DG, Boda IT, Philip RB, et al: Effects of in vitro aspirin on blood platelets of gastrointestinal bleeders. Clin Pharmacol Therap 15:187–192, 1974

6. Seaman WE, Plotz PH: Effect of aspirin on liver tests in patients with RA or SLE and in normal volunteers. Arthritis Rheum 19:155–160, 1976

7. Rich PR, Johnson JS: Salicylate hepatotoxicity in patients with juvenile rheumatoid arthritis. Arthritis Rheum 16:1–9, 1973

8. Lewis JR: New antirheumatic agents. JAMA 237:1260–1261, 1977

9. Willkins RF, Segre EJ: Combination therapy with naproxen and aspirin in rheumatoid arthritis. Arthritis Rheum 19:677–682, 1976

10. Buckingham RB: Interactions involving antirheumatic agents. Bull Rheum Dis 28:960–965, 1977–78

11. Sigler JW, Bluhm GB, Duncan H, et al: Gold salts in the treatment of rheumatoid arthritis: a double-blind study. Ann Intern Med 80:21–26, 1974

12. Tornroth T, Skrifvars B: Gold nephropathy; prototype of membranous glomerulonephritis. Am J Pathol 75:573–584, 1974

13. Kean WF, Dwosh IL, Anastassiades TP, Ford PM, Kelly HG: The toxicity pattern of D-penicillamine therapy: a guide to its use in rheumatoid arthritis. Arthritis Rheum 23:158–164, 1980

14. Bird HA, Ring EFJ, Bacon PA: A thermographic and clinical comparison of three intraarticular steroid preparations in rheumatoid arthritis. Ann Rheum Dis 38:36–39, 1979

15. Russell AS, Ansell BM: Septic arthritis. Ann Rheum Dis 31:40–44, 1972

16. Tenenbaum J, Urowitz MB, Keystone EC, et al: Leucapheresis in severe rheumatoid arthritis. Ann Rheum Dis 38:40–44, 1979

17. Kotzin BL, Strober S, Engleman EG et al: Treatment of intractible rheumatoid arthritis with total lymphoid irradiation. N Engl J Med 30S:969–976, 1981

13. Systemic lupus erythematosus

Systemic lupus erythematosus (SLE) is a chronic inflammatory disease of unknown origin which may affect many different organs (1,2). The clinical manifestations of this disease, which are remarkably diverse, include fever, an erythematous rash, polyarthralgia and arthritis, polyserositis (especially pleurisy and pericarditis), anemia, thrombocytopenia, and renal, neurologic, and cardiac abnormalities.

The disease was named after a form of facial rash (Fig 13-1) that occurs in some cases and was originally considered akin to cutaneous tuberculosis (lupus vulgaris). The term *lupus* is derived from the erosive nature of the condition, which was likened to the damage wrought by a hungry wolf.

SLE has a strong predilection for women, especially adolescents and young adults, who are affected about 8 times as often as men. A retrospective analysis of members of the San Francisco Kaiser Permanente Health Plan covering 1965–1973 revealed an annual incidence of 7.6 cases per 100,000, a figure similar to the 6.4 cases per 100,000 reported for Rochester, Minnesota (3,4). The prevalence rates were also similar: 1 case in 1,960 for San Francisco and 1 case in 2,400 for Rochester. The prevalence rate for women between the ages of 15 and 64 is 1 per 700. The disease affects members of all races, and in the United States the prevalence rate for black females is nearly 3 times that for white females.

SLE can be fulminating and rapidly fatal but this has now become an unusual occurrence, and in most cases the disease pursues a chronic irregular course in which episodes of disease activity are interspersed with long periods of complete or near-complete remission. Although SLE may exist in the form of a mild disorder, some patients eventually die as a result of vascular lesions affecting the kidneys, central nervous sytem, or other vital organs; others die of complicating secondary infections.

Pathology

In patients dying in the early stages of fulminating lupus (a rarity nowadays), there may be few, if any, histologic lesions found on ordinary microscopic examination. As a rule, however, there are alterations in the connective tissue of various organs. Among the most characteristic findings is the presence of "hematoxylin bodies," which consist of homogeneous globular masses of nuclear material that stain bluish-purple with hematoxylin and are morphologically and histochemically identical to the inclusion body of the LE cell (Fig 13–2). Other early pathologic features include a variably severe vasculitis marked by cellular infiltration of small arteries; portions of the arterial walls may become necrotic and can contain fibrinoid deposits.

It should be emphasized that the term *fibrinoid* is purely a descriptive device that indicates that staining of a given material with various dyes, e.g., eosin reveals tinctorial properties similar to those of fibrin. As such, fibrinoid has been found to vary in composition in different conditions. In SLE these deposits have been found to contain immune complexes consisting in part of DNA, anti-DNA (IgG), and complement components. In the spleen these vascular lesions take the form of concentric periarterial fibrosis of the penicillary vessels (*onion-skin* lesion) (Fig 13–3).

Lymph nodes in SLE patients with clinical evidence of active disease may show nonspecific changes consisting of follicular hyperplasia occasionally associated with areas of necrosis. In a few instances, these changes resemble giant follicular lymphoma.

Changes in the brain are either minimal or consist of focal perivascular infiltrates or microhemorrhages. Correlation of the clinical manifestations of organic brain disease with the pathologic findings is imperfect (5). The thymus shows a variable degree of atrophy and contains plasma cells and, occasionally, germinal centers. Examination of the synovium in patients with arthritis reveals a synovitis that tends to be less severe than that encountered in rheumatoid arthritis. Pannus and erosion of bone and cartilage occur rarely. Muscle biopsy usually reveals a nonspecific perivascular mononuclear infiltrate, but polymyositis with muscle necrosis can occur.

Verrucous endocarditis is present in nearly all autopsied patients. The lesions are usually microscopic, but the typical macroscopic vegetations are observed in nearly half of patients at autopsy (Fig 13–4). Typical verrucous endocarditis is a pathologic diagnosis and does not correlate with the presence of cardiac murmur. The verrucae are usually present near the edge of the valve and occur less commonly on the chordae tendinae, papillary muscles, and the mural endocardium. Mitral valve injury due to severe scarring of the leaflet and ruptured chordae tendinae is a rare occurrence. Superimposed subacute bacterial endocarditis occasionally occurs. Death from myocardial infarctions due to coronary atherosclerosis may occur late in the course of steroid treated patients.

The histologic appearance of skin lesions varies greatly. Vasculitis and leukocytoclastic angiitis may be present in skin lesions that are purpuric or hive-like. Perivascular infiltrates of lymphocytes in the upper dermis may be the only abnormalities noted in macular papular skin lesions.

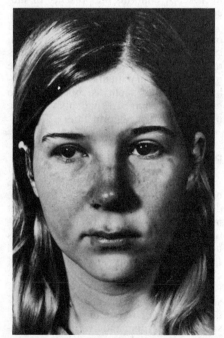

Fig 13–1. Face of a 19-year-old girl with acute systemic lupus erythematosus. Note the classic butterfly eruption over the bridge of the nose and the malar regions.

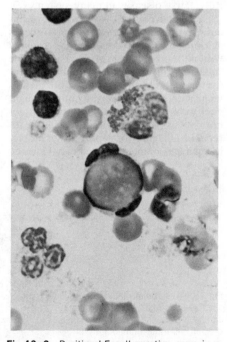

Fig 13–2. Positive LE cell reaction seen in a peripheral blood preparation obtained from a woman with procainamide-induced lupus-like syndrome.

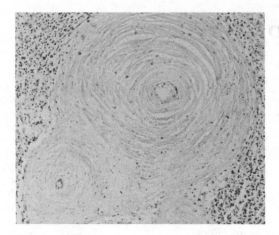

Fig 13–3. Periarterial fibrosis of the spleen in systemic lupus erythematosus. Concentric onion skin laminations of collagen surround 2 central arterioles in the spleen. A thin outer rim of lymphocytes is all that remains of the malpighian body (H&E, medium power). (From the Revised Clinical Slide Collection on the Rheumatic Diseases)

Lesions typical of chronic discoid lupus are present in 15% of SLE patients and have the typical characteristics of hyperkeratosis, follicular plugging, loss of dermal appendages, and widening and degeneration of the basal layer of the epithelium (Fig 13–5). The area between the dermis and epidermis is widened and homogenous. Deposits of immunoglobulins and complement proteins are usually found in this area (dermoepidermal junction) of the skin lesions.

In lesions of vasculitis, additional deposits of immunoglobulins and complement proteins are noted in the dermal capillaries and small vessels. The membrane attack complex of complement is specifically localized to lesional skin (6). Nonlesional skin, which is clinically and histologically normal, may contain IgG and C3 deposits in the dermoepidermal junction, especially in patients with clinically active diseases in many systems (7).

Nearly all patients with SLE have immunopathologic or electron microscopic abnormalities in their kidneys (8). Patients without urinary abnormalities may have small deposits of immunoglobulins or electron-dense deposits located in the mesangium without any changes noted by light microscopy. In patients with urinary abnormalities with or without evidence of renal insufficiency or nephrotic syndrome, the changes in the glomeruli may be noted by appropriate histologic study using light microscopy.

Four main types of lupus nephritis have been identified histologically (9):

1. **Mesangial (minimal) lupus nephritis** is characterized by glomeruli which appear normal or merely show a slight irregular increase in mesangial cells and matrix. The diagnosis depends on the demonstration of IgG and C3 in the mesangium and occasionally along the capillary walls. Electron dense deposits may be noted in the mesangium.

2. **Focal (mild) lupus nephritis** is characterized by segmental proliferation of some glomerular tufts while others appear normal (Fig 13–6). Mesangial proliferation may be present in some glomeruli. Immunofluorescence reveals immunoglobulins and C3 in the mesangium of all glomeruli with fine granules along the capillary loops which are scattered and not evenly distributed (Fig 13–7). Electron dense deposits are noted in the mesangium and scattered deposits may be found in the subendothelial, subepithelial, and intrabasement membrane areas (Fig 13–8).

3. **Diffuse (severe) proliferative lupus nephritis** is characterized by abnormalities of more than 50% of the total area of the glomerular tufts. Although the proliferation is irregular, all glomeruli are involved and usually most of each glomerulus is abnormal. Sclerosis may be present (Fig 13–9). The activity of the proliferative lesion may be graded. The following are considered active glomerular lesions: fibrinoid necrosis, endocapillary proliferation, epithelial crescents, nuclear debris, hematoxylin bodies, wire-loops, and hyaline thrombi. Active interstitial lesions include interstitial cell infiltrations and acute tubular epithelial lesions. Necrotizing angiitis is also considered an active lesion.

Chronicity may also be graded, based on the presence of fibrous crescents, periglomerular fibrosis, sclerotic glomeruli, tubular atrophy, and interstitial fibrosis. Renal biopsy scoring systems, based on activity and chronicity of lesions, provide prognostic information (10).

The immunofluorescence findings are usually striking with granules or clumps of immunoglobulins and complement proteins noted along the peripheral capillary wall and in the mesangium. Interstitial deposits and deposits along the tubular basement membrane may also be noted. Electron dense deposits are found in the mesangium, in the subendothelial and subepithelial areas, and within the basement membrane. Deposits are located all over each glomerulus, but are not evenly distributed.

4. **Membranous lupus nephritis** appears to be histologically similar to idiopathic membranous glomerulonephritis. Although no proliferation is noted, slight irregular increases in mesangial cells and matrix may be present. Immunofluorescence is striking and unlike that of the other forms of lupus nephritis. Immunoglobulins protrude on the epithelial side of the peripheral capillary loops and electron microscopy confirms the presence of subepithelial deposits.

Interstitial abnormalities such as focal or diffuse infiltrates of inflammatory cells, tubular damage, and interstitial fibrosis may be noted. These abnormalities are more common in patients with diffuse proliferative lupus nephritis, but have also been described in SLE patients with little or no glomerular abnormalities.

Pathogenesis

Examination of the renal lesions of SLE has revealed amorphous electron-dense deposits within and around the basement membrane, as well as thickening and splitting of this structure (8). These deposits have been found to contain IgG, IgM, and IgA immunoglobulins and proteins of the classical and alternative complement pathways (11,12). Fibrinogen may also be present. Deposits similar to those in the kidney have been found in vessels of the spleen, heart, lung, and liver (13). Perivascular immunoglobulin deposits have not been seen in the brain but have been noted in the choroid plexus (14). Deposits of immunoglobulins and complement pro-

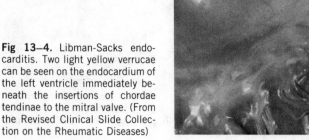

Fig 13–4. Libman-Sacks endocarditis. Two light yellow verrucae can be seen on the endocardium of the left ventricle immediately beneath the insertions of chordae tendinae to the mitral valve. (From the Revised Clinical Slide Collection on the Rheumatic Diseases)

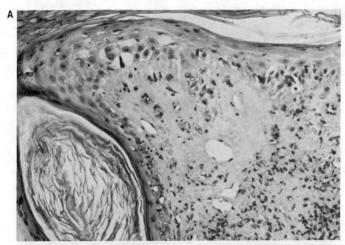

A

B

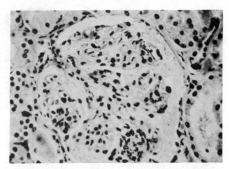

Fig 13–6. Focal glomerulonephritis. In 1 glomerular tuft there is marked hypercellularity and obliteration of capillary lumina; another tuft shows similar but less pronounced changes. The remainder of the glomerulus is normal or minimally altered (H&E, high power). (From the Revised Clinical Slide Collection on the Rheumatic Diseases)

Fig 13–5. A, Dermatitis. The characteristic changes include vacuolar alteration at the dermoepidermal junction, plugging of a hair follicle, and perivascular and perifollicular inflammatory infiltrates including histiocytes, lymphocytes, and plasmacytes. (From the Revised Clinical Slide Collection on the Rheumatic Diseases). **B,** IgG deposition in skin in discoid lupus. The typical fluorescent band is seen at the dermoepidermal junction of this patient with discoid lupus. Granular deposits may be more densely or sparsely packed than those in this example. (From the Revised Clinical Slide Collection on the Rheumatic Diseases)

teins also occur at the dermoepidermal junction in the skin (Fig 13–5B).

The glomerular and other vascular deposits are strikingly similar to those in rabbits which develop glomerulonephritis and other evidence of immune complex disease after the injection of foreign proteins such as bovine serum albumin (15).

The parallel between the findings in this experimental model and the human disease and the occurrence of a wide range of autoantibodies against tissue and nuclear antigens in SLE and the presence of circulating immune complexes in sera from patients with SLE have provided strong support for an immunologic basis of SLE.

Certain of these antibodies, such as antibody to native (double-stranded) DNA, appear and disappear sometimes together with DNA, in close and direct relation to disease activity (16). In the experimental model of immune complex nephritis in rabbits, the injected foreign antigen is present in the glomerulus, and antibody to it can be eluted from this location. The demonstration that the immunoglobulin deposits in the kidneys of patients contain DNA, anti-DNA, and other autoantibodies has further reinforced the concept that SLE is an example of immune complex disease involving autoantibodies (11,15,17).

SLE is, in part, a genetic disease, with prevalence in first-degree relatives of patients with SLE of 1.5% and a concordance for overt SLE in monozygotic twins of approximately 70%. There is a much higher than expected frequency of the major histocompatibility complex alleles DRw2 and DRw3. This genetic relationship is probably of fundamental importance to the basic pathogenetic mechanisms leading to induction of autoantibodies. SLE also is associated with various inherited complement deficiency states, including C2, C1q, C1r, C1s, C4, C5, C8, and C1 esterase inhibitor.

There is increasing evidence that hormones play an important role. Experiments in mice with an SLE-like disease indicate that estrogens potentiate disease expression whereas androgens are protective in this regard. Relative hyperestrogenemia has been identified in both male and female patients with SLE.

The idea that SLE may be due to a defective host response to an exogenous infectious agent (possibly viral) has been discussed for many years. Despite a considerable research effort, there is still no solid evidence for persistent viral infection. For example, all attempts to isolate type C viruses from SLE tissues have been unsuccessful as have studies to demonstrate viral antigen or specific antibody in the circulation using competitive radioimmunoassay procedures.

The most prominent humoral immunologic abnormalities in SLE are hypergammaglobulinemia, the development of multiple autoantibodies, and hypocomplementemia. The hypergammaglobulinemia is associated with B cells in the circulation which spontaneously proliferate and secrete exaggerated amounts of immuno-

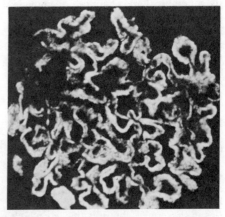

Fig 13–7. IgG deposition in the glomerulus. The basement membrane of the glomerulus is partly outlined by irregular "lumpy and bumpy" deposits of antigen–antibody complex. (From the Revised Clinical Slide Collection on the Rheumatic Diseases)

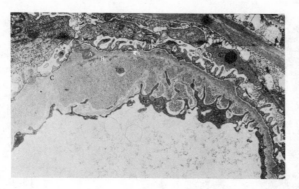

Fig 13—8. This electron micrograph of a glomerular capillary wall of a patient with SLE shows a large granular subendothelial deposit. A few small discrete subepithelial and intramembranous deposits are also seen. The basement membrane itself is lighter gray than the deposits. Some of the epithelial foot processes are broadened ("fused"). (From the Revised Clinical Slide Collection on the Rheumatic Diseases)

globulin. Patients with active SLE generally exhibit cutaneous anergy to antigens such as candida and mumps, and T cells from patients with SLE proliferate poorly in vitro in response to simulation with antigens and mitogens. As a rule, most of these humoral and cellular immunologic abnormalities reverse almost completely during periods of remission.

Although expectations for more complete understanding of the fundamental mechanisms involved here are high, at present concepts are largely speculative. Current thinking is moving away from unifying concepts applicable to all patients with SLE. Indeed, it is likely that SLE is not a single disease, but rather a limited number of closely related but, nevertheless, distinct illnesses with different genetic, immunologic, and pathogenetic bases. For example, patients with SLE and homozygous C2 deficiency are characterized clinically by an unusual rash, absence or low-levels of anti-DNA antibodies, and mild glomerulonephritis. A second SLE subset might be defined serologically by the presence of antibodies to Sm as the sole or dominant autoantibody present, and clinically by indolent, nonprogressive glomerulonephritis.

Although SLE may not be a single disease entity, the patients given this diagnosis generally share a number of immunologic features. T cells are decreased, and there is evidence that certain T cell subsets that regulate the immune response may be particularly involved in this regard. Both circulating immune complexes and anti-lymphocyte autoantibodies have been implicated in the cause of T-cell abnormalities, but an intrinsic T-cell defect has not been excluded.

Considerable information has come from study of New Zealand and other strains of mice that develop an illness both clnically and serologically similar to human SLE. There is evidence for a variety of different immunoregulatory abnormalities in these mice, but it is unclear which, if any, of these abnormalities exists in humans. At the present time it is impossible to determine whether the primary problem in human SLE lies with defective genetic control of immune responses, defi-

cient suppressor T cell function, abnormal macrophage function, an intrinsic B cell defect, a deficient host response to an exogenous infectious agent, an inherited enzyme deficiency, or a combination of such elements.

A detailed summary of current thinking on the etiology and immunopathogenesis of SLE can be found in 2 recent symposia (18,19).

Clinical features

There is no characteristic pattern of clinical features at the onset of SLE nor any consistency in the course of the illness. At the beginning only a single organ may be involved or many systems may be affected simultaneously. Constitutional symptoms—fever, weakness, fatigability, or weight loss—may be the first evidence of illness and are often insidious. In some patients it is the cumulative combination of clinical and laboratory abnormalities that arouses suspicion of the disease. In other patients with the characteristic butterfly blush and arthritis or nephritis, the diagnosis is more obvious.

General systemic complaints are very

frequent at the onset of the disease. Moderate to severe fatigue is noted in 75% of patients, loss of weight in 67%, and fever in 80% at the time of diagnosis. During the course of the disease, these constitutional symptoms may return as the disease becomes active and disappear during periods of remission. It should be noted that fever in patients with the diagnosis of SLE should suggest the presence of infection. Infection was a major cause of death in SLE patients before 1949 when corticosteroids were introduced (2) and remains an important complication to rule out.

Joints. Joint involvement is the most common manifestation of SLE (20). Joint pain or swelling may precede the onset of multisystem disease for many years. In children, the diagnosis of acute rheumatic fever may be made before the diagnosis of SLE.

Arthritis with objective evidence of pain on motion, tenderness, or effusion is present in 75% of SLE patients at the time of diagnosis. Some patients develop arthritis later during the course of the disease. Other patients have joint pain without objective evidence of arthritis. Arthritis or arthalgia is present in 95% of SLE patients. The joints most commonly involved are the proximal interphalangeal joints, knees, wrists, and metacarpophalangeal joints. The joint involvement is remarkably symmetrical. Morning stiffness is present in about 50% of patients.

Deforming arthritis without x-ray evidence of erosions occurs in about 15% of patients after 4 years of disease. Swan neck deformities may be seen but are largely reducible, an important distinction between this and similar deformities in rheumatoid arthritis. Rheumatoid nodules occur in 7% of SLE patients and are histologically similar to those of rheumatoid arthritis. Nodules in an individual SLE patient are usually noted at times of

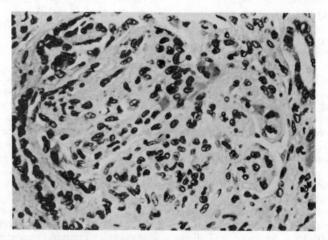

Fig 13—9. Diffuse proliferative glomerulonephritis. Although its circular outline is still discernible, the architecture of the glomerulus is largely obliterated. Note marked hypercellularity and loss of capillary lumina. The small foci of intense eosinophilia probably represent fibrin deposition. *Diffuse* refers primarily to the large number of glomeruli involved, although total involvement of each glomerulus (as seen here) is more common in diffuse than in focal glomerulonephritis (H&E, high power). (From the Revised Clinical Slide Collection on the Rheumatic Diseases)

systemic disease activity and disappear as the disease is suppressed (21). Tenosynovitis occurs in about 8% of patients. Rupture of the achilles and patellar tendons has been reported. Septic arthritis may occur in SLE patients.

Aseptic necrosis (osteonecrosis) occurs in 5–8% of SLE patients treated for at least 5 years. Aseptic necrosis and infectious arthritis are the most common causes of monarticular arthritis in a treated SLE patient. The joint most often involved is the hip. It is suggested that aseptic necrosis occurs more frequently in patients who ingest a large dose of corticosteroids over a brief interval than in patients who take smaller doses over prolonged periods (22).

Myalgia occurs in about 25% of SLE patients and myositis may be noted occasionally, especially in the proximal muscles. True polymyositis with evidence of muscle weakness, typical electromyographic changes, vacuolar myopathy, and necrosis has been reported in untreated SLE patients.

Lesions. Abnormalities of the skin, hair, or mucous membranes are the second most common manifestations of SLE, occurring in 85% of patients. The classic butterfly blush is helpful diagnostically, but is present in a minority of patients seen today. A nonspecific maculopapular erythematous rash similar to a drug eruption may be located anywhere on the body, but is most frequent on the face and chest. Scattered macules may also occur on the palms and fingers or on the soles of the feet.

Lesions of chronic discoid lupus occur in about 15% of patients and may precede the development of multisystemic disease, occur at the time of diagnosis, or erupt later in the course of the disease. Discoid lesions begin as an erythematous plaque or papule and spread outward, leaving a central area of hyperkeratosis, follicular plugging, and atrophy. The edge of the lesion is edematous and erythematous when the lesion is active. A healed discoid lesion may show central depigmentation with atrophy and hyperpigmentation at the margin. Discoid lesions commonly involve the scalp, external ear, and face. In some SLE patients, discoid lesions may be widespread involving the chest and arms.

Vasculitic lesions with ulceration may occur on the extensor surface of the forearm or purpuric palpable lesions on the legs. Less commonly, vasculitic lesions occur on the back of the hands or as blotchy purpuric lesions on the palms and tender erythematous nodules on the fingertips and toes. Periungual erythema is noted in about 10% of patients. Splinter hemorrhages occur in patients with other evidence of vasculitis. Livedo reticularis is very common in SLE patients with active systemic disease and may precede the occurrence of gangrene. Leg ulcers over the malleoli, bullous lesions, periorbital edema, urticaria, ecchymoses and petechiae, gangrene of the fingers or toes, lupus profundus (panniculitis), and dystrophic nail changes are noted in some SLE patients.

Alopecia occurs in nearly 67% of SLE patients during periods of active systemic disease. Because scarring does not usually occur, hair regrows completely at remission. Mucosal ulcers on the hard or soft palate occur in nearly half of SLE patients and are an important index of systemic disease activity (23). Similar ulcerations may be noted on the nasal septum. A rash that follows exposure to the sun (photosensitive rash) is common in these patients.

Other manifestations. Pleural effusions occur in about 40% of patients. Abnormalities of pulmonary function are common even in asymptomatic patients. Tests reveal a combination of pulmonary restriction, vascular obstruction, and airway obstruction. Acute lupus pneumonitis occurs in less than 5% of patients and is characterized by dyspnea, fever, nonproductive cough, rales, and patchy infiltrates with a predilection for basilar areas. The diagnosis of acute lupus pneumonitis should be made only after a rigorous search for an infectious agent since pneumonia due to bacterial and fungal agents is common in SLE patients. Massive pulmonary hemorrhage in SLE may be life-threatening. Chronic lupus pneumonitis is indistinguishable from idiopathic pulmonary fibrosis (fibrosing alveolitis).

The most frequent cardiovascular manifestation is pericarditis which occurs in 25% of patients and varies from a transient friction rub to a massive pericardial effusion. Transient electrocardiographic abnormalities due to myocardial ischemia may be seen and such patients may have persistent tachycardia. Myocardial disease usually occurs with pericarditis. Valvular lesions are usually asymptomatic. Raynaud's phenomenon occurs in 15% of patients.

Although enlargement of the liver is not uncommon, there are no specific lesions of SLE in the liver, and jaundice is rare. Splenomegaly is found in 10% of adult patients and 30% of children (24). Fifty percent of patients have local or generalized enlargement of lymph nodes.

Recurrent abdominal pain occurs in a majority of patients in association with evidence of disease activity in other systems. The cause of the abdominal pain is usually not clear. Mesenteric arteritis may be noted rarely on arteriography and ileal and colonic ulcers and perforations may occur (25). Other gastrointestinal manifestations include ascites, protein-losing enteropathy, and aspirin-induced hepatotoxicity. Pancreatitis may be due to arteritis of the pancreatic artery.

Lupus nephritis is present in approxi-mately one-half of SLE patients. Involvement of the kidney usually occurs early in the disease and its manifestations include microscopic hematuria, proteinuria, and cylinduria, including red cell casts. Proteinuria is present in at least one-half of patients at the time of diagnosis, hematuria in one third, and casts in one-fourth of the patients. Several types of renal lesions, of varying extent and severity and with different prognoses can be identified. Renal biopsy material from SLE patients without urinary abnormalities usually reveals minimal (mesangial) nephritis.

If the patient is free of urinary abnormalities when first seen or if biopsy reveals lesions of minimal or mild (focal) lupus nephritis, progressive renal insufficiency is less likely but can still occur (26,27). Severe basement membrane thickening (membranous lupus nephritis) is associated with profuse proteinuria and the nephrotic syndrome; this may persist for many years and is not necessarily accompanied by serious functional impairment. If, however, the glomeruli have widespread involvement or significant sclerosis, the prospect of progression to renal failure is high. Arterial hypertension is common during the uremic phase, but since this represents a relatively short segment in the evolution of the disease, it is present in only a small fraction of patients with lupus nephritis. Renal disease may progress rapidly but more often deterioration is slow.

The neurologic manifestations of SLE are exceedingly varied (5,28). Psychosis may be evidenced as a schizophreniform reaction. Organic brain syndromes with inability to perform simple calculations and loss of orientation to time and place may be accompanied by seizures or psychosis. Cranial nerve palsies, major motor weakness, and various peripheral neuropathies occur frequently. Chorea, transverse myelopathy, and aseptic meningitis are found in small numbers of SLE patients. Migraine headache is recognized as a symptom of active lupus (29).

Other central nervous system manifestations bear little relationship to extra–central nervous system disease activity status, either clinically or serologically (30). With the exception of progressive dementia, transverse myelopathy, and major strokes, most manifestations are frequently reversible.

Brain scan abnormalities may be associated with central nervous system manifestations and, if present, disappear after the central nervous system manifestations are no longer present. Intracerebral hemorrhages account for a small number of deaths in most series of patients.

A small number of SLE patients have small ovoid or circular white spots in the retina. These patches contain cytoid bodies that consist of aggregates of swollen nerve fibers and the products of proliferating and degenerating axonal structures. These lesions disappear gradually as the disease becomes inactive. Occasionally patients with SLE have evidence of Sjögren's syndrome.

Menstrual abnormalities are common in patients during the early, active phase of the disease. Stillbirths and miscarriages are common in untreated patients with active disease but normal full-term deliveries are the rule in well-controlled patients (31). Complete heart block and an unusual neonatal rash associated with transient appearance of antinuclear antibodies have been noted in offspring.

Drug-related lupus-like syndromes

Ever since the first observations in 1953 and 1954 of the so-called hydralazine syndrome, there has been a steady accumulation of reports describing the induction of lupus-like syndromes by various drugs (32–36). The list of agents implicated in this manner continues to grow and includes: procainamide (now the most commonly recognized offender), isoniazid, aminosalicylic acid, diphenylhydantoin, methphenylethylhydantoin, trimethadione, penicillin, penicillamine, sulfonamides, tetracycline, propylthiouracil, and alphamethyl dopa.

In reviewing this subject one finds that the evidence linking drug to disease is often highly circumstantial and that in some cases symptoms suggestive of SLE have antedated the use of the agent in question. The syndromes most extensively investigated and most firmly established have been those following the use of hydralazine, procainamide, and anti-seizure medication.

When hydralazine was more widely used in the treatment of arterial hypertension, it was noted that approximately 10% of patients who received this substance in relatively large amounts over a prolonged period developed a peculiar illness referred to as the hydralazine syndrome. This occurred in men and women with about equal frequency and consisted mainly of polyarthralgia or arthritis, which subsided after discontinuation of the medication. A minority of patients, however, developed additional complaints including fever, pleurisy, pericarditis, hepatosplenomegaly, erythematous rash, leukopenia, hypergammaglobulinemia, and various serologic abnormalities including positive LE cell reactions and biologic false-positive tests for syphilis. As noted in drug-induced lupus associated with other agents, renal and central nervous system involvements were notably rare. When hydralazine was stopped, these abnormalities disappeared, only to recur promptly on its readministration.

The pathogenesis of the hydralazine syndrome and the question of its relationship to SLE remain obscure. In some patients, there has been a history suggestive of a predetermined susceptibility to SLE or subclinical disease, but this is not the usual situation. A prospective study has revealed that antinuclear antibodies developed in 15 of 25 patients after 2 years of drug ingestion (35). However, only 3 of the patients had a titer of 1:10 or greater. Clinical symptoms of SLE developed in only 1 of the 25 patients. The antinuclear antibodies that develop in these hydralazine-treated patients are directed against nucleoprotein, especially the histone portion, or against single-stranded DNA. Antibodies to native double-stranded DNA are not found.

Prospective studies have revealed that procainamide-induced antinuclear antibodies occur in about 50% of individuals and that half of these individuals develop a lupus-like syndrome (34). Procainamide is therefore the most common agent implicated in producing a lupus-like syndrome. Patients with procainamide-induced lupus syndrome typically have joint pains and swelling, rashes, pleurisy, pericarditis, and pulmonary atelectasis. The disease clinically resembles the "spontaneous" disease in elderly individuals. Renal disease does not occur, and antibodies against native DNA are absent (32). Withdrawal of procainamide gradually leads to disappearance of the clinical syndrome and eventually disappearance of the antinuclear antibodies from the serum.

A prospective study of 102 patients receiving isoniazid for 1 year revealed isoniazid-induced antinuclear antibodies in 20%, but no patients developed evidence of a drug-induced lupus syndrome (36).

The phenotype of acetylating enzyme in the individual receiving procainamide, hydralazine, or isoniazide has been shown to influence the development of antinuclear antibodies. Antinuclear antibodies occur primarily in slow acetylators (37).

Diagnosis

The patient with classic multisystem disease and a positive LE cell test or positive test for antinuclear antibodies poses no diagnostic problem. However, this is not the usual mode of presentation. In general, SLE unfolds as a series of episodes. At the beginning and for some time thereafter, only one manifestation may dominate the illness. Clearly, some features such as the butterfly rash are more significant diagnostically than others. In general the diagnosis is based on an appropriate constellation of clinical features and is confirmed by serologic, histopathologic, and other laboratory findings. Testing for antinuclear antibodies (ANA) has become well established as particularly useful, especially in helping to rule out the disease, since one or more of these antibodies is found in nearly all patients with SLE.

A positive LE cell reaction also strengthens the diagnosis, but because repeatedly negative LE cell tests are seen in as many as 20% of patients, the failure to demonstrate LE cells clearly does not rule out SLE. Although the LE cell phenomenon is positive in the great majority of patients with SLE, it cannot be regarded as entirely specific. Positive reactions occur not only in patients with rheumatoid arthritis, but in other connective tissue diseases as well, including progressive systemic sclerosis, dermatomyositis, and polyarteritis nodosa.

The occurrence of antibodies to native DNA or to the Sm nuclear antigen appears to provide the strongest confirmatory serologic evidence of SLE because of their rarity in other situations. On the other hand, antibody to native DNA is present in only 80% of clinically active SLE patients (38), and anti-Sm occurs in less than 50% of patients. Thus, the failure to demonstrate antibodies to native DNA or to Sm does not rule out SLE. Immunofluorescent study of skin biopsies may prove of diagnostic value in some patients.

Preliminary criteria for the classification of systemic lupus erythematosus were prepared by the ARA Diagnostic and Therapeutic Criteria Committee in 1971 and revised in 1982 (39) (see Appendix 6). They were designed to have high specificity against rheumatoid arthritis and a variety of other nonrheumatic diseases. These criteria have been used primarily by investigators who study large groups of SLE patients. The application of the criteria for diagnosis of an individual patient is of some value if used with additional serologic and immunopathologic evaluations, such as serum CH50, C3, and C4 levels and immunopathologic studies of nonlesional skin. Also, the absence of antinuclear antibodies by the indirect fluorescent antibody technique in an untreated patient with multiple system disease generally militates strongly against a diagnosis of SLE, although "ANA negative" lupus has been described.

The distinction between SLE and rheumatoid arthritis is not always clear, especially in the early stages of the disease, since many features overlap between these 2 conditions. Articular involvement is very common in SLE and frequently resembles that of early rheumatoid arthritis. A fifth of patients with SLE have a positive test for rheumatoid factor, usually in low titer; in many of these individuals joint complaints are prominent. Conversely, the extraarticular features of rheumatoid arthritis may simulate SLE. In addition, the 15–20% of patients with rheumatoid arthritis and LE cells, compared with those with negative LE cell tests, have a slightly higher incidence of extraarticular disease compatible with rheumatoid arthritis, disease of longer duration, a higher frequency of rheumatoid nodules, and higher titers of rheumatoid factor. Many exceptions to this are seen, however.

Antinuclear antibodies may be present in about two-thirds of rheumatoid arthritis patients. In nearly all instances, titers are much lower than those found in patients with clinically active SLE, but are not lower than those found in SLE patients who have remained in remission for prolonged periods. The antinuclear antibodies in rheumatoid arthritis patients are found in high titers in those individuals with more severe disease.

Most of the patients with rheumatoid arthritis and positive LE cell tests or antinuclear antibodies can be expected to have a course similar to patients without these abnormalities and should not be considered to have SLE in the absence of appropriate clinical findings.

Clinical and serologic overlap between SLE and other rheumatic diseases such as dermatomyositis, progressive systemic sclerosis, and rheumatoid arthritis is not infrequent. A small percentage of patients with SLE have keratoconjunctivitis sicca and xerostomia (Sjögren's syndrome).

Discoid lupus erythematosus, consisting of red scaling plaque with follicular plugging and central atrophy, is a common dermatologic disorder. It occurs in twice as many females as males and has its peak age of onset between 35–45 years. Thus, more males and older individuals develop the disease than develop SLE. The lesions are present predominantly on the face and scalp and less often on the neck. Some of these individuals develop clear-cut SLE with LE cells, antinuclear antibodies, anti-DNA antibodies, and low serum complement levels. In general, discoid lupus erythematosus is a benign skin disease which can be distinguished from SLE by the absence of clinical extracutaneous manifestations and laboratory abnormalities (40).

Discoid lesions may occur in patients with SLE and may be present at the time of onset of multisystem disease or the lesions may occur for the first time during an exacerbation of disease years after diagnosis of SLE.

1. Dubois EL: Lupus Erythematosus. Ed 2. Los Angeles, University of Southern California Press, 1976
2. Ropes MW: Systemic Lupus Erythematosus. Cambridge, Harvard University Press, 1976
3. Fessel WJ: Systemic lupus erythematosus in the community. Arch Intern Med 134:1027–1035, 1974
4. Nobrega FT, Ferguson RH, Kurland LT, et al: Lupus erythematosus in Rochester, Minnesota, 1950-1965, Population Studies in the Rheumatic Diseases. PH Bennett, PHN Weed, eds. New York, Excerpta Medica, 1968, p 259
5. Johnson RT, Richardson EP: The neurological manifestations of systemic lupus erythematosus. Medicine 47:337–369, 1968
6. Biesecker G, Lavin L, Ziskind W, Koffler D: Cutaneous localization of membrane attack complex in discoid and systemic lupus erythematosus. N Engl J Med 306:264–270, 1982

7. Schrager MA, Rothfield NF: The lupus band test. Clin Rheum Diseases 3:597–611, 1975
8. Comerford FR, Cohen AS: The neuropathy of systemic lupus erythematosus: an assessment of clinical, light, and electron microscopic criteria. Medicine 46:425-473, 1967
9. Pirani CL, Pollak VE: Systemic lupus erythematous, Immunologically mediated Renal Disease: Criteria for Diagnosis. GA Andres, RT, McCLusky, eds. New York, Dekker, 1978
10. Decker JL, et al: Systemic lupus erythematosus: evolving concepts. Ann Intern Med 91:587–604, 1979
11. Koffler D, Kunkel HG: Mechanisms of renal injury in systemic lupus erythematosus. Am J Med 45:165–169, 1968
12. Koffler D, et al: Variable patterns of immunoglobulin and complement deposition in the kidneys of paients with systemic lupus erythematosus. Am J Pathol 56:305–316, 1969
13. Svec KH, Allen ST: Antibody to nuclear material eluted from isolated spleen vessels in systemic lupus erythematosus. Science 170: 550–551, 1970
14. Atkins CJ, et al: The choroid plexus in systemic lupus erythematosus. Ann Intern Med 76:65–72, 1972
15. Christian CL: Immune complex disease. N Engl J Med 280:878–884, 1969
16. Tan Em, Schur PH, Carr RI, Kunkel HG: DNA and antibodies to DNA in the serum of patients with systemic lupus erythematosus. J Clin Invest 45:1732, 1966
17. Koffler D, Agnello V, Kunkel HG: Polynucleotide immune complexes in serum and glomeruli of patients with systemic lupus erythematosus. Am J Pathol 74:109, 1974
18. Winchester RJ, ed: Proceedings of the ARA Conference on New Directions for Research in Systemic Lupus Erythematosus. Arthritis Rheum 21(suppl), 1978
19. Koffler D, ed: Proceedings of the Conference on Current Perspectives on the Immunology of Systemic Lupus Erythematosus. Arthritis Rheum 25: no. 7, 1982
20. Rothfield NF: Systemic lupus erythematosus: clinical and laboratory aspects, Arthritis and Allied Conditions. Ed 9. DJ McCarty, ed, Philadelphia, Lea & Febiger, 1979
21. Hahn BH, Yardley JH, Stevens MB: "Rheumatoid" nodules in systemic lupus erythematosus. Ann Intern Med 72:49–58, 1970
22. Abeles M, Urman JD, Rothfield NF: Aseptic necrosis of bone in systemic lupus erythematosus. Arch Intern Med 138:750–754, 1978
23. Urman JD, Lowenstein MB, Abeles M, et al: Oral mucosal ulcers in systemic lupus erythematosus. Arthritis Rheum 21:58, 1978
24. Meislin AG, Rothfield N: Systemic lupus erythematosus in childhood: analysis of 42 cases with comparative data on 200 adult cases followed concurrently. Pediatrics 42:37–49, 1968
25. Zizic TM, Shulman LE, Stevens MB: Colonic perforations in systemic lupus erythematosus. Medicine 54:411–426, 1975
26. Baldwin D, et al: The clinical course of the proliferative and membranous forms of lupus nephritis. Ann Intern Med 73:929–942, 1970
27. Morel-Maroger L, Mery JPH, Droz D, et al: The course of lupus nephritis: contribution of serial renal biopsies. Adv Nephrol 6:79–118, 1976
28. Klippel JH, Zvaifler NJ: Neuropsychiatric abnormalities in systemic lupus erythematosus. Clin Rheum Dis 1:621–638, 1975
29. Brandt KD, Lessel S: Migrainous phenomena in systemic lupus erythematosus. Arthritis Rheum 21:7-16, 1978
30. Winfield JB, Brunner CM, Koffler D: Serologic studies in patients with systemic lupus erythematosus and central nervous system dysfunction. Arthritis Rheum 21:289–294, 1978
31. Zurier RB: Systemic lupus and pregnancy. Clin Rheum Dis 1:613–620, 1975
32. Winfield JB, Davis JS, IV: Anti-DNA antibodies in procainamide-induced lupus erythematosus. Arthritis Rheum 17:97–110, 1974
33. Hahn BH, et al: Immune responses to hydralazine and nuclear antigens in hydralazine-induced lupus erythematosus. Ann Intern Med 76:365–374, 1972

34. Blomgren SE, Condemi JJ, Vaughan JH: Procainamide-induced lupus erythematosus. Am J Med 5:338–348, 1972
35. Hess EV, Loggie JM, Foad BS, et al: Prospective study of immunologic effects of hydralazine in hypertensive patients. Arthritis Rheum 21:565, 1978
36. Rothfield NF, Bierer WF, Garfield JW: Isoniazid induction of antinuclear antibodies: a prospective study. Ann Intern Med 88:650–652, 1978
37. Woosley RL, Drayer DE, Reidenberg MM, et al: Effect of acetylator phenotype on the rate at which procainamide induces antinuclear antibodies and the lupus syndrome. N Engl J Med 298:1157–1159, 1977
38. Weinstein A, Bordwell B, Rothfield N: Antinative DNA antibodies and serum C3 levels: candidates for the ARA Preliminary Criteria for the Classification of Systemic Lupus Erythematosus (abstract). Arthritis Rheum 21:602, 1978
39. Tan EM, Cohen AS, Fries JF, Masi AT, McShane DJ, Rothfield NF, Schaller JG, Talal N, Winchester RJ: 1982 Revised Criteria for the Classification of Systemic Lupus Erythematosus. Arthritis Rheum 25:1271–1277, 1982
40. Schrager MA, Rothfield NF, Pathways of complement activation in chronic discoid lupus: serologic and immunofluorescence studies. Arthritis Rheum 20:637–645, 1977

Laboratory abnormalities

Anemia occurs in many patients with SLE and is generally mild, normochromic, or normocytic. Severe hemolytic anemia is uncommon. Leukopenia occurs in about half of SLE patients. The differential white count is usually normal, although neutrophils may predominate. There may be some increase in B and a decrease in T lymphocytes including suppressor T cells (1). Infections and corticosteroids may induce a relative leukocytosis. Thrombocytopenia with or without purpura is common. The erythrocyte sedimentation rate is usually elevated.

Serum albumin levels are low, especially in patients with the nephrotic syndrome. Gamma globulin levels are frequently elevated, but may be low in patients with nephrotic syndrome. Renal dysfunction occurs in over half the patients. Mild disease may result in only some impairment of concentrating ability, a few red and/or white blood cells in the urine, and some proteinuria. Some patients have a nephrotic syndrome with only proteinuria and without cells or casts. Others may have a glomerulonephritis characterized by hematuria, pyuria ($>$5 cells/hpf), casts, a decreasing glomerular filtration rate, and proteinuria. Significant hematuria and pyuria are rarely seen in lupus nephritis in patients in remission.

The synovial fluid is generally clear or slightly cloudy. The WBC is usually $\geq$3000/mm^3 but is sometimes much less. The total protein is 2–3 gm%, but complement levels are usually quite low. The cerebrospinal fluid is abnormal in about half the patients with neurologic manifestations. The protein content may be somewhat elevated; there may be a few lymphocytes. Levels of C4 in cerebrospinal fluid are usually normal but tend to be lower in patients with active neurologic disease than in those with inactive disease. The electroencephalogram is commonly abnormal; CT scans often show cortical atropy.

A consistent and characteristic feature of SLE is the presence of numerous immunologic abnormalities, especially autoantibodies. The Coombs test is often positive even in the absence of hemolytic anemia. Antibodies to lymphocytes are common and associated with lymphopenia. Antibodies to neutrophils and platelets can be demonstrated. Rheumatoid factors occur in 15% of patients and their presence varies with clinical activity.

Biologic false positive (BFP) tests for syphilis occur in 15% of patients, especially in those with circulating anticoagulants. Antibodies to clotting factors may prolong clotting, prothrombin, and/or partial thromboplastin time—and may rarely be associated with bleeding. Antibody titers to some viruses may be elevated, as in other chronic conditions. Tests for cell-mediated immunity have yielded variable results, but generally skin tests and in vitro responses of lymphocytes to antigens or lectins have been either normal or reduced (1).

Most characteristic of SLE are the large number of antibodies that react with nuclear and cytoplasmic constituents. The first such antibody described was that causing the LE phenomenon. The LE cell is formed in vitro, as follows: some leukocytes are traumatized to release nucleoprotein (DNA-histone), the nucleoprotein reacts with an IgG antibody, and the complex is phagocytosed by the remaining viable leukocytes.

If performed repeatedly, the LE cell test is eventually positive in most SLE patients. The test may be positive in patients with other disorders (such as rheumatoid arthritis or liver disease).

The best screening test for SLE is one that detects antinuclear antibodies (ANA). Serum is incubated with tissue sections or cells rich in nuclear material. After washing to remove nonbound immunoglobulins, the antibodies bound to nuclei are demonstrated with a fluorescein tagged anti-immunoglobulin. Slides are examined under ultraviolet light to determine which portion of the nucleus fluoresces, that is, has bound antibody (Fig 13–10). ANA are found in ≥ 95% of patients with SLE, often in high titer; however, ANA may be found occasionally in normals and sometimes in patients with rheumatoid arthritis, scleroderma, Sjögren's syndrome, chronic liver disease, infectious mononucleosis, and other disorders (including drug-related lupus), but usually in low titer.

The subject of the individual antinuclear antibody patterns is well reviewed in references 2–4. The most common ANA pattern, **diffuse (homogeneous)**, represents antibodies to nucleoprotein. It may be

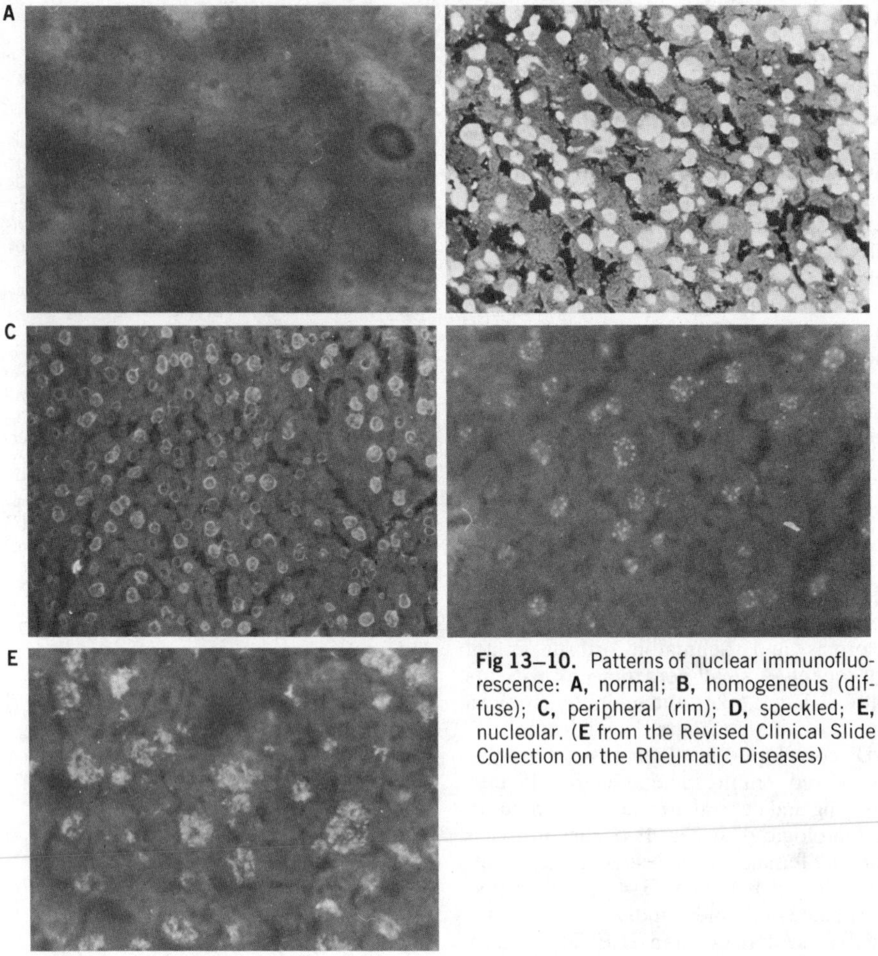

Fig 13–10. Patterns of nuclear immunofluorescence: **A**, normal; **B**, homogeneous (diffuse); **C**, peripheral (rim); **D**, speckled; **E**, nucleolar. (**E** from the Revised Clinical Slide Collection on the Rheumatic Diseases)

found in all diseases mentioned here. The **peripheral (rim, ring, shaggy) pattern** represents antibodies to DNA. It is found predominantly in SLE patients, although not all SLE patients have it. The **speckled pattern** represents antibodies to a group of substances that can be easily extracted from nuclei with saline (for example, extractable nuclear antigens such as Sm, RNP, SS-A/Ro, SS-B/La) and other less well characterized substances. These antibodies are found predominantly in patients with SLE, scleroderma, or some combination of these diseases (mixed connective tissue diseases). The **nucleolar pattern** is rare and represents antibodies to a nuclear RNA. These antibodies are found in patients with Raynaud's phenomenon, SLE, and scleroderma. Titers of ANA do not correlate with clinical activity in most patients.

Although the immunofluorescent method is an excellent screening test for ANA and SLE, more specific immunologic methods are available and useful in differentiating SLE from other disorders associated with ANA. Antibodies to native (i.e., double-stranded) DNA and Sm are found almost exclusively in patients with SLE, albeit in only 75% and 25% of patients, respectively. The level of anti-DNA antibodies correlates with clinical activity in

many but not all patients (5). Table 13–1 shows antibodies found in various diseases.

These ANA and in particular anti-DNA may bind to antigen to form immune complexes. Such complexes can be detected by direct assays such as binding to C1q or Raji cells, formation of cryoglobulins, or indirectly by serum complement levels (6).

Serum complement levels are depressed to varying degrees in most patients with SLE at some time during their illness, especially when disease activity is present (7). CH50 and C4 levels are the most frequently depressed, often in association with mild (e.g., skin, joint, hematologic) disease. Markedly depressed complement levels including CH50, C4, and C3 are seen primarily in patients with active lupus nephritis. The low levels probably reflect in vivo activation and fixation of complement components by circulating immune complexes. Serial determination of CH50 or individual complement components (especially C4 and C3) may be useful in following and managing patients with SLE; falls in complement often precede clinical flares. Some patients may have low complement levels without apparent clinical activity. Many of these patients have congenital deficiencies of complement components, particularly C2.

Table 13-1. Antinuclear antibodies in several diseases*

	ANA (% positive)	ANA pattern			Antibodies				
		Diffuse	Peripheral	Speckled	DNA	Sm	ssDNA	NP	RNP
Normal	<5	+			0	0	0	0	0
Systemic lupus	>95	++	+++++	++	75	25	>75	45	46
Rheumatoid arthritis	~35	+	±		Rare	Rare	15–50	5	8
Scleroderma	~40			+++	0	Rare		0	31
Sjögren's	~75	+		+	Rare	Rare	14	2	17
Liver disease	~15	+			Rare	Rare	Rare	Rare	Rare
Drug-related lupus		+	±		0	Rare	Common	+	Rare

*Source: References 2–4.

1. Rosenthal CJ, Franklin EC: Depression of cellular-mediated immunity in systemic lupus erythematosus. Arthritis Rheum 18:207–217, 1975
2. Reichlin M, Mattioli M: Antigens and antibodies characteristic of systemic lupus erythematosus. Bull Rheum Dis 24:756–760, 1974
3. Notman DD, Kurata N, Tan EM.: Profiles of antinuclear antibodies in systemic rheumatic diseases. Ann Intern Med 83:464–469, 1975
4. McDuffie FC, Bunch TW: Immunologic tests in the diagnosis of rheumatic diseases. Bull Rheum Dis 27:900–911, 1976–77
5. Lloyd W, Schur PH: Immune complexes, complement, and anti-DNA in exacerbations of systemic lupus erythematosus. Medicine 60:208–217, 1981
6. Nydegger UE, Lambert PH, Gerber H, et al: Circulating immune complexes in the serum in systemic lupus erythematosus and in carriers of hepatitis B antigen: quantitation by binding to radiolabeled Clq. J Clin Invest 54:297-309, 1974
7. Schur PH: Complement in lupus. Clin Rheum Dis 1:519–543, 1975

Treatment

No treatment is absolutely "indicated" in the management of systemic lupus erythematosus; a therapeutic program is developed and ordered as required by the specific problems of a specific patient. The somewhat nebulous concept of "disease activity" is the principal guide.

Symptoms such as arthralgias, chest pain, either pleuritic or steady, easy fatigue, muscle weakness, and morning stiffness or findings such as synovitis, pleural or pericardial inflammation, evolving rash, fever occasionally with chills, mouth ulcers, or falling hair are all features of active disease. Nephritis is asymptomatic save for the edema that may accompany nephrotic syndrome. Activity is estimated by the formed elements in the urine, the degree of proteinuria (if it is not "fixed"), and evolving renal function.

Changing states of consciousness, a series of seizures, chorea, impaired vision, any form of paralysis, and organic psychoses are all taken as signs of disease activity in the central nervous system. Although normal findings are common and do not exclude central nervous system lupus, the cerebrospinal fluid should be examined with the onset of any of these features.

Involvement of multiple body systems (e.g., integumentary, articular, renal, or central nervous) is taken to represent more disease activity than involvement of only one or two. The duration of findings is critical; several new features developing within a few weeks or days represent more significant activity as far as treatment urgency is concerned than those same features in a patient who has developed them progressively over many months or a year.

Increased antibodies to native DNA, falling serum complement, circulating immune complexes, and anemia are typical of active disease. Leukopenia, positive LE cell test, the titer of antinuclear antibody, and the erythrocyte sedimentation rate are less good indices on repeated reexamination over years of illness. Laboratory studies, helpful in assessing the picture, should not by themselves dictate treatment decisions.

Aspirin should be used in full antiinflammatory dosage (4 gm daily or more) as the first line drug for fever, arthralgia, or arthritis, and even serosal disease. The duration of a trial on aspirin depends on the intensity of the symptoms. In flaring SLE, the patient should be admitted to the hospital and tried on full dosage aspirin for several days or a week. In these circumstances, the drug may well result in increased serum transaminase and creatinine levels, both expected and nonthreatening findings usually dealt with by decreasing the dose.

None of the newer nonsteroidal antiinflammatory drugs (NSAID) are labeled as indicated for SLE, but they are widely used as a substitute for aspirin if it proves to be poorly tolerated. None is particularly advantageous; ibuprofen performed less well than aspirin in one of the few available trials.

The **antimalarials,** chloroquine or hydroxychloroquine, or some combination thereof, often used for discoid lupus erythematosus, can also be given for SLE (1). They have a slow onset of action over 1–8 weeks and are considered to be of benefit, especially in patients with dermatologic or articular complaints.

The major unwanted effect of the antimalarials is on the retina—a progressive retinopathy capable of inducing blindness. Regular ophthalmologic examination, including red target visual fields, is required to detect early toxicity but has not, in fact, been demonstrated to prevent loss of vision. The lesion can progress even after the drug is stopped. The great majority of the rare patients with retinal damage have taken large doses for several years; thus doses should be restricted (no more than 250 mg of chloroquine or 400 mg hydroxychloroquine daily) and duration of treatment should probably be confined to 2 or 3 years. If disease activity recedes, the physician is advised to reduce drug administration to every other day or twice weekly.

Adrenal corticosteroids, especially when administered for the first time, have a dramatic effect on the symptoms and signs of the disease, so dramatic, in fact, that their initiation is unduly attractive to the attending physician who must attempt to measure the relief expected today against the problems of 2 or 3 years hence. If hospitalization and NSAID have been inadequate to control activity and antimalarials are not yet expected to be effective, adrenal corticosteroid treatment at the level of prednisone 0.5–1.0 mg/kg/day (or its equivalent) should be started, using divided doses. Dose reduction should not start until the disease has been nearly asymptomatic for 2 weeks or more.

Reduction plans vary. The first step is to change to once daily dosage, usually in the morning. The withdrawal of 10 mg weekly down to 30 mg daily, then 5 mg weekly to 15 mg daily, and then even slower constitutes a rapid reduction program. Slower plans, always guided by symptoms, findings, and laboratory measures, are widely used.

After several months of followup and with knowledge of the patient's reactivity, reductions to alternate day doses are good practice. For example, with the patient well on 30 mg each morning, one can withdraw 5 mg on the alternate day weekly until the patient is receiving 30 mg one morning and none the next. The alternate day method can preserve or restore the hypothalamic-pituitary-adrenal axis and seems to produce less osteoporosis, cushingoid facies, and proclivity to infection than is seen on the same total dose given daily. Another potential advantage of every other day medication is the ability to detect symptoms of persistent disease activity, usually just before the next morning dose is taken; their appearance constitutes a useful suggestion to the physician that further reductions should not be attempted at once.

Many physicians go on to withdraw steroids entirely. Others prefer to continue a possibly "homeopathic" dose, 5 or 10 mg every other morning, indefinitely. In any event, every effort should be made to get the dose down to or below 10 mg daily. It is in this range and sometimes at even higher levels that NSAID and antimalarials can be of importance; alternate day fever, for example, can often be abated by suitably timed, moderate doses of aspirin.

Persistent proteinuria, sediment abnormalities, and/or deteriorating renal function ascribable to glomerular inflammation and appearing as a new finding, are usually considered an indication for somewhat higher doses of prednisone, for example, 1.0–1.5 mg/kg/day. Some continue the medication at that level until the antibody to double-stranded DNA and complement measures have returned to normal (2). Others will begin reduction on normalization of the urine and reversals of elevations of serum creatinine. If none of these favorable events occurs, there is little justification for increasing the dose and, after 2 or 3 months of such treatment, regardless of "success" or "failure," side effects usually mandate reduction.

The failure of this plan to normalize the findings in all patients has lead to much study of other modes of therapy. Persistent signs of active renal disease are today a debated indication for renal biopsy. Recent evidence strongly suggests that findings of chronic change in the biopsy specimens are predictive of an unfavorable outcome and more meaningful in that respect than is the classification scheme of the World Health Organization.

Bolus steroid treatment (methylprednisolone 1 gm intravenously each day for 3 days) has been suggested and does appear to reverse the rapid decline of function in disease of recent onset (3). Plasmapheresis is under study in renal disease although the failure of that mode to alleviate symptomatic lupus in a controlled study (4) makes its utility in slowly developing renal disease rather doubtful.

Steroid dosage is usually temporarily increased in dealing with serial seizures. More dangerous and rarer are alterations of consciousness, dementia, chorea, aseptic meningitis, transverse myelitis, and the like. These are usually treated with higher doses, for example, methylprednisolone 3 mg/kg/day intravenously. Some suggest that, in the absence of change for the better over 2 or 3 days, the dose should be doubled repeatedly up to a gram or more daily. The great variability and relative rarity of these states have not permitted controlled trials, but the risks associated with these doses over a week or more are high. The cytotoxic drugs play little role in the management of central nervous system lupus.

Psychosis in active lupus is usually treated with substantial steroid dose increases, but the psychologic effects of the adenal corticosteroids themselves regularly confuse the issue. Many patients note derangement of thought patterns, difficulty in controlling emotions, insomnia, bad dreams, and rarely, hallucinations due to steroid therapy itself. These can constitute, with the unfortunate facial changes of Cushing's syndrome, a major cause for patient aversion to the medications. Frank psychosis can result. The only useful distinguishing feature is the chronologic sequence; bizarre behavior or complaints within 15 days of a major increase in steroid dosage is probably due to the medication rather than to central nervous system lupus.

Hemolytic anemia and thrombocytopenic purpura, but not leukopenia, are indications for steroid therapy. If tolerable doses do not prevent purpura, the spleen is sometimes removed after accelerated destruction of platelets has been demonstrated by survival studies.

Cytotoxic drugs, particularly the purine analog, azathioprine, are often advised; both oral cyclophosphamide and oral azathioprine appear to prevent or delay the onset of renal functional decline in a subset of patients (5). Intermittent intravenous cyclophosphamide may also preserve function and certainly reduces the amount of extrarenal disease activity observed in trial patients (6). However, the high frequency of urinary bladder disease in the wake of cyclophosphamide administration greatly inhibits its use in nonmalignant disease.

With renal failure and superimposed infection leading the list, central nervous system disease is the third ranked cause of death in SLE. Convulsive seizures are by far the most common feature and, unless abruptly appearing at close intervals or in association with status epilepticus, should be treated with **anticonvulsants** such as diphenylhydantoin and phenobarbital.

Other complications. Although the great majority of patients with SLE do not give a history of heliosensitivity, it may appear at any time. Accordingly, undue exposure to sunlight should always be avoided but total proscription is not required. The patient should be gently encouraged to test herself in ordinary social activities requiring some sun exposure. Patients with adverse reactivity to sunlight should always be fully clothed and should use sunscreening lotions or ointments such as those containing paraaminobenzoic acid.

Advice on conception and pregnancy will be needed. It is safest for the patient with SLE to avoid pregnancy, but pregnancy is not absolutely contraindicated when the woman is interested in raising a family. When proliferative nephritis is part of the picture, pregnancy constitutes a major, though rather unpredictable, hazard for the mother. In the absence of renal disease, pregnancy or delivery may be associated with disease flares, including the onset of proliferative nephritis. Nevertheless with appropriate intra- and postpartum attention, pregnancy is not as risky as was earlier thought; this is particularly true if the lupus is inactive or quiescent at the time of conception. Mechanical modes of contraception are preferred to female sex hormones.

Antihypertensive therapy is more critical than in essential hypertension, given the frequency of steroid maintenance treatment, nephritis, and eventual renal failure in lupus. Benzothiadiazide diuretics, methyldopa, apresoline, propanolol, and guanethidine have been used to good effect just as they are in uncomplicated hypertension.

Other therapies. Antacids should be used liberally in the patient taking antiinflammatory drugs. Iron is sometimes needed and should be given by mouth. Transfusions are not contraindicated. General anesthesia and surgery can be carried out without undue difficulty. For example, severe symptoms often justify replacement of the hip damaged by avascular necrosis of the femoral head.

Any drug may be used in SLE but none should be unless clearly indicated. Drug-related lupus syndrome is no more likely to occur in a patient with SLE than it is in the general population. Despite their similarities, the 2 conditions, drug-related and idiopathic SLE, appear to be distinct and separate processes.

Educating the patient. The final—or perhaps the first—element of the management of SLE is information. As a rule the patient is in desperate need of sensible and realistic information. Many still reach physicians, perhaps having checked an ancient encyclopedia, with the feeling that they have contracted an exotic and mysterious illness with an invariably fatal outcome. It is the physician's duty and privilege to lead the patient to a more accurate and reasonable understanding of her illness and its problems. Attention devoted to this issue will be of much more significance over the years than the exact doses or types of medications.

The educational process is not a matter for the first appointment or even the fifth; rather it is achieved gradually over repeated contacts made in sickness and in health. It is crucial to fit the information to the level of the patient's understanding, a level usually underestimated. It is critically important for the physician to be realistic and open with the patient and especially to avoid "sparing" the patient while informing the family.

Some physicians prefer to do all of this themselves, whereas others depend on specially trained health educators, nurses, or social workers. Lupus discussion groups encouraging patients, with skilled professional guidance, to talk together about their worries, problems, and plans have been extremely successful. There is also a burgeoning library of books, pamphlets, tapes, and slide shows designed to instruct and assist the patient. These should not be handed out without prior review by the patient's doctor and the opportunity to deal with questions or uncertainties arising from them must be provided.

1. Dubois EL: Antimalarials in the management of discoid and systemic lupus erythematosus. Semin Arthritis Rheum 8:35–51, 1978
2. Urman JD, Rothfield NF: Corticosteroid treatment in systemic lupus erythematosus; survival studies. JAMA 238:2272–2276, 1977
3. Kimberly RP, Lockshin MD, Sherman RL, McDougal JS, Inman RD, Christian CL: High dose intravenous methylprednisolone pulse therapy in systemic lupus erythematosus. Am J Med 70:817–824, 1981
4. Wei N, Klippel JH, Huston DP, Hall RP, Lawley TJ, Balow JE, Steinberg AD, Decker JL: Randomized trial of plasma exchange in mild systemic lupus erythematosus. Lancet i:17–22, 1983
5. Carette S, Klippel JH, Decker JL, Austin HA, Plotz PH, Steinberg AD, Balow JE: Controlled studies of oral immunosuppressive drugs in lupus nephritis; a long-term followup. Ann Intern Med (in press)
6. Dinant HJ, Decker JL, Klippel JH, Balow JE, Plotz PH, Steinberg AD: Alternative modes of cyclophosphamide and azathioprine therapy in lupus nephritis. Ann Intern Med 96 (Part 1):728–736, 1982

14. Progressive systemic sclerosis and related disorders

Progressive systemic sclerosis (PSS) is a generalized disorder of connective tissue characterized by fibrosis and degenerative changes in the skin (**scleroderma**), synovium, digital arteries, and in the parenchyma and small arteries of certain internal organs, notably the esophagus, intestine, lungs, heart, kidney, and thryoid (1,2). The spectrum of severity for PSS ranges from a form marked by restricted skin involvement—often confined to the fingers and face—and the passage of a prolonged period of time (often several decades) before full expression of characteristic internal manifestations (PSS with CREST syndrome) to a form in which there is widespread thickening of the skin (PSS with diffuse scleroderma) and often rapidly progressive visceral involvement (1,2) (Table 14–1).

The origin of PSS is obscure. The demonstration of a variety of serologic abnormalities and cellular immune reactions indicates that immunologic mechanisms are important in its pathogenesis (1,3).

Clinical and pathologic features. Progressive systemic sclerosis has been described in people of all races and its distribution is global. Women are affected approximately 3–4 times as often as men. Initial symptoms usually appear in the third to fifth decade of life. The disease is relatively uncommon in childhood. Only rarely is more than 1 member of a family affected (4). The disease occurs with particularly high frequency in coalminers and it has been suggested that silicosis is a predisposing factor.

In most patients, the initial complaint is either Raynaud's phenomenon, swelling and puffiness of the hands (and sometimes the feet), or gradual thickening and tightening of the skin of the fingers (1). Approximately one-third of patients first experience polyarthralgia and joint stiffness; a few have frank polyarthritis. In others the onset of PSS is heralded by severe muscle weakness that may be indistinguishable from polymyositis (sclerodermatomyositis). In a small proportion of patients, the clinical presentation is dominated by neither cutaneous nor musculoskeletal complaints but by symptoms referable to visceral involvement (PSS without scleroderma).

Skin. In the early edematous phase of scleroderma, painless, bilateral, symmetrical pitting edema of the hands and fingers occurs which may also involve the forearms as well as the feet and legs. The appearance of the tightly swollen fingers is often compared to sausages. In patients destined to develop diffuse scleroderma, the edema typically lasts from a few weeks to several months and is gradually replaced by the indurative phase (thickening, tightening, and hardening of the skin) that begins in the fingers and first gave the disease the name scleroderma. In the CREST (calcinosis, Raynaud's phenomenon, esophageal dysmotility, sclerodacty-

Table 14–1. Classification of scleroderma

I. Progressive systemic sclerosis
  A. *PSS with diffuse scleroderma*—Symmetric, diffuse involvement of the skin (scleroderma) affecting trunk, face, proximal and distal portions of the extremities; relatively early appearance of disease of the esophagus, intestine, heart, lung, and kidney
  B. *CREST syndrome*—relatively limited involvement of the skin, often confined to the fingers and face; prominence of calcinosis, Raynaud's phenomenon, esophageal dysfunction, sclerodactyly, telangiectasia, and prolonged delay in appearance of distinctive internal manifestations (including severe pulmonary arterial hypertension and biliary cirrhosis)
  C. Overlap syndromes, including *sclerodermatomyositis* and *mixed connective tissue disease*
II. Eosinophilic fasciitis
III. Congenital fascial dystrophy
IV. Localized (focal) forms of scleroderma
  A. Morphea
    1. Plaque-like
    2. Guttate
    3. Generalized
    4. Less typical forms: subcutaneous morphea, keloid morphea
    5. Possibly superficial primary atrophic morphea (atrophoderma Pasini-Pierini)
  B. Linear scleroderma, with or without melorheostosis
  C. Scleroderma en coup de sabre, with or without facial hemiatrophy
V. Chemically induced scleroderma-like conditions

  A. Vinylchloride disease
  B. Pentazocine-induced fibrosis
  C. Bleomycin-induced fibrosis
  D. Possibly trichloroethylene-induced fibrosis
  E. Scleroderma-like illness after use of L-5-hydroxytryptophan and carbidopa
VI. Digital sclerosis and joint contractures associated with juvenile onset diabetes mellitus
VII. Diseases with skin changes resembling scleroderma (pseudoscleroderma)
  A. Edematous
    1. Scleredema adultorum of Büschke
    2. Scleredema related to diabetes mellitus
    3. Scleromyxedema (papular mucinosis)
  B. Indurative and/or atrophic
    1. Lichen sclerosus et atrophicus
    2. Porphyria cutanea tarda
    3. Acromegaly
    4. Myeloma-associated and primary amyloidosis
    5. Skin thickening associated with plasma cell neoplasia with peripheral polyneuropathy
    6. Phenylketonuria
    7. Carcinoid syndrome
    8. Localized lipoatrophy, including Gower's panatrophy, lipoatrophy of ankles, orbicular lipoatrophy
    9. Congenital poikiloderma, including Rothmund's syndrome, Rothmund-Thompson syndrome
    10. Werner's syndrome
    11. Progeria
    12. Acrodermatitis chronica atrophicans

ly, and telangiectasia) variant of PSS, the early edematous phase, with swollen puffy fingers, may persist for an indefinitely prolonged period. The symmetrically distributed skin changes may remain confined to the distal portions of the upper extremities or spread to involve the forearms, arms, upper anterior chest, abdomen, back, and face (Fig 14–1).

As the disease progresses, the skin becomes taut and shiny. There is a loss of normal wrinkles and skin folds and the development of the characteristic pinched, immobile, expressionless face. The lips become thin and tightly pursed and the mouth narrows. These changes are accompanied or, in some instances, preceded by generalized melanotic hyperpigmentation. Small macular telangiectases appear on the fingers, face, lips, tongue, and forearms. Subcutaneous calcifications (*calcinosis circumscripta*) appear most commonly in the finger tips. These calcifications vary in size from tiny punctate deposits to large masses over the knees and elbows as well as other bony eminences. Calcinosis tends to be especially abundant and telangiectasia especially profuse in individuals with CREST syndrome.

Once altered, the skin remains thickened for many years (5). In some patients, however, the skin eventually softens and

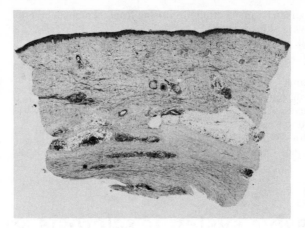

Fig 14–2. Photomicrograph of skin (forearm) of a 42-year-old woman with PSS and diffuse scleroderma. The dermis is thickened as a result of the deposition of dense collagenous connective tissue, thinning of the epidermis, and loss of the normal dermal appendages. Note numerous aggregates of cells identified as lymphocytes in the deeper portions of the dermis.

reverts toward normal thickness or may atrophy. Skin biopsy specimens obtained during the active indurative phase disclose a striking increase of compact collagen fibers in the reticular dermis, thinning of the epidermis with loss of rete pegs, atrophy of dermal appendages, and hyalinization and fibrosis of arterioles (Fig 14–2).

Raynaud's phenomenon. Paroxysmal interruption of blood flow to the fingers (Raynaud's phenomenon) occurs in approximately 98% of patients with PSS. In the majority, this reaction begins with the development of skin changes and/or rheumatic complaints. On occasion, however, Raynaud's phenomenon antedates other evidence of PSS by an interval of many years. In addition to the fingers, cold-induced blanching (cyanosis-reactive hyperemia) may occur in the toes and other acral locations including the tip of the nose, tip of the tongue, lips, and earlobes.

Angiographic studies of digital arteries of patients with PSS and Raynaud's phenomenon disclose fixed narrowing and obliteration in these vessels. The finding of diminished capillary blood flow in the fingers in both warm and cool environments and the inability to rewarm the fingers after cold exposure constitute evidence of a persistent structural defect in the blood vessels.

Histologic examination of digital arteries reveals variably severe intimal hyperplasia leading to narrowing or occlusion of the lumen (6) (Fig 14–3). Adventitial fibrosis is also found in these vessels. Changes also occur in the microcirculation. There is loss of capillaries (evident on examination of the nailfold) with tortuosity and dilatation of the remaining vessels (7,8).

Joints. Polyarthralgia and joint stiffness affecting both small and large peripheral joints are frequent complaints during the initial phases of PSS and in its subsequent course (9). In a few patients, there is evidence of frank arthritis including synovial effusions containing small numbers of mononuclear cells. Synovial biopsy specimens reveal inflammation marked by infiltration of lymphocytes and plasma cells

present in focal aggregates or scattered diffusely throughout the tissue.

In many patients, coarse leathery friction rubs, accompanied at times by audible creaking, are found over the joints (particularly the knees) as well as the distal portions of the forearms, legs, and other tendinous areas, and large bursae. These rubs (common in patients with diffuse scleroderma but rare in those with CREST syndrome) have been traced to fibrinous deposits on the surfaces of the joints, the tendon sheaths, and overlying fascia. Later in the course of PSS, there is increasing stiffness of the joints and intense fibrosis of the synovium that may encompass and obliterate the vascular structures. Many patients develop severe flexion contractures of the fingers.

Radiographic examination often reveals absorption of the tufts of the terminal phalanges, frequently accompanied by at-

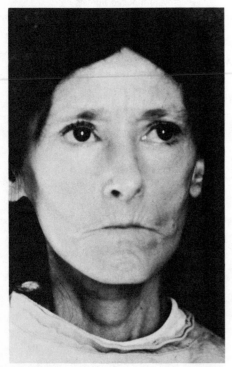

Fig 14–1. The face of this young woman demonstrates many features of systemic sclerosis including drawn pursed lips, shiny skin over the cheeks and forehead, and atrophy of muscles of the temple, face, and neck. These changes in the face are known as *Mauskopf* (mousehead). (From the Revised Clinical Slide Collection on the Rheumatic Diseases)

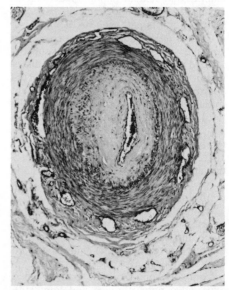

Fig 14–3. Photomicrograph of finger artery from a 55-year-old woman with PSS and diffuse scleroderma who died of renal failure (scleroderma kidney). Note intimal hyperplasia that led to severe narrowing of the lumen. In addition there is striking fibrosis of the adventitia and telangiectasia of the vasa vasorum.

rophy of the soft tissue and subcutaneous calcinosis. Although usually limited to the tufts, the erosion of bone (more severe in patients with CREST syndrome) may ultimately lead to complete dissolution of the terminal and, rarely, the middle phalanx. Other areas of bone resorption include the distal portions of the radius and ulna, the ribs (notching), and angle of the mandible.

Atrophy of the muscle in many patients with PSS is secondary to disuse, but on occasion a severe inflammatory myopathy occurs (10).

Esophagus. Esophageal dysfunction develops in the great majority of patients with PSS and constitutes the most common manifestation of internal involvement. In addition to complaints referable to esophageal reflux and peptic esophagitis (the result of a disturbance in the action of the gastroesophageal sphincter), some patients experience difficulty in swallowing since food tends to remain lodged in the lower esophagus.

Roentgenographic abnormalities are found in over 75% of patients with PSS, including many who are free from esophageal symptoms. Peristaltic activity ranges from diminution to total absence, and later dilatation (less often narrowing) of the lower one-half or two-thirds of the esophagus occurs. Gastroesophageal reflux is noted, and in many cases, a small hiatal hernia of the sliding variety is present. On occasion, peptic esophagitis is complicated by ulceration and stricture (Fig 14–4) (more common in individuals with CREST syndrome than in those with diffuse scleroderma). Histologic changes, most notable in the lower two-thirds of the esophagus, include increased quantities of collagen in the lamina propria and submucosa and atrophy of the muscularis, which, in the severest cases, may be almost totally replaced by collagen.

Lungs. Clinical and/or radiographic evidence of pulmonary involvement develops in the majority of patients. Interstitial, peribronchial, and alveolar fibrosis are found at postmortem examination in nearly all. The most prominent symptom is exertional dyspnea. A few patients experience one or more bouts of pleurisy, sometimes associated with strikingly intense friction rubs. Many remain asymptomatic, however, despite evidence of severe fibrosis, presumably because of sharply restricted physical activity.

Chest roentgenograms frequently disclose a reticular pattern of linear, nodular, and lineonodular densities most pronounced in the lower two-thirds of the lung fields, and in some patients, this pattern assumes the appearance of diffuse mottling or honeycombing.

The most sensitive and usually the earliest physiologic abnormality consists of a subnormal diffusing capacity. This change is often found in the absence of any significant alteration in ventilation or any roent-genographic evidence of fibrosis. Later there is evidence of restrictive and/or obstructive disease.

There have been several reports of the development of alveolar or bronchiolar cell carcinoma. These neoplasms are believed to arise as a result of intense bronchiolar epithelial proliferation that accompanies pulmonary fibrosis. There may be extensive sclerosis of the small pulmonary arteries, particularly in patients with CREST syndrome who are prone to develop severe pulmonary arterial hypertension (11).

Heart. The nature and severity of the cardiac disease that develops in patients with PSS depends on the degree of myocardial fibrosis, a primary component of this disorder, and on the extent to which concurrent fibrosis of the lung and thickening and fibrosis of the small pulmonary arteries place an added burden on the circulation (12). Cardiac arrhythmias, conduction disturbances, and other electrocardiographic abnormalities have been noted in a high percentage of patients, as would be expected in a disease marked by the presence of cardiomyopathy (13).

Sophisticated studies have revealed evidence of left ventricular dysfunction in many patients. Pulmonary arterial hypertension may develop as widespread fibrosis gradually obliterates the small blood vessels of the lung. In CREST syndrome, pulmonary hypertension, often severe, is due to widespread narrowing and occlusion of small pulmonary arteries rather than to pulmonary fibrosis, which may be minimal or absent (11). Pericarditis and pericardial effusion have been found with increasing frequency.

Intestinal tract. The pathologic changes in the intestine are similar to those in the esophagus and lead to such complaints as severe bloating, cramps, and episodic diarrhea. Many patients experience serious malabsorption. Hypomotility of the small intestine, the cardinal abnormality, favors the overgrowth of intestinal microorganisms that interfere with normal fat absorption, presumably as a result of the deconjugation of bile salts. Dramatic improvement has been observed after the administration of tetracycline or other broad spectrum antibiotics. Hypomotility also leads to prolonged retention of barium in the second and third portions of the duodenum, which are often atonic and widely dilated (loop sign).

In the remainder of the small intestine, irregular flocculation of the barium meal and localized areas of dilatation and hypersegmentation exist. The persistence of the close proximity of the valvulae conniventes in the distended jejunum is believed to result from fibrosis of the submucosa (Fig 14–5). Atrophy of the muscularis mucosae occasionally permits entry of air into the wall of the intestine and the development of pneumatosis intestinalis.

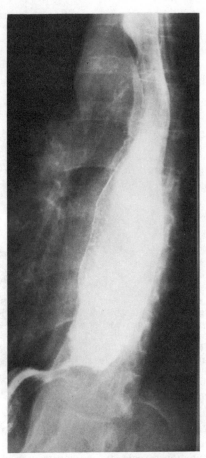

Fig 14–4. Roentgenogram of esophagus of a 52-year-old woman with PSS and CREST syndrome who had had increasing difficulty with acid reflux and dysphagia to the point that she had become unable to swallow any solid material. Note stricture involving several centimeters of the distal esophagus.

Patchy atrophy of the muscularis of the large intestine leads to the development of characteristic wide-mouthed diverticula, usually located along the antimesenteric border of the transverse and descending colon. These sacculations, unique to PSS, also occur in the jejunum and ileum.

Kidney. Renal disease, an important component of PSS, is a major cause of death in individuals with PSS and diffuse scleroderma (14,15). Typically renal disease is manifested by the abrupt development of malignant arterial hypertension which, if not treated soon, is associated with rapidly progressive and irreversible renal insufficiency. Occasionally the blood pressure may remain within normal limits, but severe elevation with extremely high plasma renin levels is the rule.

Before the advent of new and highly effective antihypertensive agents and other improvements in the management of advanced renal disease, survival for longer than 3–6 months was almost unknown. The kidneys of those who die of renal failure usually contain numerous small infarcts. Focal vascular lesions consisting of intimal hyperplasia and fibrinoid necrosis

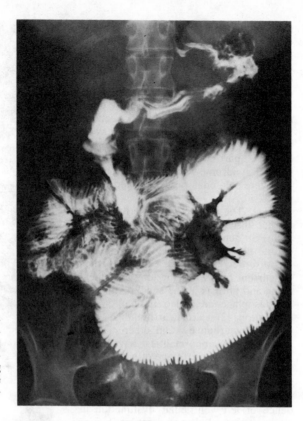

Fig 14—5. Roentgenogram of upper gastrointestinal tract of a 36-year-old woman with PSS and CREST syndrome who had intestinal malabsorption. Note striking dilatation of jejunum; the valvulae conniventes remain in close approximation.

of the arcuate and interlobular arteries and arterioles are evident. Angiographic examination reveals striking constriction of the interlobular arteries and a sharp decrease in cortical blood flow (1).

Other organs. Fibrosis of the thyroid has been observed and there is an increased frequency of Hashimoto's thyroiditis. These complications may be associated with frank hypothyroidism (16). Biliary cirrhosis is found in some women with CREST syndrome, but hepatic involvement is otherwise rare.

Trigeminal sensory neuropathy or other cranial neuropathies have been described, usually in association with CREST syndrome or mixed connective tissue disease (17). Sjögren's syndrome, confirmed by the presence of lymphocytic infiltrates in the minor salivary glands is found in 17–65% of patients with PSS (18).

Laboratory findings. Initially the blood count for PSS patients is normal except for a mild lymphopenia, affecting T-dependent cells (19). Later there may be anemia associated with visceral involvement and complications including microangiopathic anemia in patients with renal involvement. Autoimmune hemolytic anemia has also been reported. Urine is normal except in individuals with arterial hypertension and other evidence of renal involvement, who show proteinuria, microscopic hematuria, and increased numbers of casts. Mild hypergammaglobulinemia (IgG) is frequently found. Between 25–35% of patients have positive tests for rheumatoid factor.

In recent studies employing a variety of sources of nuclear antigen including HEp-2 cells, antinuclear antibodies have been found in nearly all patients with PSS (20). At least 4 separate antibodies have been identified (Table 14–2). One of these, anticentromere antibody, is found with particularly high frequency in association with CREST syndrome (20). Nucleolar immunofluorescence has been observed in 10–54% of patients and is seen more often in PSS than in any other connective tissue disease. Antibodies to double-stranded DNA have been notably rare.

Course and prognosis. The natural course of PSS varies considerably. It is difficult to determine prognosis early in the illness, especially in patients with diffuse scleroderma. In many patients, steadily progressive sclerosis of the fingers leading to crippling flexion contractures occurs. Nearly all patients eventually show evidence of visceral involvement. Esophageal, intestinal, and other internal changes may occur with minimal skin disease and may or may not progress with the scleroderma. The prognosis is significantly worse when there is clinical evidence of involvement of the kidney, heart, or lung at the time that PSS is first recognized (21).

Pathogenesis. There is convincing evidence that the fibrosis of the skin and internal organs in PSS is the result of the overproduction of collagen. Measurement of the weight and hydroxyproline content of skin biopsy cores confirmed clinical and histologic evidence of an increase in dermal thickness and has shown a concomitant and proportional increase in the collagen content of the skin (5). Dermal fibroblasts of patients with PSS, when propagated in tissue culture, accumulate abnormally large quantities of collagen and other connective tissue components (22).

Evidence of both increased humoral immune activity and abnormal cellular immune function is summarized in Table 14–3 (1,3,23,24). These findings led to the hypothesis that fibrosis of the tissues results in part from the action of a lymphokine released from activated T lymphocytes that promotes the synthesis of collagen by dermal and other fibroblasts (23).

A modest increase in the frequencies of HLA–A9 and B8 antigens has been reported. In some studies, however, the distribution of HLA–A and B antigens has been normal (25). Moderately increased frequencies of HLA–DR1 and DR3 have also been claimed, the latter associated with CREST syndrome.

Localized scleroderma. The term scleroderma has traditionally been applied not only to the cutaneous changes of PSS, but to a heterogeneous group of conditions in which there is more circumscribed or patchy or linear sclerosis of the skin (Table 14–1) (26,27). The hardening and inelasticity of the integument may be indistinguishable from that observed in PSS, but certain pathologic and clinical differences exist between these conditions and PSS. In particular, there is little convincing evidence of internal involvement in the localized forms of scleroderma or of overlap between these conditions and PSS.

Morphea. This variety of localized scleroderma begins with one or more areas of erythematous or violaceous discoloration of the skin, which take the form of

Table 14—2. Antinuclear antibodies found in progressive systemic sclerosis (20)

Nature of reactive antigen	Immunofluorescence pattern	Antibody specificity	
		PSS—diffuse scleroderma	PSS—CREST syndrome
Scl-70, a nonhistone nuclear protein of 70,000 daltons MW	Diffuse fine speckles	+ +	+
Unknown	Discrete coarse speckles	+ +	+ +
Multiple antigens, including 4–6S nucleolus-specific RNA	Nucleolar	+ +	+ +
Protein bound to centromere DNA	Centromere	+	+ + +

Table 14–3. Immunologic abnormalities in progressive systemic sclerosis

I. B cell activity
  A. Serologic abnormalities
    1. Rheumatoid factor
    2. Antinuclear antibodies (see Table 14–2) (20)
    3. Immune complexes
  B. Serum proteins—increase, usually mild, in serum IgG concentration (19)
  C. Deposition of immunoglobulin (IgM) and complement components (including C3) in kidney
II. Cellular immune (T cell) reactivity
  A. Peripheral lymphopenia, affecting T lymphocytes (19)
  B. Presence of T lymphocyte infiltrates in dermis and other tissues (1)
  C. Disturbance in immunoregulation (19)
  D. Stimulation of peripheral blood lymphocytes by cutaneous antigen(s) and collagen (1)
  E. Lymphokine stimulation of collagen production by dermal fibroblasts (23)
III. Occurrence of PSS- and Sjögren's syndrome–like disease in individuals with graft-versus-host reaction after bone marrow transplantation (24)
IV. Association of PSS with Sjögren's syndrome and Hashimoto's thyroiditis (16,18)

small or large plaques or, less often, discrete drop-like spots (*guttate morphea*). As the lesions evolve, the skin becomes sclerotic and waxy or ivory-colored. During the active phase of the disease, the plaques, which may increase to a diameter of many centimeters, are surrounded by a violaceous border of inflammation. After several months or years, spontaneous softening of the skin occurs. At this time, the smaller plaques may return to normal. Disease onset occurs at any age, affects any site, and is confined to the skin and subcutaneum. The major histologic changes consist of new collagen deposition in the dermis and septa of the subcutaneous tissue and inconsistently heavy (often intense) infiltrations of lymphocytes, plasma cells, and histiocytes.

Linear scleroderma. In this form of localized scleroderma, which usually develops during childhood, a linear streak or band of sclerosis appears in the upper or lower extremities or in the frontoparietal area of the forehead and scalp (*scleroderma en coup de sabre*). The band may eventually extend the entire length of the extremity and may affect more than 1 part. Localized scleroderma en coup de sabre is often associated with hemiatrophy of the face on the side of the skin lesion. Severe fibrosis and inflammation exist in the dermis, subcutis, and deep fascia and extend into the underlying muscle, resulting in severe damage. Infrequently, linear scleroderma coexists in the same extremity with *melorheostosis*, a peculiar linear fibrotic hyperostosis of bone.

There is considerable overlap between morphea and linear scleroderma and patches of morphea are often found in individuals with linear scleroderma. Antinuclear antibodies, including large amounts of antibody to single-stranded DNA, and rheumatoid factor are found in the sera of patients with linear scleroderma. These serologic abnormalities, accompanied by a modest degree of peripheral eosinophilia, are noted during clinically active phases of the disease.

Treatment. The management of the patient with progressive systemic sclerosis involves the judicious use of agents that may inhibit the processes that give rise to overgrowth of collagenous connective tissue, in addition to supportive and symptomatic measures designed to compensate for the damage done to the skin, joints, and internal organs. Before any form of treatment is considered, however, it is essential that the physician discuss the nature of PSS with the patient and family, who are often frightened by reports of the seriousness of the disease and fearful of the worst. It is important to stress the relatively good prognosis for survival in individuals with CREST syndrome.

Evaluation of the effectiveness of treatment is difficult because of the slowly progressive nature of PSS, the tendency in some patients toward spontaneous improvement or remission, the influence of psychophysiologic factors on many of the symptoms, and the limitations in objective criteria for ascertaining improvement (or deterioration) in the patient's condition, particularly relative to the visceral changes of the disease.

No single drug or combination has been demonstrated to be of value in adequately controlled studies or is generally accepted as useful. The corticosteroids have been disappointingly ineffective and their use is restricted to those patients who have disabling myositis or who are critically ill with mixed connective tissue disease.

Attention has been focused on D-penicillamine, an agent known to interfere with the intermolecular crosslinking of collagen. It has been reported (in uncontrolled studies) that the prolonged use of D-penicillamine in doses of 1–2 grams/day is associated with a decrease in skin thickening, a reduction in the rate of new visceral involvement, and prolongation of survival (28). This drug can often be toxic and must be administered with extreme caution.

The use of colchicine has been advocated (1). This ancient remedy has been found to inhibit the accumulation of collagen by blocking the conversion of procollagen to collagen, probably through interference with microtubule-mediated transport or perhaps via stimulation of collagenase production. It is too early to tell whether this effect can be translated into a meaningful therapeutic use. The

possible role of immunosuppressive agents in the treatment of PSS is also under study.

Supportive measures. Nearly all patients with PSS have Raynaud's phenomenon and, to the extent that it is precipitated by low temperatures, this may be prevented by dressing warmly and avoiding undue exposure to cold. Tobacco should be avoided. A variety of vasodilating drugs has been prescribed including reserpine, phenoxybenzamine, methyldopa, guanethidine, and prazosin (29). In general, these agents have proved disappointing in PSS. Perhaps this is only to be expected in view of the morphologic changes in the vessels which underlie the Raynaud's phenomenon in these patients.

Numerous drugs and hormones have been administered without success in the treatment of the calcinosis associated with PSS (1). On occasion, the combination of probenecid (which induces hypophosphatemia) with a low calcium diet proves effective. The use of diphosphonates (compounds that inhibit crystallization of calcium phosphate and are capable of preventing various types of experimental calcinosis) are usually ineffective.

Patients who have difficulty in swallowing learn to masticate carefully and to avoid foods that are likely to cause dysphagia. The development of esophageal stricture may require periodic dilatation; esophageal hiatal hernia and peptic esophagitis demand additional measures. Successful excision of strictures and correction of gastroesophageal reflux by gastroplasty have been reported (30). The dramatic improvement in steattorhea and other signs of intestinal malabsorption that often follow the administration of tetracycline and other broad spectrum antibiotics has been mentioned previously.

In recent years, the availability of new and more potent antihypertensive agents and of improved hemodialysis procedures has modified the earlier hopeless prognosis for individuals with PSS who developed malignant arterial hypertension and rapidly progressive renal failure because of renal vascular involvement (scleroderma kidney) (31). Now blood pressure can often be controlled and kidney function stabilized and improved in some cases by prompt and vigorous treatment with various drugs including hydralazine, methyldopa, minoxidil, guanethidine, diazoxide, prazosin, propranolol, and, most dramatically, captopril, which inhibits the angiotensin-converting enzyme (32).

A reduction in the severity of dermal thickening has been observed in some of patients; the explanation of this phenomenon and particularly the question of a relationship to antihypertensive treatment is being pursued. This reaction would appear to lend strong support to the hypothesis that abnormalities in microcirculation play a prime role in the pathogenesis of

PSS. A few instances of successful renal transplantation have been reported (31).

1. Rodnan GP: Progressive systemic sclerosis (scleroderma), Arthritis and Allied Conditions, ed 9. McCarty DJ Jr, ed. Philadelphia, Lea & Febiger, 1979, pp 762–809

2. LeRoy EC: Scleroderma (systemic sclerosis), Textbook of Rheumatology. WN Kelley, ED Harris Jr, S Ruddy, CB Sledge, eds. Philadelphia, Saunders, 1981, pp 1211–1230

3. Haynes DC, Gershwin ME: The immunopathology of progressive systemic sclerosis (PSS). Semin Arthritis Rheum 11:331–351, 1982

4. Gray RG, Altman RD: Progressive systemic sclerosis in a family: case report of a mother and son and review of the literature. Arthritis Rheum 20:35–41, 1977

5. Rodnan GP, Lipinski E, Luksick J: Skin thickness and collagen content in progressive systemic sclerosis and localized scleroderma. Arthritis Rheum 22:130–140, 1979

6. Rodnan GP, Myerowitz RL, Justh GO: Morphologic changes in the digital arteries of patients with progressive systemic sclerosis (scleroderma) and Raynaud's phenomenon. Medicine 59:393–408, 1980

7. Maricq HR, LeRoy EC: Progressive systemic sclerosis: disorders of the microcirculation. Clin Rheum Dis 5:81–101, 1979

8. Maricq HR, LeRoy EC Jr, D'Angelo WA, Medsger TA Jr, Rodnan GP, Sharp GC, Wolfe JF: Diagnostic potential of in vivo capillary microscopy in scleroderma and related disorders. Arthritis Rheum 23:183–189, 1980

9. Rodnan GP, Medsger TA Jr: The rheumatic manifestations of progressive systemic sclerosis (scleroderma). Clin Orthop 57:81–93, 1968

10. Clements PJ, Furst DE, Campion DS, Bohan A, Harris R, Levy J, Paulus HE: Muscle disease in progressive systemic sclerosis: diagnostic and therapeutic considerations. Arthritis Rheum 21:62–71, 1978

11. Salerni R, Rodnan GP, Leon DF, Shaver JA: Pulmonary hypertension in the CREST syndrome variant of progressive systemic sclerosis (scleroderma). Ann Intern Med 86:394–399, 1977

12 Bulkley BH: Progressive systemic sclerosis: cardiac involvement. Clin Rheum Dis 5:131–149, 1979

13. Clements PJ, Furst DE, Cabeen W, Tashkin D, Paulus HE, Roberts N: The relationship of arrhythmias and conduction disturbances to other manifestations of cardiopulmonary disease in progressive systemic sclerosis (PSS). Am J Med 71:38–46, 1981

14. Cannon PJ, Hassar M, Case DB, Casarella WJ, Sommers SC, LeRoy EC: The relationship of hypertension and renal failure in scleroderma (progressive systemic sclerosis) to structural and functional abnormalities of the renal cortical circulation. Medicine 53:1–46, 1974

15. Kovalchik MT, Guggenheim SJ, Silverman MH, Robertson JS, Steigerwald JC: The kidney in progessive systemic sclerosis: a prospective study. Ann Intern Med 89:881–887, 1978

16. Gordon MB, Klein I, Dekker A, Rodnan GP, Medsger TA Jr: Thyroid disease in progessive systemic sclerosis: increased frequency of glandular fibrosis and hypothyroidism. Ann Intern Med 95:431–435, 1981

17. Teasdall RD, Frayha RA, Shulman LE: Cranial nerve involvement in systemic sclerosis (scleroderma): a report of 10 cases. Medicine 59:149–159, 1980

18. Cipoletti JF, Buckingham RB, Barnes EL, Peel RL, Mahmood K, Cignetti FE, Pierce JM, Rabin BS, Rodnan GP: Sjögren's syndrome in progressive systemic sclerosis (scleroderma). Ann Intern Med 87:535–541, 1977

19. Inoshita T, Whiteside TL, Rodnan GP, Taylor FH: Abnormalities of T lymphocyte subsets in patients with progressive systemic sclerosis (scleroderma). J Lab Clin Med 97:264–277, 1981

20. Tan EM, Rodnan GP, Garcia I, Moroi Y, Fritzler MJ, Peebles C: Diversity of antinuclear antibodies in progressive systemic sclerosis. Anti-centromere antibody and its relationship to CREST syndrome. Arthritis Rheum 23:617–625, 1980

21. Medsger TA Jr, Masi AT, Rodnan GP, Benedek

TG, Robinson H: Survival with systemic sclerosis (scleroderma): a life-table analysis of 309 patients. Ann Intern Med 75:369–376, 1971

22. Uitto J, Bauer EA, Eisen AZ: Scleroderma. Increased biosynthesis of triple-helical type I and type III procollagens associated with unaltered expression of collagenase by skin fibroblasts in culture. J Clin Invest 64:921–930, 1979

23. Johnson RL, Ziff M: Lymphokine stimulation of collagen accumulation. J Clin Invest 58:240–252, 1976

24. Shulman HM, Sullivan KM, Weiden PL, McDonald GB, Striker GE, Sale GE, Hackman R, Tsoi M-S, Storb R, Thomas ED: Chronic graft-versus-host syndrome in man: a long-term clinicopathologic study of 20 Seattle patients. Am J Med 69:204–217, 1980

25. Birmbaum NS, Rodnan GP, Rabin BS, Bassion S: Histocompatibility antigens in progressive systemic sclerosis (scleroderma). J Rheumatol 4:425–428, 1977

26. Jablonska S: Scleroderma and Pseudoscleroderma. Ed 2. Warsaw, Polish Medical Publishers, 1975

27. Jablonska S, Rodnan GP: Localized forms of scleroderma. Clin Rheum Dis 5:215–241, 1979

28. Rodnan GP: Progressive systemic sclerosis and penicillamine. J Rheumatol 8 (supplement 7):116–120, 1981

29. Coffman JD: Vasodilator drugs in peripheral vascular disease. Med Intell 300:713–717, 1979

30. Orringer MB, Orringer JS, Dabich L, Zarafonetis CJD: Combined collis gastroplasty-fundoplication operations for scleroderma reflux esophagitis. Surgery 90:624–630, 1981

31. LeRoy EC, Fleischmann RM: The management of renal scleroderma. Experience with dialysis, nephrectomy and trasplantation. Am J Med 64:974–978, 1978

32. Whitman HH III, Case DB, Laragh JH, Christian CL, Botstein G, Maricq H, LeRoy EC: Variable response to oval angiotensin-converting-enzyme blockade in hypertensive scleroderma patients. Arthritis Rheum 25:241–248, 1982

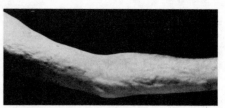

Fig 14–6. The arm of this patient demonstrates the "puckered" or "orangepeel" appearance of the skin which may occur in eosinophilic fasciitis. The skin feels firm and is bound to the underlying structures. In contrast to scleroderma, the fingers are spared and the ability to make fine wrinkles in the superficial skin is usually maintained. (From the Revised Clinical Slide Collection on the Rheumatic Diseases)

Eosinophilic fasciitis

Eosinophilic fasciitis (EF) is a recently recognized scleroderma-like disorder characterized by symmetrical and often widespread inflammation and sclerosis of the deep fascia, subcutis, and dermis (1–4). EF occurs in children but the great majority of patients are middle-aged and older adults.

Clinical features. The disorder usually begins with pain, swelling, and tenderness of the hands, forearms, feet, and legs. This is soon followed by signs of inflammation and hardening of the skin and subcutaneous tissues of these parts. Striking contractures of the fingers may develop within a few weeks. Carpal tunnel syndrome is an early feature in approximately a third of patients (2–4). Polyarthralgia and mild polyarthritis, occurring early in the course of illness and involving both small and large peripheral joints, are often noted (2,3). At the onset of illness, fever may be as high as 40°C. Constitutional complaints, including fatigue and weight loss, are common.

Induration and thickening of the skin and subcutaneum may remain confined to the distal parts or may spread to the proximal portions of the extremities and to extensive areas of the trunk and face. The fingers are often spared in eosinophilic fasciitis, as compared with the constancy of involvement in progressive systemic sclerosis (PSS). In eosinophilic fasciitis

the skin is often warm and erythematous (later hyperpigmented) and subcutaneous tissues (often described as woody) and the dermis are indurated. Retraction of the fibrotic subcutis produces a nodular irregularity of the skin surface, and when the arm or leg is elevated, deep grooves or furrows appear over the course of the superficial veins (groove sign) (Fig 14–6).

With the exception of an uncommon and minor elevation in serum glutamicoxaloacetic transaminase and/or creatine phosphokinase activity, there is no clinical evidence of myopathy, and muscle strength is unimpaired. The lack of Raynaud's phenomenon in EF and the conspicuous absence of the characteristic internal manifestations of PSS constitute additional evidence separating these disorders.

Laboratory findings. Striking peripheral eosinophilia is found during the early stage of EF. Eosinophils usually account for 20–30% of the total white blood cell count (which is most often normal, but may be mildly elevated) and may number several thousand per cubic millimeter (2–4). Serum eosinophil chemotactic activity is uniformly and markedly increased (5).

Hypergammaglobulinemia (IgG) is a common finding, with levels of IgG as high as 4.0 gm/dl. Erythrocyte sedimentation rate is usually elevated. Rheumatoid factors and antinuclear antibodies are absent and the levels of serum complement components are normal. Synovial fluids obtained from patients with arthritis can contain 1,000–4,000 cells/mm³, almost all lymphocytes.

The diagnosis of EF is confirmed by means of a deep biopsy that includes skin, subcutis, fascia, and muscle. Wound healing proceeds normally. During the first several months of the disease, inflammation and fibrosis are found in all layers, including the dermis, but are most conspicuous in the deep fascia, which may be thickened many-fold (2). Large numbers of lymphocytes, plasma cells, eosinophils, and histiocytes are present in the affected areas.

Later when peripheral eosinophilia

abates (spontaneously, or as a result of the administration of corticosteriods) eosinophils are no longer encountered in the tissues, which remain thickened and fibrotic for as long as several years. During this later phase, the inflammatory reaction ceases and it may be difficult or impossible to distinguish the tissue changes from those found in PSS. Biopsies of articular synovium have revealed infiltrations of lymphocytes and plasma cells. In those individuals with carpal tunnel syndrome, there is inflammation of the tenosynovium of the flexor tendon sheaths, marked by heavy accumulation of lymphocytes, plasma cells, and eosinophils (2).

Treatment. Some patients with EF have developed aplastic anemia or thrombocytopenic purpura (6). In the great majority, however, EF appears to be a self limited and uncomplicated disorder. As a rule, complete or nearly complete resolution

(including loss of contractures) occurs after 2–5 years. Spontaneous remission has been observed in a number of instances. On occasion, fibrosis of the skin and deeper structures persists for a longer time. Recurrence appears to be rare.

Early on, small doses of corticosteroids (10–15 mg prednisone/day) often provide substantial symptomatic relief and can readily eradicate the eosinophilia. These compounds appear to have no effect on the fibrosis of EF, however, and little or no benefit is to be expected from their continued use after the initial inflammatory phase of the disease has subsided.

The etiology of eosinophilic fasciitis is unknown, although it has been noted that in men, at least, the illness is often preceded by unusually strenuous physical exertion. The presence of eosinophilia, raised serum IgG levels, and identification in some cases of immunoglobulins and C3 in

the inflamed fascia raise the possibility that a humoral immune mechanism may be involved in the pathogenesis. This theory is supported by the demonstration of circulating immune complexes during the early phase of the disease (7).

1. Shulman LE: Diffuse fasciitis with eosinophilia: a new syndrome. Arthritis Rheum 20: S205–S215, 1977
2. Barnes EL, Rodnan GP, Medsger TA Jr, Short D: Eosinophilic fasciitis: a pathologic study of 20 cases. Am J Pathol 96: 493–518, 1979
3. Moore TL, Zuckner J: Eosinophilic fasciitis. Semin Arthritis Rheum 9: 228–235, 1981
4. Rodnan GP: Eosinophilic fasciitis, Internal Medicine. JH Stein, ed. Boston, Little Brown, 1982
5. Wasserman SI, Seibold JR, Medsger TA Jr, Rodnan GP: Serum eosinophilotactic activity in eosinophilic fasciitis. Arthritis Rheum 25: 1352–1356, 1982
6. Hoffman R, Dainiak N, Sibrack L, Pober JS, Waldron JA Jr: Antibody-mediated aplastic anemia and diffuse fasciitis. N Engl J Med 300: 718–721, 1979
7. Seibold JR, Rodnan GP, Medsger TA Jr, Winkelstein A: Circulating immune complexes in eosinophilic fasciitis. Arthritis Rheum 25: 1180–1185, 1982

15. Mixed connective tissue disease

Mixed connective tissue disease (MCTD) is a term for a syndrome characterized by an admixture of clinical features found in systemic lupus erythematosus (SLE), progressive systemic sclerosis (PSS), and polymyositis and by unusually high titers of a circulating antibody with specificity for a nuclear ribonucleoprotein antigen (1). Considerable controversy exists regarding whether MCTD represents a distinct entity, is instead a variant of SLE, PSS, or polymyositis, or is one aspect of a heterogeneous group of overlap syndromes. This question will be resolved with certainty only when pathogenic mechanisms in the connective tissue diseases are better understood.

The prevalence of MCTD is unknown, but it appears to be more common than polymyositis and less frequent than SLE. The age range extends from 4–80 years with a mean of 37 years. Approximately 80% of the patients are female.

Clinical features. The typical clinical features of MCTD consist of Raynaud's phenomenon, polyarthralgia or arthritis, puffiness of the hands, esophageal hypomotility, diminished pulmonary diffusing capacity, and inflammatory myopathy. Raynaud's phenomenon, present in approximately 85% of patients, may precede other disease manifestations by months or years (1–3).

More than two-thirds of the patients have sausage-like swelling of the fingers with edema and increased collagen content in the dermis. Diffuse sclerodermatous changes and ischemic necrosis or ulceration of the fingertips are infrequent in MCTD. Other frequent cutaneous find-

ings include lupus-like rashes, erythematous patches over the knuckles, violaceous discoloration of the eyelids, diffuse nonscarring alopecia, and periungual telangiectasia.

Almost all patients have polyarthralgias and three-fourths have frank arthritis (1–4). Although the arthritis is usually nondeforming, in some cases changes are indistinguishable from rheumatoid arthritis, including erosions and subcutaneous nodules. Proximal muscle weakness with or without tenderness is common (1–3).

Levels of serum creatine phosphokinase and aldolase activity may be elevated and electromyograms show typical inflammatory myopathy. Muscle fibers degenerate and interstitial and perivascular infiltrates of lymphocytes and plasma cells are seen.

Systemic manifestations. Radiographic and manometric studies have revealed evidence of esophageal dysfunction in 80% of patients, including many who are asymptomatic (5). The characteristic abnormalities include a decreased amplitude of peristalsis in the distal two-thirds of the esophagus, and a decrease in both upper and lower sphincter pressure.

Abnormalities in pulmonary function including decreased diffusing capacity and, less often, reduced lung volume have been found in 80% of patients tested (6). Roentgenograms of the chest often reveal diffuse interstitial infiltrates and, less frequently, evidence of pleural disease. In occasional patients, involvement of the lung is the predominant clinical problem, leading to exertional dyspnea and/or pulmonary hypertension.

Although cardiac involvement appears

to be less common than pulmonary disease in the adult, nearly two-thirds of children with MCTD in one study had evidence of heart disease, including pericarditis, myocarditis leading to congestive heart failure, and aortic insufficiency (4).

Renal disease, indicated by proteinuria, hematuria, and/or an abnormal kidney biopsy specimen (usually mesangial hypercellularity and/or focal glomerulitis) occurs in only about 10% of patients with MCTD and is often mild (1–3). On occasion, however, kidney involvement becomes a major clinical problem and patients have died because of progressive renal failure (2–3).

Serious neurologic abnormalities are noted in only 10% of patients with MCTD (1–3). Neurologic findings have included trigeminal sensory neuropathy, organic mental syndrome, "vascular" headaches, aseptic meningitis, seizures, cerebral thrombosis or hemorrhage, and multiple peripheral neuropathies.

Moderate anemia and leukopenia occur in 30–40% of cases (1–3). Clinically significant Coombs positive hemolytic anemia and thrombocytopenia are rare except in children (4). Other findings include fever, lymphadenopathy (often of massive proportions), splenomegaly, hepatomegaly, intestinal involvement similar to that of PSS, Sjögren's syndrome, and Hashimoto's thyroiditis.

Serologic characteristics. Almost all patients with MCTD have high titers (frequently >1:1,000) of antinuclear antibodies (ANA), which produce a speckled pattern of immunofluorescence. Utilizing the technique of passive hemagglutination, one typically finds extremely high titers (frequently >1:100,000) of antibody to a nuclear ribonucleoprotein antigen (1) that is extractable in isotonic buffer—**extractable nuclear antigen (ENA)**.

Immunodiffusion studies have shown that ENA consists of at least 2 distinct antigens. One, sensitive to ribonuclease and trypsin, is the nuclear ribonucleoprotein (RNP) to which antibodies are found in MCTD. The other, resistant to RNASe and trypsin, is the previously described Sm antigen to which antibodies are found in systemic lupus erythematosus (7–9). Antibodies to RNP, Sm, and several other nuclear acidic protein antigens all produce speckled ANA patterns (10) (Fig 13–10D). Patients with MCTD characteristically have high titers of antibody to RNASe-sensitive ENA by hemagglutination and antibody to only RNP and not to Sm by immunodiffusion. High titers of circulating RNP antibody usually persist during periods of remission as well as disease activity. Rarely, patients with clinical features of MCTD lack RNA antibody or have antibodies to both RNP and Sm.

Other frequent serologic findings in MCTD include an elevated erythrocyte sedimentation rate, diffuse hypergammaglobulinemia, and positive tests for rheumatoid factor. In contrast, antibodies to native DNA and positive LE cell reactions are infrequent; serum complement levels are slightly to moderately reduced in about 25% of patients.

The finding of high titers of antibody to RNP alone is much more frequently associated with clinical features of MCTD than with other individual rheumatic diseases in most studies (1,2,4,7,11,12). One recent report, however, showed that only half of 44 patients with anti-RNP in the absence of anti-Sm had any overlap type features typical of MCTD (13).

Immunologic characteristics. Although the etiology and pathogenesis of MCTD are unknown, various immunologic abnormalities have been observed, for example, persistence over many years of extremely high titers of RNP antibody; marked hypergammaglobulinemia; mild to moderate hypocomplementemia; presence of circulating immune complexes during active disease (14); specific deposition of IgG, IgM, or complement in the walls of blood vessels or muscle fibers, along the glomerular basement membrane, and at the dermoepidermal junction (3,15,16); and infiltrations of lymphocytes and plasma cells in many tissues (3,15,16).

A recent indication that MCTD may be unique is provided by the findings of abnormalities of immunoregulatory T cell circuits in MCTD which are quite different from those found in SLE, PSS, and rheumatoid arthritis (17).

One of the major findings in patients with fatal disease is a proliferative intimal and/or medial vascular lesion that results in narrowing of the lumen of large vessels (e.g., aorta, coronary, pulmonary, and renal) and small arterioles of many organs, (3,16) often associated with pulmonary hypertension (18).

Treatment. Although no controlled studies have been performed, many of the manifestations of MCTD appear to respond to corticosteroid therapy (1–3). Mild disease is often controlled by nonsteroidal antiinflammatory drugs or low doses of corticosteroids. When more severe involvement of major organs supervenes, larger doses, e.g., 1 mg/kg/day of prednisone, are employed. Improvement in scleroderma-like skin changes and in esophageal and pulmonary function has been noted after corticosteroid therapy (1,5,6). In general, however, the scleroderma-like features of MCTD are least likely to respond.

When one collects the recent observations on MCTD-related morbidity and mortality, it is necessary to modify early predictions of a generally favorable prognosis. In 5 series with sequential evaluations (2,16,18–20), the combined frequency of 24 deaths in 186 patients (13%) suggests that the prognosis for MCTD is similar to that of SLE and somewhat better than that of PSS.

1. Sharp GC, Irvin WS, Tan EM, Gould RG, Holman HR: Mixed connective tissue disease—an apparently distinct rheumatic disease syndrome associated with a specific antibody to an extractable nuclear antigen (ENA). Am J Med 52:148–159, 1972
2. Sharp GC, Irvin WS, May CM, Holman HR, McDuffie FC, Hess EV, Schmid FR: Association of antibodies to ribonucleoprotein and Sm antigens with mixed connective tissue disease, systemic lupus erythematosus and other rheumatic diseases. N Engl J Med 295:1149–1154, 1976
3. Wolfe JF, Kingsland L, Lindberg D, Sharp GC: Disease pattern in patients with antibodies only to nuclear ribonucleoprotein (abstract). Clin Res 25:488A, 1977.
4. Singsen BH, Bernstein BH, Kornreich HK, King KK, Hanson V, Tan EM: Mixed connective tissue disease in childhood. J Pediatr 90:893–900, 1977
5. Winn D, Gerhardt D, Winship D, Sharp GC: Esophageal function in steroid treated patients with mixed connective tissue disease (abstract). Clin Res 24: 545A, 1976.
6. Harmon C, Wolfe JF, Lillard S, Heid C, Cordon R, Sharp GC: Pulmonary involvement in mixed connective tissue disease (abstract). Arthritis Rheum 19:801, 1976
7. Northway JD, Tan EM: Differentiations of antinuclear antibodies giving speckled staining patterns in immunofluorescence. Clin Immunol Immunopathol 1:140–154, 1972
8. Sharp GC, Irvin WS, Northway JD, Tan EM: Specificity of antibodies to extractable nuclear antigens in mixed connective tissue disease and systemic lupus erythematosus (abstract). Arthritis Rheum 15:125, 1972
9. Reichlin M, Mattioli M: Correlation of a precipitin reaction to an RNA protein antigen and low prevalence of nephritis in patients with systemic lupus erythematosus. N Engl J Med 286:908, 1972
10. Tan EM, Christian C, Holman HR, Homma M, Kunkel HG, Reichlin M, Sharp GC, Ziff M, Barnett EV: Antitissue antibodies in rheumatic disease: standardization and nomenclature. Arthritis Rheum 20:1419–1420 1977
11. Parker MD: Ribonucleoprotein antibodies: frequencies and clinical significance in systemic lupus erythematosus, scleroderma, and mixed connective tissue disease. J Lab Clin Med 82:769–775, 1973
12. Notman DD, Kurata N, Tan EM: Profiles of antinuclear antibodies in systemic rheumatic diseases. Ann Intern Med 83:464–469, 1975
13. Lemmer JP, Curry NH, Mallory JH, Waller MV: Clinical characteristics and course in patients with high titer anti-RNP antibodies. J Rheumatol 9:536–542, 1982
14. Halla JT, Volanakis JE, Schrohenloher RE: Circulating immune complexes in mixed connective tissue disease. Arthritis Rheum 22:484–489, 1979
15. Oxenhander R, Hart M, Corman L, Sharp GC, Adelstein E: Pathology of skeletal muscle in mixed connective tissue disease. Arthritis Rheum 20:985–988, 1977
16. Singsen BH, Swanson VL, Bernstein BH, Heuser ET, Hanson V, Landing BH: A histologic evaluation of mixed connective tissue disease in childhood. Am J Med 68:710–717, 1980
17. Alarcón-Segovia D, Palacios R: Human postthymic precursor cells in health and disease. IV. Abnormalities in immunoregulatory T cell circuits in mixed connective tissue disease. Arthritis Rheum 24:1486–1494, 1981
18. Esther JH, Sharp GC, Agia G, Hurst DJ: Pulmonary hypertension in patients with mixed connective tissue disease and antibody to nuclear ribonucleoprotein. Arthritis Rheum 24:S105, 1981
19. Grant KD, Adams LE, Hess EV: Mixed connective tissue disease: a subset with sequential clinical and laboratory features. J Rheumatol 8:587–598, 1981
20. Nimelstein SH, Brody S, McShane D, Holman HR: Mixed connective tissue disease: a subsequent evaluation of the original 25 patients. Medicine (Baltimore) 59:239–248, 1980

16. Polymyositis and dermatomyositis

Polymyositis and dermatomyositis are diffuse inflammatory disorders of striated muscle which cause symmetrical weakness and, to a lesser degree, atrophy of muscles principally of the limb girdles, neck, and pharynx. These are perplexing disorders of unknown cause which occur in all age groups and are usually grouped with the connective tissue diseases. Such inclusion appears to be warranted since overlapping clinical and laboratory features commonly occur, especially with rheumatoid arthritis and scleroderma, and less frequently with systemic lupus erythematosus or polyarteritis nodosa. In addition, a link seems to exist between certain cases of myositis and malignant neoplasms.

Classification. The classification of polymyositis and dermatomyositis (1,2) has perplexed all who had attempted to deal with this problem, since the origins of these conditions are unknown. The following classification is useful (3):

Group 1. Primary idiopathic polymyositis

Group 2. Primary idiopathic dermatomyositis

Group 3. Dermatomyositis (or polymyositis) associated with neoplasia

Group 4. Childhood dermatomyositis (or polymyositis) associated with vasculitis

Group 5. Polymyositis or dermatomyositis associated with collagen-vascular disease (overlap group)

Clinical features. Polymyositis and dermatomyositis may occur at any age. Females are affected twice as commonly as males. The general frequency is difficult to assess, so only estimates are possible. However, this condition is not rare. One group of authors saw 89 cases during a 12-year span from an estimated regional population of 3.3 million persons and calculated an approximate incidence of 1 case per 280,000 population per year. Another survey estimates 1:200,000 population per year. Among the primary myopathies affecting the pelvis, shoulder girdle, and proximal portions of the extremities, polymyositis is about as common as muscular dystrophy in adult life, whereas in childhood it is much less common.

Polymyositis is varied not only in its mode of onset but also in rate of progression of symptoms, whether muscular, dermal, articular, or other. Moreover, in some patients the clinical course is one of spontaneous remissions and exacerbations. This variability makes it difficult to provide a unified clinical portrait of the disease. The extremes include acute polymyositis, with or without an edematous skin rash, severe constitutional symptoms and rapid weight loss, and the gradual appearance of weakness in the pelvic girdle musculature over a period of 5 or more years with few or no other features.

Muscular weakness is present in nearly all patients with all types of polymyositis except for a very few with characteristic dermal manifestations in the absence of clinical, histologic, or electromyographic evidence of myositis. In subacute or chronic cases, the weakness develops slowly and first affects the lower extremities, closely resembling muscular dystrophy. The individual experiences difficulty in arising from the floor or getting out of a bathtub. It may become impossible to climb up a high bus step, and soon difficulty is encountered when arising from a low chair and then from a higher chair. Stairs can be ascended only with the assistance of a handrail and the gait becomes clumsy and waddling. Shortly after pelvic girdle weakness occurs, strength is lost in the shoulder girdle. Combing the hair or keeping the arms elevated for a few moments is impossible. Weakness of the anterior neck muscles is shown by the inability to raise the head from the pillow while in bed. Involvement of the posterior pharyngeal muscles accounts for dysphagia and dysphonia (nasal voice).

In a few patients, muscular pain, tenderness, and induration are present in the early stages; these features are usually accompanied by the rash of dermatomyositis. Contractures or shortening of muscles rarely occur early and instead are features of advanced or long-standing disease.

The classic rash of dermatomyositis occurs in about 40% of patients with inflammatory myopathy. The eruptions, consisting of dusky-red patches slightly elevated and smooth or slightly scaly, are found on the elbows, over the dorsum of the proximal interphalangeal and metacarpophalangeal joints, over the knees, and on the medial malleoli at the ankles. At times linear hyperemic streaks are seen on the dorsum of the hands and fingers with accentuation over the joints. Hyperemia may be present at the base and sides of the fingernails and fingertips. These areas sometimes become shiny, red, and atrophic. Frequently there is a coexistent dusky erythematous eruption on the face, especially in the "butterfly" and periorbital areas. Occasionally this is present on the forehead as well as on the neck, shoulders, and front and back of the upper chest area. On the upper eyelids, a peculiar dusky lilac suffusion is sometimes seen. This is called the **heliotrope rash** and is typical of dermatomyositis (Fig 16–1). In addition, periorbital edema may occur.

Raynaud's phenomenon is another symptom. Polyarthritis or polyarthralgia is usually early and transitory (4). A small percentage of patients develop intestinal disturbances and pulmonary infiltrates or fibrosis (5). Myocarditis and conduction abnormalities can occur (6). Dysphagia is usually due to weakness or paralysis of the posterior pharyngeal striated musculature, but manometric studies will also demonstrate hypomotility of the esophagus, similar to that found in scleroderma in some cases. Some patients with dermatomyositis, particularly children and young adults, develop widespread calcification of the skin, subcutaneous, and periarticular tissues, as well as muscle (*calcinosis universalis*).

Children with dermatomyositis may have abdominal pain and hematemesis and melena as a result of widespread gastrointestinal ulceration which occasionally leads to perforation with complicating mediastinitis and peritonitis.

Coexistence of malignant disease. Malignant neoplasms are found in patients with polymyositis and dermatomyositis more often than in the general population (7),

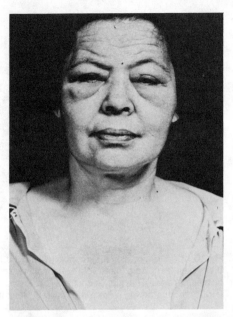

Fig 16–1. This patient has periorbital edema and a purplish (heliotrope) discoloration of the eyelids. Both findings occur in dermatomyositis but are not necessarily diagnostic. Note also the erythema over the upper sternum and the V area of the neck. (From the Clinical Slide Collection on the Rheumatic Diseases)

nearly always in adults beyond the age of 40 years. Internal malignancies were found in 27% of adults over age 55 with polymyositis or dermatomyositis (8).

Some studies suggest that adult dermatomyositis is more likely to be related to tumors. The most common malignancies are carcinoma of the lung, prostate, ovary, uterus, breast, or large intestine. Less commonly, the stomach, gall bladder, parotid gland, tonsil, and other organs have been the source of the tumor. Lymphoma, Hodgkin's disease, or benign or malignant thymoma have also been described in conjunction with dermatomyositis. Treatment or removal of the malignancy may be followed by remarkable improvement in the muscle disease.

Pathology. The location for muscle biopsy should be carefully judged in accordance with the electrical abnormalities noted below. The (proximal) muscle selected should be one that is slightly weakened but not yet completely atrophic. The quadriceps femoris and the deltoid usually yield the most fruitful results (Fig 16–2). The pathologic alterations include: 1) focal or extensive primary degeneration of muscle fibers; 2) basophilia of some fibers with prominent central positioning of nuclei (features of regeneration); 3) necrosis of parts or entire groups of muscle fibers; 4) focal or diffuse infiltrates of chronic inflammatory cells (chiefly small lymphocytes and lesser numbers of plasma cells); when focal, these infiltrates are usually located around or near blood vessels or between individual muscle fibers; 5) interstitial fibrosis which varies in severity,

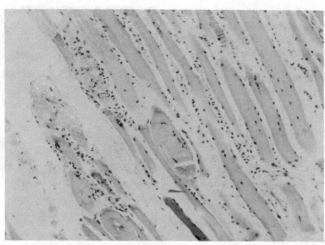

Fig 16–2. Acute myositis. Lymphocytes and histiocytes have infiltrated the muscle fibers. Many of these skeletal muscle fibers appear normal. Two are necrotic and another is fragmented and invaded by macrophages. The muscle changes in polymyositis are identical to those found in dermatomyositis (H&E, medium power). (From the Revised Clinical Slide Collection on the Rheumatic Diseases)

especially with the duration of the disease and to some extent with the type of disease; and 6) a variation in cross-sectional diameter of fibers, especially in disease of relatively long duration.

In children with dermatomyositis, there may be an impressive degree of inflammation and thickening of small arteries and veins in the gastrointestinal tract, muscles, and small nerves. Occlusion of these vessels may lead to infarction.

Laboratory findings. Results of most of the routine laboratory tests are normal with the exception of an elevation of the erythrocyte sedimentation rate and an alteration of some of the serum acute-phase reactive proteins. In acute cases, a neutrophilic leukocytosis may occur, but anemia is rare unless severe debility or accompanying neoplasm coexists. Antinuclear antibodies or positive LE cell tests are rarely found, even when the facial rash resembles that of systemic lupus. Elevated titers of tests for rheumatoid factor were found in 40% of cases in 1 series.

Although not pathognomonic, elevation of serum levels of various enzymes that normally reside within skeletal muscle fibers is of considerable diagnostic and prognostic assistance. Transaminase, creatine phosphokinase, and aldolase are sensitive indicators of muscle injury and these enzymes can also be used to prognosticate a beneficial therapeutic effect when a decrease occurs in the course of treatment or during a spontaneous remission.

Myoglobinemia and more often myoglobinuria of mild degree are common, particularly in patients with dermatomyositis. On rare occasions, the occurrence of severe myoglobinuria has been associated with the development of (reversible) renal failure.

Electromyographic findings are helpful in establishing the diagnosis. Some features are common to both denervation and primary muscle disease. Generally, the characteristic triad of findings in polymyositis consists of 1) spontaneous fibrillations and positive "saw-toothed" (spike) potentials, 2) complex polyphasic or short-duration potentials which appear on voluntary contraction, and 3) salvos of repetitive high frequency action potentials (*pseudomyotonia*).

Prognosis. It is generally agreed that prognosis is better in children than in adults and that younger adult patients survive longer than older ones. In one series that used life-table methods, the overall cumulative survival after a 7-year follow-up period was 53% but 90% for children. Adults under 50 years at diagnosis survived significantly longer than those 50 or older, even excluding those with associated malignancy.

Origin. The origins of polymyositis and dermatomyositis are not known. A multitude of infectious agents has been suspected but none proved. Increased titers of antibodies against toxoplasma have been described in up to 35% of patients, but isolation of toxoplasma from muscles in typical polymyositis has not been achieved and polymyositis generally does not respond to therapy against toxoplasma (9).

One explanation for the concurrence of dermatomyositis and malignant tumors is that the neoplasm induces the muscle disease through an immunologic or hypersensitivity reaction. In this view, the myositis may be the result of an autoimmune reaction, perhaps directed against a similar or common antigen in the tumor and muscle.

Search for the presence of circulating antibody directed against muscle tissue has been unrewarding. However, deposits of IgG, IgM, and C3, alone or in combination, were found in the blood vessel walls of skeletal muscle of 17 of 39 patients with polymyositis. These deposits were particularly common in children. A more recent study in children identified vascular IgM, C3d, and fibrin but not IgG and C3 (10), and the authors considered this evidence against typical immune complex–mediated injury. Lymphocytic and noninflammatory vascular injury seemed more prominent in this study.

Other studies suggest that certain types of polymyositis may be due to cell-mediated immune reactions. In one investigation, lymphocytes from patients with polymyositis were incubated with whole-muscle homogenates and showed a significantly higher uptake of tritiated thymidine (indicating activation of the cells) than did lymphocytes from patients with other diseases, with and without muscle wasting. Activated lymphocytes from patients with polymyositis have been found to be cytotoxic to fetal muscle cells in culture. This has been traced to the production of a lymphotoxin, whose action is inhibited by the addition of methylprednisolone.

Picornavirus-like structures have been visualized in muscle cells of a few patients with polymyositis; in many more, tubular inclusions (considered not be be actual viruses but often associated with virus infection) have been found in muscle and endothelial cells of vessels in skin, muscle, and synovium (4,11).

Treatment. Treatment of polymyositis is now moderately satisfactory. This consists of supportive therapy, corticosteroids, and in some cases, immunosuppressive or cytotoxic agents. Sustained improvement usually occurs in patients with straightforward polymyositis or dermatomyositis, whereas in some children and in adults with coexistent malignancy or with Sjögren's syndrome, the response will often be poor or only temporarily beneficial.

Adults should receive prednisone, 50–60 mg per day. Serial analysis of serum enzyme levels provides the best early guide to the effectiveness of this treatment. If enzyme levels fall toward normal, return in strength will probably soon occur. The prednisone dosage is then reduced slowly, while the serum enzyme levels are continually monitored. Rapid lowering of the dose or attempts to discontinue therapy abruptly have generally been met with recurrent elevation of serum enzyme levels and the reappearance of symptoms several weeks later. Long-term maintenance therapy with 7.5–20 mg of prednisone daily is often necessary to control the disease.

It has become apparent that a number of adult patients respond poorly to corticosteroids but improve when such treatment is supplemented with either weekly intravenous methotrexate (12) or azathioprine (13).

A search for malignant neoplasm should be undertaken in individuals over 40 years. Extensiveness of such a search depends on clinical clues and findings from less invasive studies. If a tumor is found and removed, complete remission of the dermatomyositis process may ensue without the need for adjunctive therapy.

1. Pearson CM: Polymyositis. Ann Rev Med 17:63–82, 1966
2. Walton JN: Classification of the neuromuscular disorders. J Neurol Sci 6:165–177, 1968
3. Bohan A, Peter JB: Polymyositis and dermatomyositis. N Engl J Med 292:344–347 1975
4. Schumacher HR, Schimmer B, Gordon GV, et al: Articular manifestations of polymyositis and dermatomyositis. Am J Med 67:287–292, 1979
5. Salmeron G, Greenberg SD, Lidsky MD: Polymyositis and diffuse interstitial lung disease. Arch Intern Med 141:1005–1010, 1981
6. Kehoe RF, Bauernfeind R, Tommaso C, et al: Cardiac conduction defects in polymyositis. Ann Intern Med 94:41–43, 1981
7. Williams RC Jr: Dermatomyositis and malignancy: a review of the literature. Ann Intern Med 50:1174–1181, 1959
8. Callen JP, Hyla JF, Bole GG, et al: The relationship of dermatomyositis and polymyositis to internal malignancy. Arch Dermatol 116:295–298, 1980
9. Phillips PE, Kassan SS, Kagen LJ: Increased toxoplasma antibodies in idiopathic inflammatory muscle disease: a case controlled study. Arthritis Rheum 22:209–214, 1979
10. Crowe WE, Bove KE, Levinson JE, et al: Clinical and pathogenetic implications of histopathology in childhood polydermatomyositis. Arthritis Rheum 25:126–139, 1982
11. Norton WL, Velayos E, Robisan L; Endothelial inclusions in dermatomyositis. Ann Rheum Dis 29:67–71, 1970
12. Metzger AL, Bohan A, Goldberg LS: Polymyositis and dermatomyositis: combined methotrexate and corticosteroid therapy. Ann Intern Med 81:182–188, 1974
13. Bunch TW: Prednisone and azathioprine for polymyositis: long term followup. Arthritis Rheum 24:45–48 1981

17. Myasthenia gravis

Myasthenia gravis is a disease of the endplates of striated muscles which affects women more than men. Incidence peaks in the third or fourth decades, but it may occur any time from childhood until well into late adult life. In older patients, men and women are equally affected.

The primary clinical features consist of progressive weakness with exertion and involvement of muscles supplied by cranial nerves, resulting in unilateral or bilateral ptosis, diplopia, dysphagia, and other bulbar signs, especially dysphonia and paralysis of the respiratory musculature. In most instances the musculature of the limbs may be affected as well, although a purely ocular form exists. The development of progressively increasing weakness later in the day with added activities is frequently noted.

In most instances an association with a pathologic thymus gland (either thymic hyperplasia or a thymoma) occurs. A progressive decline in the amplitude of recruited motor units, as determined by repetitive nerve stimulation at low frequency (2–10 seconds) of stimulation, is frequently observed.

It seems clear that myasthenia gravis (MG) represents an autoimmune disorder which involves an immunologic response toward one or more proteins at the neuromuscular junction (1). Myasthenia gravis appears to occur with increased frequency in individuals with various connective tissue diseases including rheumatoid arthritis and systemic and discoid lupus erythematosus (2). In 1973 Patrick and Lindstrom observed that a disorder resembling MG developed in rabbits injected with purified postsynaptic acetylcholine receptor protein (AChR) (3). Circulating antibodies directed against AChR are present in significant quantities in most patients with MG (1,4). There is also evidence of a cellular immune response to AChR in individuals with MG. However, this mechanism appears to be of lesser pathogenetic importance than the circulating antibodies. Antibodies to skeletal muscle are also found in patients with MG, as well as in a large number of persons with thymoma, even those without MG (5).

Antibody to receptor has been identified at the neuromuscular junction (4,6). Further support of this hypothesis is the observation that newborn children of mothers with MG develop a myasthenic syndrome responsive to neostigmine which remits spontaneously after 2–3 weeks. Presumably, this is caused by AChR antibodies originating in the mother and entering the fetal bloodstream (4). Moreover, serum immunoglobulin from myasthenia is capable of passively transferring disease to mice (7).

The development of a myasthenia gravis–like syndrome has also been reported in a small number of patients with rheumatoid arthritis, Wilson's disease, or progressive systemic sclerosis who are under treatment with D-penicillamine (8). These individuals have been shown to have high titers of anti-AChR in their sera. The muscle disorder subsides after discontinuation of the drug.

Treatment. Surgical resection of the thymus is frequently successful in inducing remission (20–40%) or improvement (20–40%). Symptoms frequently respond to anticholinesterase agents such as neostigmine or pyridostigmine. Plasmapheresis has proved successful in treating patients with life-threatening disease (9). Corticosteroids or immunosuppresive agents may be useful in certain patients (4).

1. Lindstrom JM, Seybold ME, Lennon VA, Whittingham, Sand Duane DD: Antibody to acetylcholine receptor in myasthenia gravis: prevalence, chemical correlates, and diagnostic value. Neurology 26:1054–1059, 1976
2. Simpson JA: Myasthenia gravis, a new hypothesis. Scot Med J 5:419–436, 1960
3. Patrick J, Lindstrom JM: Autoimmune response to acetylcholine receptor. Science 180:871–872, 1973
4. Lisak RP, Barch RL: Myasthenia Gravis. Philadelphia, WB Saunders Co, 1982
5. Strauss AJC, Seegal BC, Hsu, KC, Burkholder PM, Nastuk WL, Osserman KE: Immunofluoresence demonstration of a muscle binding complement fixed serum globulin fraction in myasthenia gravis. Proc Soc Exp Biol Med 105:184–195, 1960
6. Lindstrom JM, Lambert EH: Content of acetylcholine receptor and antibodies bound to receptor in myasthenia gravis: experimental autoimmune myasthenia gravis and Eaton Lambert syndrome. Neurology 28:130–138, 1978
7. Toyka KV, Drachman DB, Pestrouk A, Koo I: Myasthenia gravis: passive transfer from man to mouse. Science 190:397–399, 1975
8. Masters CL, Dawkins RL, Zilko PJ, Simpson JA, Leedman RJ, Lindstrom J: Pencillamine-associated myasthemia gravis, antiacetylcholine receptor and antistriational antibodies. Am J Med 63:689–694, 1977
9. Pinching AJ, Peters DK, Newsom-Davis J: Remission of myasthenia gravis following plasma-exchange. Lancet 2:1373–1376, 1976

18. Systemic necrotizing vasculitis and other forms of vasculitis

The generic term, **systemic necrotizing vasculitis** will be used in this section to denote a clinically widely diverse group of syndromes related by the presence of a necrotizing inflammatory process of the blood vessels (1–4). This term is preferred over previously popular designations, such as polyarteritis and necrotizing arteritis, since in several of these disorders the vascular lesions involve not only the arteries and arterioles but the veins, capillaries, and sometimes the lymph vessels.

At present there is no standard classification of vasculitides. Earlier attempts to subclassify these syndromes on the basis of histopathologic changes resulted in the creation of a confusing system of overlapping clinical syndromes. The differential diagnosis of the systemic necrotizing vasculitides is based on a constellation of clinical and pathologic findings. It is important that the correct diagnosis be established as early as possible to institute appropriate therapeutic regimens. Current therapies often result in dramatic remissions of what were previously catastrophic disorders.

A useful classification of the necrotizing vasculitides for diagnostic, prognostic, and therapeutic purposes is tabulated in Table 18–1.

Pathogenesis. Although no specific etiologic factors have yet been found which would unify these disorders, the pathogenesis in a number of these syndromes appears to lie in a disordered immune response to an antigenic stimulus, which results in the development of circulating immune complexes that deposit in blood vessels. This deposition leads to inflammatory changes and fibrinoid necrosis of the vessel walls.

In some of these syndromes a specific antigen has been recognized. In 25% or more of patients with classic polyarteritis nodosa, evidence of hepatitis B virus surface antigen (HBsAg) circulating with its antibody has been found in the plasma and in deposits in the arteritic lesions (5). Indeed, a variety of vasculitic syndromes may occur in response to hepatitis B virus infection, ranging from classic polyarteritis nodosa with severe, multiple organ involvement to localized vasculitis in patients with essential mixed cryoglobulinemia (see Section 23).

A variety of other antigenic substances (i.e., infectious agents, drugs) have been

Table 18–1. Varieties of systemic necrotizing vasculitis and other vasculitides

Classic polyarteritis (nodosa)
Allergic granulomatous angiitis
Systemic necrotizing vasculitis—overlap syndrome
Cogan's syndrome
Hypersensitivity vasculitis
   Serum sickness
   Schönlein-Henoch purpura
   Cutaneous vasculitis, including hypocomplementemic vasculitis
   Essential mixed cryoglobulinemia
   Vasculitis associated with other connective tissue diseases
   Subacute bacterial endocarditis
   Benign hyperglobulinemic purpura
   Vasculitis associated with malignancies
Goodpasture's syndrome
Wegener's granulomatosis
Giant cell arteritis
   Temporal arteritis
   Takayasu's arteritis
Kawasaki disease (acute febrile mucocutaneous lymph node syndrome)
Miscellaneous vasculitides

implicated in some cases of vasculitis, but these syndromes are almost certainly multifactorial in origin, with environmental and genetic factors playing a role in determining the type and severity of the vasculitic syndromes.

Polyarteritis

This is the term now assigned to the classic syndrome of periarteritis nodosa described by A Kussmaul and R Maier in 1866 and characterized by involvement of medium-sized and small muscular arteries (Fig 18–1). The disease varies in extent and severity from a relatively benign form of cutaneous vasculitis that may resolve spontaneously to a much more serious, often fatal, disorder affecting blood vessels in many organs.

When it was learned that all 3 layers of the blood vessel wall were involved (rather than a perivasculitis), the syndrome was more appropriately called *polyarteritis nodosa*. The appellative *nodosa* was subsequently deleted when clinically detectable nodular lesions were found to occur in only 10–15% of cases.

The polyarteritic lesion tends to be segmental, with a predilection for bifurcations and branching of arteries with distal spread involving arterioles. Venous involvement occurs solely through contiguity. The early lesion is marked by necrosis in the media and intima followed by infiltration of the vessel walls first with neutrophils and later with mononuclear cells and fibroblasts. Attempts at repair result in fibrosis of the arterial wall and intimal proliferation, often leading to thrombosis, ischemia, and infarction. Only a portion of the circumference of the vessel wall may be affected, leading to aneurysmal dilatation and rupture. Characteristically, the vascular changes are found in all phases of development.

Polyarteritis can affect the vessels of any organ but involvement of the pulmonary and splenic vessels is uncommon. Multiple organs are involved and the variable clinical picture reflects the sites and degree of severity of vascular damage.

Clinical features. Polyarteritis predominantly affects men in middle life (6) but also occurs in children (7). The onset may be acute or insidious. Presenting symptoms and clinical findings are so protean that a unified clinical picture is difficult to portray. Polyarteritis may begin as fever of unknown origin, since fever, weakness, malaise, and weight loss are commonly present.

The kidney is the most frequently affected site (80%). In terms of prognosis, it is the key organ since renal failure is the most common cause of death. Polyarteritis of the renal arteries or necrotizing glomerulonephritis may occur, simultaneously or independently. Arterial hypertension, present more often than not, is

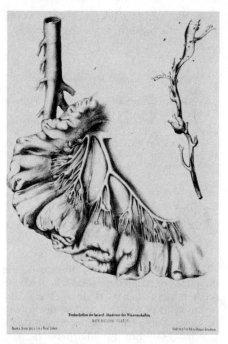

Fig 18–1. First case of polyarteritis nodosa examined at autopsy (K von Rokitansky, 1852), illustrating aneurysms of mesenteric arteries.

the result of healed arteritis of the kidney vessels (even of a single branch of the renal arteries). Perirenal hematoma or retroperitoneal hemorrhage may result from rupture of aneurysms in the kidney.

Cardiac involvement (70%) is the second most common cause of death. Congestive heart failure may result from myocardial infarction due to coronary arteritis or hypertension secondary to renal polyarteritis. Pericarditis occurs more frequently than is recognized antemortem.

Gastrointestinal involvement (65%) may give rise to symptoms of an "acute abdomen," hematemesis, melena, gastric or intestinal ulceration, perforation, infarction, intestinal obstruction, intussusception, or rupture of a mesenteric arterial aneurysm.

In addition, there may be signs of liver involvement, especially in those individuals with hepatitis B virus infection. When seropositive (HBsAg) patients with polyarteritis are compared with seronegative patients, the only significant clinical difference is the liver disease.

Involvement of the gall bladder occurs with notable frequency. Acute pancreatitis and acute appendicitis result from inflammation of the vessels of these organs. Peripheral neuropathy (50%) is frequently bilateral, but tends to be asymmetric and more pronounced in the lower extremities (mononeuritis multiplex). Less commonly, cerebral arteritis may produce convulsions, hemiparesis, or subarachnoid hemorrhage.

Arthralgias are more common than arthritis and are due to arterial lesions rather than synovitis. Muscle weakness may result from involvement of the arterial blood supply or from a peripheral neuropathy. Testicular pain, tenderness, swelling, or atrophy may occur. In a few patients, tender subcutaneous nodules, the result of aneurysms of superficial blood vessels, appear in crops along the course of arteries. Other cutaneous findings include subcutaneous hemorrhage, livedo reticularis, superficial ulcerations, gangrene, and splinter hemorrhages.

Laboratory findings. Leukocytosis with neutrophilia is commonly noted, but eosinophilia is rare. Anemia, when present, is due to blood loss or renal insufficiency. The sedimentation rate is usually elevated, serum immunoglobulin levels are frequently increased, and thrombocytosis may be present. Proteinuria, microscopic hematuria, and cylindruria are common. Antinuclear and rheumatoid factors are rarely found; when detected they are usually present in low titer.

Biopsy of an appropriate organ is the preferred means of definitive diagnosis. When signs and symptoms are present in the skin, testes, or peripheral nerve tissue, biopsy of these sites is frequently rewarding. Renal biopsy is hazardous (because of the risk of perinephric bleeding), and rectal and muscle biopsy results are often disappointing. The segmental distribution of the arteritis makes examinations of multiple biopsy sections mandatory. In the absence of an appropriate site for biopsy, angiographic study of the renal, hepatic, or mesenteric arteries is often helpful, even if there is no evidence of visceral involvement detectable by other means (4,6).

The angiographic findings consist of microaneurysms and/or sharply segmental narrowing (or pruning) of medium-sized arteries (Fig 18–2). Aneurysms may evolve, rupture, or resolve. They are not specific and may also occur in Wegener's granulomatosis, allergic granulomatous angiitis, and thrombotic thrombocytopenic purpura (6). Although these angiographic abnormalities are highly characteristic of polyarteritis, they are not indispensable for the diagnosis.

Treatment. Prolonged survival has been demonstrated with the use of corticosteroid therapy, especially when instituted early in the course of the disease (8,9). In patients with severe necrotizing angiitis unresponsive to high doses of corticosteroids alone, the addition of immunosuppressive agents i.e., cyclophosphamide (3) or azathioprine (8), has appeared to be beneficial. Survival with combination therapy of corticosteroids and immunosuppressive agents has been demonstrated to be longer than that following the use of corticosteroids alone (8). Treatment with immunosuppressive agents should be reserved, however, for patients with an established diagnosis and grave prognosis who can be monitored regularly for side effects or infection.

Allergic granulomatous angiitis

Originally described by J Churg and L Strauss in 1951, this systemic necrotizing angiitis has clinicopathologic manifestations similar to polyarteritis but with certain distinguishing features (10). This uncommon disorder is usually heralded by months to years of intractable asthma or other allergic manifestations such as hay fever, drug sensitivity, or sinusitis. Those with asthma often also have arterial hypertension. Pulmonary involvement is the rule and takes the form of a migratory and variable pneumonitis resembling Loeffler's syndrome. This is frequently accompanied by a striking leukocytosis (up to $50,000/mm^3$) with eosinophilia (up to 90%) and elevated IgE levels. Palpable granulomatous nodules and cutaneous nonthrombocytopenic purpura are common.

Distinguishing pathologic findings are vascular and extravascular granulomatous lesions involving small (capillaries and venules) and medium-sized vessels. The granulomas are composed of an eosinophilic core surrounded by giant cells. An eosinophilic infiltrate is often found in the lungs. Gastrointestinal involvement is well recognized, but renal disease is uncommon (10). The etiology is unknown.

In patients treated with corticosteroids early in the course of illness, disease has been suppressed and survival extended (10). The addition of cytotoxic agents, including cyclophosphamide or azathioprine, has been shown to promote long lasting remission (1). Some patients with systemic necrotizing vasculitis have features of both this disorder and classic polyarteritis and represent a true overlap syndrome.

Cogan's syndrome

This is a rare disease of young adults who develop nonsyphilitic interstitial keratitis and vestibuloauditory dysfunction (tinnitus, vertigo, and hearing loss) over a period of weeks or months (11,12). Long-term followup observation often reveals an underlying systemic necrotizing vasculitis. Fever, lymphadenopathy, arthralgias, abdominal pain, gastrointestinal hemorrhage, splenomegaly, and cardiac manifestations are common. Approximately 10% of patients develop disease of the aortic valve which is now amenable to valvular replacement. Leukocytosis, elevated sedimentation rate, and hypereosinophilia may be found. The course is variable; occular and vestibular symptoms are self-limited but sensorineural deafness has been permanent.

Corticosteroid therapy has proved helpful in suppressing the systemic manifestations, especially when instituted early in the course of the syndrome. Since sensorineural deafness associated with vasculitis in a recently described "autoimmune" syndrome responded to long-term treatment with corticosteroids and cyclophosphamide (13), this combination is worthy of further trial in Cogan's syndrome.

Hypersensitivity vasculitis

The most common form of vasculitis, hypersensitivity vasculitis, gives rise to a heterogeneous group of syndromes. That

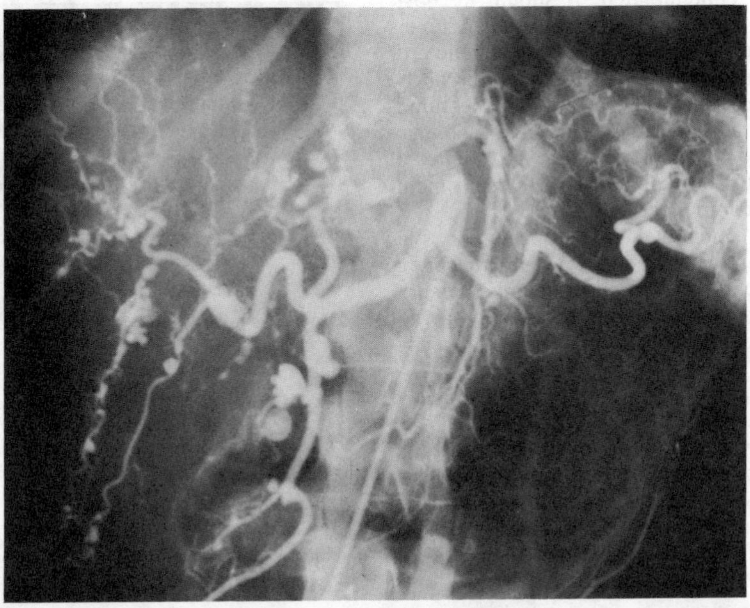

Fig 18–2. Selective celiac arteriogram of woman with polyarteritis demonstrates numerous small and large aneurysms at sites of bifurcation of the intrahepatic, gastroduodenal, and left gastric arteries. Microaneurysms are also present in the pancreatic vessels. (Illustration reproduced with permission of Citron BP et al: Necrotizing angiitis associated with drug abuse. N Engl J Med 283:1003-1011, 1970)

hypersensitivity vasculitis is mediated by immune mechanisms is suggested by its similarity to experimental serum sickness and the demonstration of circulating and/or deposited immune complexes at the site of vascular injury (1). The sensitizing agent may be recognizable as a drug or infectious particles; in some patients, an endogenous antigen such as a tumor antigen may be responsible. Usually no precipitating antigen can be identified.

These syndromes have been variously referred to as allergic vasculitis or leukocytoclastic vasculitis and their characteristic lesion is an inflammatory infiltrate in the postcapillary venule, consisting of polymorphonuclear leukocytes with leukocytoclasis (nuclear debris), fibrinoid necrosis, and extravasation of erythrocytes. The lesions are found in the same stage of development, suggesting an episodic exposure to inciting antigens, in contradistinction to classic polyarteritis where lesions are found in various stages of evolution, suggesting a more continuous exposure to sensitizing antigens.

The skin, the organ most frequently involved in hypersensitivity vasculitis, is the site of palpable purpura or hemorrhagic infarcts, often in the legs. This postcapillary venulitis may also become manifest in the form of nodules, papules, bullae, necrotic ulcers, or chronic urticaria, with or without attendant hemorrhagic lesions. Other organs may be involved, but usually not to the degree found in the more severe systemic necrotizing vasculitides.

There are many clinical syndromes classified under hypersensitivity vasculitis which display clinicopathologic features sufficiently distinct to permit their classification as subvarieties of this disorder (see Table 18–1).

In cases where the inciting antigen is known, e.g., bacterial endocarditis or drug hypersensitivity, elimination of that antigen is often sufficient to arrest the disease. Other therapeutic decisions are influenced by the pattern of organ involvement. When confined to the skin, the syndrome is often self-limiting. When the disease affects vital organs, i.e., kidney, gastrointestinal tract or nervous system, corticosteroid therapy in large doses is frequently helpful (1).

Goodpasture's syndrome

After the 1918 influenza pandemic, EW Goodpasture described an acute fulminating illness characterized by glomerulonephritis and pulmonary hemorrhage (1,14). This uncommon disorder is associated with circulating antibodies to human renal glomerular basement membrane (GBM) and human pulmonary alveolar basement membrane. The binding of this anti-GBM antibody to kidney and lung leads to an inflammatory reaction involving complement activation, polymorphonuclear leu-

kocyte chemotaxis, and platelet-coagulation cascade activation. Anti-GBM antibodies can be demonstrated in the circulation (especially after nephrectomy) and deposited in the renal glomerulus and lung.

A flu-like illness heralds the onset in most but not all patients. Men are affected 4 times as often as women. The typical patient is a man about age 30, who develops rapidly progressive acute nephritis (leading to renal failure) or acute life-threatening pulmonary hemorrhage. Both of these conditions can occur with equal frequency.

Other characteristics include microcytic hypochromic anemia, low serum iron concentration, sequestered erythrocytes in the lung, proteinuria, hematuria, and red cell casts. Serum complement levels are usually unaffected. Diffuse proliferative glomerulonephritis is found and immunohistologic study reveals the distinct but not absolutely pathognomonic pattern of linear or ribbon-like deposition of anti-GBM antibody throughout the glomerulus.

Tubular basement membrane staining is common. Anti-GBM antibodies can be eluted from the kidney or lung or may be measured directly in serum, using radioimmunoassay techniques. Circulating products of complement activation have been used to monitor disease activity. Alveolar hemorrhage and hemosiderosis are prominent in the lung.

Therapy usually includes hemodialysis, large doses of corticosteroids, and careful management of cardiac output and circulating volume. Nephrectomy, cytotoxic drugs, and plasmapheresis have been used with success (15,16). If renal transplantation is contemplated, it should be postponed until circulating anti-GBM levels subside to avoid abrupt recurrence of acute nephritis (14). Patients who can be stabilized and survive beyond the fulminating acute phase of the disease may recover in proportion to the subsidence of the antibody response to basement membrane components.

The etiology of Goodpasture's syndrome remains unclear. The inciting event may be infection, toxic inhalant exposure, or both. The perpetuating antigen has not been identified definitively, but most evidence pinpoints the noncollagen, heteropolysaccharide-containing portions of basement membranes.

Early recognition of these acutely ill patients and aggressive support have permitted a substantial proportion to return to a useful and functional state. The precise immunologic mechanisms involved remain to be elucidated.

Wegener's granulomatosis

This distinct syndrome is characterized by granulomatous vasculitis of the upper

and lower respiratory tract, by disseminated vasculitis which may affect both arteries and veins, and by a necrotizing glomerulonephritis with glomerular destruction (17). It is compelling to distinguish Wegener's granulomatosis from other forms of necrotizing vasculitis, both local and diffuse, because of its remarkable response to cytotoxic therapy.

Clinical features. Involvement of the upper respiratory passages leads to purulent rhinorrhea, erosion of the nasal septum, saddle nose deformity (Fig 18–3), epistaxis, nasal obstruction, chronic necrosing sinusitis, and otitis media. Disease of the lower tract is marked by cough with purulent sputum, nasopharyngeal or tracheobroncial ulcerations, or pneumonitis.

Constitutional complaints, which are common, include fever and malaise. There may be polyarthralgia. Over 90% of patients have sinus involvement. Approximately one-half of patients with Wegener's granulomatosis develop ocular signs, including proptosis, conjunctivitis, episcleritis, and scleritis; palsy of eye muscles, uveitis, and retinal-optic nerve disease are less frequent (18). Involvement of the skin, peripheral nervous system (mononeuritis multiplex), and heart including pericarditis and intractable arrhythmias (19) has been documented.

The patient with Wegener's granulomatosis is usually very seriously ill; secondary bacterial infection is common.

Laboratory findings. Laboratory study reveals elevated sedimentation rate, anemia which may be microangiopathic, leukocytosis with or without eosinophilia, microscopic hematuria with or without proteinuria, and azotemia if the nephritis

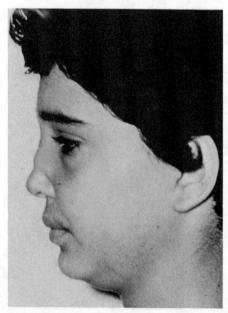

Fig 18–3. Deformity of the nose secondary to granulomatous disease is shown in this patient with Wegener's granulomatosis. (From the Revised Clinical Slide Collection on the Rheumatic Diseases)

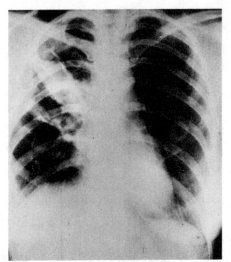

Fig 18–4. Roentgenogram of the chest of a man with Wegener's granulomatosis showing bilateral pulmonary infiltrates and a solitary cavitary nodule in the left midlung field (From the Revised Clinical Slide Collection on the Rheumatic Diseases)

has progressed. Serum IgA levels may be increased. Tests for rheumatoid factor and antinuclear antibodies give negative results. Chest roentgenograms show infiltrates or nodular lesions which represent granulomata and may cavitate (Fig 18–4).

Tissue diagnosis is essential. The hallmark of Wegener's granulomatosis is granulomatous and necrotizing vasculitis, with leukocytes and lymphocytes and giant cells in major organ sites (Fig 18–5). A sinus biopsy is often the safest means to a definitive diagnosis.

The classic renal lesion is a focal necrotizing glomerulitis. Fibrinoid necrosis of one or more glomerular capillary loops is a characteristic finding. Later there is epithelial crescent formation in Bowman's capsule. Granulomatous inflammation may be found around affected glomeruli, together with interstitial nephritis of varying degree. The small and medium-sized renal arteries are the site of necrotizing vasculitis.

The etiology of Wegener's granulomatosis is unknown. Circulating and deposited immune complexes have been observed (20). However, most classic immune complex–mediated syndromes are *not* granulomatous in character. Studies of cell-mediated immunity have shown reduced skin test and lymphocyte transformation reactivity. It is usually possible to distinguish Wegener's granulomatosis from local midline granuloma on clinical grounds and from lymphomatoid granulomatosis by histologic criteria. Characteristic involvement of the respiratory tract alone has been termed *limited* or *incomplete Wegener's syndrome* (21).

Treatment. Cytotoxic therapy has changed the life expectancy of patients with Wegener's granulomatosis from an average survival of 5 months before gluco-

corticoids (with 80% of patients dead in 1 year), to 12 months with glucocorticoids alone, to 36 months and indefinitely longer with cytotoxic agents (1,3). Cyclophosphamide, with or without glucocorticoids, is the treatment of choice at this time.

Successful renal transplantation has been accomplished in individuals who have not received therapy in time to avert kidney failure (22). Dramatic responses to current therapeutic regimens have changed the prognosis of Wegener's granulomatosis from a disease of almost uniform fatality to one of consistent treatability and perhaps ultimate curability. This degree of success is virtually unique to Wegener's granulomatosis in the area of necrotizing vasculitis. It supports the potential for precise description of clinical syndromes and careful evaluation of empirical therapeutic regimens.

Schönlein-Henoch purpura

This disorder, also known as anaphylactoid or allergic purpura, is a form of hypersensitivity vasculitis that occurs most often in children and young adults, slightly more often in boys than in girls. It is characterized by nonthrombocytopenic purpura, fever, abdominal complaints, arthralgia, and renal involvement (1,23).

Clinical features. Although any feature of the syndrome may occur alone, a typical patient has the signs and symptoms of an upper respiratory illness followed in 1–3 weeks by a symmetrical urticarial rash

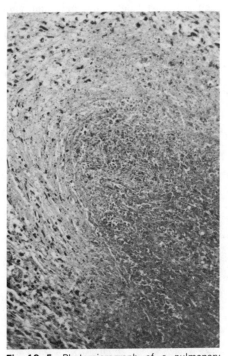

Fig 18–5. Photomicrograph of a pulmonary nodule from a patient with Wegener's granulomatosis showing characteristic granuloma formation (hematoxylin and eosin, original magnification ×50). (Courtesy of G Godman)

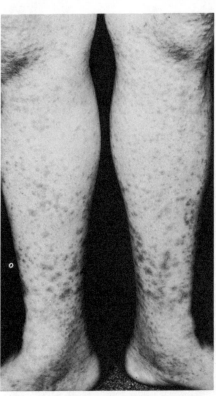

Fig 18–6. The legs of this person with Schönlein-Henoch purpura are covered by slightly raised, palpable purpuric lesions. In Schönlein-Henoch syndrome the lesions are characteristically more prominent distally in the lower half of the body. (From the Revised Clinical Slide Collection on the Rheumatic Diseases)

on the lower extremities (Fig 18–6) and trunk (especially the buttocks) as well as the extensor surfaces of the hands and elbows. This may be plentiful or sparse and in a matter of hours evolves to macular purpuric lesions that may become raised and may coalesce to form ecchymoses or bullae or may ulcerate. The lesions generally resolve in 1–2 weeks and fade without trace. At times colicky abdominal pain or polyarthralgia is the dominant complaint. Frank arthritis is much less common.

Evidence of renal involvement in the form of microscopic hematuria and proteinuria is detectable in a majority of patients 4–8 weeks after the onset of illness. The pancreas, heart, lungs, brain, and testes are involved only rarely. Any portion of the gastrointestinal tract may be affected, but the jejunum and ileum are involved most frequently. Hematemesis and/or melena are common and the blood loss may be severe. Other complications include intestinal obstruction (later stricture), intestinal infarction and perforation, intussusception, and protein-losing enteropathy. Epistaxis and bleeding gums are common. The polyarthralgia, usually of the knees and ankles, is accompanied by mild warmth and effusion.

The renal disease usually resolves spontaneously, but may progress and prove fatal. Nephrotic syndrome may develop (24). Although these attacks usually end in 1–4 months, recurrences have been noted in up to 40% of patients.

Laboratory findings. In addition to those already noted, laboratory findings include mild anemia and leukocytosis, a normal platelet count, elevated sedimentation rate, an increase in serum immune complexes containing IgA and IgG (25), and no antinuclear antibodies. Rheumatoid factor may be present in low titer (23).

The distinctive histopathologic lesion at all sites of involvement is a perivasculitis in which polymorphonuclear leukocytes are prominent and often fragmented—hence the term **leukocytoclastic angiitis**, the hallmark of all immunogenic vasculitides. Small coalescing hemorrhages are found in the synovium. There is variably severe focal segmental and less often diffuse proliferative glomerulonephritis, which includes epithelial crescents in Bowman's capsule (24,26).

IgA, IgG, and C3 are deposited in the glomeruli (26). Deposits of IgA present, at least in part, in the form of an immune complexes and deposits of C3 and C4 or only C3 have also been detected in capillary walls in the skin lesions. The finding of C3 and properdin in the absence of C1q provides evidence that the C3 in the mesangium of these patients is the result of activation of the alternate complement pathway.

Exposure to infectious agents (especially the streptococcus), foods, drugs, and other physical agents has been implicated, but the etiology of this disease remains unknown.

Although spectacular recoveries have been reported, conclusive evidence of a favorable effect of corticosteroids, cytotoxic agents, or anticoagulants alone or in combination is unconfirmed (27).

Takayasu's arteritis

Takayasu's arteritis is a chronic nonspecific obliterative arteritis which classically affects the branches of the aortic arch at their origin. It is also well known as **pulseless disease** because all the arm as well as the carotid pulses may become impalpable. It was first described by M Takayasu, a Japanese ophthalmologist, in 1908. Pulseless disease and aortitis syndrome are recognized as single disease entities for which the designation of **Takayasu's truncoarteritis** is recommended. Giant cell arteritis appears to be a different but closely related form of vasculitis.

Vascular lesions have a characteristic distribution that corresponds to clinical findings (1). Inflammatory reaction is found frequently in the media and less frequently the adventitia of elastic type arteries. The intima becomes sclerotic and thickened as a secondary change. Inflam-

matory aneurysms and aortic insufficiency are not rare complications.

Microscopic findings of the truncoarteritis are classified into 3 major categories. The first is marked by a granulomatous inflammation which is predominant in approximately 25% of autopsies. The granuloma, with or without necrotic foci, is occasionally accompanied by giant cells. In the second type there is a diffuse infiltration of lymphocytes and a proliferation of connective tissue cells. It is found in approximately 15% of cases. The third, or fibrotic, is found in the majority (60%) of cases at the time of autopsy. The fibrotic change is followed by sclerosis with calcification, the final picture resembling atherosclerosis.

Takayasu's truncoarteritis is a rare disease. The annual rate of occurrence is one case per million population in Japan, where the disease incidence is the greatest. The same or an indistinguishable disease has been described in Malaysia as the middle aortic syndrome and also occurs in other parts of the Middle and Far East as well as South Africa where blacks are affected. The condition is rare in whites. The disease occurs 8 times more frequently in women than men. The peak age of onset is in the twenties.

The cause of the disorder is unknown. The higher incidence in Japanese and aggregation in families may reflect a genetic predisposition. A high frequency of HLA–DR4 and MB3 has been reported.

Clinical features. Clinical manifestations include constitutional symptoms and ischemic features (28). Moderate fever, fatigue, polyarthralgia, and muscular pain are common. Signs and symptoms due to ischemic change depend on the site of vascular lesion (Table 18–2) (29). Diminished or abnormally weak arterial pulsation, low blood pressure, and muscular weakness in the arms are important physical signs in the aortic arch syndrome. Pulsation in the left arm is often weaker than in the right since the left subclavian artery is likely to have more severe obstructive change.

Table 18–2. Takayasu's arteritis: frequency and distribution of arterial lesions among 76 autopsies*

Changes found	Site
More than 75% of patients	Ascending aorta, aortic arch, brachicephalic trunk, subclavian arteries, common carotid arteries
50–75%	Thoracic and abdominal aorta
25–50%	Pulmonary and renal arteries
Less than 25%	Coronary, mesenteric, and iliac arteries

* Modified by the permission of Prof Nasu (29).

Transient visual disturbance, syncope, and vertigo correspond to cerebral ischemia. Hypotensive ophthalmoangiopathy is an early and frequent sign. The presence of arterial hypertension suggests involvement of the renal artery. Intermittent claudication is a symptom related to disease of the iliac arteries. Vascular murmurs and local tenderness indicate areas of stenosis.

Laboratory findings. Laboratory findings include an elevated sedimentation rate, leukocytosis, and hypergammaglobulinemia with elevation in IgA and IgM. Rheumatoid factors, antinuclear factors, and antiaortic antibody are found in a minority of cases. Angiography, especially cineangiography, has proved extremely useful in establishing the diagnosis. Biopsy of peripheral arteries is of limited value.

No specific treatment is generally agreed to be effective. However, corticosteroids are recommended as a supportive measure, especially during early stages (28). Immunosuppressive drugs are under study. It is possible to prolong life by successful management of arterial hypertension. The survival rate at 10 years in a recent study was 77%.

Kawasaki disease

Also known as the mucocutaneous lymph node syndrome, Kawasaki disease is a systemic disorder of unknown etiology; some form of infection is suspected (30,31). Eighty percent of patients are under 5 years of age. Male to female ratio is 1.5:1.

Clinical features. The disease is triphasic, consisting of an acute febrile phase (days 1–14), a subacute phase (days 10–25), and a convalescent phase (days 25–60).

During the acute febrile phase the child initially appears acutely ill and is irritable because of a high, spiking fever unresponsive to antibiotics. There is bilateral conjunctival injection frequently associated with an asymptomatic iridocyclitis disclosed on slit-lamp examination. Oropharyngeal manifestations include a diffusely red throat, a strawberry tongue (Fig 18–7), and red, dry lips. Cervical lymphadenopathy and rash also occur during the acute febrile phase. The rash is intensely erythematous, varying from a generalized scarlatiniform eruption to an erythema multiforme that begins on the extremities and spreads to the trunk.

There is an indurative edema of the hands and feet together with pronounced erythema of the palms and soles. As the edema subsides, there is desquamation of the skin, occasionally diffuse but more typically confined to the tips of the fingers and toes. Finally, during the convalescent period, transverse grooves appear in the finger and toenails.

Half the patients have heart involvement, with manifestations ranging from nonspecific T-wave and S-T segment electrocardiographic changes to murmurs, gallop rhythm, pericarditis, myocarditis, and heart failure. Most deaths are cardiac in origin, accounting for the 1–2% mortality, and are due primarily to coronary thromboarteritis and aneurysms that may occur months and even years after onset. Angiographic studies show up to a 20% incidence of coronary arteritis.

During the subacute phase of the illness, arthralgia and arthritis occur in up to half the patients. The knees or other large joints are most often involved and the synovial fluid is typically inflammatory. Other less common manifestations include meningitis, encephalitis, otitis media, and hydrops of the gall bladder.

Laboratory findings. Initial laboratory findings include a neutrophilic leukocytosis, anemia, elevated sedimentation rate, thrombocytosis, sterile pyuria, proteinuria, and hepatic function abnormalities that resolve by the convalescent period when neutropenia develops, which often persists for 6 months or more. IgE levels are often elevated.

Diagnostic criteria for Kawasaki disease are shown in Table 18–3.

Patients generally recover in 4–6 weeks. Treatment with corticosteroids is currently contraindicated. Aspirin in large amounts is effective in suppressing the high fever. Subsequently, aspirin is often prescribed in the hope of preventing coronary thrombosis, but the value of such treatment is not established.

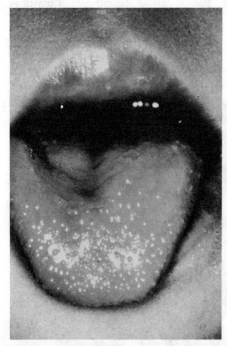

Fig 18–7. This is the *strawberry tongue* characteristic of Kawasaki disease. Papillae are enlarged and the tongue is red. Note erythematous lips. (From the Revised Clinical Slide Collection on the Rheumatic Diseases)

Table 18–3. Diagnostic criteria for Kawasaki disease:, 5 of the 6 criteria are required for definitive diagnosis

1. Spiking fever, 5 days or more
2. Bilateral conjunctival injection
3. One of the following oropharyngeal manifestations:
   a. Diffuse oropharyngeal erythema
   b. Strawberry tongue
   c. Redness, dryness, and fissures of lips
4. One or more of the following signs in the extremities:
   a. Indurative edema of hands and feet
   b. Erythema of palms and soles
   c. Desquamation of fingers and toes (about 2 weeks after onset)
   d. Transverse grooves in finger- and toenails (second to third months)
5. Variable erythematous rash
6. Cervical lymphadenopathy

Cutaneous vasculitis

Some individuals develop necrotizing angiitis that involves and is limited to the vessels of the skin (32–34). This is manifested typically as urticaria or palpable purpura; less often there is bulla formation, necrotic ulceration, or livedo reticularis.

Histologic examination of the skin reveals 2 distinct cellular patterns of angiitis involving the venules of individuals with clinically identical cutaneous lesions (32). In those individuals who are found to have serum hypocomplementemia, there is a perivascular infiltrate composed predominantly of neutrophilic leukocytes with fibrin deposition and nuclear debris (leukocytoclastic angiitis). In patients with normal serum complement levels, in addition to an infiltrate of neutrophils and fibrin deposition, perivenular lymphocytes in various stages of activation are prominent. In one study 9 of 10 patients with hypocomplementemia had complement abnormalities compatible with activation of the classical pathway; in the remaining individual activation appeared to have occurred by the alternative pathway (32).

The changes observed in the tissues of the patients with hypocomplementemia were similar to immune complex–induced cutaneous lesions in experimental animals, a conclusion supported by the demonstration of immunoglobulin and complement-containing deposits in affected blood vessel walls in some instances. In patients with normocomplementemia the histologic changes bore a resemblance to findings observed in experimental contact hypersensitivity. Degranulation of mast cells was noted in both of the cellular patterns of cutaneous vasculitis.

Individuals with hypocomplementemic cutaneous vasculitis may also have arthralgia, abdominal pain, and glomerulonephritis (34). This syndrome has been described in the members of a family with inherited partial deficiency of C3 (34).

See also erythema elevatum diutinum in Section 84.

1. Cupps TR, Fauci AS: The Vasculitides. Philadelphia, WB Saunders Co, 1981
2. Alarcon-Segovia D: The necrotizing vasculitides: a new pathogenetic classification. Med Clin N Am 61:241–260, 1977
3. Fauci AS, Haynes BF, Katz P: The spectrum of vasculitis: clinical, pathologic, immunologic, and therapeutic considerations. Ann Intern Med 89:660–676. 1978
4. Fan PT, Davis JA, Somer T, Kaplan L, Bluestone R: A clinical approach to systemic vasculitis. Semin Arthritis Rheum 9:248–304, 1980
5. Fye KH, Becker MJ, Theofilopoulos AN, Moutsopoulos H, Feldman J-L, Talal N: Immune complexes in hepatitis B antigen–associated periarteritis nodosa: detection by antibody-dependent cell-mediated cytotoxicity and the Raji cell assay. Am J Med 62:783–791, 1977
6. Travers RL, Allison DJ, Brettle RP, Hughes GRV: Polyarteritis nodosa: a clinical and angiographic analysis of 17 cases. Semin Arthritis Rheum 8:184–199, 1979
7. Ettlinger RE, Nelson AM, Burke EC, Lie JT: Polyarteritis nodosa in childhood: a clinical pathologic study. Arthritis Rheum 22:820–825, 1979
8. Leib ES, Restivo C, Paulus HE: Immunosuppressive and corticosteroid therapy of polyarteritis nodosa. Am J Med 67:941–947, 1979
9. Cohen RD, Conn DL, Ilstrup DM: Clinical features, prognosis, and response to treatment in polyarteritis. Mayo Clin Proc 58:146–155, 1980
10. Chumbley LC, Harrison EG Jr, DeRemee RA: Allergic granulomatosis and angiitis (ChurgStrauss syndrome): report and analysis of 30 cases. Mayo Clin Proc 52:477–484, 1977
11. Cheson BD, Bluming AZ, Alroy J: Cogan's syndrome: a systemic vasculitis. Am J Med 60:549–555, 1976
12. Haynes BF, Kaiser-Kupfer MI, Mason P, Fauci AS: Cogan syndrome: studies in 13 patients, long-term follow-up, and a review of the literature. Medicine 59:426–441, 1980
13. McCabe BF: Autoimmune sensorineural hearing loss. Ann Otol Rhinol Laryngol 88:585–590, 1979
14. Bergrem H, Jervell J, Brodwall EK, Flatmark A, Mellbye O: Goodpasture's syndrome: a report of 7 patients including long-term follow-up of 3 who received a kidney transplant. Am J Med 68:54–58, 1980
15. Rosenblatt SG, Knight W, Bannayan GA, Wilson CB, Stein JH: Treatment of Goodpasture's syndrome with plasmapheresis: a case report and review of the literature. Am J Med 66:689–696, 1979
16. Johnson JP, Whitman W, Briggs WA, Wilson CB: Plasmapheresis and immunosuppressive agents in antibasement membrane antibody-induced Goodpasture's syndrome. Am J Med 64:354–359, 1978
17. Fauci AS, Wolff SM: Wegener's granulomatosis: studies in 18 patients and a review of the literature. Medicine 52:535–561, 1973
18. Haynes BF, Fishman ML, Fauci AS, Wolff SM: The ocular manifestations of Wegener's granulomatosis: fifteen years experience and review of the literature. Am J Med 63:131–141, 1977
19. Forstot JZ, Overlie PA, Neufeld GK, Harmon CE, Forstot SL: Cardiac complications of Wegener's granulomatosis: a case report of complete heart block and review of the literature. Semin Arthritis Rheum 10:148–154, 1980
20. Howell SB, Epstein WV: Circulating immunoglobulin complexes in Wegener's granulomatosis. Am J Med 60:259–268, 1976
21. Schechter SL, Bole GG, Walker SE: Midline granuloma and Wegener's granulomatosis: clinical and therapeutic considerations. J Rheumatol 3:241–250, 1976
22. Fauci AS, Balow JE, Brown R, Chazan J, Steinman T, Sahyoun AI, Monoaco AP, Wolff SM: Successful renal transplantation in Wegener's granulomatosis. Am J Med 60:437–440, 1976
23. Cream JJ, Gumpel JM, Peachey RDG: Schönlein-Henoch purpura in the adult: a study of 77 adults with anaphylactoid or Schönlein-Henoch purpura. Q J Med 39:461–484, 1970

24. Meadow SR, Glasgow EF, White RHR, Moncrieff MW, Cameron JS, Ogg CS: Schönlein-Henoch nephritis. Q J Med 41:241–258, 1972

25. Kauffmann RH, Herrmann WA, Meyer CJLM, Daha MR, Van Es LA: Circulating IgA–immune complexes in Henoch-Schönlein purpura: a longitudinal study of their relationship to disease activity and vascular deposition of IgA. Am J Med 69:859–866, 1980

26. Nakamoto Y, Asano Y, Dohi K, Fujioka M, Iida H, Kida H, Kibe Y, Hattori N, Takeuchi J: Primary IgA glomerulonephritis and Schönlein-Henoch purpura nephritis: clinicopathological and immunohistological characteristics. Q J Med 47:495–516, 1978

27. Meadow SR: The prognosis of Henoch-Schoenlein nephritis. Clin Nephrol 9:87–90, 1978

28. Fraga A, Mintz G, Valle L, Flores-Izquierdo G: Takayasu's arteritis: frequency of systemic manifestations (study of 22 patients) and favorable response to maintenance steroid therapy with adrenocorticosteroids (12 patients). Arthritis Rheum 15:617–624, 1972

29. Nasu T: Pathology of Takayasu's truncoarteritis: a statistical observation of 76 autopsy cases in Japan, Vascular Lesions of Collagen Diseases and Related Conditions. Tokyo, University of Tokyo Press, 1977, pp 149–160

30. Kawasaki T, Kosaki F, Osawa S, Shigematsu I, Yanagawa H: A new infantile acute febrile mucocutaneous lymph node syndrome (MLNS) prevailing in Japan. Pediatrics 54:271–276, 1974

31. Yanagihara R, Todd JK: Acute febrile mucocutaneous lymph node syndrome. Am J Dis Child 134:603–614, 1980

32. Soter NA, Mihm MC, Gigli I, Dvorak HF, Austen KF: Two distinct cellular patterns in cutaneous necrotizing angiitis. J Invest Dermatol 66:344–350, 1976

33. Callen JP, Chanda JJ, Voorhees JJ: Cutaneous angiitis (vasculitis). Dermatology 17:105–113, 1978

34. McLean RH, Weinstein A, Chapitis J, Lowenstein M, Rothfield NF: Familial partial deficiency of the third component of complement (C3) and the hypocomplementemic cutaneous vasculitis syndrome. Am J Med 68:549–558, 1980

19. Polymyalgia rheumatica and temporal arteritis (giant cell arteritis)

Although an association between polymyalgia rheumatica and giant cell arteritis has been recognized for over 25 years, the nature of this relationship is still incompletely understood.

Polymyalgia rheumatica is a relatively common clinical syndrome characterized by severe aching and stiffness in the neck, shoulder girdle, or pelvic girdle muscle areas, which lasts for a month or longer (1,2). The stiffness is usually more prominent in the morning or after periods of rest. Polymyalgia rheumatica usually occurs in persons over 50 years, and women predominate in a ratio of 2:1. In one study the average annual incidence in persons over age 50 years was 54/100,000 and the prevalence of active and recovered cases was approximately 500/100,000 (2).

The myalgias and arthralgias sometimes begin abruptly but tend to evolve gradually. Systemic symptoms including low grade fever, malaise, and weight loss are present in the majority of patients. Because the erythrocyte sedimentation rate is elevated in nearly all patients to more than 40 or 50 mm in 1 hour (Westergren), this finding is considered an important diagnostic feature.

There is little on physical examination to explain the severe proximal musculoskeletal discomfort. However, synovial biopsies have revealed lymphocytic inflammation in some patients and suggest that the condition may be a form of proximal synovitis (3). Synovitis in polymyalgia rheumatica has also been implicated by the results of synovial fluid analyses and joint scintiscans (4). In most cases of polymyalgia rheumatica no other illness is found, although occasionally patients with infections, neoplasms, or other connective tissue diseases may have similar symptoms. When an associated process can be identified, giant cell arteritis is by far the most common.

Giant cell arteritis (also known as cranial arteritis, temporal arteritis, and granulomatous arteritis) affects the same groups as polymyalgia rheumatica. Epidemiologic surveys show incidence rates of giant cell arteritis of 12–17/100,000 and prevalence of 133/100,000 in persons 50 years and older (active and inactive disease included) (5,6). Autopsy studies in Sweden point to an even higher frequency.

In giant cell arteritis the branches of the arteries originating from the arch of the aorta are involved most prominently (7). The vessels are frequently affected in a discontinuous fashion. Histologic sections of inflamed areas show infiltration of lymphocytes, macrophages, histiocytes, and multinucleated giant cells (Fig 19–1). The changes are often centered around the elastic laminae, but a panarteritis may be present which causes disruption of the vessel wall layers. Fibrous thickening of the intima results in further narrowing or occlusion of the lumen.

The onset of the arteritis may be sudden, but in many instances symptoms are present for months before the diagnosis is established. Constitutional symptoms usually include fever, malaise, and weight loss. Most patients have clinical findings related to the arteries. Headaches, often localized to the regions of the temporal or occipital arteries, occur in the majority. Tenderness or enlargement of involved portions of the arteries of the head and neck are often found (Fig 19–2).

Sudden loss of vision is a dread complication of this disease. Once established, a visual deficit is permanent. According to recent reports permanent visual loss occurs in approximately 5–15% of patients (1,8–10).

Pain occurs in the muscles of mastication during chewing and occasionally in other groups. An aortic arch syndrome may result from narrowing or dissection of the aorta or its primary branches. Other possible consequences include myocardial

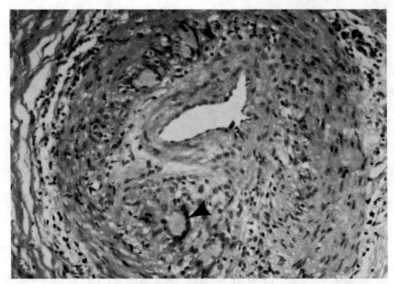

Fig 19–1. Photomicrograph of a small branch of a temporal artery illustrates changes of giant cell arteritis. Multinucleated giant cells (**arrowhead**) are present at the junction of the media and intima. There is extensive disruption of all layers of the vessel wall.

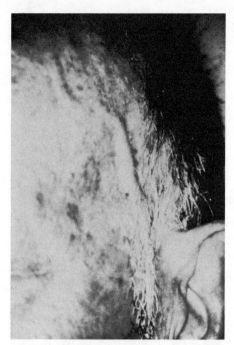

Fig 19–2. A dilated artery can be seen in this patient with temporal arteritis (giant cell arteritis). It is tender and indurated, but pulsations can still be felt. These signs are not always present even when biopsy of the temporal artery is abnormal. (From the Revised Clinical Slide Collection on the Rheumatic Diseases)

infarction, mesenteric infarction, and cerebral thrombosis.

Polymyalgia rheumatica occurs in half or more patients with giant cell arteritis and may appear in any phase of the disease (5). Because temporal artery biopsies reveal the existence of giant cell arteritis in some patients with polymyalgia rheumatica who have no symptoms or signs of arterial disease, it has been suggested that all patients with polymyalgia rheumatica have arteritis and that the musculoskeletal symptoms are due to vasculitis. However, only a minority (perhaps 15% or less) of patients with polymyalgia rheumatica without evidence of arteritis on initial examination (including temporal artery biopsy) ever develop overt arteritis.

Laboratory studies reflect the underlying inflammatory processes in these conditions. The erythrocyte sedimentation rate is nearly always highly elevated (often over 100 mm in 1 hour, Westergren) in both polymyalgia rheumatica and giant cell arteritis. Other common findings are moderate anemia, decreased serum albumin, and increased alpha$_2$-globulin concentrations, and mild hepatic dysfunction.

Giant cell arteritis can usually be distinguished from Takayasu's arteritis (see Section 18) and other forms of vasculitis by differences in clinical manifestations, age, and affected populations.

The etiology of giant cell arteritis and polymyalgia rheumatica is unknown, but reports of their presence in first-degree relatives and the strong predominance in whites have suggested a genetic predisposition. Since the internal elastic membrane appears to be the focus of the inflammatory reaction in giant cell arteritis, the presence of an antigen (perhaps autoantigen) in this structure has been considered. Identification of immunoglobulin deposits in the walls of inflamed temporal arteries has supported the concept that an immunologic mechanism is involved in the pathogenesis of giant cell arteritis (11).

Corticosteroids are highly effective in the treatment of giant cell arteritis, and their efficacy in the prevention of blindness is well documented. An initial daily dose of 40–60 mg of prednisone, or the equivalent, is adequate in nearly all cases (9). All reversible symptoms and findings usually remit within a month, and laboratory test results revert to normal. Thereafter, the dose should be gradually lowered to the minimum amount of corticosteroid that suppresses the symptoms and laboratory abnormalities. In patients with polymyalgia rheumatica alone, smaller doses of prednisone such as 5–20 mg daily relieve the aching and stiffness, but may not control an underlying arteritis if present.

Both of these conditions tend to run a self-limited course lasting several months to several years.

1. Calamia KT, Hunder GG: Clinical manifestations of giant cell arteritis. Clin Rheum Dis 6:389–403, 1980
2. Chuang T-Y, Hunder GG, Ilstrup DM, Kurland LT: Polymyalgia rheumatica: a 10-year epidemiologic and clinical study. Ann Intern Med 97:672–680, 1982
3. Henderson DRF, Tribe CR, Dixon AStJ: Synovitis in polymyalgia rheumatica. Rheumatol Rehab 14:244–250, 1975
4. O'Duffy JD, Hunder GG, Wahner HW: A follow-up study of polymyalgia rheumatica: evidence of chronic axial synovitis. J Rheumatol 7:685–693, 1980
5. Huston KA, Hunder GG, Lie JT, Kennedy RH, Elveback LR: Temporal arteritis: a 25-year epidemiologic clinical and pathologic study. Ann Intern Med 88:162–167, 1978
6. Bengtsson B-Å, Malmvall B-E: The epidemiology of giant cell arteritis including temporal arteritis and polymyalgia rheumatica. Arthritis Rheum 24:899–904, 1981
7. Wilkinson IM, Russell RW: Arteries of the head and neck in giant cell arteritis: a pathologic study to show the pattern of arterial involvement. Arch Neurol 27:378–391, 1972
8. Fauchald P, Rygvold B, Øystease B: Temporal arteritis and polymyalgia rheumatica: clinical and biopsy findings. Ann Intern Med 77:845–852, 1972
9. Hunder GG, Allen GL: Giant cell arteritis: a review. Bull Rheum Dis 29:980–987, 1978
10. Healey LA, Wilske KR: Manifestations of giant cell arteritis. Med Clin N Am 61:261–270, 1977
11. Liang GC, Simkin PA, Mannik M: Immunoglobulins in temporal arteritis: an immunofluorescent study. Ann Intern Med 81:19–24, 1974

20. Sjögren's syndrome

Sjögren's syndrome, a chronic inflammatory disorder, is characterized by diminished lacrimal and salivary gland secretion (*sicca complex*), resulting in **keratoconjunctivitis sicca** (KCS) and xerostomia. The glandular insufficiency also affects other exocrine glands and is associated with lymphocytic and plasma cell infiltration as well as features of autoimmunity (1–3).

As originally described, the syndrome consisted of a triad of dry eyes, dry mouth, and rheumatoid arthritis. We now know that other connective tissue diseases (e.g., systemic lupus erythematosus, progressive systemic sclerosis, and polymyositis) may be present in place of rheumatoid arthritis, and that the sicca complex can exist as a primary pathologic entity with no associated disorder. Moreover, lymphoproliferation, pseudolymphoma, or even lymphoid malignancy may appear in some patients.

More than 90% of patients are women, with a mean age of 50 years at diagnosis; only rarely are children affected. The disease occurs in all races.

Clinical features. The most common early symptoms include insidious, slowly progressive development of the sicca complex in a patient with rheumatoid arthritis or the more rapid development of a severe oral and ocular dryness, often accompanied by episodic parotitis, in an otherwise healthy individual.

KCS develops in 10–15% of patients with rheumatoid arthritis. The most frequent ocular complaint is that of foreign body sensation: the eye is described as feeling "gritty" or "sandy." Other symptoms include burning, accumulation of thick ropy strands at the inner canthus (particularly upon awakening), decreased tearing, redness, photosensitivity, eye fatigue, itching, and a "filmy" sensation that interferes with vision.

The Schirmer filter paper test provides a crude measure of tear formation. More reliable diagnostic signs are obtained using rose bengal dye and biomicroscopy. Grossly visible or microscopic staining of the bulbar conjunctiva or cornea indicates the presence of small superficial erosions. Biomicroscopy may reveal increased amounts of corneal debris and attached filaments of corneal epithelium (*filamentary keratitis*). Ocular complications include corneal ulceration, vascularization, and opacification, followed rarely by perforation.

The distressing symptoms of salivary insufficiency include difficulty with chewing, swallowing, and phonation; adherence of food to buccal surfaces; fissures and ulcers of the tongue, buccal membranes, and lips (particularly at the corners of the mouth); the need for frequent ingestion of liquids (particularly at mealtimes); and rampant dental caries. Dryness may also involve the nose, the posterior pharynx, the larynx, and the tracheobronchial tree, and may lead to epistaxis, hoarseness, and recurrent otitis media, bronchitis, or pneumonia. One-half of the patients have parotid and/or submandibular salivary gland enlargement (Fig 20–1). This symmetrical, often recurrent, condition may be accompanied by fever, tenderness, or erythema.

Superimposed infection is rare. Rapid fluctuations in gland size are not unusual. A particularly hard or nodular gland may suggest a neoplasm. Salivary gland function can be evaluated by measuring the volume of parotid saliva and by salivary scintigraphy. In this latter procedure, the uptake, concentration, and excretion of intravenously injected ^{99m}Tc-pertechnetate by the major salivary glands is measured by means of a sequential scintiphotographic technique.

Biopsy of the minor salivary glands in the lower lip (Fig 20–2) permits histopathologic confirmation of destructive lymphocytic infiltration (4). Multiple aggregations of lymphocytes, replacing and

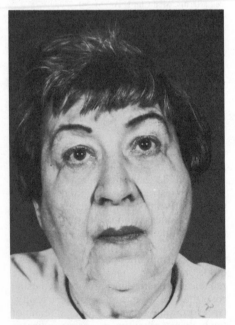

Fig 20–1. Bilateral parotid gland enlargement in a 70-year-old woman who had Sjögren's syndrome for 6 years. Her serum contained a monoclonal rheumatoid factor (titer > 1:8,192) that formed a cryogel with IgG. A malignant lymphoid nodule was removed from her lung.

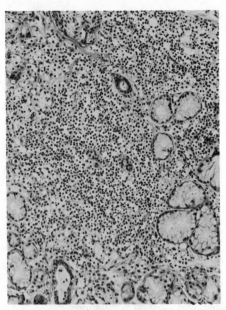

Fig 20–2. Photomicrograph of portion of minor salivary gland (lip biopsy specimen) of 26-year-old woman with Sjögren's syndrome (associated with mixed connective tissue disease). There is an intense infiltration of lymphocytes and destruction of most of the acinar tissue.

destroying the acinar tissue, characterize the lesion. An aggregate of more than 50 lymphoid cells is called a focus. A focus score greater than 1 (i.e., more than 1 focus per 4 mm^2 of glandular tissue) is characteristic of Sjögren's syndrome and is found in less than 1% of lip biopsy specimens obtained from either living or autopsy control patients of all ages.

Only 50% of patients referred for suspected Sjögren's syndrome have an autoimmune disease. Other frequent causes of oral and ocular dryness are local glandular disorders, anxiety-depression syndromes, and parasympathetic drugs.

Because Sjögren's syndrome appears to represent an immunologic attack on exocrine organs, the term **autoimmune exocrinopathy** has been proposed to describe an expanded concept of the syndrome. The diagnosis of this disorder depends upon the presence of at least 2 of the following 3 criteria: characteristic lymphocytic infiltrates in the salivary gland (i.e., a focus score greater than 1), definite KCS, and an associated extraglandular connective tissue or lymphoproliferative disorder.

Associated disorders. Splenomegaly and leukopenia (suggestive of Felty's syndrome), vasculitis with leg ulcers, and peripheral neuropathy may appear even in the absence of rheumatoid arthritis. Raynaud's phenomenon occurs in 20% of patients. Nonthrombocytopenic purpura, generally accompanied by hypergammaglobulinemia, may be present, sometimes in association with renal tubular acidosis. Chronic thyroiditis of the Hashimoto type is found in approximately 5% of

patients. Hepatomegaly, chronic active hepatitis or biliary cirrhosis, gastric achlorhydria, acute pancreatitis, and adult celiac disease have also been reported in association with Sjögren's syndrome. Neuromuscular abnormalities include polymyositis and myopathy, peripheral or cranial (particularly trigeminal) neuropathy, and cerebral vasculitis.

Several patients with Sjögren's syndrome of 2–26 years' duration have developed generalized lymphomas, pseudolymphoma with pulmonary lymphoid infiltration, or primary macroglobulinemia. Some have died of lymphoid malignancies that show great histologic variability. Several of these malignant lymphomas have been found to contain cytoplasmic IgM, κ-type immunoglobulin (5). This observation constitutes evidence that the lymphomas are of B cell origin, regardless of their histologic type or extent of differentiation. The benign lymphocytic salivary gland infiltrates preceding the malignant tumor expressed both κ and λ light chains. Thus, in some patients, lymphoproliferative lesions may progress from a polyclonal infiltrate to a monoclonal B cell neoplasm.

HLA antigens. Sjögren's syndrome is one of several autoimmune diseases associated with histocompatibility antigens HLA–B8 and Dw3 (6). This genetic predisposition is seen in organ-specific autoimmune diseases such as celiac disease, dermatitis herpetiformis, myasthenia gravis, Graves' disease, chronic active hepatitis, idiopathic Addison's disease, and insulin-dependent diabetes mellitus. Furthermore, patients with Sjögren's syndrome also have an abnormally high frequency of certain B lymphocyte antigens that may be similar to immune response–associated (Ia) antigens in the mouse (7). These findings suggest an underlying genetic predisposition that may operate through a disordered state of immunologic regulation.

Laboratory findings. A mild normocytic, normochromic anemia occurs in about 25% of patients, leukopenia in 30%, mild eosinophilia (about 6% eosinophils) in 25%, and an elevated erythrocyte sedimentation rate (>30 mm/hour, Westergren) in over 90%.

Half of the patients have hypergammaglobulinemia with a diffuse elevation of all immunoglobulin classes; this is most notable in patients without rheumatoid arthritis but who have polymyopathy, purpura, or renal tubular acidosis. Monoclonal IgM may be seen. Cryoglobulinemia (often of the mixed IgM–IgG type) may be present, particularly in patients with glomerulonephritis or pseudolymphoma. Hyperviscosity associated with IgG rheumatoid factor and intermediate complexes has been reported. Some patients with malignant lymphoma have hypogammaglobulinemia. A mild hypoalbuminemia is common.

Rheumatoid factor is detected in over 90% of sera when pooled human F II gamma globulin is used as antigen and in 75% when rabbit gamma globulin is used. Thus, many patients have rheumatoid factor without having rheumatoid arthritis. Rheumatoid factor may disappear or diminish noticeably in titer when lymphoid malignancy develops.

The LE cell phenomenon occurs in 20% of patients with Sjögren's syndrome who also have rheumatoid arthritis. It is otherwise rare unless systemic lupus erythematosus is also present.

Antinuclear factors, giving immunofluorescent homogeneous or speckled patterns, are seen in approximately 70% of patients. Antibodies to native DNA in low titer are occasionally present. In 50% of patients, an antibody specific for salivary duct epithelium has been observed by indirect immunofluorescence. Thyroglobulin antibodies, detected by hemagglutination, are present in 35%.

Precipitating antibodies to tissue antigens extracted from a human lymphocyte culture line are present in a majority of patients (8,9). A high percentage of individuals with only the sicca complex have antibodies reactive with the nuclear antigen SS-B(Ha). Antibodies to another nuclear antigen, SS-A, are less common and less specific.

The number of peripheral blood T lymphocytes are decreased in approximately 33% of patients but increase toward normal following incubation with thymosin. Immunoglobulin-positive lymphocytes (B cells) in peripheral blood may be increased slightly. Most patients have an impaired lymphocyte response to phytohemagglutinin, particularly when stimulated with a suboptimal concentration of the mitogen. A diminished capacity to develop delayed hypersensitivity to dinitrochlorobenzene may also be present.

An increase in salivary $beta_2$-microglobulin concentration correlates with the degree of lymphocytic infiltration found on labial biopsy specimens. Serum $beta_2$-microglobulin levels may be increased, particularly in patients with associated renal or lymphoproliferative complications.

Treatment. Treatment is largely symptomatic. Artificial tears or 0.5% methylcellulose eye drops are useful. Sugar-free lozenges can stimulate saliva.

Corticosteroids or immunosuppressive drugs may be prescribed for patients with severe functional disability or life-threatening complications. The use of cyclophosphamide (75–100 mg daily) has led to a diminution in extraglandular lymphoid infiltrates and restoration of salivary gland function in some patients.

1. Mason AM, Gumpel JM, Golding PL: Sjögren's syndrome—a clinical review. Semin Arthritis Rheum 2:301–331, 1973
2. Shearn MA: Sjögren's Syndrome. Philadelphia, WB Saunders Company, 1971
3. Talal N: Sjögren's syndrome and connective tissue disease with other immunologic disorders, Arthritis and Allied Conditions. Ed 9. DJ McCarty Jr, ed. Philadelphia, Lea and Febiger, 1979, pp 810–824
4. Greenspan JS, Daniels TE, Talal N, Sylvester RA: The histopathology of Sjögren's syndrome in labial salivary gland biopsies. Oral Surg 37:217–229, 1974
5. Zulman J, Jaffe R, Talal N: Evidence that the malignant lymphoma of Sjögren's syndrome is a monoclonal B-cell neoplasm. N Engl J Med 299:1215–1220, 1978
6. Fye KH, Terasaki PI, Michalski JP, Daniels TE, Opelz G, Talal N: Relationship of HLA–Dw3 and HLA–B8 to Sjögren's syndrome. Arthritis Rheum 21:337–342, 1978
7. Moutsopoulos HM, Chused TM, Johnson AH, Knudsen B, Mann ÐL: B lymphocyte antigens in sicca syndrome. Science 199:1441–1442, 1978
8. Alspaugh MA, Talal N, Tan EM: Differentiation and characterization of autoantibodies and their antigens in Sjögren's syndrome. Arthritis Rheum 19:216–222, 1976
9. Akizuki M, Boehm-Truitt MJ, Kassan SS, Steinberg AD, Chused TM: Purification of an acidic nuclear protein antigen and demonstration of its antibodies in subsets of patients with sicca syndrome. J Immunol 119:932–938, 1977

21. Amyloidosis

Amyloidosis is a disorder characterized by the accumulation of an unusual extracellular fibrous protein (*amyloid*) in the connective tissue of the body (1). The term amyloid originated with Virchow (1854), who mistakenly believed that this substance was akin to starch. Amyloid protein has now been found to have unique ultrastructural (Figs 21–1 and 2), x-ray diffraction, and biochemical characteristics. The deposition of amyloid may be widespread, involving major organs and leading to serious clinical consequences, or it may be very limited in extent with little effect on health.

Amyloidosis has been classified as: 1) *primary amyloidosis*—no evidence for pre-exisiting or coexisting disease; 2) amyloidosis associated with *multiple myeloma*; 3) *secondary amyloidosis*—associated with a) chronic infections (e.g., osteomyelitis, tuberculosis, leprosy), b) chronic inflammatory disease (e.g., rheumatoid arthritis, ankylosing spondylitis, regional enteritis, etc), or c) neoplasms (e.g., medullary carcinoma of the thyroid); 4) *heredofamilial amyloidosis*—the amyloidosis associated with familial Mediterranean fever and a variety of heritable neuropathic, renal, cardiovascular, and other syndromes; 5) *local amyloidosis*—local, often tumorlike, deposits in isolated organs without evidence of systemic involvement; 6) amyloidosis associated with *aging*.

Immunochemical findings. With the recent studies delineating the chemical composition of the protein in the various types of amyloidosis, a more exact immunochemical classification is available in part: 1) amyloid associated with tissue deposition of protein AA, a newly defined tissue protein (2,3) (secondary amyloidosis and the amyloid of familial Mediterranean fever); 2) amyloid associated with tissue deposition of protein AL, a protein consisting primarily of the amino-terminal variable segment of the light chain of homogeneous immunoglobulins, or in a few instances the whole light chain (3–6) (primary amyloid and amyloid associated with multiple myeloma). Other chemical types also exist, i.e., those associated with medullary carcinoma of the thyroid, "senile" cardiac deposition, and the neuropathic Portuguese type (7).

Antisera to protein AA type react with an antigenically related serum component, SAA, of higher molecular weight than AA, that some regard as a precursor. SAA behaves as an acute phase reactant and is elevated in concentration in infection, inflammation, and with aging. SAA is increased in amyloid-resistant animals, suggesting that amyloid resistance is related to the processing and catabolism of SAA. It has been suggested that an SAA-like material is produced by fibroblasts and is a normal constituent of developing extracellular connective tissue. SAA appears to suppress antibody response, suggesting that it may act as a regulator of such responses.

A second component of amyloid, P-component (plasma component or pentagonal unit) with different ultrastructure, x-ray diffraction pattern, and chemical characteristics, has been isolated from amyloid and shown to be identical with a circulating alpha globulin present in minute amounts (8). P-component is not responsible for the characteristic tinctorial properties or ultrastructure of amyloid (Fig 21–3). It has certain similarities to C-reactive protein (CRP) but does not behave as an acute phase protein and has biophysical and immunologic distinctions from CRP.

Clinical features. Clinical and pathologic investigations reveal a remarkable overlap among the different types of amyloid with regard to organ distribution and tinctorial characteristics (Table 21–1). As viewed by electron microscopy, all types of amyloid

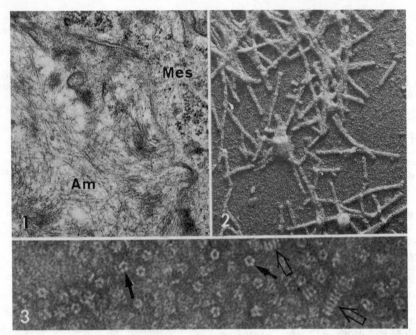

Fig 21–1. Electron micrograph of a portion of glomerulus from a patient with secondary amyloidosis, showing a portion of a mesangial cell (**Mes**) and extracellular amyloid fibrils. (**Am**) (original magnification ×24,000). **2**, Isolated human secondary amyloid fibrils; shadow-casted with platinum-palladium (original magnification ×70,000). **3**, Purified amyloid P-components, from spleen of a patient with secondary amyloidosis, are seen as pentagonal structures of about 100 A in diameter (**solid arrows**) or short rods with clear banding (probably side views of stacking of several pentagonal units) (**open arrows**); negatively stained with phosphotungstate (original magnification ×320,000).

examined consist chiefly of fine fibrils, 100 A in diameter in tissue section (Fig 21–1) or 70–100 A on isolation, depending upon the type of contrast stain used (Fig 21–2).

Since any organ may be involved, the clinical manifestations of amyloidosis are extremely varied (1). Infiltration of and about peripheral nerves, skin (9), tongue, joints, and heart (10) is most frequent in the primary forms (Fig 21–4), while in secondary amyloidosis, the liver, spleen, and kidney are the major sites of deposits.

Carpal tunnel syndrome (median neuropathy), resulting from local deposition of amyloid, is a frequent finding in certain types of primary amyloidosis and in the amyloidosis associated with multiple myeloma. Amyloid of the primary variety and that which occurs in association with myeloma may infiltrate the synovium and the periarticular and subcutaneous tissue. This form of amyloid arthropathy is easily mistaken for rheumatoid arthritis.

Less commonly, joint disease may occur when replacement of subchondral bone marrow by large tumefactions of amyloid is complicated by fracture. Some patients with primary amyloidosis develop a coagulation disorder in which there is a deficiency of factor X and occasionally factor IX. This condition has been traced to the binding of these proteins to amyloid fibrils (11).

Amyloid in the heredofamilial forms is responsible for peripheral neuropathy in certain kindreds in Portugal, Japan, and Sweden; upper limb neuropathy in certain families of German or Swiss ancestry in the United States; cranial nerve neuropathy in a group of Finnish ancestry; and for renal disease and cardiovascular disease in others (12). All of the above conditions are inherited as autosomal dominant traits except for the amyloid associated with familial Mediterranean fever which is inherited in an autosomal recessive manner.

Features that should alert the clinician to the diagnosis of primary amyloidosis include *unexplained* proteinuria, peripheral neuropathy, enlargement of the tongue, cardiomegaly, intestinal malabsorption, bilateral or familial carpal tunnel ,syndrome, or orthostatic hypotension. Symptoms frequently exist for several years before the correct diagnosis is made.

All patients with suspected primary amyloidosis should be thoroughly investigated for evidence of an underlying disease to rule out possible inflammatory disorders and malignant tumors. In patients with chronic infectious or inflammatory diseases, secondary amyloid should be suspected if unexplained proteinuria, hepatomegaly, or splenomegaly is present.

The diagnosis is established by means of microscopic examination of appropriate biopsy specimens. Rectal tissue has proved to be particularly useful, and in selected cases, skin (9), gingival, renal, and liver biopsy specimens are valuable. Since a biopsy specimen may contain only a small quantity of amyloid, it is important to stain the specimen with Congo red and/or thioflavine T and to view it in polarized light for birefringence.

Laboratory findings. Laboratory abnormalities are nonspecific and may or may not include proteinuria and an elevated erythrocyte sedimentation rate. Elevated or depressed serum immunoglobulin (IgG, IgA, IgM) levels may be encountered in patients with secondary amyloidosis as well as in patients with idiopathic (primary) disease and multiple myeloma (3). Serum and/or urine M-components are regularly detectable in the latter patients and are often seen in primary amyloidosis as well.

Treatment. There is no specific treatment for amyloidosis. Some patients with secondary renal amyloidosis have improved after cure of a predisposing disease such as active tuberculosis or chronic osteomyelitis, but histologic confirmation of improvement is rare. Therapy is difficult to assess since nephrotic syndrome secondary to amyloidosis may sometimes remit spontaneously. Renal transplants have been carried out successfully in a few patients with renal failure. Colchicine has

Table 21–1. Characteristics of amyloid

1. Homogeneous, eosinophilic extracellular substance when stained with hematoxylin and eosin
2. Green birefringence after Congo red stain when viewed in polarizing microscope
3. Fine, nonbranching fibrils 70–100 A in diameter seen with electron microscopy
4. Cross beta pattern on x-ray diffraction
5. Amino acid sequence studies demonstrate protein AA, or protein AL, or possibly new moieties

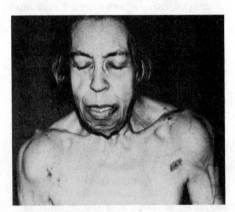

Fig 21–4. This patient with primary systemic amyloidosis exhibits advanced macroglossia, resulting in inability to close her mouth. Purpura are present around the eyelids, lips, and anterior thorax. Solid firm masses of amyloid have caused prominence of both shoulders (shoulder pad sign). Over 100 cc of noninflammatory fluid containing Bence-Jones protein was aspirated from her right shoulder. (From the Revised Clinical Slide Collection on the Rheumatic Diseases)

been shown to relieve the acute attacks of familial Mediterranean fever and may decrease the formation of amyloid. Clinical trials of colchicine in amyloidosis are currently in progress.

1. Cohen AS: Amyloidosis. N Engl J Med 277:522–530, 574–583, 628–638, 1967
2. Benditt EP, Eriksen N, Hermodson MA, Ericsson LH: The major properties of human and monkey amyloid substance: common properties including usual N-terminal amino acid sequences. FEBS Lett 19:169–173, 1971
3. Amyloidosis. O Wegelius, A Pasternack, eds. New York, Academic Press, 1976
4. Glenner GG, Terry W, Harada M, Isersky G, Page D: Amyloid fibril proteins: proof of homology with immunoglobulin light chains by sequence analyses. Science 172:1150–1151, 1971
5. Franklin EC: Amyloidosis. Bull Rheum Dis 26:832–837, 1975
6. Cohen AS, Cathcart ES, Skinner M: Amyloidosis: current trends in its investigation. Arthritis Rheum 21:153–160, 1978
7. Glenner GG: Amyloid deposits and amyloidosis: the B-fibrilloses. N Engl J Med 302:1283–1292, 1333–1343, 1980
8. Skinner M, Cohen AS, Shirahama T, Cathcart ES: P-component (pentagonal unit) of amyloid: isolation, characterization and sequence analysis. J Lab Clin Med 84:604–614, 1974
9. Rubinow A, Cohen AS: Skin involvement in generalized amyloidosis: a study of clinically involved and uninvolved skin in 50 patients with primary and secondary amyloidosis. Ann Intern Med 88:781–785, 1978
10. Case Records of the Massachusetts General Hospital (Case 27-1981). N Engl J Med 305:33–40, 1981
11. Furie B, Voo LA, McAdam KPWJ, Furie BC: Mechanism of factor X deficiency in systemic amyloidosis. N Engl J Med 304:827–830, 1981
12. Cohen AS, Benson MD: Amyloid peripheral neuropathy, Peripheral Neuropathy. PT Dyck, KP Thomas, EH Lambert, eds. Philadelphia, WB Saunders Co, 1975, pp 1076–1091

22. Serum sickness and drug reactions

Serum sickness was originally defined as an adverse reaction to heterologous serum (usually horse serum) administered to humans as vaccine. Since heterologous antisera are rarely used today except in treatment of snake bite and clostridium infection, serum sickness has virtually disappeared. In some instances, however, drug hypersensitivity reactions may be identical to serum sickness.

Adverse drug reactions of all types account for approximately 5% of hospital admissions. Drug reactions are sometimes the result of immunologic mechanisms that mimic serum sickness but are also due to pharmacologic effects of the drugs. These include: 1) overdose (too much drug or undermetabolism); 2) intolerance (adverse reactions to small dose); 3) idiosyncrasy (an abnormal susceptibility to a drug peculiar to an individual); 4) side effects (undesirable pharmacologic effects); and 5) secondary reactions occasionally resulting from pharmacologic effects, e.g., osteonecrosis following use of corticosteroids (1).

Clinical and laboratory findings. When it occurs, serum sickness or drug hypersensitivity normally follows parenteral administration of antitoxin or drug 1–2 weeks after first exposure or a few days after re-exposure. Itching begins at the injection site and is followed by fever, malaise, abdominal pain, nausea, vomiting, myalgia, or generalized swelling. A rash that is usually urticarial, but sometimes petechial or purpuric, appears early in the course.

In both serum sickness and hypersensitive reaction to a drug, the joints frequently become painful and stiff 2–3 days after onset of skin inflamation. Large joints (knees, ankles, and wrists) are most likely to be affected. While considerable swelling and effusion are common, increased heat or erythema is unusual. The joint fluid may contain as many as 20,000 white cells/mm^2. These are predominantly polymorphonuclear cells.

Both diseases are characteristically mild and self-limited, disappearing in 2–3 weeks. Occasionally, more prolonged and severe reactions do occur; rarely, these may prove fatal. Severe glomerulonephritis, involvement of the central and peripheral nervous systems, carditis, and other manifestations of diffuse vasculitis may all be part of the clinical spectrum (2).

The erythrocyte sedimentation rate is often normal in these patients. Eosinophilia does occur in drug hypersensitivity, but israre in serum sickness. Complement levels, frequently decreased in serum sickness, are often normal in drug hypersensitivity.

Diagnosis, etiology, and treatment. A history of serum or drug administration is of prime diagnostic importance. Skin tests are useful in ascertaining allergy to penicillin, but are of little or no value in determining hypersensitivity to other drugs. Serum sickness–like reactions are also caused by aminosalicyclic acid, diphenylhydantoin, iodinated dyes, streptomycin, sulfonamides, and thiouracils (3).

Serum sickness is a classic example of an immune complex disease (4). Approximately 1 week after administration of heterologous protein, antibody to the foreign protein is formed while antigen is still present in the circulation. Under such conditions of antigen excess, circulating (soluble) immune complexes develop. Increased vascular permeability (probably secondary to vasoactive amine release by platelets) is followed by localization of the complexes in the vessel wall where complement chemotactic factors are generated. These immune complexes then attract polymorphonuclear leukocytes (PMN). Inflammation and reversible tissue damage are the result of phagocytosis of the complexes by PMN. The type of clinical symptoms depend on the organs or cell membranes in which the immune complexes localize.

At the first indication of drug hypersensitivity, the offending agent should be discontinued and the patient should be warned against taking this or related compounds in the future. No treatment other than relief of symptoms may be necessary in patients with mild reactions, but in more severe cases of serum sickness, corticosteroids may be prescribed. Drug-induced lupus-like syndromes are discussed in Section 13.

1. deWick AL: Drug reactions, Immunologic Diseases. Ed 3. M Samter, ed. Boston, Little, Brown & Co, 1978, pp 413–439
2. Von Pirquet CE, Schick B: Serum Sickness. Baltimore, Williams & Wilkins, 1951
3. Parker CW: Drug allergy. N Engl J Med 292:511–514, 732–736, 957–960, 1975
4. Cochrane CG, Dixon FJ: Immune complex injury, Immunologic Diseases. Ed 3. M Samter, ed. Boston, Little, Brown & Co, 1978, pp 210–229

23. Cryoglobulinemia

Cryoglobulins are immunoglobulin molecules that have the unusual property of reversibly precipitating at low temperatures. Since their discovery more than 45 years ago (1), it has become apparent that cryoglobulins are found not only in patients with multiple myeloma, macroglobulinemia, and other proliferative disorders of plasma cells and lymphocytes, but occur with even higher frequency in the other diseases listed in Table 23–1. In these latter diseases, cryoglobulins are frequently found at low serum concentrations (2–8).

Classification. Cryoglobulins can be classified on the basis of their constituent molecules. Approximately one-third of cryoglobulins are composed of a monoclonal protein (most often IgG or IgM and very rarely IgA). These are usually associated with multiple myeloma and related diseases. Bence-Jones proteins also infrequently behave as cryoglobulins.

Cryoglobulins composed of 2 or more classes of immunoglobulins are much more common and constitute at least two-thirds of cold insoluble globulins (2–4,8). These mixed cryoglobulins are most frequently composed of IgM and IgG, occasionally IgM and IgA, or IgM, IgG and IgA, and in rare instances, other combinations of immunoglobulins.

Studies of many mixed cryoglobulins show that cryoprecipitability is generally dependent on the presence of an IgM molecule. By itself, the IgM may behave as a rheumatoid factor, but it is not cryoprecipitable without the concomitant presence of another immunoglobulin, usually IgG or its Fc fragment (3,6,8). The IgM component may be either monoclonal (almost invariably with κ light chains) or polyclonal. Most commonly, mixed cryoglobulins develop in diseases other than plasmacytic or lymphocytic neoplasms (2–4,8).

Tests. The test for cryoglobulins is performed by incubating serum at 0–4°C and then by determining the quantity of cold insoluble protein. This is done by means of a cryocrit or, alternatively, by isolating the cryoglobulin and determining the amount of protein precipitated. The type of immunoglobulin and the presence of other molecules such as complement components can then be detected by use of specific antisera.

When testing for cryoglobulins, it is important to draw the blood in a warm syringe, to both clot the blood and separate the serum at a warm temperature, and then to incubate the serum at 0–4°C for at least a week. The serum, not plasma, should be tested for cryoglobulins. This avoids confusion with various types of cold precipitable fibrinogen in the plasma of patients with other illnesses. Special attention should be paid to small amounts of cryoglobulins since these are often responsible for major clinical problems.

The amount of cryoglobulin in the serum may vary from several gm/dl (most often in patients with myeloma and macroglobulinemia) to a few mg/dl (in some disorders in Table 23–1 and occasionally in normal individuals).

Clinical features. The frequency with which large amounts of cryoglobulins may be present in the circulatory system without giving rise to symptoms, especially in individuals with monoclonal proteins, is surprising (2,4,7). Symptoms, when present with monoclonal cryoglobulins, include cold-induced urticaria, Raynaud's phenomenon, cutaneous ulcers (usually on the lower extremities), and gangrene of the fingers and toes on exposure to cold.

Mixed cryoglobulins cause some symptoms such as polyarthralgia and dependent purpura by immune complex deposition. About 50% of patients with mixed cryoglobulinemia develop immune complex nephritis that can be mild and at times reversible or can rapidly progress to renal failure. Hepatomegaly, splenomegaly, and moderate lymphadenopathy are common. Other less common manifestations include Raynaud's phenomenon, cutaneous ulcers, cold-induced urticaria, pericarditis, thyroiditis, Sjögren's syndrome, and other connective tissue diseases (2,3,8).

Laboratory findings. Laboratory examination generally reveals mild to moderate hypergammaglobulinemia and the absence of a monoclonal spike. Tests for rheumatoid factor are positive in virtually all patients with mixed cryoglobulinemia and serum complement levels are generally depressed. Antinuclear antibodies are sometimes present. Abnormalities in liver function tests can occur.

The prognosis for patients with symptomatic mixed cryoglobulinemia is unpredictable and depends on the severity of renal involvement. When the latter is absent, the course is usually of long duration. However, once renal disease develops, the disease may progress rapidly and prove fatal in a period of months to years. At autopsy, vasculitis, involving many organs, is usually found and evidence of sepsis is frequent (2,3,8).

There is little doubt that mixed cryoglobulins result from circulating immune complexes, and the associated symptoms are a consequence of immune complex deposition in the small vessels. In many instances, both the antigen and the antibody can be identified. Most commonly, perhaps because they are readily detectable, hepatitis B virus and its antibody have been recognized. Other agents such as Epstein-Barr (EB) virus have also been found, and it seems likely that other infectious agents and other types of antigens can give rise to circulating immune complexes (3,8).

Most mixed cryoglobulins contain rheumatoid factors, and at times, some of the components of complement may also be present.

A major role for the cryoglobulins in disease pathogenesis is indicated by the following: 1) circulating immune complexes composed of immunoglobulins and identified or unidentified antigens are present in the serum; 2) depressed levels of total hemolytic complement and individual complement components are common, especially during the acute state of the disease; 3) the vasculitic lesions in the glomeruli or the small vessels in the skin contain immunoglobulins, rheumatoid factors, complement components, and in rare instances, other antigens such as hepatitis B surface antigen; 4) the isolated cryoglobulins can interact with complement in vitro.

Although the IgM component may be

Table 23–1. Cryoglobulinemia: clinical associations

Monoclonal cryoglobulins
Myeloma, macroglobulinemia, other lymphoproliferative disorders
Mixed cryoglobulins
Infections
  Viral: infectious mononucleosis, hepatitis, rubella, cytomegalic virus
  Bacterial: subacute bacterial endocarditis, leprosy, post-streptococcal nephritis, intestinal bypass, visceral abscess
  Parasitic: kala-azar, schistosomiasis, malaria
Collagen diseases
  systemic lupus erythematosus, rheumatoid arthritis, polyarteritis nodosa, Sjögren's syndrome, progressive systemic sclerosis
Lymphoproliferative diseases (usually monoclonal)
  chronic lymphocytic leukemia, macroglobulinemia, immunoblastic lymphadenopathy
Miscellaneous
  essential mixed cryoglobulinemia, chronic liver disease, glomerulonephritis, sarcoidosis

either monoclonal or polyclonal, clinically and pathologically there is little difference in the patients with either form of mixed cryoglobulinemia (2,3,8).

A careful search for cryoglobulins should be part of the workup for all patients suspected of having immune complex diseases, since the presence of cryoglobulins provides strong evidence for the presence of these complexes. Although somewhat less sensitive as a test for immune complexes, cold insoluble immune complexes permit the ready isolation and subsequent characterization of the antigen and antibody.

Treatment, if required, should be directed toward the underlying disease. Benefit

has been reported in uncontrolled studies with corticosteroids, immunosuppressive agents, and with plasmapheresis in individuals with mixed cryoglobulinemia (9).

1. Wintrobe MM, Buell MV: Hyperproteinemia associated with multiple myeloma. Bull Johns Hopkins Hosp 52:156–165, 1933
2. Brouet J-C, Clauvel J-P, Danon F, Klein M, Seligmann M: Biological and clinical significance of cryoglobulins. Am J Med 57:755–788, 1974
3. Gorevic PD, Kasab HJ, Levo Y, Kohn R, Meltzer M, Prose P, Franklin EC: Mixed cryoglobulinemia: clinical aspects and long-term follow-up of forty patients. Am J Med 69:287, 1980
4. Grey HM, Kohler PF: Cryoimmunoglobulins. Semin Hematol 10:87–112, 1973

5. Levo Y, Gorevic PD, Kassab HJ, Zucker-Franklin D, Franklin EC: Association between hepatitis B virus and essential mixed cryoglobulinemia. N Engl J Med 296:1501–1504, 1977
6. LoSpalluto J, Dorward B, Miller W Jr., Ziff M: Cryoglobulinemia based on interaction between a gamma macroglobulin and 7S gamma globulin. Am J Med 32:142–147, 1962
7. Meltzer M, Franklin EC: Cryoglobulinemia. I. A study of 29 patients: IgG and IgM cryoglobulins and factors affecting cryoprecipitability. Am J Med 40:818–836, 1966
8. Meltzer M, Franklin EC, Elias K, McCluskey RT, Cooper N: Cryoglobulinemia: a clinical and laboratory study. II. Cryoglobulins with rheumatoid factor activity. Am J Med 40:837–856, 1966
9. Geltner D, Kohn RW, Gorevic P, Franklin EC: The effect of combination therapy (steroids, immunosuppressives, and plasmapheresis) on 5 mixed cryoglobulinemia patients with renal, neurologic, and vascular involvement. Arthritis Rheum 24:1121–1127, 1981

24. Relapsing polychondritis

Relapsing polychondritis is a relatively rare disease characterized by episodic inflammation and progressive destruction of cartilage. Systemic vasculitis is often present. There is no sex predilection and the peak of onset appears to be in the fifth decade.

A review of this disorder (1) suggests the following diagnostic criteria:

1. Recurrent chondritis of the auricles
2. Inflammation of ocular structures including conjunctivitis, keratitis, scleritis/episcleritis, and/or uveitis
3. Chondritis of the laryngeal and/or tracheal cartilage
4. Cochlear and/or vestibular damage manifested by neurosensory hearing loss, tinnitus, and/or vertigo

When 3 or more of these criteria are present, with biopsy confirmation, the diagnosis is considered "certain."

Cardiovascular involvement is also relatively common; aortic insufficiency may occur due to loss of elastic fibrils and resultant dilatation of the aortic ring. Patients may die from airway obstruction due to collapse of the tracheal and bronchial cartilage.

About half of the patients present with either inflammation of the external ears or arthritis. The inflammation is characterized by the sudden onset of intense pain with redness and swelling of one or both helices (Fig 24–1). The arthritis is usually an oligo- or polyarthritis involving both large and small joints (1). At the outset, the arthritis is often migratory and may resemble rheumatoid arthritis. Some patients present with the other manifestations listed here.

The frequency of specific organ system involvement at any time during the disease course is approximately as follows: auricular chondritis, 89%; arthritis, 81%; nasal chondritis, 72%; eye involvement, 65%; respiratory tract disease, 56%; inner ear disease, 46%; cardiovascular system involvement, 24%; and skin lesions, 17% (1). Renal disease may occur (2,3).

There are no diagnostic laboratory findings although the sedimentation rate is often extremely high. Rheumatoid factors and antinuclear antibodies are usually absent. In many instances, there is a mild to moderate anemia and moderate leukocytosis.

The pathologic changes in cartilage include loss of basophilic staining of the matrix, inflammatory cell infiltration, loss of distinction at the borders with other tissues, vacuolization of chondrocytes, phagocytosis of chondrocytes by macrophages, and total destruction of cartilage with fibrous replacement. Electron microscopy has revealed alterations of chondrocytes as well as degradation of elastic and collagen fibers (4,5).

The origin of relapsing polychondritis is unknown, but the demonstration of antibodies to type II collagen (6) and of cell-mediated immunity to proteoglycan suggests that immunologic mechanisms are involved in pathogenesis.

Relapsing polychondritis has been associated with other diseases in about 30% of cases, often leading to diagnostic confusion. Associated disorders include rheumatic diseases (especially rheumatoid arthritis and Sjögren's syndrome), thyroid disease, ulcerative colitis, malignancies, sinusitis, mastoiditis, and diabetes mellitus.

Treatment has been primarily symptomatic, although the use of corticosteroids during active inflammatory episodes appears to be helpful, especially in cases of life-threatening involvement of the respiratory tract. There is no evidence, however, that corticosteroids halt the progression of the disease.

Relapsing polychondritis has been likened to hypervitaminosis A, a condition in which chondroitin sulfate is destroyed by lysosomal enzymes. Since dapsone inhibits this destruction in rabbits, the drug has been administered to patients with relapsing polychondritis with apparent success (3,7,8). This innovative approach warrants further study.

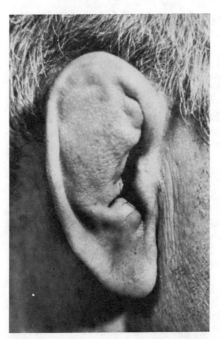

Fig 24–1. Thickened ear of a 61-year-old man with relapsing polychondritis.

1. McAdam LP, O'Hanlan MA, Bluestone R, Pearson CM: Relapsing polychondritis: prospective study of 23 patients and a review of the literature. Medicine 55:193–215, 1976
2. Ruhlen JL, Huston KA, Wood WG: Relapsing polychondritis with glomerulonephritis: improvement with prednisone and cyclophosphamide. JAMA 245:847–848, 1981
3. Espinoza LR, Richman A, Bocanegra T, Pina I, Vasey FB, Rifkin SI, Germain BF: Immune complex-mediated renal involvement in relapsing polychondritis. Am J Med 71:181–183, 1981

4. Dryll A, Lausarman J, Meyer O, Bardin T, Rychewaert A: Relapsing polychondritis: an ultrastructural study of elastic and collagen fibres, degradation revealed by tannic acid. Virchows Arch [Pathol Anat] 390:109–119, 1981

5. Shaul SR, Schumacher HR: Relapsing polychon-dritis: electron microscopic study of ear cartilage. Arthritis Rheum 18:617–625, 1975

6. Foidart JM, Abe S, Martin GR, Zizic TM, Barnett EV, Lawley TJ, Katz SI: Antibodies to type II collagen in relapsing polychondritis. N Engl J Med 299:1203–1207, 1978

7. Martin J, Roenigk HH Jr, Lynch W, Tingwald FR: Relapsing polychondritis treated with dapsone. Arch Dermatol 112:1272–1274, 1976

8. Barranco VP, Minor DB, Solomon H: Treatment of relapsing polychondritis with dapsone. Arch Dermatol 112:1286–1288, 1976

25. Thrombotic thrombocytopenic purpura

Thrombotic thrombocytopenic purpura is included among the rheumatic disorders because it has many features found in systemic lupus erythematosus and is sometimes associated with other multisystem diseases.

The major clinical manifestations include: thrombocytopenia with purpura, hemolytic anemia, fever, neurologic dysfunction, and renal abnormalities (1). Bleeding is sometimes severe and the disease may begin with hemorrhage from the gastrointestinal, urinary, or vaginal tracts. Neurologic involvement is characteristically wavering and migratory with a broad spectrum of manifestations including mental changes, convulsions, hemiplegias, cranial nerve palsies, and aphasia. The disease affects women more often than men; the peak incidence is in the third decade.

Characteristic laboratory findings in the blood are severe thrombocytopenia and anemia; red cells show a wide variety of sizes and shapes. In a typical smear, small cell fragments, bizarre forms, and large young cells are seen. There is often a moderate leukocytosis (20,000–30,000 cells/mm^3). Fibrin split products may be detected at times, suggesting diffuse intra-vascular coagulation. The urine may show moderate proteinuria and hematuria. Bone marrow biopsy is often diagnostically helpful, but gingival biopsies have recently been advocated as more reliable, simple, and safe (2).

The essential pathologic feature is eosinophilic hyaline thrombi in small arterioles and capillaries with associated endothelial damage. These vascular lesions may be seen in almost every organ. There may be characteristic aneurysmal dilatation of vessels.

Controversy continues regarding whether primary vascular inflammation leads to the platelet aggregation and thrombus formation. The platelets have been found to be coated with increased amounts of IgG, possibly the result of direct antibody or immune complex attachment (3). It has been speculated that these platelets clump and occlude vessels.

The typical course of untreated thrombotic thrombocytopenic purpura is that of a fulminant disease with death of 80% of patients in 3 months. Chronic relapsing or recurrent illnesses have also been reported.

Treatment has improved the prognosis, but no single reliable approach has been established. Almost all patients have been treated with moderate to large doses of corticosteroids. Recently splenectomy (4), plasma infusion (5), or exchange transfusions (6), or vincristine (7) have been used in patients with severe disease; dramatic improvement and indeed total remissions have been reported.

1. Amorosi EL, Ultmann JE: Thrombotic thrombocytopenic purpura: report of 16 cases and review of the literature. Medicine 45:139–159, 1966

2. Goldenfarb PM, Finch SC: Thrombotic thrombocytopenic purpura: a 10 year survey. JAMA 226:644–647, 1973

3. Morrison J, McMillan R: Elevated platelet-associated IgG in thrombotic thrombocytopenic purpura. JAMA 238:1944–1945, 1977

4. Reynolds PM, Jackson JM, Brine JA, Vivian AB: Thrombotic thrombocytopenic purpura–remission following splenectomy: report of a case and review of the literature. Am J Med 61:439–447, 1976

5. Byrnes JJ, Khurana M: Treatment of thrombotic thrombocytopenic purpura with plasma. N Engl J Med 297:1386–1389, 1977

6. Rossi EC, del Greco F, Kwan HC et al: Hemodialysis-exchange transfusion for treatment of thrombotic thrombocytopenic purpura. JAMA 244:1466–1468, 1980

7. Gutterman LA, Stevenson TD: Treatment of thrombotic thrombocytopenic purpura with vincristine. JAMA 247:1433–1435, 1982

26. Chronic active liver disease

Regardless of the initial cause of liver damage, some patients continue to have active liver necrosis beyond the stage of acute hepatitis, even when they may have already developed cirrhosis. Chronic active liver disease is often marked by multisystem extrahepatic manifestations, autoantibodies, and disease associations that suggest a relationship to the connective tissue diseases.

There are 3 main forms of chronic active liver disease: 1) chronic active hepatitis (CAH), 2) primary biliary cirrhosis (PBC), and 3) cryptogenic cirrhosis. The first two can usually be distinguished by the predominant hepatocyte (CAH) or cholangitic (PBC) damage and their resulting clinical and laboratory features, whereas cryptogenic cirrhosis seems to be the end stage of a variety of liver diseases including the previous two (1).

Diagnostic features of chronic active hepatitis include a persistent (> 6 months) and significant (> 4-fold) elevation in the activity of liver enzymes in the serum, hypergammaglobulinemia, and histologic changes that include piecemeal necrosis of hepatocytes, lobular distortion, and lymphocytic and plasma cell infiltrates. Cirrhosis may be present (2). Two-thirds of patients with CAH have hepatitis B–associated surface antigen in their serum, indicating the probable original cause of liver disease. That genetic factors are implicated in the development of CAH is suggested by its association with haplotype HLA–A1+B8, a haplotype that may also be associated with other autoimmune diseases.

Serologic findings include cryoglobulinemia, anti-smooth muscle and antinuclear antibodies (ANA) each present in 60% of patients, and rheumatoid factor in 20% (1,3). The finding of positive LE cell reactions in up to 40% of patients with CAH gave rise to the term *lupoid hepatitis* (1).

CAH patients with LE cells and/or a high titer of ANA may have multisystem features akin to and sometimes indistinguishable from those of systemic lupus erythematosus.

Articular manifestations occur in one-third of patients with chronic active hepatitis and in nearly two-thirds of those with lupoid hepatitis (3). They may involve both large and small joints, are often associated with periarticular swelling, are seldom erosive, and their course may coincide with that of the liver disease (3). Sjögren's syndrome occurs in at least one-third of patients with CAH, and many more may have some clinical evidence of salivary or lacrimal gland damage. Articular manifestations usually respond to treatment of CAH with low doses of corticosteroids or azathioprine.

Pruritus, jaundice, xanthomata, skin hyperpigmentation, and liver failure are the main clinical features of primary biliary cirrhosis. About 5% of the patients have articular involvement akin to that of CAH (4), and 70–90% of patients with PBC have evidence of Sjögren's syndrome (5). The association of PBC with progressive systemic sclerosis (see Section 14) is frequent enough to have been considered a distinct syndrome that also associates with HLA–A1+B8. Occasional association with lupus erythematosus has also been described (6).

The histologic changes in the liver in primary biliary cirrhosis have been staged from the initial acute cholangitis (I), to cholangiolar proliferation (II), to scarring (III), and finally portal cirrhosis (IV). Anti-mitochondrial antibodies are found in the serum of nearly all patients with PBC. One-third of these patients have ANA and one-fourth have rheumatoid factor (3).

That liver disease in some patients with cryptogenic cirrhosis represents an end stage of CAH or PBC is indicated by the occasional finding of arthritis, Sjögren's syndrome, ANA, anti-mitochondrial or anti-smooth muscle antibodies (3).

1. MacKay IR, Weiden S, Hasker J: Autoimmune hepatitis. Ann NY Acad Sci 124:767–780, 1965

2. Czaja AJ: Current problems in the diagnosis and management of chronic active hepatitis. Mayo Clin Proc 56:311–323, 1981
3. Golding PL, Smith M, Williams R: Multisystem involvement in chronic liver disease: studies on the incidence and pathogenesis. Am J Med 55:772–782, 1973
4. Clarke AK, Galbraith RM, Hamilton EBD, Williams R: Rheumatic disorders in primary biliary cirrhosis. Ann Rheum Dis 37:42–47, 1978
5. Alarcon-Segovia D, Diaz-Jouanen E, Fishbein E: Features of Sjögren's syndrome in primary biliary cirrhosis. Ann Intern Med 79:31–36, 1973
6. Iliff GD, Naidoo S, Hunter T: Primary biliary cirrhosis associated with features of systemic lupus erythematosus. Digest Dis Sci (NS) 27:274–278, 1982

27. Ankylosing spondylitis

Once considered a rare, predominantly male disease that progresses relentlessly to spinal fusion, ankylosing spondylitis (AS) is now recognized as affecting both sexes, with males having more symptomatic and severe disease. AS is the prototype of the seronegative spondylarthropathies, a group of interrelated disorders that includes psoriatic arthropathy, Reiter's syndrome, the reactive arthropa-thies, and juvenile chronic polyarthropathy (1–3). All these disorders are associated with HLA–B27, absence of rheumatoid factor in the serum, and lack of rheumatoid nodules. They are enthesopathic (develop inflammation at the site of the enthesis or ligamentous insertion into bone) and have a marked degree of familial aggregation (Table 27–1).

The term *ankylosing spondylitis* derives from the Greek *ankylos* (bent or crooked) and *spondylos* (vertebra). Past names have included von Bechterew's disease, Marie-Strumpell's disease, and more recently rheumatoid spondylitis. This last was inappropriate since AS may be distinguished from rheumatoid disease on clinical and nonclinical grounds (2) (Table 27–2). Likewise, the related seronegative spondylarthritides should not be consid-

Table 27–1. Comparison of seronegative spondylarthropathies*

	Ankylosing spondylitis	Reiter's syndrome	Psoriatic arthropathy	Intestinal arthropathy	Juvenile chronic arthropathy	Reactive arthropathy
Sex distribution	Male ≥ female	Male ≥ female	Female ≥ male	Female = male	Male ≥ female	Male = female
Age at onset (yrs)	≥ 20	≥ 20	Any age	Any age	<25	Any age
Uveitis	+	++	+	+	++	+
Prostatitis	+	+	−	−	−	?
Peripheral joints	Lower limb, often	Lower limb, usually	Upper > lower limb	Lower > upper limb	Upper or lower limb	Lower > upper limb
Rheumatoid nodules	<1%	<1%	<1%	<1%	<1%	<1%
Sacroiliitis	Always	Often	Often	Often	Often	Often
Plantar spurs	Common	Common	Common	?	?	?
Rheumatoid factor	<5%	<5%	<5%	<5%	<10%	<5%
HLA–B27 positive	90%	90%	20% (50% with sacroiliitis)	5% (50% with sacroiliitis)	20% (50% with sacroiliitis)	90%
Enthesopathy	+	+	+	?+	+	?
Aortic regurgitation	+	+	?+	?	?	+
Familial aggregation	+	+	+	+	+	+
Response to therapy (indomethacin, phenylbutazone)	+++	+	++	+	+	+
Risk for HLA–B27 positive individual	~20%	~20%	?	?	?	~20%
Onset	Gradual	Sudden	Variable	Peripherally: sudden; axial: gradual	Variable	Sudden
Urethritis	−	+	−	−	−	+
Conjunctivitis	+	+++	+	+	+	+
Skin involvement	−	+	+++	−	−	−
Mucous membrane involvement	−	++	−	+	−	−
Spine involvement	+++	+	+	+	+	+
Symmetry	+	−	−	+	±	±
Self-limiting	−	±	±	±	±	±
Remissions, relapses	−	±	±	±	±	±

* Modified from Calin A: Spondylarthritis. Medicine. Sci Am 1982, pp 15, III, 6.

Table 27–2. Comparison of ankylosing spondylitis and rheumatoid arthritis*

	Ankylosing spondylitis	Rheumatoid arthritis
History	Evidence in animals and humans dating from 3,000 BC	Documented in humans since 19th century
Distribution	Racial	Worldwide
Prevalence	1–2%	1–2%
Etiology	Unknown	Unknown
Positive family history	Frequent	Rare
Sex distribution	More frequently diagnosed in males	More common in females
Age group	Peak at 20–30 years	All ages; peak at 30–50 years
Joint involvement	Oligarthropathy; asymmetric; large joints; lower limbs more than upper limbs	Polyarthropathy; symmetric; small and large joints; upper and lower limbs
Sacroiliac involvement	Yes	No
Spine involvement	Total (ascending)	Cervical
Nodules	No	Yes
Aortic regurgitation	Yes	No
Eyes	Conjunctivitis, uveitis	Sicca syndrome, scleritis, scleromalacia perforans
Lungs	Upper lobe pulmonary fibrosis	Caplan's syndrome, effusions
Rheumatoid factor	No	Yes
HLA–B27	≈90%	≈6% (normal distribution)
HLA–Dw4	≈20% (normal distribution)	≈60%
Pathology	Enthesopathy	Inflammatory synovitis
Radiology	Asymmetric erosive arthropathy, new bone formation, ankylosis, sacroiliitis	Symmetric erosive arthropathy
Therapy	Indomethacin, phenylbutazone	Aspirin, gold, penicillamine

* Modified from Calin A: Spondylarthritis. Medicine. Sci Am 1982, pp 15, III, 3.

ered "rheumatoid variants." Ankylosing spondylitis is not an ideal name since few patients progress to a "bent" spine, total "ankylosis" is rare, and extrapelvic spread occurs in a minority of patients.

Criteria for diagnosis have been developed (4). The disease is *primary* if no other rheumatologic disorder is present or *secondary* if the sacroiliitis is related to one of the other spondylarthropathies.

Prevalence. Many patients with a diagnostic label of "seronegative rheumatoid arthritis," mechanical back pain, or even "neurosis" do have ankylosing spondylitis. Unfortunately patients with AS are still inappropriately receiving myelograms, bed rest, and even surgery.

About 20% of HLA–B27 positive individuals develop AS or another seronegative spondylarthropathy (5,6), resulting in a prevalence of about 1% in whites, a figure similar to that for rheumatoid arthritis. The sex ratio of saroiliitis is about equal (5,6), but men have more progressive spinal disease, giving a clinical ratio of about 3:1 (7). The geographic distribution of disease mirrors that of HLA–B27. Thus AS occurs less frequently in African blacks, Japanese, and American blacks but more frequently in Pima and Haida Indians. (The prevalence of B27 ranges from near zero to 50% in these populations.)

Primary AS usually develops during the second and third decade, but juvenile AS (7) (a subset of juvenile chronic polyarthropathy) may occur in younger individuals and the secondary forms may occur at any age.

Clinical features and diagnosis. Many people with ankylosing spondylitis remain undiagnosed. Symptoms may be mild with minimal early morning stiffness or can be severe and progressive.

In the differential diagnosis of inflammatory and mechanical (nonspecific) spinal disease (9) (Table 27–3), the following features suggest inflammation: 1) insidious onset of discomfort over weeks or months, 2) age of onset below 40 years, 3) more or less persistent discomfort for months, 4) association with morning stiffness, 5) improvement with exercise.

Any patient with a history suggestive of spondylitis should be evaluated by pelvic radiography. Family history of psoriasis, arthropathy, back disease, eye disease, and other features may be relevant. Extraspinal symptoms include enthesopathic features (a pleuritic-like chest pain, achilles tendinitis, plantar fasciitis, dactylitis, and iliac crest discomfort), inflammatory eye disease, peripheral arthropathy (especially hips), and nonspecific symptoms such as weight loss, malaise, fatigue, and mood change.

Examination may reveal muscle spasm, loss of lumbar lordosis, and decreased spinal mobility in all directions (Fig 27–1). The modified Schober test measures the distraction on anterior flexion of 10 cm measured vertically above the level of the posterior iliac spines. Lateral spinal flexion measures the distraction of an arbitrary 20 cm line drawn in the midaxillary plane. On anterior or contralateral flexion, a distraction of 5–10 cm is considered normal. Finger-to-floor measurement reflects general fitness and hip status rather than spinal mobility per se.

Chest expansion is difficult to measure especially in women and is decreased only late in the disease. Evidence for psoriasis, urethritis, and bowel disease must be sought.

The sine qua non for diagnosis is sacroiliitis, a radiologic diagnosis that requires experience and the appreciation that early change may be subtle. The apparent rarity of the disease in the past was related to the fact that radiologists and physicians were reluctant to diagnose it unless marked

Table 27–3. Contrasting features of mechanical (nonspecific) and inflammatory (ankylosing spondylitis) spinal disease

Clinical features	Mechanical	Inflammatory
Clinical history*	Episodic, related to exercise	Persistent
Family history	Negative	Possibly positive
Onset*	Acute	Insidious
Age* (yrs)	15–90	<40
Sleep disturbance	Variable	Variable
Morning stiffness*	+	+++
Involvement of other systems	Absent	Eyes, joints
Effect of exercise*	Worse	Better
Effect of rest	Better	Worse
Radiation of pain	Anatomic (S1,L5)	Diffuse (thoracic, buttock)
Sensory symptoms	Present	Absent
Motor symptoms	Present	Absent
Scoliosis	Present	Absent
Decreased range of movement	Asymmetrically	Symmetrically
Tenderness	Local	Diffuse
Muscle spasm	Local	Diffuse
Straight leg raising	Decreased	Normal
Sciatic nerve stretch	Positive	Absent
Hip involvement	Absent	Present
Neurodeficit	Present	Absent

* Important historical differences.

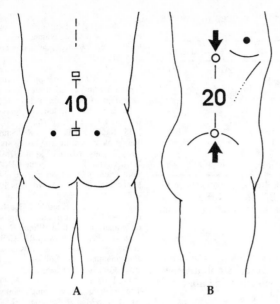

Fig 27–1. A, Note the 10 cm line between 2 points, the lower at level of post-iliac spines. **B**, Note 20 cm line in midaxilliary plane. (Illustration provided by Dr A Calin)

radiologic changes were present. Pelvic radiographs are graded (0–IV) according to the New York criteria (4). The grading depends on the degree of juxtaarticular sclerosis, blurring of the joint margin, narrowing of the joint space, erosions, and finally fusion. A single anteroposterior view of the pelvis is generally sufficient. Additional oblique views are rarely helpful.

A diagnosis depends on history, examination, and radiologic confirmation. The erythrocyte sedimentation rate may be increased. HLA–B27 typing is unnecessary as a routine clinical test (9–11). About 90% of white patients and 60% of black patients with AS are HLA–B27 positive in contrast to about 7% of white controls and 4% of black controls. Thus, the presence of B27 is not diagnostic and its absence does not exclude the diagnosis. Radionuclide scanning may show sacroiliitis before radiologic change (12), but because of its lack of specificity and expense, it is of limited value. Computerized tomography will no doubt have its enthusiasts but cost will hopefully preclude widespread use.

Some findings (e.g., peripheral joint involvement, eye disease, and plantar fasciitis) may occur at any time whereas others such as aortic regurgitation (13), cord compression, upper lobe pulmonary fibrosis (14), and amyloid deposition are late disease manifestations.

Asymmetric (often, lower limb) peripheral arthropathy occurs in about 20% of patients at presentation and in a third at some stage of disease. Iritis, unrelated to disease severity, occurs in up to 25% of patients. Episodes are usually self-limiting, but may require local or even systemic corticosteroid therapy. B27-associated uveitis may occur as a forme fruste in the absence of rheumatic disease.

Patients with upper lobe pulmonary fibrosis (14), have cough, sputum, and dyspnea. Radiographic changes mimic tuberculosis. Invasion with *Aspergillus* may cause hemoptysis and death. A rigid chest wall may result from fusion of thoracic joints but pulmonary ventilation is maintained by the diaphragm. Excessive deaths from nonradiotherapy causes are now recognized (15–17).

Cardiovascular involvement (aortic incompetence, cardiomegaly, and conduction defects) may affect up to 3% of patients with long-standing, severe disease. Cardiac disease may be silent (18) or dominate the picture. A rare complication is the cauda equina syndrome (19), which presents with leg and buttock pain, bowel and bladder symptoms, and evidence of a neurodeficit. Diverticulae may be seen on myelography. There appears to be no impairment of renal glomerular function (20), despite the recognized pathologic changes.

Relatively few patients progress to a classic bamboo spine. Trivial injury to the fused cervical spine may result in fracture and cord compression (21). Because of deformity, radiographic visualization of the fracture site may be difficult. Conservative management with halo traction and body cast is often adequate, although surgical intervention may be required. Vertebral endplate destruction (*spondylodiscitis*) may result from minimal trauma and is managed by rest.

Radiologic evaluation. Sacroiliitis must be differentiated from Paget's disease of bone, metastatic disease, infection, and other rarer causes. Osteitis condensans ilii is an idiopathic sclerotic condition of one or both iliacs, occurring in females. The iliac sclerosis increases demarcation of the joint margin in contrast to the blurring

seen in sacroiliitis. Patients may have bilateral grade IV sacroiliitis in the absence of extrapelvic disease. In contrast, some with relatively minimal sacroiliac involvement develop spinal disease. Squaring of the vertebral body due to enthesopathic disease at the site of insertion of the disc anulus fibrosis is an early spinal change resulting in loss of the normal anterior vertebral concavity. The bony reaction to this destructive lesion results in syndesmophyte formation. Progressive ossification (Fig 27–2) may result in the typical but not invariable bamboo spine. Spinal changes in primary ankylosing spondylitis and inflammatory bowel disease mimic each other whereas changes occurring in psoriatic arthropathy and Reiter's syndrome tend to be asymmetric with skip lesions (22).

Extraspinal changes include a typical erosive destructive arthropathy of the hip and to a lesser extent other joints and new bone formation at the site of enthesopathic lesions. Examples include plantar spurs and calcaneal periostitis at the site of the achilles tendon insertion.

The unique pathology (enthesopathy) of ankylosing spondylitis and the other seronegative spondylarthritides is now recognized (23). Ossification occurs in the region of discs, the apophyseal and sacroiliac joints, and extraspinal sites, initiated by lesions at the site of ligamentous insertions.

Laboratory abnormalities. The erythrocyte sedimentation rate, alkaline phosphatase, and creatinine phosphokinase (24) are often elevated. Ankylosing spondylitis in HLA–B27 positive and negative patients is similar. AS was long considered

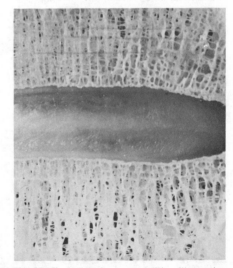

Fig 27–2. Ankylosing spondylitis, illustrating ossification of the anulus fibrosus. (Illustration provided by Dr L Sokoloff and reproduced with permission from Sokoloff L: The pathology of rheumatoid arthritis and allied disorders, in Hollander JL, McCarty DJ Jr, eds: Arthritis and Allied Conditions. Ed 8, Philadelphia, Lea & Febiger Publishers, 1972, pp 309–332)

an immunologically silent disease. Now, recognition of raised levels of complement inactivation products, antiglobulins of the IgG class, C4 and IgA in the sera, and circulating immune complexes (25) as well as the link with HLA–B27 suggest immunologic activity.

Ankylosing spondylitis in women. The diagnosis is often delayed or missed in women. Sacroiliitis may be equally prevalent in both sexes but progressive disease is more common in men. Women tend to have more peripheral joint involvement and are sometimes misdiagnosed as having "seronegative rheumatoid arthritis" (26). Disease manifestations by gender are shown in Table 27–4. A recent study reviewed the experience of 87 pregnancies in 50 women with disease. The course was largely unaffected by pregnancy and the newborns were unharmed (27).

AS and rheumatoid arthritis are not mutually exclusive disorders. Since 1% of the population may develop either disease, both will be seen in 1:10,000 subjects.

Etiology. Twenty percent of B27 positive people develop AS after an unknown event (5,6) or Reiter's syndrome after a specific infection (28). What protects the remaining 80% remains unknown. Since identical twins may be discordant for ankylosing spondylitis, an environmental factor is required. It is likely that the putative organisms are ubiquitous. *Klebsiella* has been incriminated (29,30), but proof is lacking.

Management. Most patients with ankylosing spondylitis function normally despite chronic discomfort for many years. Antiinflammatory medication (indomethacin 25–50 mg 3–4 times per day, or if not efficacious, phenylbutazone 100 mg 3–4 times per day) enables the patient to follow an adequate exercise program, maintain good posture, and pursue normal activities. A hard bed at night, extension exercises directed toward maintaining erect posture and normal height, and hydrotherapy are appropriate. One uncontrolled retrospective study (31) suggested that phenylbutazone is associated with decreased skeletal ossification. Other nonsteroidal antiinflammatory drugs such as sulindac 150–200 mg twice a day may be used for patients who cannot tolerate the above agents.

Radiotherapy has fallen into disrepute because of the risk of leukemia (32). Surgi-

Table 27–4. Sex differences in ankylosing spondylitis*

	Males	Females
% HLA–B27 positive	90	90
Delay in diagnosis (yrs)	3	10
Progression	+++	+
Severity	+++	+
Peripheral joint disease		
initial	+	++
subsequent	+	+++
Spinal ankylosis	++	+
Cervical spine symptoms	++	+†

* Modified from Calin A: Spondylarthritis. Medicine. Sci Am 1982, pp 15, III, 9.
† Not necessarily including thoracic and lumbar spine.

cal treatment is occasionally indicated, and a vertebral wedge osteotomy performed. Gold and penicillamine appear to have little part to play.

At present, routine family HLA typing is not advised since the disease cannot be prevented and adequate function is usually maintained with simple treatment.

Outcome for the individual patient is often difficult to assess. Most will enjoy a normal professional and social existence (33), despite concerns to the contrary (16,17).

1. Wright V, Moll JMH: Seronegative Polyarthritis, Amsterdam, North Holland Publishing Co, 1976
2. Calin A, Fries JF: Ankylosing spondylitis: discussions in patient management. Garden City, NY, Medical Examination Publishing Co, 1978, pp 1–117
3. Calin A: Ankylosing spondylitis, Textbook of Rheumatology. WN Kelley, ED Harris, S Ruddy, CB Sledge, eds. Philadelphia, WB Saunders Co, 1981, pp 1017–1032
4. Moll JMH, Wright V: New York criteria for ankylosing spondylitis: a statistical evaluation. Ann Rheum Dis 32:354–358, 1973
5. Calin A, Fries JF: The striking prevalence of ankylosing spondylitis in "healthy" W27 positive males and females: a controlled study. N Engl J Med 293:835–839, 1975
6. Editorial: HLA–B27 and the risk of ankylosing spondylitis. Br Med J 2:650–651, 1978
7. Marks SH, Calin A: A case control study of juvenile and adult onset disease. J Rheumatol 9:739–747, 1982
8. Hill HFH, Hill AGS, Bodmer JG: Clinical diagnosis of ankylosing spondylitis in women and relation to presence of HLA B27. Ann Rheum Dis 35:267–270, 1976
9. Calin A, Porta J, Fries JFF: The clinical history as a screening test for ankylosing spondylitis. JAMA 237:2613–2614, 1977
10. Calin A: HLA–B27: to type or not to type? Ann Intern Med 92:208–211, 1980
11. Calin A: HLA–B27 in 1982: reappraisal of a clinical test. Ann Intern Med 96:114–115, 1982

12. Russel AS, Lentle BC, Percy JS: Investigation of sacroiliac disease: comparative evaluation of radiological and radionuclide techniques. J Rheumatol 2:45–51, 1975
13. Buckley BH, Roberts WC: Ankylosing spondylitis and aortic regurgitation: description of the characteristic cardio-vascular lesion from study of 8 necropsy patients. Circulation 18:1014–1027, 1973
14. Editorial: The lungs in ankylosing spondylitis. Br Med J 3:492–493, 1971
15. Radford EP, Doll R, Smith PG: Mortality among patients with ankylosing spondylitis not given x-ray therapy. N Engl J Med 297:572–576, 1977
16. Carter ET, McKenna CH, Brian DD, et al: Epidemiology of ankylosing spondylitis in Rochester, Minnesota, 1935–1973. Arthritis Rheum 22:365–370, 1979
17. Khan MA, Khan MK, Kushner I: Evidence of decreased survival in ankylosing spondylitis by life-table analysis. Arthritis Rheum 22:628, 1979
18. Tucker CR, Fowles RE, Calin A, et al: Aortitis in ankylosing spondylitis: early detection of aortic root abnormalities with 2-dimensional echocardiography. Am J Cardiol 9:680–686, 1982
19. Russell ML, Gordon DA, Ogryzlo MA, et al: The cauda equina syndrome of ankylosing spondylitis. Ann Intern Med 78:551–554, 1973
20. Calin A: Renal glomerular function in ankylosing spondylitis. Scand J Rheumatol 4:241–242, 1975
21. Murray GC, Persellin RH: Cervical fractures complicating ankylosing spondylitis: a report of 8 cases and review of the literature. Am J Med 70:1033–1041, 1981
22. McEwen C, DiTata D, Ling C, et al: Ankylosing spondylitis and spondylitis accompanying ulcerative colitis, regional enteritis, psoriasis in Reiter's disease. Arthritis Rheum 14:291–318, 1971
23. Ball J: Enthesopathy of rheumatoid and ankylosing spondylitis. Ann Rheum Dis 30:213–223, 1971
24. Calin A: Creatine phosphokinase in ankylosing spondylitis. Ann Rheum Dis 34:244–248, 1975
25. Corrigal V, Panayi GS, Unger A, et al: Detection of immune complexes in serum of patients with ankylosing spondylitis. Ann Rheum Dis 37:159–163, 1978
26. Calin A, Marks SH: The case against seronegative rheumatoid arthritis. Am J Med 70:992–994, 1981
27. Ostensen M, Romberg O, Husby G: Ankylosing spondylitis and motherhood. Arthritis Rheum 25:140–143, 1982
28. Calin A, Fries JF: An "experimental" epidemic of Reiter's syndrome revisited: follow-up evidence on genetic and environmental factors. Ann Intern Med 84:564–566, 1976
29. Seager K, Bashir HV, Geczy AF, et al: Evidence for a specific B27-associated cell surface marker on lymphocytes of patients with ankylosing spondylitis. Nature 277:68–69, 1979
30. Eastmond CJ, Calguneri M, Shinebaum R, et al: A sequential study of the relationship between faecal Klebsiella aerogenes and the common clinical manifestations of ankylosing spondylitis. Ann Rheum Dis 41:15–20, 1982
31. Boersma JW: Retardation of ossification of the lumbar vertebral column in ankylosing spondylitis by means of phenylbutazone. Scand J Rheumatol 5:60–64, 1976
32. Smith RG, Doll R: Mortality among patients with ankylosing spondylitis after a single treatment course with x-rays. Br Med J 284:449–460, 1982
33. Calin A: Ankylosing spondylitis, Prognosis. JF Fries, GE Ehrlich, eds. Maryland, The Charles Press, 1981, pp 357–359

28. Reiter's syndrome

The first description of the syndrome of arthritis and ocular inflammation following sexually acquired urethritis, which now bears the eponymous title of Reiter, was made in 1818 by Sir Benjamin Brodie.

In 1916 Hans Reiter described a Prussian cavalry officer who developed an acute febrile illness characterized by arthritis, urethritis, and conjunctivitis 8 days after an episode of abdominal pain and blood-

stained diarrhea (1). Feissinger and LeRoy in France also reported a case in 1916 similar to that described by Reiter.

Etiology. In the United Kingdom and North America, most cases of Reiter's

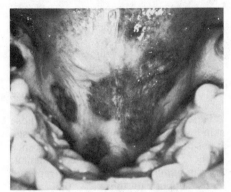

Fig 28–1. Ulcerations on undersurface of tongue in a man with Reiter's syndrome. (Illustration provided by Dr WW Buchanan)

syndrome appear to follow venereal exposure, whereas in Europe, Africa, and the Middle and Far East, the postdysenteric form appears to be more common (2). *Chlamydia trachomatis* has been isolated from the urethra, conjunctiva, synovial fluid, and synovial membrane of patients with Reiter's syndrome, and complement-fixing antibodies and lymphocyte transformation to chlamydia antigens have also been demonstrated. *Chlamydia trachomatis* cannot be isolated in all patients, however, and there is as yet no definite evidence that it causes the venereally acquired syndrome.

The postdysenteric form of Reiter's syndrome usually follows infection with *Shigella flexneri* and rarely occurs after Salmonella infection. A reactive arthritis, i.e., one in which the joint fluid is sterile, may follow Shigella, Salmonella, and *Yersinia enterocolitica* intestinal infection and may represent a partial form of the disease (3).

Synovial fluid mononuclear cells have recently been shown to respond with increased thymidine incorporation after stimulation with either chlamydia or ureaplasmal antigens in venereally acquired

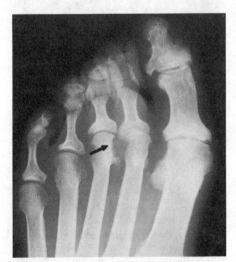

Fig 28–2. Left foot of a 45-year-old man with Reiter's syndrome. Note erosion of the heads of the second and third metatarsal bones (**arrow**).

Reiter's syndrome but only after stimulation with enteric pathogens in Reiter's syndrome following enteric infection (4).

The occasional familial aggregation of Reiter's syndrome and the increased prevalence of sacroiliitis, ankylosing spondylitis, and psoriasis among relatives suggest a genetic basis for the disorder. This has been confirmed by the findings of the HLA–B27 phenotype in 75% or more of patients (5). HLA–B27 is present with equally high frequency in venereally acquired and postdysenteric disease. HLA–B27 is not associated with nongonococcal urethritis or dysentery per se, but patients who are positive for the antigen with these conditions appear particularly prone to develop Reiter's syndrome (6).

Reiter's syndrome is widespread throughout the world. It has been estimated that 1% of patients with nongonococcal urethritis develop the syndrome. In outbreaks of *Shigella flexneri* dysentery, 0.2% of patients subsequently experienced Reiter's syndrome (2). Reiter's syndrome is being recognized more frequently as a relatively common cause of arthritis in young adult males. The disease is rare in women, children, and elderly persons, in whom it usually is of the postdysenteric form.

Clinical features. The illness begins most often with symptoms of urethritis, followed by conjunctivitis and arthritis. The urethral discharge is usually scanty and serous, but may be profuse, purulent, and blood-stained. Conjunctivitis is usually bilateral, mild, and fleeting, but may also be purulent. Arthritis begins in both the venereal and postdysenteric forms 1–3 weeks after the initial symptom and may dominate the clinical picture. The full attack may be accompanied by fever and other constitutional complaints, including anorexia with considerable weight loss, and may prove highly debilitating.

In the past many have insisted on the triad of urethritis, arthritis, and conjunctivitis for the diagnosis of Reiter's syndrome. However, it is now recognized that circinate balanitis and keratodermia blennorrhagicum are of at least equal significance, and most would agree that the presence of any combination of 3 of these features (which may appear asynchronously) or even 2, if characteristic, warrants a presumptive diagnosis.

Urethritis occurs in both sexually acquired and dysenteric forms of the disease. Usually it is accompanied by dysuria and frequency of micturition but may be asymptomatic and detected only by "milking" the urethra before urination in the morning or by finding shreds of mucus in the first sample of urine voided in the morning (2-glass test).

Painless superficial moist ulcerations, beginning as small vesicles, often perimeatal, may involve the entire glans, undersurface of the prepuce, and even the shaft

of the penis and scrotum. These superficial circinate lesions may coalesce into large serpiginous patches and cover the entire glans, which may be intensely red but not tender.

The occurrence of **circinate balanitis** is independent of the presence or severity of urethritis. The balanitis usually clears within days or at most a few weeks, but rarely may last a few months. Prostatitis is often present in the acute disease. Other uncommon urologic problems include urethral stricture, prostatic abscess, seminal vesiculitis, hemorrhagic cystitis, and ureteral stenosis complicated by hydronephrosis and glomerulonephritis.

Conjunctivitis is usually mild and evanescent, and hence frequently overlooked. The inflammation, which is generally bilateral, usually subsides in a day or two, but may recur and last several weeks. Anterior uveitis (iridocyclitis) is the second most common ocular manifestation. Others that have been reported include superficial punctate keratitis, corneal ulceration, episcleritis, optic and retrobulbar neuritis, and complete destruction of the eye by panophthalmitis.

Oral lesions in Reiter's syndrome are often overlooked because, unlike aphthous and herpetic ulcers, they are painless. They may be found on the buccal mucosa (Fig 28–1), palate, tongue, and pharynx. The lesions start as tiny vesicles or slightly elevated erythematous papules which break down into superficial ulcers coated with a greyish membrane. Red atrophic bald patches with slightly raised white curving borders may give rise to the appearance of a "geographic" tongue.

The onset of **arthritis** is often abrupt. Most commonly affected are the weight-bearing joints, especially the knees and ankles. However, any joint may be affected. The arthritis is usually oligarticular and asymmetrical, but rarely may be monarticular. The involved joints are often acutely inflamed and swollen with effusion. Muscle wasting around the affected joint is often evident, especially in the

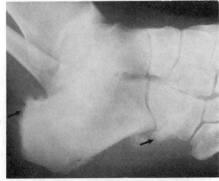

Fig 28–3. Roentgenogram of left heel of same patient whose foot is shown in Fig 28–2. Note fluffy new bone formation on posterior and inferior margins of calcaneus and on cuboid.

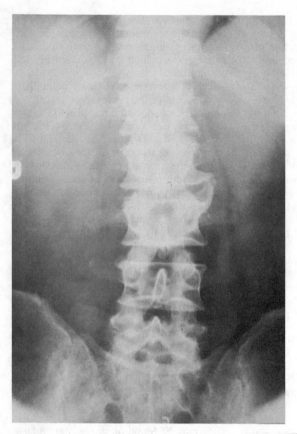

Fig 28-4. Lumbar vertebrae of 50-year-old man with Reiter's syndrome. Note bridge of nonmarginal syndesmophytes between bodies of second and third vertebrae.

quadriceps muscles. Back pain from sacroiliitis is not uncommon during the acute episode. Tenosynovitis is rare with the exception of the achilles tendon.

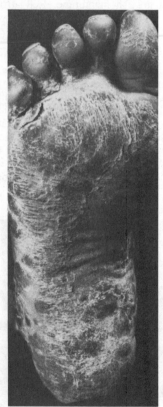

Fig 28-5. Keratodermia blennorrhagicum in a 49-year-old man with Reiter's syndrome. These lesions subsequently healed without scarring.

Recurrences of Reiter's syndrome are common and bouts of arthritis may last for a few weeks to several years, with intervals varying from weeks to years. Although complete recovery is the rule after each acute episode, patients with multiple recurrences are prone to develop residual joint damage, particularly in the feet (metatarsal heads) (Fig 28-2), sacroiliac joints, and vertebral column. Periostitis involving the inferior and posterior aspects of the os calcis may be associated with painful heels ("lover's heel") and calcaneal spurs (Fig 28-3). Sacroiliitis, often asymmetrical, is often associated with both marginal and nonmarginal syndesmophytes (Fig 28-4) (7).

The histologic changes in the synovium are the nonspecific changes of an acute, subacute, or chronic inflammation. The synovial fluid changes reflect this inflammation, but, unlike rheumatoid arthritis, synovial fluid complement levels are not reduced.

Keratodermia blennorrhagicum is the characteristic cutaneous manifestation of the syndrome and has been reported in 10–30% of patients. Those with the post-dysenteric form appear to be less frequently affected with this complication. The lesions begin on the soles of the feet 4–6 weeks after the onset of the urethritis. They first appear as small red to yellowish brown vesicles or papules, firm on palpation and nontender. The lesions may become confluent (Fig 28-5) and may also appear on the palms and other areas of the body, where the appearances may be in-

distinguishable from psoriasis. Histologically, the lesions are identical to pustular psoriasis (Fig 28-6).

Nail dystrophy may simulate that of the grosser changes in psoriasis. **Hyperkeratosis** with heaping of cornified material under the nail is very typical and may cause loss of the nail (Fig 28-7).

Patients have been described whose skin lesions progressed to frank psoriasis. It has been suggested that the concurrence of the 2 diseases is merely coincidental, but the number of patients now reported lends support to the view that a true association exists.

Other associated disorders. Cardiac involvement is now well documented, but uncommon (8,9). Some patients have pericardial friction rubs, heart block, and various other cardiac abnormalities that have been attributed to pericarditis and myocarditis. A small number eventually develop aortic insufficiency as a result of mesoaortic disease and dilatation of the root of the aorta (8).

Neurologic complications are rare and include peripheral neuropathy, transient hemiplegia, meningoencephalitis, and cranial nerve palsies (9).

Pleurisy and pulmonary infiltrates have occasionally been reported during the acute illness. Secondary amyloidosis may

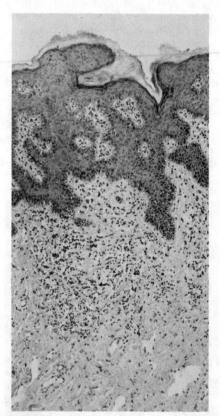

Fig 28-6. Photomicrograph of abdominal skin from a 50-year-old man with Reiter's syndrome and extensive keratodermia blennorrhagicum. Note parakeratosis, elongation and hypertrophy of rete pegs, and lymphocytic infiltration of the papillary dermis.

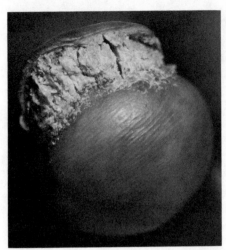

Fig 28–7. Hyperkeratosis beneath fingernail in a man with Reiter's syndrome.

rarely occur after only a few years. Purpura, thrombophlebitis, and severe gastrointestinal hemorrhage have also been reported but are rare.

A mild normocytic, normochromic anemia is common. Moderate to marked elevation of the erythrocyte sedimentation rate (>100 mm/hour, Westergren) often occurs. A polymorphonuclear leukocytosis as high as 25,000–30,000/mm³ is frequently present during acute episodes. Tests for rheumatoid and antinuclear factors are negative.

Treatment. Treatment is essentially symptomatic. Nonsteroidal antiinflammatory drugs are useful in reducing joint pain. A period of bedrest in the hospital with splinting of acutely inflamed joints may be indicated. The value of tetracycline for urethritis and prostatitis and for prevention of recurrences has not been substantiated.

Corticosteroids may relieve pain and swelling of the joints, but do not shorten the course of the disease and are often quite ineffective. Local injection of corticosteroid in the plantar fascia and around the achilles tendon may help reduce pain. The use of cytotoxic and immunosuppressive drugs has not been evaluated in controlled studies, but methotrexate has been used to treat the severe arthritis and generalized psoriaform lesions.

Conjunctivitis usually responds well to local symptomatic therapy. Ocular complications require prompt consultation with the ophthalmologist. Oral ulceration and circinate balanitis usually require no therapy but, if persistent, may heal with local application of a hydrocortisone preparation.

1. Wright V, Moll JMH: Seronegative Polyarthritis. Amsterdam, North-Holland, 1976
2. Ford DK: Reiter's syndrome. Bull Rheum Dis 20:588–591, 1970
3. Dumonde DC: Infection and Immunology in the Rheumatic Disease. Oxford, Blackwell Scientific Publications, 1976
4. Ford DK, daRoza DM, Schulzer M: The specificity of synovial mononuclear cell responses to microbiological antigens in Reiter's syndrome. J Rheumatol 9:561–567, 1982
5. Morris R, Metzger AL, Bluestone R, Terasaki PI: HL-A W27: a clue to the diagnosis and pathogenesis of Reiter's syndrome. N Engl J Med 290:554–556, 1974
6. Calin A, Fries J: An "experimental" epidemic of Reiter's syndrome revisited: follow-up evidence on genetic and environmental factors. Ann Intern Med 84:564–566, 1976
7. McEwen C, DiTata D, Lingg C, Porini A, Good A, Rankin T: Ankylosing spondylitis and spondylitis accompanying ulcerative colitis, regional enteritis, psoriasis, and Reiter's disease: a comparative study. Arthritis Rheum 14:291–318, 1971
8. Paulus HE, Pearson CM, Pitts W: Aortic insufficiency in 5 patients with Reiter's syndrome: a detailed clinical and pathologic study. Am J Med 53:464–472, 1972
9. Good AE: Reiter's disease: a review with special attention to cardiovascular and neurologic sequelae. Semin Arthritis Rheum 3:252–286, 1974

29. Psoriatic arthritis

The association of psoriasis and arthritis was recorded over 150 years ago and the concept of psoriatic arthritis as a distinct clinical entity is generally accepted (1,2). It appears that as many as 7% of patients with psoriasis have some type of inflammatory joint disease (3,4).

Clinical features. Classically the term *psoriatic arthritis* has been used for an arthritis affecting the distal interphalangeal joints (Fig 29–1). It is now clear, however, that the disease has a wide spectrum. Three other major clinical groups with peripheral arthritis have been identified: 1) patients with arthritis mutilans, often complicated by "telescoping" of the digits, 2) patients with asymmetric arthritis often involving only 2–3 joints at a time, and 3) patients with a pattern of symmetric polyarthritis clinically indistinguishable from rheumatoid arthritis. There is a closer temporal relationship between nail and joint involvement than skin and joint disease. In some patients psoriatic arthropathy long precedes cutaneous disease.

The metatarsophalangeal joints and the interphalangeal joints of the fingers and toes are frequently affected. Apart from the uncommon arthritis mutilans, psoriatic arthritis tends to cause less pain and less disability than rheumatoid arthritis.

Involvement of the nails is seen in 80% of patients with psoriatic arthritis compared with 30% in psoriatic individuals without arthritis. There is topographic relationship between involvement of distal joints and adjacent nails. Subcutaneous nodules are not seen. Histologically the synovitis is similar to that of rheumatoid arthritis although fibrosis may be more prominent.

Involvement of joints other than the distal interphalangeals does not differ appreciably from that of rheumatoid arthritis, especially in patients with bilaterally symmetrical arthritis. This has led some to

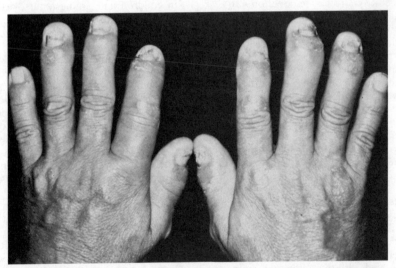

Fig 29–1. Swelling and deformity of distal interphalangeal joints are present together with typical psoriatic involvement of the skin and nails. Nail changes associated with psoriasis may include discoloration, fragmentation, pitting, and lifting up of the distal portion of the nail (onycholysis). Several digits, including the left thumb and index finger, are diffusely swollen suggesting a "sausage-like" appearance. (From Perlman SG, Barth WF: Comprehensive Therapy 5:60–66, 1979)

consider such cases as examples of rheumatoid arthritis coincidentally associated with psoriasis. Occasionally patients also have subcutaneous nodules or positive tests for rheumatoid factor and thus seem to have coincidental rheumatoid arthritis. It appears that rheumatoid arthritis occurs in psoriatic patients no more often than would be expected and these cases probably represent chance occurrence of 2 relatively common diseases.

In addition to arthritis of peripheral joints, psoriatic patients are also subject to spondylitis. This differs from ankylosing spondylitis in a number of respects, most notably in the tendency for many of the syndesmophytes to arise not at the margins of the vertebral bodies but from the lateral and anterior surfaces of the bodies (5). This type of syndesmophyte is also seen in Reiter's syndrome.

Laboratory findings. There are no specific laboratory tests for psoriasis or the arthritis associated with it. Anemia, raised erythrocyte sedimentation rate, and increased levels of alpha$_2$ globulin, are nonspecific.

The more characteristic radiographic features of psoriatic arthritis include the following (3,5,6): 1) gross destructive changes of isolated small joints; 2) arthritis mutilans, showing marked osteolysis and ankylosis, and "pencil-in-cup" appearance resulting from severe bony erosion (5); 3) "fluffy" periositis, including involvement of shafts of long bones (6); 4) atypical spondylitis with nonmarginal as well as marginal syndesmophytes.

Treatment. Most patients require no more than aspirin or other nonsteroidal antiinflammatory drugs plus appropriate measures for the skin disease. Corticosteroids may produce marked improvement in both skin and joints, but such large doses are usually required that this form of treatment often leads to undesirable side effects. Intraarticular injections of corticosteroids may be used for temporary help. Gold has recently been shown to be effective and well tolerated in many patients with polyarthritis (7). Hydroxychloroquine may also be used although there is still some question of whether it causes exacerbations of psoriasis in some patients (8).

Methotrexate and other of the so-called immunosuppresive drugs appear to be the most effective agents currently available for both cutaneous and articular manifestations (9). However, the potential hazard (in the case of methotrexate, the risk of serious liver damage) justifies their use only in extremely severe cases. Reconstructive operations and arthrodeses have the same indications as in rheumatoid arthritis.

1. Reed WB: Psoriatic arthritis: a complete clinical study of 86 patients. Acta Derm Venereol 41:396–403, 1961
2. Baker H, Golding DN, Thompson M: Psoriasis and arthritis. Ann Intern Med 58:909–925, 1963
3. Wright V: Seronegative polyarthritis: a unified concept. Joseph J Bunim Memorial Lecture. Arthritis Rheum 21:619–633, 1978
4. Baker H: Epidemiological aspects of psoriasis and arthritis. Br J Dermatol 78:249–261, 1966
5. McEwen C, et al: Ankylosing spondylitis and spondylitis accompanying ulcerative colitis, regional enteritis, psoriasis and Reiter's disease: a comparative study. Arthritis Rheum 14:291–318, 1971
6. Wright V: Psoriatic arthritis: a comparative radiographic study of rheumatoid arthritis and arthritis associated with psoriasis. Ann Rheum Dis 20:120–132, 1961
7. Dorwart BB, Gall EP, Schumacher HR: Chrysotherapy in psoriatic arthritis: efficacy and toxicity compared to rheumatoid arthritis. Arthritis Rheum 21:513–518, 1978
8. Luzar MJ: Hydroxychloroquine in psoriatic arthropathy: exacerbation of psoriatic skin lesions: J Rheumatol 9:462–464, 1982
9. Weinstein GD, Frost P: Methotrexate for psoriasis: a new therapeutic schedule. Arch Dermatol 103:33–38, 1971

30. Arthritis associated with chronic inflammatory disease of the intestine

Arthritis occurs in association with a number of diseases that affect the bowel: ulcerative colitis, Crohn's disease, the various forms of bacillary dysentery, Whipple's disease (see Section 31), and Behçet's syndrome (see Section 42).

There are 2 forms of arthropathy associated with Crohn's disease and ulcerative colitis: enteropathic arthritis and ankylosing spondylitis.

Enteropathic arthritis. Synovitis affecting the peripheral joints occurs in approximately 11% of patients with ulcerative colitis (1,2) and approximately 21% of those with Crohn's disease (3). The features are similar (2). The synovitis is acute and monarticular in many cases. Occasionally a polyarthritis develops, sometimes accompanied by erythema nodosum. This usually involves the larger joints, particularly the knees and the ankles, and resolves in a period of weeks. Residual damage is rare.

The peripheral arthritis that develops in patients with ulcerative colitis is closely associated with the bowel condition, generally occurring after its onset. This arthritis is more common when the colitis is chronic and extensive; or when it is associated with local complications such as pseudopolyps, massive hemorrhage, and perianal disease, or with systemic complications such as oral ulceration or skin lesions such as erythema nodosum, pyoderma gangrenosum, and uveitis.

In children and young adults, arthritis may appear before the onset of intestinal complaints (4). Proctocolectomy cures the arthritis. In Crohn's disease, too, arthritis may occasionally antedate the bowel symptoms. Synovitis is no more frequent when complications of the bowel disease occur. Surgery produces a remission of the synovitis in only a small number of patients—almost certainly because of the difficulty in removing all the diseased intestine.

There are no characteristic laboratory features. Nonspecific inflammatory changes are found in the synovial fluid along with poor mucin clot formation. Cell counts are usually 5,000–7,000/mm^3 but can range to 40,000/mm^3 (4); the majority of the cells are polymorphonuclear leukocytes. Synovial tissue shows nonspecific inflammatory changes.

Rheumatoid factor is absent from the blood and synovial fluid. Roentgenograms of peripheral joints reveal no abnormality.

The synovitis is self-limiting and nonde-forming. The best therapy lies in control or cure of the underlying bowel disease. Analgesic and antiinflammatory drugs may be given in short courses to control the joint inflammation, but the patient's response should be monitored very carefully because of the gastrointestinal side effects of many of these drugs.

Ankylosing spondylitis. This occurs in about 7% of patients (5). The spondylitis frequently precedes the bowel disease (6). Radiologic evidence of sacroiliitis occurs in about 17% of patients and may be asymptomatic. The spinal disease does not differ from idiopathic "primary" ankylosing spondylitis and follows a course independent from the bowel disease. Family studies have shown an increased prevalence of bowel disease and spondylitis among first degree relatives of patients with ulcerative colitis and with Crohn's disease (7). There are features that demonstrate interrelationship of diseases encompassed in the concept of seronegative spondylarthritis (8).

Roentgenograms of the axial skeleton disclose the changes of idiopathic ankylosing spondylitis (9). Anemia and a raised erythrocyte sedimentation rate may be associated with the bowel disease. HLA antigen distribution is normal in patients with bowel disease uncomplicated by arthritis, but B27 is found in the majority of patients with ankylosing spondylitis (10).

1. Wright V, Watkinson G: Articular complications of ulcerative colitis. Am J Proctol 17:107–115, 1966

2. McEwen C: Arthritis accompanying ulcerative colitis. Clin Orthop 57:9–19, 1968

3. Haslock I, Wright V: The arthritis associated with intestinal disease. Bull Rheum Dis 24:750–754, 1973

4. Ament E: Inflammatory diseases of the colon: ulcerative colitis and Crohn's colitis. J Pediatr 86:322–334, 1975

5. Wright V, Watkinson G: Sacro-iliitis and ulcerative colitis. Br Med J 2:675–680, 1965

6. Acheson ED: An association between ulcerative colitis, regional enteritis and ankylosing spondylitis. Q J Med 29:489–499, 1960

7. Macrae I, Wright V: A family study of ulcerative colitis, with particular reference to ankylosing spondylitis and sacro-iliitis. Ann Rheum Dis 32:16–20, 1973

8. Moll JMH, Haslock I, Macrae I, Wright V: Associations between ankylosing spondylitis, psoriatic arthritis, Reiter's disease, the intestinal arthropathies, and Behcet's syndrome. Medicine 53:343–364, 1974

9. McEwen C, DiTata D, Lingg C, Porini A, Good A, Rankin T: A comparative study of ankylosing spondylitis and spondylitis accompanying ulcerative colitis, regional enteritis, psoriasis and Reiter's disease. Arthritis Rheum 14:291–318, 1971

10. Morris RI, Metzger AL, Bluestone R, Terasaki PI: HL-A-W27: a useful discriminator in the arthropathies of inflammatory bowel disease. N Engl J Med 290:1117–1119, 1974

31. Whipple's disease

Whipple's disease was originally recognized as a chronically progressive, ultimately fatal disorder, occurring chiefly in men. It is characterized by fever, anemia, steatorrhea, wasting, and other evidence of intestinal malabsorption, hyperpigmentation, lymphadenopathy, polyserositis, abdominal pain, and polyarthralgia. In the past 20 years, it has been realized that arthralgia and/or arthritis occurs in approximately 90% of patients and usually antedates other manifestations of the disorder, often by more than 10 years. Polyarthritis tends to be migratory and episodic but residual deformity does not occur (1). Spinal pain with or without radiographic evidence of sacroiliac involvement has been noted occasionally, but only a few well-documented cases of Whipple's disease associated with ankylosing spondylitis have been reported (2).

Synovial biopsy and synovial fluid analyses have shown mild nonspecific inflammatory changes; tests for rheumatoid factor and antinuclear antibodies give negative results.

The pathognomonic feature of this disease is the presence of sickle-shaped particles in the cytoplasm of macrophages which stain with the periodic acid-Schiff (PAS) reagent. Under electron microscopy, these particles consist of heterophagic vacuoles containing clumps of bacilliform bodies measuring $0.2\mu \times 2\mu$ with a trilaminar cell wall. The bacilli are in various stages of digestion but the bacterial cell walls appear partially resistant to lysosomal degradation. Efforts to isolate the organism or transmit the disease have been unsuccessful, but after antibiotic treatment, the bacilliform bodies disappear in association with regression of disease manifestations.

Jejunal biopsy nearly always reveals diagnostic changes with the lamina propria of the short clubbed villi being extensively infiltrated by free bacilli and numerous macrophages packed with ingested bacilli (PAS-positive particles). Peripheral or mesenteric lymph nodes may also contain such PAS-positive material. In one instance, characteristic morphologic changes were found in an axillary node of a patient in whom repeated small bowel biopsies proved negative (3).

The characteristic macrophages have also been occasionally noted in the synovium (4). These recent observations suggest that joint manifestations of Whipple's disease result from the colonization of synovial tissue by the organism and thus represent an unusual form of chronic nondestructive infectious arthritis.

Inflammatory myopathy has also been reported in Whipple's disease. Intrafascicular PAS-positive macrophages containing bacillary bodies (5) have been described.

The rarity of this disorder and its lack of contagiousness have led to consideration of abnormal host responsiveness as a factor in disease susceptibility. Humoral immune functions prove normal, but defective cell-mediated immunity has been demonstrated frequently. T cell lymphopenia and cutaneous anergy, described in active disease, sometimes revert to normal with treatment. On the other hand, lymphocyte responsiveness to mitogens has usually been found to be impaired during and after treatment (6). Some have interpreted these results as being indicative of an acquired immune impairment in response to an unusual microorganism.

Treatment with tetracycline, 1 gram per day for 3–12 months, usually leads to complete resolution of all manifestations of disease. Occasionally relapses occur and at times treatment with other antibiotics such as erythromycin has been necessary.

1. LeVine ME, Dobbins WO III: Joint changes in Whipple's disease. Semin Arthritis Rheum 3:79–93, 1973

2. Canoso JJ, Saini M, Hermos JA: Whipple's disease and ankylosing spondylitis: simultaneous occurrence in HLA–B27 positive male. J Rheumatol 5:79–84, 1978

3. Mansback CM II, Shelburne JD, Stevens RD, Dobbins WO III: Lymph-node bacilliform bodies resembling those of Whipple's disease in a patient without intestinal involvement. Ann Intern Med 89:64–66, 1978

4. Hawkins CF, Farr M, Morris CJ, Hoare AM, Williamson N: Detection by electron microscope of rod-shaped organisms in synovial membrane from a patient with the arthritis of Whipple's disease. Ann Rheum Dis 35:502–509, 1976

5. Swash M, Schwartz MS, Vandenburg MJ, Pollock DJ: Myopathy in Whipple's disease. Gut 18:800–804, 1977

6. Haeney MR, Ross IN: Whipple's disease in a female with impaired cell-mediated immunity unresponsive to cotrimoxazole and levamisole therapy. Postgrad Med J 54:45–50, 1978

32. Yersinial arthritis

Infections due to *Yersinia* are widely distributed but reported most commonly from Scandinavia, Northern Europe, Canada, and Japan. Children or adults of both sexes can be infected. These Gram negative organisms previously classified as *Pasteurella* include *Y enterocolitica*, commonly associated with a reactive arthritis, *Yersinia pseudotuberculosis*, occasionally reported with arthritis, and *Yersinia pestis*, the agent of bubonic plaque (1).

Yersinia enterocolitica infection can be acquired from contaminated food and water or occasionally from small domestic animals or humans infected by fecal contamination of hands or foodstuffs. Initial infection is usually manifested by fever, gastroenteritis which can be followed by terminal ileitis or mesenteric lymphadenitis mimicking appendicitis, and less often by other systemic features including myocarditis or septicemia (2).

An aseptic polyarthritis begins 4–10 days after the diarrhea. Arthritis occurred in 4 of 28 infected patients in 1 series (3). Joint disease is self-limited, generally subsiding in 1–4 months (4–7). A few patients have had more prolonged arthritis (1). Fever, tendinitis, and erythema nodosum can occur with the arthritis. Most commonly involved joints have been knees and ankles although wrists, hands, feet, and other sites have also been affected. Pain may be severe. Arthritis is often additive, not usually migratory. Full blown Reiter's syndrome has also been reported after yersinial infection (7,8).

A presumptive diagnosis is usually made by demonstration of elevated agglutinating antibody titers against *Yersinia* with a subsequent fall during convalescence (4). Because there is some cross reaction of agglutination with *Brucella*, absorption studies should be done. Culture of the organism is difficult but occasional positive stool cultures have been obtained with special cultures at 4°C (1). Blood cultures are rarely positive. Other laboratory tests are nonspecific with frequent elevations of sedimentation rates and leukocytosis.

HLA–B27 has been found in a number of patients. This antigen was present in 43 of 49 patients with yersinial arthritis in one series (9). Another found 14 of 25 HLA–B27 positive (11). One study suggested that arthritis was more severe in HLA–B27 positive patients (5). Synovial effusions studied have been mildly to markedly inflammatory with leukocyte counts from 4,310–58,000 mm³ with 13–95% polymorphonuclear leukocytes (5,10). Antibodies to *Yersinia* and immune complexes have been reported in joint fluid (10).

Organisms have not been cultured from the joint except in a single reported case of actual septic arthritis (2). X-rays have not shown erosions. A few patients have been reported with sacroiliitis, but this aspect has not been systematically studied.

There is no evidence that antibiotics help either the self-limited gastroenteritis or arthritis but chloramphenicol and other antibiotics have been used with apparent success in patients with severe systemic infections and septic arthritis (2). Nonsteroidal antiinflammatory agents, intraarticular depot corticosteroids, and occasionally systemic corticosteroids have been used for symptomatic relief of the arthritis (2,6).

The aseptic polyarthritis now being increasingly seen after yersinial infections seems to behave in many ways like the other seronegative reactive spondylarthropathies with pathogenetic mechanisms possibly similar to those being considered in Reiter's syndrome, anklosing spondylitis, and the arthritis after intestinal bypass surgery.

1. Kohl S: Yersinia enterocolitica: a significant "new" pathogen. Hosp Practice :81–85, 1978
2. Spira TJ, Kabins SA: Yersinia enterocolitica septicemia with septic arthritis. Arch Intern Med 136:1305–1308, 1976
3. Ford DK, Henderson E, Price G, Stein HB: Yersinia related arthritis in the Pacific Northwest. Arthritis Rheum 20:1226–1230, 1977
4. Ahvonen P, Sievers K, Aho K: Arthritis associated with Yersinia enterocolitica infection. Acta Rheum Scand 15:232–253, 1969
5. Laitinen O, Leirisalo M, Skylv G: Relation between HLA-B27 and clinical features in patients with Yersinia arthritis. Arthritis Rheum 20:1121–1124, 1977
6. Laitinen O, Tuuhea J, Ahvonen P: Polyarthritis associated with Yersinia enterocolitica infection: clinical features and laboratory findings in 9 cases with severe joint symptoms. Ann Rheum Dis 31:34–39, 1972
7. Chalmers A, Kaprove RE, Reynolds WJ, Urowitz MB: Post diarrhea arthropathy of Yersinia pseudotuberculosis. Can Med Assoc J 118:515–516, 1978
8. Raison G, Guillien P, Mage B, et al: Syndrome de Fiessinger-LeRoy-Reiter associe à une serologie positive pour Yersinia pseudotuberculosis. Rev Rhum 48:637–638, 1981
9. Aho K, Ahvonen P, Lassus A, Sievers K Tiilikainen A: HLA 27 in reactive arthritis. Arthritis Rheum 17:521–26, 1974
10. Sheldon JHS, Mair RNS, Fox E: Yersinia arthritis: a clinical, immunological and family study of 2 cases. Ann Rheum Dis 41:153–158, 1982
11. Dequeker J, Jamar R, Walravens M: HLA B27, arthritis and Yersinia enterocolitica infection. J Rheumatol 7:706–710, 1980

33. Rheumatic fever and Jaccoud's syndrome

Acute rheumatic fever is an inflammatory disease characterized clinically by fever, polyarthritis, and carditis; histologically by a specific granuloma in the myocardium; and bacteriologically by an antecedent group A beta-hemolytic streptococcal infection (1).

Epidemiology. Rheumatic fever occurs worldwide and is considered the most common cause of heart disease in persons under age 40. In countries with adequate therapy for streptococcal infections, both the frequency and severity of rheumatic fever and rheumatic heart disease are decreasing (2). Nevertheless, acute rheumatic fever (ARF) and rheumatic heart disease continue to be significant health problems wherever the predisposing factors of inadequate primary medical treatment, crowded living conditions, close person-to-person contact, inadequate nutritional intake, and lowered host defenses exist.

The epidemiology of rheumatic fever is the epidemiology of the streptococcus (3). Group A streptococci alone are rheumatogenic and rheumatic fever follows only infections of the throat, not of the skin. Although it is uncertain whether all pharyngeal strains of group A beta-hemolytic streptococci carry the same risk of eliciting ARF, it appears that most strains are rheumatogenic.

The incidence of streptococcal disease in the economically developed countries of the world has been declining progressively. This has been accompanied by a comparable decrease in the incidence of the nonsuppurative complications of streptococcal infection such as acute rheumatic fever and acute glomerulonephritis. Nevertheless, in the United States it is estimated that approximately 100,000 new cases of acute rheumatic fever occur each year (3). The attack rate of rheumatic fever after epidemic streptococcal pharyngitis is approximately 3%. The frequency of ARF after sporadic streptococcal disease is considerably lower.

Both sexes are equally affected although some of the manifestations of the acute illness have a striking sex predilection. ARF does not exhibit a preference for any racial or ethnic group. The age distribution coincides with the peak frequency of streptococcal infections and is greatest between 7–14 years. Attacks are rare in children under the age of 2. Although the frequency of first attacks declines after puberty, rheumatic fever is still relatively common in young adults (4).

The occurrence of ARF fluctuates with seasons, paralleling streptococcal pharyngitis. Thus, in colder climates the peak occurrence is in the late winter and early spring months; in more temperate areas and in the tropics, the illness may occur year-round. Because of a familial tendency for the development of ARF, genetic factors have been considered to play a role.

Studies thus far have failed to document strong associations between acute rheumatic fever and the HLA antigens from either the A or B loci (5). Recently, however, a B-cell alloantigen has been found with significantly increased frequency in ARF patients from Bogota, Colombia, and from New York City (6).

Pathogenesis. Although firmly established as a sequel to group A streptococcal infection, the exact pathogenetic mechanism responsible for the development of rheumatic fever remains unknown. The risk of developing rheumatic fever is dependent on the length of time the streptococcus is present in the pharynx, and the attack rate correlates with the magnitude of the humoral immune response to the infecting organism (1).

Why streptococcal pharyngitis is rheumatogenic and impetigo is not is unknown (7). The organisms responsible for skin infections may differ antigenically from those responsible for throat infections. The titers of anti-streptolysin O after pharyngitis are usually greater than those found in skin infections. Perhaps this is due to the suppression of the antigenicity of the streptococcus by skin lipids (8).

Three main hypotheses concerning the pathogenesis of rheumatic fever have been developed: 1) streptococcal products have a direct toxic effect on tissue, 2) streptococcal antibody reacts with streptococcal antigens bound to the target tissues, and 3) streptococcal antibodies and sensitized lymphocytes cross-react with tissue antigens.

Much evidence favors an exaggerated cellular or humoral immune reaction as responsible for the disease. In favor of this argument are the latent period after the pharyngitis before the development of ARF—suggesting a period of sensitization, the correlation of attack rate with the magnitude of the humoral response, the presence of serum antibodies that react with antigens in the organs commonly involved in ARF, the cross-reactivity of some of these antibodies with certain streptococcal antigens, and the finding of cell-mediated immune reactions to both streptococcal and host tissue antigens.

A variety of antigens from streptococci have been found to be immunologically similar to certain tissue antigens, including those from the joint capsule, the neuronal cytoplasm, and especially the myocardium and heart valves. Antibodies arising as a consequence of the streptococcal infection might then cause a cytotoxic reaction in these organs. Consistent with this hypothesis are the findings of focal deposits of immunoglobulin as well as complement in the myocardium and the detection of massive deposits of antibody in the hearts of patients dying with severe acute rheumatic heart disease (9). Approximately one-half of patients with rheumatic chorea have circulating IgG antibody that reacts with the cytoplasm of caudate and subthalamic neuronal nuclei, a reaction that can be prevented by absorption with group A streptococcal cell walls (10).

Additional evidence implicating immunoglobulins (immune complexes) in the pathogenesis of ARF is the finding of local consumption of several complement components in the synovial fluids of patients with ARF (11). Since total serum complement concentrations are generally either normal or elevated in acute rheumatic fever, the finding of decreased levels at inflammatory sites suggests activation by immune complexes. Approximately 90% of patients with ARF have been reported

to have circulating immune complexes (12). Titers diminished markedly after subsidence of the acute illness, but did not correlate with the extraarticular manifestations of ARF.

Individuals positive for HLA–B5 demonstrated a significantly more pronounced immune response as measured by circulating immune complexes. In many patients with ARF, however, no anti-tissue antibodies can be found, and neither immunoglobulin nor complement has been detected in the Aschoff nodule, the hallmark of rheumatic myocarditis.

Evidence has been presented that cell-mediated immune mechanisms may account for the manifestations of ARF. Lymphocytes from ARF patients exhibit enhanced reactivity to streptococcal antigens (13). The potential pathogenetic significance of these observations is increased by the finding that T lymphocytes from animals sensitized to streptococcal antigens are cytotoxic for mammalian cardiac cells in vitro (14).

Viable streptococci are not found at the site of rheumatic fever lesions, although mucopeptide remnants of the bacterial cell wall may be present. The diffuse proliferative and exudative inflammatory reactions seen in multiple organs are not unique.

The unique and pathognomonic alteration is the myocardial **Aschoff nodule**. Developing after 2 weeks of acute illness, these characteristic localized granulomas tend to persist and do not, in general, correlate with inflammatory disease activity. The Aschoff nodule is marked by swelling and fragmentation of collagen fibers and by fibrinoid degeneration.

Rheumatic valvulitis leads to the most serious cardiac damage. Initially the valve cusps are edematous and the inflammatory exudate is predominantly lymphocytic. Later, the cusps become thickened and fibrotic and adhesions of the valve commissures and chordae tendinae may occur. The mitral valve, either alone or in combination with the aortic, is the valve most often involved, sometimes leading to severe stenosis and regurgitation.

Clinical manifestations. The usual presentation of rheumatic fever is in the form of an acute febrile illness with polyarthritis (15). The description by Thomas Sydenham in 1686 remains valid: "The synovitis of rheumatic fever is transient, migratory, and reversible. The patient is troubled with a violent pain, sometimes in this, sometimes in that joint; in the wrist and shoulders, but commonly in the knees, it now and then changes places."

The sequence of development of the major manifestations of ARF after streptococcal pharyngitis is predictable. Inflammation of the heart, joints, and skin occurs early and is often associated with fever. Chorea and subcutaneous nodules usually become apparent as the arthritis and carditis are subsiding.

Arthritis is the most common feature of rheumatic fever and becomes increasingly frequent with age (Fig 33–1). Usually accompanied by fever, the joint symptoms reported are generally out of proportion (greater) to the signs of inflammation. The onset of arthritis is abrupt and initially involves the joints of the lower extremities in 85% of patients. Articular inflammation in the affected joint reaches a maximum intensity in 12–24 hours after onset and then gradually subsides over several days. During this time additional joints become inflamed. In addition to the knee and ankle, other commonly affected joints are the shoulder, elbow, wrist, and the metacarpal and metatarsophalangeal joints; frequently bursae and tendon linings are also inflamed. The mean number of joints involved in a large group of adults with ARF was 7 (4).

The usual duration of the inflammatory migratory polyarthritis varies from 1–4 weeks. Permanent deformities of the joints are very rare.

Carditis occurs almost as frequently as arthritis in younger patients (Fig 33–1). Approximately 90% of young children develop carditis in their initial attacks as compared with only 15% of adults. The first clinical manifestation is usually the appearance of a new heart murmur, especially of mitral and/or aortic regurgitation. Signs and symptoms of pericarditis and congestive heart failure may develop but are uncommon in the absence of detectable valve abnormalities. Often rheumatic carditis is asymptomatic and diagnosed only during the course of examination of a patient with arthritis or chorea.

The prognosis for permanent cardiac damage is related primarily to the severity of the valvular involvement. Valve lesions may heal, remain stationary, or undergo progressive sclerosis and calcification. First degree heart block and other electrocardiographic (ECG) changes are common. ECG changes alone have a benign prognosis and are not considered a diagnostic criterion of acute rheumatic fever (16).

Erythema marginatum, another of the early clinical manifestations, is detected in only 10% of children and even fewer adults. This evanescent, erythematous dermatitis is painless, nonpruritic, and blanches on pressure. Easily overlooked, the rash appears on the trunk and proximal parts of the extremities and can be made more evident with heat. The subcutaneous nodules of rheumatic fever are pea-sized, painless swellings located over bony prominences. Usually lasting only several days to a week, nodules appear in crops and are found more frequently in patients with severe disease.

Sydenham's chorea is now an infrequent manifestation of ARF. This involuntary movement disorder generally develops 2 or more months after the initial strepto-

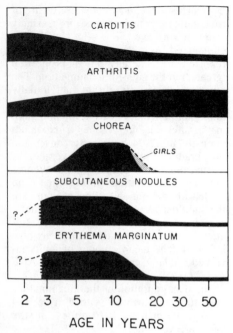

Fig 33-1. The variations with age of the occurrence of the major manifestations of acute rheumatic fever. The maximum height of each curve indicates the age at which a given manifestation has its highest frequency. (Reprinted with permission, from Arthritis and Allied Conditions, 9th edition) (15)

coccal infection, at a time when other manifestations of rheumatic fever have subsided. This major manifestation is rare after puberty in boys and does not occur in adult men. The presence of choreiform movements in adult females should suggest disorders other than acute rheumatic fever such as systemic lupus erythematosus. Sydenham's chorea, like subcutaneous nodules and erythema marginatum, is usually found only in individuals with carditis.

Less noteworthy manifestations of ARF include epistaxis, abdominal pain, pleurisy, and rheumatic pneumonitis. These features are observed in children.

Course. The acute episode of rheumatic fever is self-limited, lasting from 1–3 months. Unlike poststreptococcal glomerulonephritis, which has little tendency to recur, repeated episodes of rheumatic fever are common, especially during the first several years after the initial attack. Recurrences are more likely to develop in patients with preexisting rheumatic heart disease. The tendency to suffer recurrences after streptococcal infection declines with the passage of years.

The clinical manifestations of rheumatic recurrences tend to resemble those of the first episode. However, this mimetic nature of rheumatic fever is not absolute, and the character of past attacks must be used with great caution in the decision to discontinue prophylaxis against recurrent streptococcal infection.

Laboratory findings. Laboratory findings are used to detect an antecedent streptococcal infection, to demonstrate an acute inflammatory reaction, and to assist in excluding other diagnostic possibilities.

Throat cultures should be obtained in patients suspected of having rheumatic fever. Since results are positive for group A beta-hemolytic streptococci in only approximately 20% of patients, streptococcal antibody determinations should also be performed.

Rheumatic fever rarely, if ever, occurs without a measurable humoral immune response. The latent period between the pharyngeal infection and the development of clinical symptoms is such that the patient presents at the time antibody titers are increasing. The humoral response peaks approximately 2 weeks after the onset of acute rheumatic fever, declining rapidly in the next several weeks. Therefore, serum antibody titers, if not initially elevated, should be measured again 1–2 weeks after the acute illness has begun.

The specific antibodies used to detect streptococcal infections are primarily anti-streptolysin O (ASO), anti-hyaluronidase, anti-streptokinase, anti-DPNase, and anti-DNAse B. At least 80% of patients will have an increased ASO titer during the course of their disease and virtually all patients will have an elevated and/or changing antibody titer to at least one of the streptococcal antigens. A highly sensitive slide agglutination test for streptococcal antibodies is now available, which utilizes sheep cells coated by a concentrate of extracellular streptococcal antigens.

Since the inciting streptococcal pharyngitis may be mild or totally asymptomatic in approximately half the patients with acute rheumatic fever, laboratory documentation of the infection becomes critical to the diagnosis.

An increase in the erythrocyte sedimentation rate (ESR) or the appearance of C-reactive protein (CRP) in the blood occurs during the acute episode in essentially all patients. The ESR (Westergren method) is usually rapid, often greater than 90 mm/hr. CRP levels and ESR return to normal after the acute illness subsides (1–2 months). A rebound will be noted after discontinuation of antiinflammatory treatment if the rheumatic process is still active. Thus, these measurements of the inflammatory reaction serve to monitor the underlying disease process. It should be remembered that numerous other inflammatory disorders and irritating stimuli (including intramuscular injections of benzathine penicillin) may cause elevations in both the ESR and CRP.

Synovial fluid from inflamed joints will reflect the variable intensity of arthritis. White blood cell counts may range from the near-normal to as high as 80,000/mm³ in markedly inflamed joints (4). The majority of the cells are polymorphonuclear leukocytes. The fluids are sterile and free of crystals. The concentrations of Clq, C4, and C3 are generally comparable to serum concentrations of these complement components, although in several individuals low synovial fluid concentrations have been detected (11).

Other laboratory abnormalities during the acute illness suggest renal and hepatic dysfunction. Approximately 50% of patients will have mild proteinuria and/or casts. Elevations in transaminase (SGOT) and alkaline phosphatase activity have also been noted. These abnormalities are mild and evanescent and not related to aspirin ingestion (4).

Diagnosis. Since no single clinical feature of the disease is pathognomic and no specific diagnostic test for acute rheumatic fever is available, criteria have been formulated to act as a guide in establishing the diagnosis (16) (Appendix 5). The diagnosis of ARF implies long-term administration of antibiotics for the prevention of streptococcal pharyngitis and portends the insidious onset of heart disease.

Several disorders can mimic the arthritis of acute rheumatic fever. This is especially true of other postinfectious diseases in which an acute reactive arthritis follows an infection elsewhere in the body. Examples are the synovitis after infections by rubella virus or *Yersinia enterocolitica* (17,18). Similarities are also found between the clinical features of viral heart disease and rheumatic carditis (19). The physician should be aware that the fortuitous association of a streptococcal infection with another disease may occur, especially in children.

Treatment. The treatment of acute rheumatic fever consists of eradication of streptococci from the pharynx, prevention of recurring streptococcal infection, and suppression of the tissue inflammation.

Acute rheumatic fever can be prevented if the respiratory tract infection caused by group A streptococci is treated early and adequately. Children with streptococcal pharyngitis should receive a single intramuscular injection of 600,000 units of benzathine penicillin G, and adults 1.2 million units. Any alternative plan of parenteral or combined parenteral and oral antibiotic therapy should provide treatment for 10 days. The prolonged duration of exposure to antibiotic is the most important factor in preventive therapy (1). Once rheumatic fever is diagnosed, treatment to eliminate group A streptococci should be administered regardless of the results of throat cultures.

The antiinflammatory agents most often used are salicylates and adrenal corticosteroids. When there is no evidence of carditis, salicylates, usually in the form of aspirin, are used by most authorities (15). Aspirin is administered in an initial daily dose of 0.1 gm/kg of body weight, ranging from 3 gm in children to 6–8 gm in adults. The desired goal is a plasma salicylate concentration in the range of 20–30 mg/dl. Young adults may fail to show a significant response when given 4 gm of aspirin per day and improve dramatically when the dose is increased to 6 gm per day. Thereafter subsidence of the acute arthritis is prompt.

Marked improvement is noted within 12–24 hours and near complete resolution of the inflammatory synovitis occurs within 48 hours of continued administration of aspirin.

Corticosteroids are more potent than salicylates in suppressing the acute inflammation and are generally given to patients with carditis. However, without conclusive evidence that their use will reduce the degree of ultimate cardiac scarring, the place of corticosteroids in the treatment of patients with mild carditis varies with the convictions of the physician. When carditis is severe, most patients are treated promptly with corticosteroids, usually prednisone 40–60 mg daily in divided doses, particularly if heart failure is evident.

The duration of treatment should be guided by the expected course of the disease and the severity of the rheumatic process in each individual case. During the acute inflammatory illness, physical activity should be limited. In individuals with heart failure, salt intake should be restricted and the use of diuretics is advocated. If antiinflammatory medications are discontinued before the subsidence of the attack, a relapse is likely. Reactivation of ARF after 1–3 months is unlikely unless a streptococcal infection has intervened.

The most efficient means of continuous prophylaxis against group A streptococci is a monthly intramuscular injection of 1.2 million units of benzathine penicillin G. Although prophylaxis can be achieved by a variety of oral antibiotic medications, compliance is not as complete as with the intramuscular route of administration.

The duration for maintenance of prophylaxis is uncertain, but several principles have been suggested (1). Prophylaxis against recurrent streptococcal infection should be administered 1) for 5 years after the last attack, 2) to all individuals under age 18 who have had rheumatic fever, 3)

indefinitely to all subjects who have rheumatic heart disease, and 4) to patients frequently exposed to streptococcal disease.

1. Stollerman GH: Rheumatic Fever and Streptococcal Infection. New York, Grune & Stratton, 1975
2. Strasser T: Rheumatic fever and rheumatic heart disease in the 1970's. WHO Chronicle 32:18–25, 1978
3. Peter G, Smith AL: Group A streptococcal infections of the skin and pharynx. N Engl J Med 297:311–317, 365–370, 1977
4. Barnert AL, Terry EE, Persellin RH: Acute rheumatic fever in adults. JAMA 232:925–928, 1975
5. Murray GC, Monteil MM, Persellin RH: A study of HLA antigens in adults with acute rheumatic fever. Arthritis Rheum 21:652–656, 1978
6. Patarroyo ME, Winchester RJ, Vejerano A, Gibofsky A, Chalem F, Zabriske J, Kunkel HG: Association of a B-cell alloantigen with susceptibility to rheumatic fever. Nature 278:173–174, 1979
7. Potter EV, Svartman M, Mohammed I, Cox R, Poon-King T, Earle DP: Tropical acute rheumatic fever and associated streptococcal infections compared with concurrent acute glomerulonephritis. J Pediatr 92:325–333, 1978
8. Kaplan EL, Anthony BF, Chapman SS, Ayoub EM, Wannamaker LW: The influence of the site of infection on the immune response to group A streptococci. J Clin Invest 49:1405–1414, 1970
9. Kaplan MH: The cross-reaction of group A streptococci with heart tissue and its relation to induced autoimmunity in rheumatic fever. Bull Rheum Dis 19:560–567, 1969
10. Husby G, Van De Rijn I, Zabriskie JB, Abdin ZH, Williams RC Jr: Antibodies reacting with cytoplasm of subthalamic and caudate nuclei neurons in chorea and acute rheumatic fever. J Exp Med 144:1094–1110, 1976
11. Svartman M, Potter EV, Poon-King T: Immunoglobulins and complement components in synovial fluid of patients with acute rheumatic fever. J Clin Invest 56:111–117, 1975
12. Toshinoya S, Pope RM: Detection of immune complexes in acute rheumatic fever and their relationship to HLA-B5. J Clin Invest 65:136–145, 1980
13. Read SE, Fischetti VA, Utermohlen V, Falk RE, Zabriskie JB: Cellular reactivity studies to streptococcal antigens. J Clin Invest 54:439–450, 1974
14. Yang LC, Soprey PR, Wittner MK, Fox EN: Streptococcal-induced cell-mediated immune destruction of cardiac myofibers in vitro. J Exp Med 146:344–360, 1977
15. Taranta A: Rheumatic fever: clinical aspects, Arthritis and Allied Conditions. Ed 9. DJ McCarty, Jr, ed. Philadelphia, Lea & Febiger, 1979, pp 825–870
16. Stollerman GH, Markowitz M, Taranta A, Wannamaker LW, Whittemore R: Jones criteria (revised) for guidance in the diagnosis of rheumatic fever. Circulation 32:664–668, 1965
17. Persellin RH: Acute rheumatic fever: changing manifestations (editorial). Ann Intern Med 89:1002–1003, 1978
18. Ahvonen P, Sievers K, Aho K: Arthritis associated with Yersinia enterocolitica infection. Acta Rheum Scand 15:232–253, 1969
19. Ward C: Observations on the diagnosis of isolated rheumatic carditis (editorial). Am Heart J 91:545–550, 1976

Jaccoud's syndrome or chronic postrheumatic fever arthropathy

Jaccoud's syndrome (1), the deformity of the hands and feet frequently mistaken for rheumatoid arthritis, is a rare consequence of repeated attacks of rheumatic fever. A very similar condition, both clinically and pathologically, is seen after repeated episodes of lupus synovitis involving the hands (2).

Over the years, after each recurrent attack of rheumatism, the hands gradually develop ulnar deviation and subluxation at the metacarpophalangeal joints. The same deformity occurs in the feet at the metatarsophalangeal joints. This easily correctable deformity is painless, and without swelling or limitation. The patient has a history of repeated attacks of rheumatic fever; examination shows the signs of inactive rheumatic heart disease, and the erythrocyte sedimentation rate is normal. Rheumatoid factor and antinuclear and anti-DNA antibody are not found (3).

This arthropathy is thought to be due to fibrosis in the capsule of the joint where rheumatic inflammatory granulomata can be seen during the active phase. A notch or "hook" is sometimes seen in the roentgenogram on the ulnar side of each metacarpal head. This follows ulnar deviation in this condition, in the similar lupus deformity, and in rheumatoid arthritis. It is not a true erosion. Transient nodules have been recorded (4).

As rheumatic fever and its recurrences disappear, this chronic but harmless condition will become rarer. Today it is seen only in countries that still have much residual rheumatic disease. Its recognition is important because it must be differentiated from rheumatoid arthritis. No specific treatment is needed.

1. Jaccoud FS: Legons de Clinique Médicale Faites à l'Hôpital de la Charité. Ed 2. Paris, Delahaye, 1869
2. Bywaters EGL: Jaccoud's syndrome, a sequel to the joint involvement of systemic lupus erythematosus. Clin Rheum Dis 1:125–148, 1975
3. Grahame R, Mitchell ABS, Scott JT: Chronic postrheumatic fever (Jaccoud's) arthropathy. Ann Rheum Dis 29:622–625, 1970
4. Ruderman JEJ, Abruzzo JL: Chronic post rheumatic fever arthritis (Jaccoud's): report of a case with subcutaneous nodules. Arthritis Rheum 9:640–647, 1966

34. Rheumatic diseases of childhood

The rheumatic diseases are not rare in children. They include most of the diseases described in this *Primer*. Though generally similar in adult and child, they differ at times in ways worthy of consideration.

Juvenile rheumatoid arthritis (JRA)

Juvenile rheumatoid arthritis is characterized by chronic synovial inflammation of unknown cause. It is a relatively common chronic childhood disease, affecting

an estimated 60,000–200,000 children in the United States (1). Overall the disease may begin at any age during childhood and girls are more often affected than boys; however, sex and age ratios appear to differ in disease subgroups.

Many children complain little of joint pain but rather limit any motion that would result in pain; severe joint pain or pain at rest are unusual. Stiffness after periods of immobility is common (morning stiffness). Affected joints are swollen, stiff, limited in motion, and sometimes warm and tender. Arthritis may affect multiple joints in a generally symmetric fashion (polyarticular distribution) or may be limited to only a few joints, predominantly large ones, asymmetrically (pauciarticular distribution).

JRA can exert several effects on growth including the generalized growth retardation of chronic childhood illness and the localized effects of inflammation on epiphyseal growth which can result in bony overgrowth or undergrowth around affected joints (2,3). Micrognathia can result from impaired growth of the mandible.

There are no diagnostic laboratory tests for juvenile arthritis, although tests such as rheumatoid factors, antinuclear antibodies, and HLA antiens may be useful in classifying patients (4,5). Joint radiographs are not diagnostic except in late disease when they may reveal characteristic articular destruction (6). There is no clear evidence of a genetic predisposition for juvenile arthritis, except in the case of late childhood pauciarticular disease which may be associated with HLA–B27 and familial spondylarthropathy (5).

The current American Rheumatism Association classification of juvenile rheumatoid arthritis is outlined in Appendix 4; three onset subtypes (systemic, polyarticular, and pauciarticular) are recognized.

Both the name of the disease and the number and classification of subtypes are currently matters of controversy which demand continuing study. The terms juvenile chronic polyarthritis and juvenile chronic arthritis have been proposed by some European investigators; these terms would also encompass childhood ankylosing spondylitis and related conditions (7,8). There is yet no general agreement concerning these proposed changes. Many American investigators continue to use the term juvenile rheumatoid arthritis and some prefer juvenile arthritis.

Subtypes of JRA

Systemic onset disease accounts for about 20% of JRA. In this subgroup the sex ratio is approximately equal, and the disease can begin at any age during childhood. Rheumatoid factor and antinuclear antibodies generally are negative. Clinical characteristics include high intermittent fevers, rheumatoid rash, polyserositis, generalized lymphadenopathy, hepatosplenomegaly, leukocytosis, and anemia. The typical rash is evanescent, pale erythematous and macular.

Systemic manifestations are generally present at disease onset and are usually self-limited to several consecutive months' duration. The systemic disease

itself is rarely life-threatening, although occasionally severe pericarditis, myocarditis, or anemia demand prompt therapeutic intervention. About half of patients have more than 1 systemic attack.

Musculoskeletal manifestations early in the disease often consist only of recurrent arthralgia, myalgia, and transient arthritis which are maximal at times of fever.

Chronic polyarthritis develops in most patients, generally within the first months of disease, but sometimes not until months or even years later. About 25% of patients ultimately have severe chronic arthritis which continues after systemic manifestations have subsided. Systemic onset disease has been described in adults, although it is rare; affected children may have recurrences of systemic manifestations of unknown frequency after they have reached adulthood. Chronic arthritis may continue with or without fever.

Polyarticular onset disease without the extraarticular manifestations of systemic onset disease occurs in approximately 40% of children with JRA. There is a female preponderance. The disease may begin at any age during childhood.

The majority of children with polyarthritis have negative results for rheumatoid factors by standard agglutination techniques; those with positive results are generally older than 8 years when the disease begins. Positive tests for antinuclear antibodies are often found in both rheumatoid factor positive and negative patients. Patients may have malaise, low-grade fever, modest organomegaly, adenopathy, anemia, and growth retardation or weight loss.

Patients with consistently positive rheumatoid factor tests are more likely to develop severe chronic arthritis and therefore have a worse prognosis than those who are rheumatoid factor negative. Destructive, disabling arthritis occurs in as many as 50% of rheumatoid factor positive patients, but in perhaps only 10–15% of rheumatoid factor negative patients. Rheumatoid nodules and rheumatoid vasculitis also occur in the rheumatoid factor positive group. Indeed, this type of disease closely resembles classic adult-onset rheumatoid arthritis.

For these reasons, some investigators propose division of polyarticular onset group into rheumatoid factor positive and rheumatoid factor negative groups. In England the term juvenile rheumatoid arthritis denotes only the rheumatoid factor positive group. Rheumatoid factors can be detected by different techniques in patients who are seronegative by classic agglutination techniques; the significance of these antibodies remains to be defined (9,10). Cervical spine disease most often at the C2–3 apophyseal joints is most common with polyarticular disease with or without systemic onset (Fig 34–1).

Pauciarticular onset JRA affects 40% or more of children with juvenile arthritis; such children have arthritis affecting only a few joints within the first 6 months of disease. Several subgroups of pauciarticular JRA have been proposed; at least 2 can presently be defined.

One subgroup is characterized by early childhood onset (generally before age 6) and female preponderance. These patients often have positive tests for antinuclear

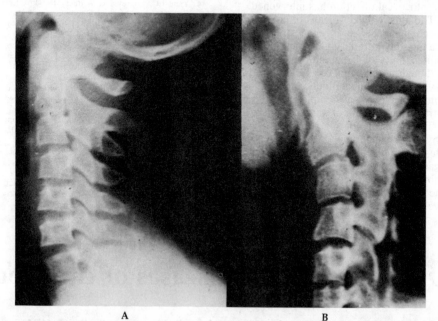

A **B**

Fig 34–1. Lateral projections of the cervical spine in juvenile arthritis. **A,** Narrowing of interspace 2–3 with obliteration of the apophyseal articulation. **B,** Extensive fusion of the posterior articulations of 2, 3, and 4. The normal cervical lordosis is lost, and some degree of kyphosis is seen at this level. There is a decrease in the anteroposterior diameter of the fifth and sixth vertebrae on the right, usually the result of disease early in life. (From the Revised Clinical Slide Collection on the Rheumatic Diseases)

antibodies, but are rheumatoid factor negative. Joints most frequently affected are some combination of the knees, ankles, and elbows; hips are generally spared and sacroiliitis is not seen. Although synovitis may be chronic, the prognosis for joint function is generally good. Systemic manifestations are not prominent.

Ten to 50% of these patients in different reports have developed inflammation of the anterior uveal tract (iridocyclitis) (11–13). This iridocyclitis occasionally precedes joint complaints, but generally begins concurrently with or as long as 10 years after onset of arthritis. Since few symptoms and signs are associated, early detection can be made only by routine slit-lamp examinations; such examinations are recommended 4 times yearly. The iridocyclitis is often chronic and insidious with great potential for ocular damage (posterior synechiae, cataract formation, band keratopathy, secondary glaucoma) and visual loss or even blindness.

A second subgroup of pauciarticular disease is characterized by older age onset and strong male preponderance. Test results for rheumatoid factors and antinuclear antibodies are negative, but more than half of patients have HLA–B27 (14,15). Family histories may be positive for spondylarthropathy.

Arthritis affects predominantly joints of the lower limbs, and early hip or hip girdle involvement is common. Patients frequently have sacroiliitis at onset or during the period of followup; such sacroiliac involvement may be either silent or symptomatic. Attacks of acute self-limited iridocyclitis may occur. Some children with this type of disease have self-limited arthritis which may represent a forme fruste of spondylarthropathy; however with longer followup, an increasing number of these patients can be expected to fulfill criteria for ankylosing spondylitis or another of the spondylarthropathies.

Differential diagnosis. A number of conditions that cause musculoskeletal complaints in children and which may closely mimic JRA must be distinguished before the physician settles on a diagnosis of any childhood rheumatic disease. These include other autoimmune diseases, joint infections of bacterial or viral origin, childhood malignancies, inherited conditions, congenital anomalies, musculoskeletal trauma, avascular necrosis, and others. A number of children with hysteria or psychogenic symptoms focus complaints on the musculoskeletal system; the growing pains (idiopathic limb pains of childhood) and hypermobility syndromes should not be mislabeled as rheumatic in origin.

A partial list of the diagnoses to be differentiated is shown in Table 34–1. Diagnosis of JRA requires *chronic* (6 or more consecutive weeks) objective synovitis. Adherence to this important criterion

along with careful evaluation of each patient will generally lead to correct diagnosis.

Treatment. The outlook for most children with JRA is good. Although the disease is often chronic, at least 75% of patients eventually enter long remissions with little or no residual disability (16). Early diagnosis and appropriate therapy are important to prevent ultimate deformity. Nonetheless, most parents and patients are alarmed by the diagnosis, and education of patients and families is important.

The major goals of therapy are relief of symptoms of active disease; maintenance of joint position, function, and muscle strength in patients seen early in their disease; and restoration of these factors in those seen later in the disease. Physical methods of therapy are as important as the medicinal (17).

The therapy of juvenile arthritis follows the general pattern described for treatment in the adult. *Aspirin* remains a basic therapy and should be started at a dosage of 80 mg/kg/day. This dosage can be increased to levels of about 120 mg/kg if good results are not obtained at the lower dosage level. Serum salicylate levels can be used to control the level and it has been

shown that serum levels above 30 mg% do not increase the therapeutic benefit but do increase side effects (18,19). The therapeutic range is therefore between 20–30 mg/100 ml.

Some children may be more tolerant of swallowing a smooth (enteric coated) tablet. Liquid choline salicylate (Arthropan) is helpful in children who are unable or unwilling to swallow tablets.

Elevated serum transaminase values are routinely found in children taking aspirin. They invariably return to normal when the aspirin is stopped (20).

Reye's syndrome has been said to appear in children who are treated with aspirin for fever accompanying certain viral infections such as smallpox and influenza (21). Children with arthritis who are treated continuously for long periods of time with high doses of salicylate have not been shown to have any increased frequency of Reye's syndrome. However, according to present recommendations, aspirin should be stopped during the presence of these specific infections.

For children who cannot tolerate aspirin therapy or who fail to show adequate response within a period of months, other drugs should be considered. For children over 14 years, any of the *nonsteroidal*

Table 34–1. Differential diagnosis of arthritis in childhood

1. Rheumatic diseases
  a. Rheumatoid arthritis
  b. Rheumatic fever
  c. Systemic lupus erythematosus
  d. Anaphylactoid purpura
  e. Systemic vasculitis
  f. Erythema nodosum
  g. Dermatomyositis
  h. Scleroderma
  i. Mixed connective tissue disease
  j. Ankylosing spondylitis
  k. Rheumatoid nodules sine arthritis
  l. Related conditions
    (1) Ulcerative colitis
    (2) Regional enteritis
    (3) Psoriasis
    (4) Sarcoidosis
    (5) Reiter's syndrome
    (6) Stevens-Johnson syndrome
    (7) Beçhet's syndrome
    (8) Sjögrens syndrome
  m. Polyarteritis nodosa
2. Septic arthritis and virus related
  a. Septic
    (1) Staphylococcus
    (2) Other common pyogens
    (3) Gonococcus
    (4) Mycobacteria
  b. Virus related
    (1) Rubella
    (2) Hepatitis
    (3) Mumps
    (4) Other
3. Osteomyelitis
4. Neoplastic diseases
  a. Leukemia
  b. Lymphoma
  c. Neuroblastoma
	5. Heritable disorders
	  a. Sickle cell disease
	  b. Marfan's syndrome
	  c. Familial Mediterranean fever
	  d. Hereditary multicentric osteolysis
	  e. Mucopolysaccharidoses
	  f. Mucolipidoses
	  g. Fabry's disease
	  h. Weill-Marchesani syndrome
	  i. Farber's disease
	  j. Epiphyseal dysplasia
	  k. Ehlers-Danlos syndrome
	  l. Homocystinuria
	  m. Hemophilia
	  n. Immune deficiency syndromes
	6. Metabolic-endocrine
	  a. Gout
	  b. Pseudogout
	  c. Hypothyroidism
	  d. Hypoparathyroidism
	  e. Progeria
	  f. Other
	7. Miscellaneous
	  a. Transient synovitis
	  b. Palindromic rheumatism
	  c. Traumatic arthritis
	  d. Popliteal cysts
	  e. Villonodular synovitis
	  f. Osteochondritis syndromes
	  g. Hypertrophic osteoarthropathy
	  h. Osteoid osteoma
	  i. Tietze's syndrome
	  j. Short bowel syndrome
	  k. Periodic fever
	  l. Histiocytoses
	  m. Juvenile osteoporosis
	  n. Reflex neurovascular dystrophy
	  o. Psychogenic rheumatism
	  p. Arthromyalgia

agents can be tried. For children under 14, tolmetin, naproxen, and fenoprofen have been approved for use and others are currently under study (22,23).

If such drugs are incompletely effective, *gold therapy* is generally considered. Gold has been reported to be as effective in the treatment of children as in adults (24). When used in the treatment of juvenile arthritis, gold is given at dosages of either 1 mg/kg weekly or 10 mg/week in children up to 19 kg; 20 mg/kg/week between 20–30 kg; 30 mg/kg/week up to 40 kg; 50 mg weekly above 40 kg.

Gold therapy must be monitored by blood counts, urinalyses, and physical examinations at weekly intervals.

Although *hydroxychloroquine* and *penicillamine* have been used in JRA (25) with results comparable to those seen in adults, neither has been approved in the United States for use in children. Studies of both these drugs and oral gold are under way.

Systemic *corticosteroids* are contraindicated except in patients with severe systemic disease, or rarely, with severe polyarthritis that has failed to respond to more conservative treatment (26). Corticosteroid therapy should be limited to once daily or alternate day therapy whenever possible.

There is no indication for corticosteroids in therapy of mild or pauciarticular JRA. Persistent inflammation of one or a few joints may occasionally be treated by intraarticular corticosteroid injections. Iridocyclitis is best managed in cooperation with an ophthalmologist. Topical steroid preparations and dilating agents, combined with close followup, often control the ocular inflammation. If not, locally injected or systemic corticosteroids may be required. Immunosuppressive agents must be considered strictly experimental in the therapy of JRA.

Muscle atrophy and joint contractures are prominent features of JRA that contribute significantly to disability. *Exercises* designed to maintain or regain both muscle strength and joint range of motion are extremely important aspects of therapy (17). Such exercises need to be adapted to the level of the child's maturity and should be performed daily by most patients.

The tendency toward increasing contractures may be reduced by night splints and adoption of the prone position for extended periods several times daily. Maneuvers such as serial splinting or soft tissue releases may be required for reduction of unyielding contractures; such treatment must always be combined with active physical therapy (27). Prolonged immobilization either by bedrest or plaster casting is contraindicated.

Synovectomy does not appear to affect the course of disease significantly in any joint, but may be helpful in rare instances. Total joint replacements may greatly improve function, but must await full bone growth near affected joints (28).

Children should be encouraged to be self-sufficient and should generally attend regular schools and lead as normal lives as possible. Adaptive devices may be helpful in achieving independence. Vocational counseling may be needed for teenagers with significant disabilities.

Juvenile ankylosing spondylitis

The diagnosis of ankylosing spondylitis presents some difficulty. The disease may begin in either central or peripheral joints (14,15). About half of preadolescent children with ankylosing spondylitis present with signs and symptoms of sacroiliac disease such as hip-girdle pain, limping, and occasional low back pain and stiffness.

Radiographs of the sacroiliac joints may be difficult to interpret in children; clear radiographic changes may not appear for some years after onset of sacroiliac symptoms. The role of radiographic scans in identifying early sacroiliitis remains to be defined.

In many children with ankylosing spondylitis the disease begins in peripheral joints, simulating pauciarticular onset JRA, with no evidence of sacroiliac or spine involvement for months or years after onset. Such patients are generally boys, older than age 8 at onset, and at times have a positive family history for spondylarthropathy. Children with ankylosing spondylitis may have attacks of acute iridocyclitis; aortitis has been rarely described during the childhood years.

Symptomatic sacroiliitis of other causes is rare in preadolescents, but occasionally occurs with sacroiliac joint infections, familial Mediterranean fever, Reiter's syndrome, or inflammatory bowel disease. Intervertebral discitis gives rise to similar symptoms affecting the low back, hips, and thighs, but is often a condition of younger children and is not associated with peripheral arthritis.

Systemic lupus erythematosus

Clinical features. Systemic lupus erythematosus (SLE) in childhood as in adult life is a multisystem disease with diverse and varied manifestations associated with antibodies to nuclear antigens. The most common presenting signs of SLE in children are fever, arthralgia, arthritis, and rash. The joint disease may be migratory or rheumatoid-like but is rarely deforming. The rashes of SLE in children are markedly varied in character and distribution and may be erythematous, maculopapular, urticarial, purpuric, bullous, or discoid. The classic butterfly rash is observed on the face in about one-third of the children at the time of diagnosis. Sixty to 80% of children have laboratory evidence of renal disease at the time of diagnosis (29,30).

In many children the presenting signs and symptoms of SLE may be referable to organ systems other than skin, joints, or kidneys. It may appear at first that only a single organ system is involved (Table 34–2). Pleural effusion, pulmonary infiltrates, pericarditis, thrombocytopenia, abdominal pain, and convulsions or other neurologic manifestations alone or in various combinations may all be presenting signs. Lymphadenopathy and hepatosplenomegaly are more prominent and common in children than in adults. The Diagnostic Criteria for SLE of the American Rheumatism Association are as applicable to SLE in children as in adults and are shown in Appendix 6.

SLE occurs in childhood from infancy onward, but the incidence is very low under 5 or 6 years of age and rises markedly as adolescence is approached but with a much lower onset before puberty. The female to male ratio is approximately 5:1. Multiple cases of SLE are found in about 10% of the families of children with this disease.

Infants born to mothers with known SLE often have placentally transmitted antinuclear antibody (31). Most do not have clinical evidence of SLE, but a few have congenital heart block; others develop transient rash or immunologic changes.

Drugs implicated in the induction of lupus-like syndromes in children are primarily the anticonvulsants (32). The resulting disease is usually mild and resolves in most of the patients after discontinuation of the specific anticonvulsant involved, but persists as classic SLE in 20–30% of the reported cases.

Antinuclear antibodies detectable by standard immunofluorescent techniques are present in all children with active SLE except in very rare instances. IgM rheu-

Table 34–2. Major systems involved at onset in 108 children with SLE*

System involvement	% of patients affected between onset and diagnosis (before treatment)
Joints: arthritis and/or arthralgia	78.7
Cutaneous	70.4
Renal	61.1
Hematopoietic†	46.3
Lymphadenopathy	38.9
Hepatosplenomegaly	27.8
Palatal exanthem	21.3
Pulmonary	19.4
Gastrointestinal	18.5
Cardiac	16.7
Central nervous system	13.0

* From King et al (29), courtesy of the Arthritis Foundation.
† Excluding anemia and leukopenia.

matoid factor is found in 5–10% of children with SLE. Depressed levels of C3 and C4 are frequently associated with exacerbations of extrarenal involvement as well as with advancing renal disease (33).

Course. The course of SLE in children treated with corticosteroids and other agents is subject to varied and unpredictible remissions and exacerbations. Approximately 5–10% have mild disease, often manifested by widely separated remissions and exacerbations without critical episodes.

The most common course is characterized by chronic low grade disease activity punctuated by irregular, often severe exacerbations in which first one organ system and then another bears the brunt of attack.

Only about one-third of the deaths in childhood SLE are attributable to lupus renal disease (29). Infection, heart failure, and pulmonary involvement are other significant causes. The reported prognosis for children with SLE has improved dramatically within the last 15 years from an estimated 75–80% mortality within the first 5 years in the 1950s and early 1960s, to an estimated 75–85% survival after 10 years of disease in the 1970s (34,35).

Treatment of children with SLE is much like that of adults (see Section 13). With mild disease, aspirin or other nonsteroidal antiinflammatory agents are used. When prednisone is needed for severe disease, it is given as 40–60 mg/meter^2/24 hours in divided doses.

Dermatomyositis and polymyositis

Dermatomyositis and polymyositis in children are characterized by symmetrical proximal muscle weakness due to a chronic inflammatory myopathy of unknown cause. Dermatomyositis is distinguished from polymyositis by the presence of a characteristic rash on the face and extremities. Dermatomyositis is reported much more frequently than polymyositis in children, whereas polymyositis is more frequent in adults.

Dermatomyositis may begin at any age in childhood; the median age at onset is 6 years (36). Females are more commonly affected than males by about 2:1.

Clinical features. The early signs of dermatomyositis are not specific and malaise and easy fatigability usually precede obvious muscle weakness. The rash is prominent around the eyes (Fig 34–2) and over the malar areas, elbows, knuckles, and knees and is characteristically violaceous or heliotrope. Periorbital edema is evident in about half the cases.

Arthritis occurs in some children but is usually transient. Daily temperature elevations to 38.5C° are reported in half to three-fourths of the children and 5% or more have high spiking fevers.

The histopathology is characterized by

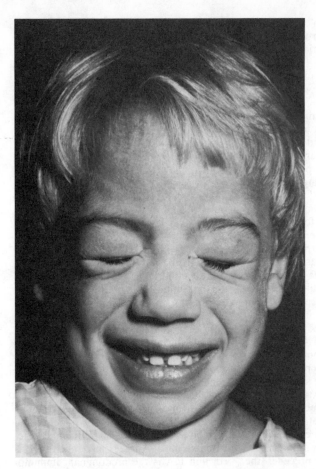

Fig 34–2. The face of this child with dermatomyositis demonstrates heliotrope discoloration of the upper eyelids, periorbital edema, malar rash, and dry shiny erythematous involvement of the upper forehead. The facial rash of this disease can resemble that seen in SLE. This rash is also frequently photosensitive and may be associated with mild alopecia as seen on this child's right side. (From the Revised Clinical Slide Collection on the Rheumatic Diseases)

a diffuse angiopathy involving the small arteries, venules, and capillaries of skin, muscle, fat, small nerves, and gastrointestinal tissue, and in this respect differs from the adult onset disease (37). Muscles show moderate to marked perivascular inflammation in some areas and in other areas diffuse inflammatory infiltrates among the muscle fibers associated with varied evidence of muscle fiber damage.

Other studies of value include electromyography and measurement of serum enzymes, particularly creatine kinase. However, there are no diagnostic laboratory tests.

Dermatomyositis in children is a potentially fatal disease, but the mortality has decreased dramatically in recent years from 38% of the cases reported prior to 1967 to 10% of those reported subsequently (38).

Course. The overall course of the disease can be divided into 3 principal types: 1) a monocyclic course of relatively short duration without relapse, 2) a relapsing form, and 3) a long persisting active disease that may endure for many years. Eighty to 90% of surviving children recover normal or near normal function if properly treated.

Calcinosis develops in 30–50% but is rarely observed before the end of the first year. It may take the form of discrete subcutaneous nodules around major joints, diffuse sheets of calcification in the

dermis and deeper tissues, or rarely flocculant deposits throughout a major muscle group. The calcific deposits are usually spontaneously reabsorbed slowly, but occasionally with dramatic suddenness.

Corticosteroid therapy sustained for an extended time is the treatment of choice although a few children with very mild disease may be treated with aspirin alone (36,38). For the small percentage of children who do not respond to steroid therapy, immunosuppressive agents have been used by some investigators (39).

It should be noted that myositis does occur in association with other diseases, e.g., SLE, scleroderma, or JRA. The muscle disease, however, does not dominate the clinical picture and the presence of other characteristic features aids in distinguishing these conditions from true polymyositis. A painful but transient myositis affecting primarily the calf muscles has been reported in association with influenza B virus infection (40).

Scleroderma

Scleroderma occurs in childhood, both as localized scleroderma and systemic sclerosis. Much more than the skin alone is involved in both these forms of scleroderma, and both are associated with various immunologic alterations and rheumatic signs and symptoms (41). The characteristic skin lesions in both forms of the disease evolve slowly through the classic stages of edema, induration, and atrophy.

Localized scleroderma is usually subdivided into 2 major subtypes: morphea and linear scleroderma (see Section 14). In children, failure of growth in areas affected by linear disease results in deformity. Arthritis occurs in one-third or more of children with linear scleroderma and may be either pauciarticular or polyarticular. There are no specific laboratory findings. Antinuclear antibodies and rheumatoid factor, often in high titer, and elevated immunoglobulin levels are found in one-fourth to one-half the children, particularly those with linear scleroderma (42). Mild elevations of CPK are occasionally seen but the sedimentation rate is usually normal. Treatment is of uncertain value.

Systemic sclerosis. The reported age of onset of systemic sclerosis in children is from 3–14 years with a peak incidence of about 10–13 years of age (41,43). Females predominate in a ratio of about 6:1.

The most commonly reported early symptom is tightening of the skin, particularly around the face and extremities, but the sausage fingers and facial swelling commonly noted in adults at the stage of edema have been reported occasionally.

Raynaud's phenomenon is found in 70% of the children and often precedes the onset of other symptoms. Dysphagia is noted in half of the children. Arthralgia and arthritis also occur but the prevalence is not known.

Cardiac and pulmonary manifestations are frequent and often of grave consequence, and cardiopulmonary disease is the major cause of death in childhood systemic sclerosis. Renal failure is rare and malignant hypertension has not been reported. The estimated mortality is approximately 25% but the prognosis of juvenile onset systemic sclerosis must be considered uncertain.

There is no specific treatment of proven value for systemic sclerosis. Many of the patients show substantial spontaneous improvement and can lead useful and productive lives.

Vasculitis syndromes of childhood

Vasculitis occurs both as primary disease and secondary to other systemic disorders of childhood. The vasculitic syndromes are often accompanied by such rheumatic signs and symptoms as arthralgia, arthritis, fever, and rash.

Small vessel vasculitis. In this category the venules, capillaries, and small arterioles are involved with prominent perivascular infiltrates that also invade the vessel walls in many areas in association with necrotic changes. The associated skin rashes vary from macules or papules, to urticaria, petechiae, purpura, or ecchymo-

ses, usually with a mixture of several forms (44).

Anaphylactoid purpura (Schönlein-Henoch purpura) is the best known and most common of the small vessel vasculitides in children. It is characterized by nonthrombopenic purpura in a characteristic distribution, arthritis with often severe arthralgia, and cramping abdominal pain (45,46). It is much more common in childhood than in adult life, occurring from infancy to adolescence with a median age of onset of about 6 years. Males are more commonly affected than females in a ratio of 2:1.

The skin lesions have a characteristic distribution, being most numerous and prominent over the buttocks and down the backs of the legs. Angioedema occurs in half the children and is more prominent on the extremities than on the face and scalp.

Intussusception is an infrequent but potentially dangerous complication. Hematuria is noted in one-fourth to half the patients during the acute phase. Mild urinary changes persist for a year or so in about one-fourth the patients, but the incidence of chronic renal disease is probably less than 5%.

The white blood cell (WBC) count is elevated in the majority of patients and may be as high as 40,000 WBC/mm^3. Elevated serum IgA levels have been reported, and IgA is the predominant immunoglobulin found in the capillary walls and the glomeruli by immunofluorescence (47,48).

The prognosis is for ultimate recovery without sequelae in 95% or more of the children, even though recurrent attacks may occur for 2 years or more after onset.

Allergic vasculitis is similar in many respects to anaphylactoid purpura with rash, fever, and frequently arthralgia, arthritis, abdominal pain, and urinary changes during the acute illness. Recurrent attacks are likewise common. The skin lesions are much more varied in type and distribution.

Polyarteritis. Classic polyarteritis nodosa (PAN) in children occurs primarily in the preadolescent and adolescent age range and is in most respects similar to the adult disease (49). The male to female ratio is 1.5:1 in children compared with 3:1 reported in adult life. Skin rashes are reported more frequently and are varied in character, suggesting small vessel involvement as well as medium sized arteries. Recently, high titers of antibody to streptococcal antigens have been reported in association with PAN in children.

Cutaneous polyarteritis is a subtype of PAN that occurs in children as well as in adults. The arteries of the skin and subcutaneous tissues are primarily involved, although deeper lesions occur in some patients. The skin often shows livedo reticularis and small painful nodules occuring in crops. The prognosis for this condi-

tion is better than for those with classic PAN.

Infantile polyarteritis (IPN) and *Kawasaki's disease* are clinically and histologically virtually indistinguishable (50–53). IPN is characterized by persistent fever, malaise, morbiliform rash, and leukocytosis. Death occurs unexpectedly about 4 weeks after onset. Death is due to coronary arteritis with prominent aneurysm formation and myocardial infarction (54,55).

Kawasaki's disease is described in detail in Section 18.

Takayasu's arteritis. Takayasu's arteritis (*pulseless disease*) involves the aorta and its branches. Twenty-five to 30% of the patients have the onset of their disease before age 16. See Section 18 for a complete description.

Allergic granulomatous angiitis. The allergic granulomatous angiitis of Churg and Strauss is clinically a syndrome of asthma, fever, hypereosinophilia, cardiac failure, renal damage, and peripheral neuropathy (56). As many as 20% of the cases occur in the preadolescent age range (see Section 18.)

Wegener's granulomatosis. Onset of Wegener's granulomatosis after 10 years of age is much more likely than before. This disorder is covered in Section 18.

1. Baum J: Epidemiology of juvenile rheumatoid arthritis. Arthritis Rheum 20(suppl):158–160, 1976
2. Bernstein BH, Stobie D, Singsen BH, et al: Growth retardation in juvenile rheumatoid arthritis (JRA). Arthritis Rheum 20(suppl):212–216, 1976
3. Ansell BM, Bywaters EGL: Growth in Still's disease. Ann Rheum Dis 15:295–319, 1956
4. Hanson V, Kornreich HK, Bernstein B, et al: Three subtypes of juvenile rheumatoid arthritis: correlations of age at onset, sex, and serologic factors. Arthritis Rheum 20(suppl):184–186, 1976
5. Levinson JE, Balz GP, Hess EV: Report of studies on juvenile arthritis. Arthritis Rheum 20(suppl):189–190, 1976
6. Cassidy JT, Martel W: Juvenile rheumatoid arthritis: clinicoradiologic correlations. Arthritis Rheum 20(suppl):207–211, 1976
7. Ansell B: Diagnostic criteria, nomenclature, classification, The Care of Rheumatoid Children. Ed 1. E Munthe, ed. Basel, Switzerland, EULAR, 1978, pp 42–46
8. Wood P: Special meeting on: Nomenclature and classification of arthritis in children, The Care of Rheumatic Children, Ed 1. E Munthe, ed. Basel, Switzerland, EULAR, 1978, pp 47–50
9. Moore TL, Dorner RW, Weiss TD, et al: Specificity of hidden 19S IgM rheumatoid factor in patients with juvenile rheumatoid arthritis. Arthritis Rheum 24:1283–1290, 1981
10. Wernick R, LoSpalluto JJ, Fink CW, et al: Serum IgG and IgM rheumatoid factors by solid phase radioimmunoassay. Arthritis Rheum 24:1501–1511, 1981
11. Chylack LT Jr: The ocular manifestations of juvenile rheumatoid arthritis. Arthritis Rheum 20(suppl):217–223, 1976
12. Cassidy JT, Sullivan DB, Petty RE: Clinical patterns of chronic iridocyclitis in children with juvenile rheumatoid arthritis. Arthritis Rheum 20(suppl):224–227, 1976
13. Schaller JG, Johnson GD, Holborow EJ, et al: The association of antinuclear antibodies with the chronic iridocyclitis of juvenile rheumatoid arthritis (Still's disease). Arthritis Rheum 17:409–416, 1974
14. Schaller J, Bitnum S, Wedgwood RJ: Ankylos-

ing spondylitis with childhood onset. J Pediatr 74:505–516, 1969

15. Albert ED: Genetic analysis of HLA–B27-associated disease, Arthritis in Childhood: Report of the Eightieth Ross Conference in Pediatrics Research. TD Moore, ed. Columbus, Ohio, Ross Laboratories, 1979, pp 75–77

16. Hanson V, Kornreich H, Bernstein B, et al: Prognosis of juvenile rheumatoid arthritis. Arthritis Rheum 20(suppl):279–284, 1977

17. Donovan WH: Physical measures in the treatment of juvenile rheumatoid arthritis. Arthritis Rheum 20(suppl):553–557, 1976

18. Baum J, Pless IB: Juvenile rheumatoid arthritis, Ambulatory Pediatrics. Ed 2, M Green, RJ Haggerty, eds. Philadelphia, W B Saunders Co, 1977, pp 139–146

19. Schaller JG: Chronic salicylate administration in juvenile rheumatoid arthritis: aspirin "hepatitis" and its clinical significance. Pediatrics 62(suppl):916–925, 1978

20. Doughty RA, Giesecke L, Athreya B: Salicylate therapy in juvenile rheumatoid arthritis. Am J Dis Child 134:461–463, 1980

21. Starko KM, Ray CG, Dominquez LB, et al: Reye's syndrome and salicylate use. Pediatrics 66:859–864, 1980

22. Gewanter HL, Baum J: The use of tolmetin sodium in systemic onset JRA. Arthritis Rheum 24:1316–1319, 1981

23. Brewer EJ: Nonsteroidal anti-inflammatory agents. Arthritis Rheum 20(suppl):513–525, 1976

24. Brewer EJ Jr, Giannini EH, Barkley E: Gold therapy in the management of juvenile rheumatoid arthritis. Arthritis Rheum 23:404–411, 1980

25. Stillman JS, Barry PE: Juvenile rheumatoid arthritis, series 2. Arthritis Rheum 20(suppl):171–175, 1976

26. Schaller JG: Corticosteroids in juvenile rheumatoid arthritis. Arthritis Rheum 20(suppl):537–543, 1976

27. Granberry GM: Soft tissue release in children with juvenile rheumatoid arthritis. Arthritis Rheum 20(suppl):565–566, 1976

28. Singsen BH, Isaacson AS, Bernstein BH, et al: Total hip replacement in children with arthritis. Arthritis Rheum 21:401–406, 1978

29. King KK, Kornreich HK, Bernstein BH, et al: The clinical spectrum of systemic lupus erythematosus in childhood. Arthritis Rheum 20(suppl):287–294, 1976

30. Meislin AG, Rothfield N: Systemic lupus erythematosus in childhood: analysis of 42 cases with comparative data on 200 adult cases followed concurrently. Pediatrics 42:37–49, 1968

31. Schaller JG: Lupus phenomena in the newborn. Arthritis Rheum 20(suppl):312–314, 1976

32. Singsen BH, Fishman L, Hanson V: Antinuclear antibodies and lupus-like syndromes in children receiving anticonvulsants. Pediatrics 57:529–534, 1976

33. Singsen BH, Bernstein BH, King KK, et al: Systemic lupus erythematosus in childhood: correlations between changes in disease activity and the serum complement levels. J Pediatr 89:358–365, 1976

34. Walraven STA, Chase H: The prognosis of childhood systemic lupus erythematosus. Am J Dis Child 130:929–933, 1976

35. Fish AJ, Blau EB, Westberg NG, et al: Systemic lupus erythematosus within the first 2 decades of life. Am J Med 62:99–117, 1977

36. Hanson V: Dermatomyositis, scleroderma, and polyarteritis nodosa. Clin Rheum Dis 2:445–467, 1976

37. Banker BQ, Victor M: Dermatomyositis (systemic angiopathy) of childhood. Medicine 45:261–289, 1966

38. Sullivan DB, Cassidy JP, Petty RE, et al: Prognosis in childhood dermatomyositis. J Pediatr 80:555, 1972

39. Jacobs JC: Treatment of dermatomyositis. Arthritis Rheum 20:338–341, 1979

40. Middleton PJ, Alexander RM, Szymanski RM: Severe myositis during recovery from influenza. Lancet 2:533–535, 1970

41. Kornreich HK, King KK, Bernstein BH, et al: Scleroderma in childhood. Arthritis Rheum 20(suppl):343–350, 1976

42. Hanson V, Kornreich HK, Drexler E: Some immunologic considerations in focal scleroderma and progressive systemic sclerosis in children. Pediatr Res 8:806–809, 1974

43. Dabish L, Sullivan DB, Cassidy JT: Scleroderma in the child. J Pediatr 85:770–775, 1974

44. Gilliam JN, Smiley JD: Cutaneous necrotizing vasculitis and related disorders. Ann Allergy 37:328–339, 1976

45. Wedgwood RJP, Klaus MH: Anaphylactoid purpura (Schonlein-Henoch syndrome). Pediatrics 16:196–205, 1955

46. Allen DM, Diamond LK, Howell DA: Anaphylactoid purpura in children (Henoch-Schonlein syndrome). Am J Dis Child 99:833–854, 1960

47. Trygstad CW, Stiehm ER: Elevated serum IgA globulin in anaphylactoid purpura. Pediatrics 47:1023–1028, 1971

48. Giangiacomo J, Tsai CC: Dermal and glomerular deposition of IgA in anaphylactoid purpura. Am J Dis Child 131:981–983, 1977

49. Blau EB, Morris RF, Yunis EJ: Polyarteritis nodosa in older children. Pediatrics 60:227–234, 1977

50. Landing BH, Jarson EJ: Are infantile periarteritis nodosa with coronary artery involvement and fatal mucocutaneous lymph node syndrome the same? Comparison of 20 patients from North America with patients from Hawaii and Japan. Pediatrics 59:651–662, 1977

51. Roberts FB, Fetterman GH: Polyarteritis nodosa in infancy. J Pediatr 63:519–529, 1963

52. Kawasaki T, Kosaki F, Okawa S, et al: A new infantile acute febrile mucocutaneous lymph node syndrome (MLNS) prevailing in Japan. Pediatrics 54:271–276, 1974

53. Melish ME, Hicks RM, Larson EJ: Mucocutaneous lymph node syndrome in the United States. Am J Dis Child 130:599–607, 1976

54. Yoshida H, Funabashi T, Nakaya S, et al: Mucocutaneous lymph node syndrome. Am J Dis Child 133:1244–1247, 1979

55. Fujiwara H, Hamashima Y: Pathology of the heart in Kawasaki disease. Pediatrics 61:100–107, 1978

56. Churg J, Strauss L: Allergic granulomatosis, allergic angiitis and periarteritis nodosa. Am J Pathol 27:277–301, 1951

35. Adult onset Still's disease

This is a rare form of seronegative polyarthritis which begins during the early years of adult life and affects both men and women (1–13). The latest onset in a total of 70 cases recorded to date is 56 years.

Clinical features. The clinical features include a systemic onset, with high daily intermittent fever accompanied by a small nonspreading salmon-colored, measles-like macular rash (often marked along pressure lines), polyarthritis, tenosynovitis, pericarditis, and sometimes splenic and lymph node enlargement. All except the rash were mentioned by GF Still in 1897 (1). Nodules over pressure points have not been described. Sore throat may also occur.

Fever and rash are characteristic and often the only the initial signs of disease. Both are maximal in the late afternoon and may be accompanied by malaise and headache, and sometimes followed by hairfall. Only rarely is the eruption raised or itchy. This stage may remit and recur for many years or it may lead rapidly to transient and recurrent, but sometimes prolonged, joint involvement.

Arthralgia or myalgia is common. Synovitis is usually mild and transient, only

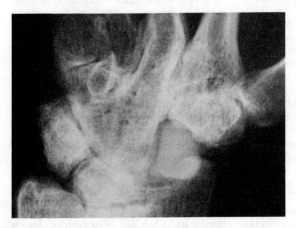

Fig 35–1. Roentgenogram illustrating carpometacarpal joint ankylosis in a patient with adult onset Still's disease. Note also the carpal prosthesis. (Illustration provided by Dr EGL Bywaters)

seldom leading to disability or erosions. Individual joints are affected with the frequency found in other types of chronic polyarthritis (i.e., knees, wrists, fingers). However, a special predilection exists for the upper cervical apophyseal joints (in children) (2,5,10), carpometacarpal joints (6,8) (Fig 35–1), and the terminal interphalangeal joints (without evidence of psoriasis). These joints tend to fuse rather than to undergo the erosion, and in the neck the subluxation seen in seropositive rheumatoid arthritis. Therefore, residual disability is often minimal.

Visceral lesions include pericarditis and pleural effusions, both mild and transient. Abdominal pain has been recorded, perhaps related to lymph node enlargement. Splenomegaly may be found, and liver failure in association with drug ingestion has been recorded (9).

Laboratory findings. The erythrocyte

sedimentation rate and white blood cell count are raised during periods of activity, but tests for rheumatoid factor and antinuclear antibody usually show negative results. Serum IgG concentration may be raised. Synovial fluid shows a polymorphonuclear leukocytosis with decreased complement. Immune complexes may be found in the serum, and reticuloendothelial clearance is impaired. Amyloidosis has developed (13). Lymphocytotoxic cold-reactive antibody may be transiently present in the early stages, suggesting a virus infection (14).

Diagnosis and treatment. Initially, many of these febrile patients are ineffectively treated for an infection with antibiotics. The rash usually suggests the correct diagnosis but must be differentiated from the annular spreading circles of erythema marginatum seen in rheumatic fever. German measles in young women is often accompanied by arthralgia or synovitis, as is viral hepatitis. Other combinations of rash, fever, and arthritis due to infection and/or immune reaction should be excluded such as meningococcal disease, mononucleosis, Lyme arthritis, Schönlein-Henoch purpura, drug allergy, systemic lupus erythematosus, and erythema multiforme.

The acute symptoms will respond to full dosage of aspirin (blood levels of 20–30 mg/dl). Other nonsteroidal antiinflammatory drugs are effective if aspirin is not tolerated. Only rarely should prednisone be necessary and then in 1 single daily dose (or alternate day dosage if possible) not greater than 10 mg per day.

Prognosis is usually excellent: most patients are able to lead a normal life. A few, however, have developed more severe joint damage, requiring hip replacement (11).

1. Still GF: On a form of chronic joint disease in childhood. Med-Chir Trans 80:47–49, 1897
2. Bywaters EGL: Still's disease in the adult. Ann Rheum Dis 30:121–133, 1971
3. Bujak JS, Aptekar RG, Decker JL, Wolff SM: Juvenile rheumatoid arthritis presenting in the adult as fever of unknown origin. Medicine 52:431–444, 1973
4. Aptekar RG, Decker JL, Bujak JS, Wolff SE: Adult onset juvenile rheumatoid arthritis. Arthritis Rheum 16:715–718, 1973
5. Fabricant MS, Chandor SB, Friou GJ: Still's disease in adult: a cause of prolonged undiagnosed fever. JAMA 225:273–276, 1973
6. Medsger TA, Christy WC: Carpal arthritis with ankylosis in late onset Still's disease. Arthritis Rheum 19:232–242, 1977
7. Gupta RC, Mills DM: Still's disease in an adult: a link between juvenile and adult rheumatoid arthritis. Am J Med Sci 269:137–144, 1975
8. Zajacsek-Grabowski A, Maldykowa H, Chwalinska-Sadowska H: Ankylosing carpal disease in adult rheumatoid arthritis. Rheumatologia 16:539–546, 1978
9. Baker DG, Schumacher HR: Fifteen patients with adult onset Still's disease: life threatening liver failure in two (abstract). Arthritis Rheum 22:590, 1979
10. Wilson W, Morgan OS, Bain B, Taylor JE: Takayasu's arteritis: association with Still's disease in an adult. Arthritis Rheum 22:684–688, 1979
11. Kaplinsky N, Pras M, Frankl O: An adult form of juvenile rheumatoid arthritis. Arch Intern Med 140:1073–1074, 1980
12. Esdaile JM, Tannenbaum H, Hawkins D: "Adult Still's disease." Am J Med 68:825–830, 1980
13. Elkon KH, Bywaters EGL, Inman RQ, Hughes GRV: Adult onset Still's disease: long term followup and immunologic studies. Ann Rheum Dis 39:187–188, 1980
14. Bresnihan B, Hughes GRV: Lymphocytotoxic antibodies in Still's disease (correspondence). Lancet 1:803, 1977

36. Osteoarthritis

Osteoarthritis (osteoarthrosis, degenerative joint disease) is the most common disease of both axial and peripheral diarthrodial joints. It is characterized pathologically by progressive deterioration and loss of articular cartilage and by reactive changes at the margins of the joints and in the subchondral bone.

Clinical manifestations are characterized by slowly developing joint pain, stiffness, enlargement with limitation of motion. Associated secondary synovitis is common.

Osteoarthritis has been divided into primary and secondary forms, depending on the absence or presence of some clearly evident underlying local or systemic etiologic factor. This classification may at times be artificial. For example, many cases of osteoarthritis of the hip, long considered primary, are probably secondary to variously expressed childhood anatomic abnormalities such as congenital hip dysplasia or slipped femoral epiphysis (1).

Pathologic and roentgenographic evidence of osteoarthritis is not rare as early as the third decade of life. Prevalence increases with age; the disease is almost universal in persons 65 years or older. Racial differences in prevalence and distribution of affected joints may be related to differences in occupation, life style, and predisposing genetic factors. The low incidence of osteoarthritis of the hip in Chinese as compared with whites may be related to protection of the joint by the more complete range of motion associated with frequent squatting (2).

Genetic factors play a role in the development of osteoarthritis of the distal interphalangeal joints of the hands (*Heberden's nodes*). The genetic mechanism appears to involve a single autosomal gene, sex influenced, dominant in females, resulting in an incidence in women 10 times that in men.

The pathogenic role of obesity remains controversial. Some studies suggest that obesity per se is not a factor in disease development (3); other studies demonstrate an increased frequency of osteoarthritis in obese patients, particularly when weight-bearing joints are evaluated (4). Obesity may also be a secondary phenomenon related to decreased physical activity brought about by joint pain and limitation of motion (3).

Pathology. Normally blue translucent cartilage takes on an opaque yellowish appearance. Surface irregularities due to fissuring and pitting are followed by erosions. These erosions, initially focal, become confluent and lead to large areas of denuded surface. Initial involvement of superficial and middle layers is followed by full-thickness loss of cartilage down to bone.

Osteophyte spur formation, a proliferative lesion, is seen most prominently at joint margins. Some studies suggest that osteophyte spur formation is not a characteristic component of the osteoarthritic process but is a separate manifestation of aging (5). These studies demonstrated that erosive cartilage loss did not inevitably follow the appearance of osteophytes, even after many years. At present, most investigators consider osteophytes a manifestation of the osteoarthritic process. Subchondral bone becomes thickened and sclerotic (eburnated).

Cyst formation in the juxtaarticular bone is common. Transmission of high forces transmitted through synovial fluid to subchondral bone may play a role in their evolution. Alternatively, cyst development may follow tissue breakdown related to focal areas of microfracture in the ischemic subchondral bone.

Secondary synovitis, seen frequently in advanced disease, may result from release of crystals from cartilage, inflammatory mediators initiated by cartilage breakdown components, or possibly from immune challenge by previously "hidden" proteinaceous materials. Eventually, gross deformity and subluxation of joints are seen.

Histologic examination reveals fibrillation of superficial cartilage layers and development of fissures that extend through various layers of cartilage (Fig 36–1). Alterations in the intracellular proteoglycan matrix lead to loss of staining with agents such as toluidine blue or safranin-O. Chondrocyte response varies, depending on disease severity and duration.

Early, there is a proliferative response

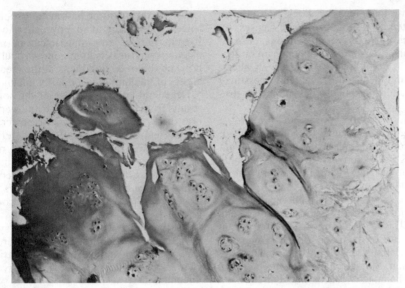

Fig 36–1. Osteoarthritic human cartilage: pathologic changes include surface fibrillation, vertical fissure formation, and clusters (clones) of proliferating cells; cartilage components are being released into the synovial cavity.

with general hypercellularity and increased numbers of chondrocytes in clusters of cells (Fig 36–1). Later, hypocellularity is noted. Osteophytes consist of proliferating new bone capped by cartilage. Subchondral bone is thickened.

Biochemical and metabolic alterations. It is now well established by histochemical and biochemical observations that the proteoglycan content of osteoarthritic cartilage is diminished and that the decrease is directly proportional to the disease severity (6,7). Although the total glycosaminoglycan (GAG) content is diminished, the depletion does not uniformly affect all species of these macromolecular materials. Specifically, the glucosamine containing amino sugars (including keratan sulfate) are more severely affected than those containing galactosamine (especially chondroitin sulfate) (8).

Studies have shown an increase in chondroitin 4–sulfate concentration, mostly at the expense of the keratan sulfate. Proteoglycan subunits are smaller in osteoarthritic articular cartilage, and aggregation is retarded (9). One theory of the pathogenesis of the disorder suggests that the apparatus for proteoglycan aggregation is somehow damaged, particularly in late stage disease (10).

The total collagen content of osteoarthritic cartilage varies little (11); some type I collagen appears around chondrocyte lacunae, but most of the collagen remains type II as in normal cartilage. Fiber diameters and orientation may show considerable variation from normal (12), and recent findings show that the collagen network in the middle zones may be very loose, allowing swelling of the cartilage (13).

The water content of osteoarthritic ar-

ticular cartilage is significantly increased and, further, freshly administered water binds more avidly than to normal tissue. Swelling of the cartilage on exposure to water is not seen in normal cartilage but is noted in osteoarthritic cartilage and may be important in progressive biomechanical disruption of the tissue with advancing disease.

Contrary to a view held for many years, cartilage in osteoarthritis is not passively eroded away, but in fact, the synthesis of all matrix components is markedly increased (14). DNA synthesis, normally

absent in adult articular cartilage, is active in osteoarthritic tissue and appears to be roughly proportional to the disease severity. Proteoglycan synthesis is increased in similar fashion, and the synthesis of collagen has recently been noted to be increased as much as 6-fold compared with normal tissues (15).

This seemingly extraordinary rapid metabolic activity suggests that the articular chondrocyte is responding to the "chronic" stress of osteoarthritis by a reparative reaction which appears to be quite brisk and in theory could, under proper circumstances, heal the disease (6,14). The fact that the process is one of "inexorable" progression with gradual erosion of the articular surface over time suggests that degradation is even more rapid than repair and implies the presence of increased activity in the enzymatic internal remodeling system.

The enzymes active in articular cartilage that show a marked increase in osteoarthritic tissue include cathepsin D and neutral proteoglycanase, proteases that attack the protein core of the proteoglycan; sugar-splitting enzymes and sulfatases, which degrade the glycosaminoglycans; and a collagenase (16,17).

Pathogenesis. These data suggest that the initiating event in osteoarthritis, although unknown, influences the cellular process in several ways (Fig 36–2). The chondrocytes under the influence of the insult either die (and release enzymes) or begin to replicate DNA, increasing the number of cells and the formation of clones. The cells synthesize increased amounts of proteoglycan and at the same time produce increased quantities of lyso-

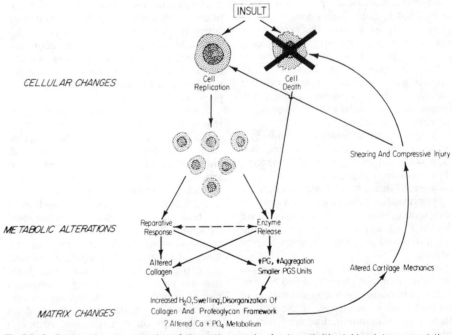

Fig 36–2. Schematic representation of the pathogenesis of osteoarthritis, taking into account the metabolic alterations and the biochemical changes in the matrix. (Illustration provided by Dr RW Moskowitz)

somal enzymes that degrade the matrix. Variations in the degree of altered synthesis and degradation produce the alterations in structure consisting of altered collagen, increased water and swelling, and a slowly diminishing concentration of proteoglycan (with decreased size of the subunits and diminished aggregation).

With advancing disease, the mechanical factors become more important, the insult is perpetuated, or possibly enhanced, and the proteoglycanases and collagenase cause even more severe degradation. Despite very active chondrocyte synthetic activities, the cartilage cannot keep pace with the disease and eventually becomes eroded and totally destroyed.

The nature of the initiating event (the insult) in this pathogenetic scheme is not known, but clearly the most likely candidate is trauma, either acute or, even more reasonably, chronic (18,19) (see Section 5).

Another factor of some importance is aging, which in itself may not be a cause of osteoarthritis but may cause changes in chondrocyte function required for the osteoarthritic process to begin or be perpetuated. Family influences are difficult to evaluate, but in such lesions as Heberden's nodes and generalized osteoarthritis some genetic alterations in chondrocyte function may predispose to the disease.

Similarly, hormonal factors may play a role, particularly since osteoarthritis appears to be more prevalent in women than men. The possible action of immune mechanisms has recently been postulated, particularly in perpetuation of the disease (20). It is possible that the initiating event is some combination of these or perhaps some other as yet unknown factor.

Another aspect of the process not well understood is time. Indications from autopsy studies show that the progress of osteoarthritis may be very slow indeed, and the initial phases may be slow or perhaps nonprogressive. However, with advancing age, presumably in susceptible individuals, the process may accelerate in almost an exponential manner to produce the clinical syndrome.

Clinical features. Symptoms and signs are usually local; generalized osteoarthritis, however, may suggest a systemic form of connective tissue disease.

Clinical symptoms and roentgenographic abnormalities generally show a positive correlation. However, in any given case the lack of correlation between joint symptoms and pathologic findings may be striking.

Pain early in the course of disease occurs after joint use and is relieved by rest. Later, pain occurs with minimal motion or even at rest; at this stage of the disease night pain is common. Cartilage has no nerve supply and is insensitive to pain. Pain arises from other intraarticular and periarticular structures.

Acute inflammatory flares may be precipitated by trauma or, in some cases, by crystal-induced synovitis in response to crystals of calcium pyrophosphate or apatite (21). Joint stiffness is relatively short-lived and localized. Local tenderness may be elicited, especially if synovitis is present.

Pain on passive motion and *crepitus*, a feeling of crackling as the joint is moved, are prominent findings. Joint enlargement results from synovitis, increased amounts of synovial fluid, or proliferative changes in cartilage and bone.

Heberden's nodes are characterized by spur formation at the dorsolateral and medial aspects of the distal interphalangeal joints of the fingers. Flexor and lateral deviations of the distal phalanx are common. Similar changes at the proximal interphalangeal joints are called *Bouchard's nodes*.

In most patients, Heberden's nodes develop slowly over months or years. In other patients, onset is rapid and associated with moderately severe inflammatory changes. Gelatinous cysts resembling ganglia may precede the appearance of the Heberden's node itself.

High intraarticular pressure may account for the frequent involvement of the distal interphalangeal joints in the osteoarthritic process (22). Involvement of the first carpometacarpal joints leads to tenderness at the base of the first metacarpal bone and a squared appearance of the hand. Common involvement of the trapezioscaphoid joint has been emphasized (23).

Osteoarthritis of the acromioclavicular joint may cause shoulder area pain. Osteoarthritis of the knee is characterized by localized tenderness over various components of the joint, and pain on passive or active motion. Crepitus can often be detected. Muscle atrophy is seen secondary to disuse. Disproportionate losses of cartilage localized to the medial or lateral compartments of the knee lead to secondary genu varus or valgus.

Chondromalacia patellae, seen most often in young adults, is associated with softening and erosion of patellar articular cartilage. More severe osteoarthritic changes often follow. Pain, localized around the patella, is aggravated by activity such as walking hills or stairs.

Osteoarthritic changes in the hip lead to an insidious onset of pain, often followed by a limp. Pain is usually localized to the groin or along the inner aspect of the thigh. The patient often complains of pain in the buttocks, sciatic region, or the knee due to pain referral along contiguous nerves. Physical examination shows loss of hip motion, initially most marked on internal rotation or extension. Although less common than osteoarthritis of the knee, hip involvement is the most disabling form of osteoarthritis.

Osteoarthritis of the first metatarsophalangeal joint is aggravated by tight shoes. Irregularities in joint contour can be palpated. Tenderness is common, particularly when the overlying bursa at the medial aspect of the joint is secondarily inflamed.

Degenerative joint disease of the spine results from involvement of the intervertebral discs, vertebral bodies, or posterior apophyseal articulations. Large anterior osteophytes in the cervical spine give rise at times to dysphagia or respiratory tract symptoms. Compression of the anterior spinal artery by large posterior spurs or discs leads to a central cord syndrome (24).

Basilar-vertebral insufficiency syndrome results when large spurs compress the vertebral arteries. Degenerative changes of the dorsal spine are relatively uncommon.

Involvement of the lumbar spine is seen most commonly at the L3–4 area. Associated symptoms include local pain and stiffness and radicular pain due to compression of contiguous nerve roots. Cauda equina syndrome with sphincter dysfunction may result.

Variant forms. Certain so-called variant forms of primary osteoarthritis have been defined. Patients with *primary generalized osteoarthritis* reveal involvement of the distal and proximal interphalangeal joints of the hands, the first carpometacarpal joint, knees, hips, and metatarsophalangeal joints. Radiologic changes often exceed clinical findings. These cases may represent a more severe form of ordinary osteoarthritis, differing only in the number and severity of joints involved.

Erosive inflammatory osteoarthritis involves primarily the distal or proximal interphalangeal joints of the hands (25). Painful inflammatory episodes are associated with eventual development of joint deformity and ankylosis. After a variable period of years of intermittent acute flares, the joints tend to become asymptomatic. Bony erosions are prominent on x-ray.

Ankylosing hyperostosis, more recently given the name diffuse idiopathic skeletal hyperostosis (DISH), is characterized by flowing ossification along the anterolateral aspect of the vertebral bodies (26). Disc narrowing does not appear to be part of the process, so that this disease is more a source of confusion with osteoarthritis than a variant (see Section 63).

Secondary osteoarthritis produces clinical findings and roentgenographic changes similar to those seen in the primary form of the disease. Underlying causes are listed in Table 36–1. A relationship between generalized joint hypermobility, osteoarthritis, and chondrocalcinosis has been noted (27).

Laboratory and x-ray findings. Laboratory evaluations other than roentgenographic study are helpful primarily in ex-

Table 36–1. Varieties of secondary osteoarthritis. Consult appropriate sections for detailed descriptions of these conditions

1. Heritable metabolic disorders
   a. Alkaptonuria
   b. Wilson's disease
   c. Hemochromatosis
   d. Morquio's disease
2. Multiple epiphyseal dysplasia
3. Slipped capital femoral epiphysis
4. Congenital dislocation of the hips
5. Neuropathic arthropathy (Charcot joints)
6. Hemophilic arthropathy
7. Acromegalic arthropathy
8. Paget's disease of bone (osteitis deformans)
9. Rheumatoid arthritis
10. Gout
11. Septic and tuberculous arthritis

cluding other joint diseases. The erythrocyte sedimentation rate, normal in most patients, may be slightly elevated in patients with erosive inflammatory or generalized forms of the disease. Minimal abnormalities are seen on synovial fluid study. Viscosity is good; the cell count is slightly increased. Calcium pyrophosphate dihydrate and/or apatite crystals are seen in many osteoarthritic joint effusions (21,28).

X-rays may be normal if pathologic changes are mild. Characteristic progressive changes include joint space narrowing, subchondral bony sclerosis (eburnation), marginal osteophyte formation, and cyst formation (Fig 36–3). Ankylosis is uncommon except in patients with the erosive inflammatory form of the disease. Osteoporosis is not a component of degenerative change.

Specialized roentgenographic views, such as x-rays of the knees with the patient standing, should be obtained when the disease is suspected and not visualized on routine anteroposterior and lateral films. X-rays of contralateral joints are helpful in evaluating the significance of observed changes.

Prognosis. The prognosis for patients with primary osteoarthritis varies. Involvement of weight-bearing joints or the spine is more likely to lead to disability. Not all patients with osteoarthritis inevitably deteriorate (29). However, severe involvement of critical joints leads to significant disability. In this sense, osteoarthritis is not always a benign disease.

Differential diagnosis. In patients with generalized or inflammatory osteoarthritis, a diagnosis of seronegative rheumatoid arthritis cannot always be excluded. Certain rheumatic diseases such as psoriatic arthritis, Reiter's syndrome, and the arthritis of chronic ulcerative colitis may lead to diagnostic confusion since distal interphalangeal joints of the hands are frequently involved.

Neurologic abnormalities due to spinal osteoarthritis are at times confused with those seen in primary neurologic disorders.

Treatment. The selection of a specific therapeutic program must be individualized. Many patients require only reassurance that they have no generalized crippling form of rheumatic disease.

Protection of joints from overuse is important, especially if weight-bearing joints are involved. Forces on the lower extremity are increased 3 to 4-fold when weight is shifted to each leg in walking. Appliances such as canes are beneficial for joint protection, when indicated.

Weight reduction should be carried out, especially in patients with marked obesity. Physical therapy relieves pain and associated muscle spasm and maintains and regains joint range of motion. Simple measures such as plain hot water soaks or warm tub baths may alleviate pain.

Isometric exercises, in which the muscles are strengthened against weight resistance while the joint is kept in a normal anatomic position, maintain muscle function and strength. Isotonic exercises, in which joints are put through a range of motion while being exercised, should be used without resistance lest the basic pathologic process be aggravated.

Pharmacologic agents. Analgesic agents such as acetaminophen, propoxyphene hydrochloride, or diflunisal may be used on a continuous or as needed basis. Narcotic preparations, required only occasionally for acute flares, should be limited in use.

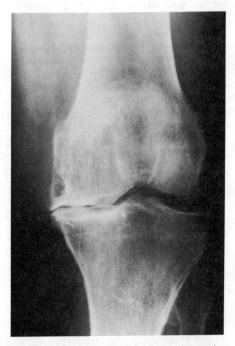

Fig 36–3. Osteoarthritis, left knee, anteroposterior view. Medial compartment changes are characterized by structural cartilage loss with joint space narrowing, and subchondral bony sclerosis. (Illustration provided by Dr RW Moskowitz)

Nonsteroidal antiinflammatory agents are often beneficial. Aspirin, which has both analgesic and antiinflammatory properties, is still generally considered the drug of first choice.

Newer nonsteroidal antiinflammatory agents are available for alternative use in patients who are allergic to or intolerant of salicylates. At present, indomethacin, ibuprofen, fenoprofen, naproxen, tolmetin, meclofenamate, piroxicam, and sulindac are available for use. These agents share a number of toxic side reactions including rash, gastrointestinal upset, peptic ulceration, occasional vague psychic reactions, and tinnitus.

Phenylbutazone and its derivative, oxyphenbutazone, are less commonly used in the treatment of osteoarthritis now that the newer less toxic nonsteroidal agents are available.

Oral or parenteral therapy with adrenal corticosteroids is contraindicated in the treatment of degenerative joint disease. These agents are generally ineffective in improving symptoms and their toxic potential makes their use risky.

However intraarticular injections of corticosteroids, judiciously used, may be beneficial in the management of acute joint flares. Injections should be infrequent, especially if given into weight-bearing joints. Joint deterioration may be accelerated due to masking of pain with subsequent joint overuse. A direct deleterious effect of these drugs on cartilage has also been described. Pericapsular and ligamentous injections in areas of tenderness around involved joints provides relief with less hazard.

Transcutaneous nerve stimulation, which involves delivery of an electrical current through the skin to a peripheral nerve, may provide pain relief in patients with osteoarthritis of the spine (30). More controlled trials of its use in osteoarthritis are needed. Studies of the effectiveness of acupuncture in the treatment of pain associated with osteoarthritis have shown inconsistent results (31).

Surgical procedures. Orthopedic surgical procedures of use in patients with osteoarthritis include arthroplasty, osteotomy, fusion, and partial or total prosthetic replacement. Angulation osteotomy is particularly helpful in correcting joint malalignment when significant varus or valgus deformities of the knee are present in unicompartmental disease. Pain is relieved by bringing healthy articular cartilages into position.

Hip replacement procedures produce striking symptomatic relief and improved range of motion. Total knee replacements are less consistently beneficial but provide significant pain relief in patients with advanced disease.

Potential benefits of prosthetic replacements must be weighed against associated complications which include infection, phlebitis, pulmonary emboli, nerve injury, and eventual failure of the prosthesis itself by loosening or fracture.

Management of specific joints. Hot soaks, paraffin wax applications, and avoidance of aggravating repetitive trauma are helpful in osteoarthritis of the *hands*. Analgesic and nonsteroidal antiinflammatory agents are useful. Local steroid injections into or around involved joints are particularly beneficial when only 1 or 2 joints are symptomatic. Relief of pain and morning stiffness can be achieved in some patients by the use of nylon-Spandex stretch gloves, especially when worn at night. Osteoarthritis of the first carpometacarpal joint responds temporarily to judicious use of intraarticular steroids. Splinting may be helpful. Joint arthroplasty or arthrodesis is necessary when conservative measures fail.

Osteoarthritis of the *hip* requires heat, rest from weight bearing, and appropriate range of motion exercises. Analgesic and antiinflammatory drugs are helpful. Stress is reduced by the use of crutches, canes, or a walker. Although hip replacement procedures are generally recommended for moderate to advanced hip osteoarthritis, arthrodesis may still be indicated in severe unilateral disease in younger patients with physically demanding occupations.

Patients with osteoarthritis of the *knee* may require elastic supports or knee cages to provide increased stability. Local steroid injections may be considered for acute flares, but more than occasional use should be avoided. Total replacements of the knee, although useful, have not been as effective as in the hip.

Cervical spine symptoms benefit from the use of a cervical collar and traction when symptoms are acute, particularly when nerve root pain is prominent. Patients with acute or subacute symptoms involving the *lumbar spine* should use a lumbosacral corset for abdominal support. A firm mattress is helpful.

Exercises to strengthen anterior abdominal muscles should be initiated when acute symptoms have resolved. Laminectomy, disc removal, and fusion can be recommended for patients with severe involvement of either the cervical or lumbar spine.

1. Solomon L: Patterns of osteoarthritis of the hip. J Bone Joint Surg 58B:176–183, 1976
2. Hoaglund FJ, Yau AGMC, Wong WL: Osteoarthritis of the hip and other joints in Southern Chinese in Hong Kong. J Bone Joint Surg 55A:545–557, 1973
3. Goldin RH, McAdam L, Louis JS, et al: Clinical and radiological survey of the incidence of osteoarthrosis among obese patients. Ann Rheum Dis 35:349–353, 1976
4. Leach RE, Baumgard S, Broom J: Obesity: its relationship to osteoarthritis of the knee. Clin Orthopedics 93:271–273, 1973
5. Hernborg J, Nilsson BE: The relationship between osteophytes in the knee joint, osteoarthritis and aging. Acta Orthop Scand 44:69–74, 1973
6. Mankin HJ: The reaction of articular cartilage to injury and osteoarthritis. N Engl J Med 291:1285–1292, 1335–1340, 1974
7. Maroudas A, Evans H, Almeida L: Cartilage of the hip joint: topographical variation of glycosaminoglycan content in normal and fibrillated tissue. Ann Rheum Dis 32:1–9, 1973
8. Mankin HJ, Johnson MT, Lippiello L: Biochemical and metabolic abnormalities in articular cartilage from osteoarthritic human hips. II. Distribution and metabolism of amino sugar containing macromolecules. J Bone Joint Surg 63A:131–134, 1981
9. Palmoski M, Brandt K: Hyaluronate binding by proteoglycans: comparison of mildly and severely osteoarthritic regions of the human femoral head cartilage. Clin Chem Acta 70:87–95, 1976
10. Inerot S, Heingard D, Arndell L, Olsson SE: Articular cartilage proteoglycans in aging and osteoarthritis. Biochem J 169:143–156, 1978
11. Lane JM, Weiss C: Current comment: review of articular cartilage collagen research. Arthritis Rheum 18:553–559, 1975
12. Weiss C: Ultrastructural characteristics of osteoarthritis. Fed Proc 32:1459–1466, 1973
13. Maroudas A, Venn M: Chemical composition and swelling of normal and osteoarthritic femoral head cartilage. II. Swelling. Ann Rheum Dis 36:399–406, 1977

14. Mankin HJ, Dorfman H, Lippiello L, et al: Biochemical and metabolic abnormalities in articular cartilage from osteoarthritic human hips. II. Correlation of morphology with biochemical and metabolic data. J Bone Joint Surg 53A:523–537, 1971
15. Lippiello L, Hall D, Mankin HJ: Collagen synthesis in normal and osteoarthritic human cartilage. J Clin Invest 59:593–600, 1977
16. Ali SY, Evans L: Enzymic degradation of cartilage in osteoarthritis. Fed Proc 32:1494–1498, 1973
17. Ehrlich MG, Mankin HJ, Jones H, et al: Collagenase and collagenase inhibitors in osteoarthritic and normal human cartilage. J Clin Invest 59:226–233, 1977
18. Radin EL: The physiology and degeneration of joints. Semin Arthritis Rheum 2:245–257, 1973
19. Radin EL: Mechanical aspects of osteoarthritis. Bull Rheum Dis 26:862–865, 1976
20. Cooke TDV, Bennett EL, Ohno O: Identification of immunoglobulins and complement components in articular collagenous tissues of patients with idiopathic osteoarthroses, The Aetiopathogenesis of Osteoarthroses. G Nuki, ed. Kent, Pitman Medical, 1980, pp 144–155.
21. Schumacher HR, Somlyo AP, Tse RL, et al: Arthritis associated with apatite crystals. Ann Intern Med 87:411–416, 1977
22. Radin EL, Parker HG, Paul IL: Pattern of degenerative arthritis. Preferential involvement of distal finger-joints. Lancet 1:377–379, 1971
23. Patterson AC: Osteoarthritis of the trapezioscaphoid joint. Arthritis Rheum 18:375–379, 1975
24. Nurick S: The pathogenesis of the spinal cord disorder associated with cervical spondylosis. Brain 95:87–100, 1972
25. Ehrlich GE: Inflammatory osteoarthritis. I. The clinical syndromes. J Chron Dis 25:317–328, 1972
26. Resnick O, Shapiro RF, Weisner KB, et al: Diffuse idiopathic skeletal hyperostosis (ankylosing hyperostosis of Forestier and Rotes-Querol). Semin Arthritis Rheum 7:153–187, 1978
27. Bird HA, Tribe CR, Bacon PA: Joint hypermobility leading to osteoarthrosis and chondrocalcinosis. Ann Rheum Dis 37:203–211, 1978
28. Schumacher HR, Gordon GV, Paul H et al: Osteoarthritis, crystal deposition and inflammation. Semin Arthritis Rheum 11:116–119, 1981
29. Siefert MH, Whiteside CG, Savage O: A 5-year follow-up of 50 cases of idiopathic osteoarthritis of the hip. Ann Rheum Dis 28:325–326, 1969
30. Loeser JD, Bloch RG, Christman A: Relief of pain by transcutaneous stimulation. J Neurosurg 42:308–314, 1975
31. Gaw AC, Chang LW, Shaw LC: Efficacy of acupuncture on osteoarthritic pain: a controlled, double-blind study. N Engl J Med 293:375–378, 1975

37. Neuropathic arthropathy (Charcot joints)

Neuropathic joint disease (Charcot joints) is a chronic progressive degenerative arthropathy affecting one or more peripheral and/or vertebral articulations. This disease develops as a result of a disturbance in sensory innervation of the affected joints (1). Thus, neuropathic arthropathy represents a *complication* of various neurologic disorders.

Diabetic neuropathy has now replaced syphilitic tabes dorsalis as the most frequent underlying disorder (2), followed by a number of less common conditions such as syringomyelia, myelomeningocele, and congenital indifference to pain (Table 37–1).

Loss of proprioception and/or pain sensation leads to instability of the joints which may be damaged by everyday repetitive longitudinal impulsive loading and injury incident to the neurologic dysfunction. Severe and/or cumulative injury results in damage to articular cartilage and subchondral bone with eventual degeneration and disorganization of the joint. On occasion affected joints may undergo relatively rapid disintegration (acute neuroarthropathy) with changes that suggest underlying linear "stress" or microfractures. This occurs most frequently in syringomyelia (shoulder).

The presence of chondrocalcinosis has been described in a number of Charcot joints, and it has been suggested that this disorder predisposes to the development of neuropathic arthropathy.

Charcot joints occur most commonly in individuals past 40. The distribution is determined by the basic neural lesion. In tabes dorsalis, the knees, hips, ankles, and vertebrae are involved (Fig. 37–1). In diabetic neuropathy, destructive changes occur in tarsal and metatarsal joints (Fig 37–2) and in syringomyelia, the shoulder or elbow is involved (Fig 37–3).

Typically, the patient notes insidious enlargement and/or instability of a single joint. This is often painful, but discomfort tends to be disproportionately mild compared with the degree of effusion and joint destruction. Pathologic fractures involv-

Table 37–1. Neurologic disorders responsible for the development of neuropathic arthropathy

Neurologic disorder	Joints most affected
Diabetic neuropathy	Tarsus, tarsometatarsal, metatarsophalangeal
Syphilitic tabes dorsalis	Knee, hip, ankle, lumbar and lower dorsal vertebrae
Syringomyelia	Shoulder, elbow, cervical vertebrae
Myelomeningocoele	Ankle, tarsus
Congenital insensitivity to pain (including familial dysautonomia)	Ankle, tarsus
Miscellaneous	
Hereditary sensory neuropathy	
Charcot-Marie-Tooth disease	
Familial intersititial polyneuropathy of Dejerine and Sottas	
Peripheral nerve injury	
Leprous neuropathy	
Late yaws	
Amyloid neuropathy	

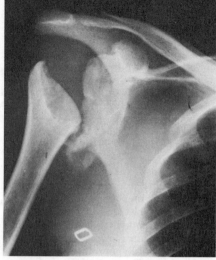

Fig 37-3. Neuropathic disease of the shoulder of a 54-year-old woman with syringomyelia. Note loss of bony substance of humeral head and cloud-like calcification in the periarticular soft tissues. The patient had first noted painless swelling of the shoulder only 2 weeks before this roentgenogram was taken. (Reproduced from Arthritis and Allied Conditions, with permission)

ing the joint surfaces are common in neuropathic joint disease and may account for a dramatic onset of symptoms of this arthropathy.

Examination reveals an unstable hypermobile joint which may be swollen, warm, and tender. Effusions often persist for months and yield large amounts of fluid, which may be bloody and usually have relatively low white blood cell counts. Later, there is increasing enlargement and crepitation as a result of loss of cartilage, overgrowth of bone, and loose bodies.

In disease associated with diabetic neuropathy, there is thickening of the foot accompanied by little or no evidence of inflammation. Some cases are complicated by infection, and osteomyelitis may account for destructive changes.

At first, roentgenograms may be normal except for effusion. Later, these reveal cartilage loss, fragmentation and absorption of subchondral bone, and marginal osteophytes which tend to be bulky and bizarre in configuration (Fig 37–2). These abnormalities are generally similar to those encountered in non-neuropathic osteoarthritis. It is the exaggerated degree of the changes that distinguishes the radiographic appearance of the Charcot joint.

The synovium exhibits only a mild inflammatory reaction and frequently contains bits of calcified cartilage and metaplastic bone.

Management includes immobilization of affected joints and restriction of weight-bearing with crutches, walking splints, and braces.

In the past, efforts at arthrodesis often proved unsuccessful because of infection and nonunion. The apparent improvement in recent years in knee fusion has been attributed to better methods of internal

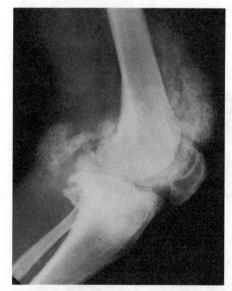

Fig 37–1. Neuropathic arthropathy of the right knee of a 60-year-old man with syphilitic tabes dorsalis, illustrating loss of articular cartilage, massive osteophyte formation, ossified masses in the suprapatellar and semimembranous bursae, and sclerosis of subchondral bone. An anteroposterior view of this knee revealed a fracture of the medial condyle of the tibia. (Reproduced from Arthritis and Allied Conditions. Ed 9, with permission of the editor, Dr Daniel J McCarty, Jr and the publishers, Lea & Febiger, Philadelphia)

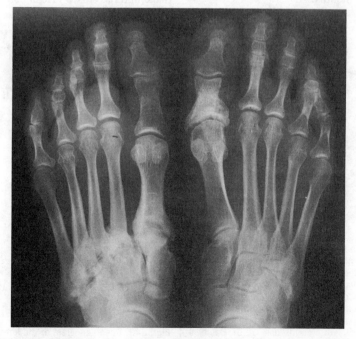

Fig 37–2. Neuropathic arthropathy involving the right first metatarsophalangeal joint and left tarsometatarsal joints of a 31-year-old woman who had developed diabetes mellitus at the age of 6.

fixation and use of a compression technique.

Total knee arthroplasty and total hip replacement have been carried out in a few instances, but recurrent dislocation and other disastrous complications occur so often that these procedures are generally considered to be contraindicated in individuals with Charcot joint disease.

1. Rodnan GP: Neuropathic joint disease (Charcot joints). Arthritis and Allied Conditions, ed. 9. DJ McCarty, Jr, ed. Philadelphia, Lea & Febiger, 1979, pp 892–904

2. Sinha S, Munichoodappa CS, Kozak GP: Neuroarthropathy (Charcot joints) in diabetes mellitus: clinical study in 101 cases. Medicine 51:191–210, 1972

38. Hemophilic arthropathy

Hemarthrosis, the most frequent (aside from skin bruises) and the most painful manifestation of hemophilia, happens in all the heritable coagulation disorders (with the exception of factor V deficiency). It may also occur as an unusual complication of hypoprothrombinemia induced by anticoagulant drugs.

Hemophilic hemarthrosis usually results from trauma, although the injury may be trivial and often inapparent. Joint bleeding usually begins before the patient reaches the age of 5 and tends to recur repeatedly during childhood, after which it diminishes sharply in frequency. The knees, elbows, and ankles (including the subtalar joints) are the parts most often affected; less commonly shoulders, hips, wrists, fingers, and toes are involved. Generally only a single joint is involved in each episode (1,2).

In acute hemarthrosis, the joint is warm and swollen and often becomes conspicuously tender and painful; when hemorrhage is severe, there may be fever and leukocytosis. When the bleeding is mild, the joint may return to normal in a few days. In severe and/or protracted hemorrhage, joint inflammation may persist for weeks or months.

Repeated hemarthroses lead to hemosiderosis of the synovium (Fig 38–1), with synovial proliferation and production of collagenase, which may lead to degeneration of the articular cartilage (4,5). There can be thickening of periarticular tissues, bony hypertrophy, and various deformities, the most common of which are flexion contractures of the elbows and knees.

Approximately one-half of those patients who suffer repeated hemarthrosis develop some permanent articular changes, although many joints remain normal or nearly so despite repeated bleeding.

In addition to hemarthrosis, there may be bleeding into muscle and bone. The terms *hemophilic pseudotumor* or *hemophilic cyst* have been applied to the destructive hematomas that result from massive muscle, subperiosteal, and/or intraosseous hemorrhages that occur most often in the thigh or leg. This bleeding may prove especially dangerous because of neurovascular compression, destruction and contracture of muscle, cyst rupture, sinus formation, or infection.

One of the most dramatic examples of hemophilic pseudotumor involves hemorrhage into the closed fascial compartment containing the iliacus muscle and femoral nerve. This gives rise to severe pain in the groin and thigh followed by the appearance of a tender mass (hematoma) in the iliac fossa and groin, flexion contracture of the hip, and signs of femoral nerve palsy.

In acute intraarticular hemorrhage, roentgenograms reveal distention of the joint capsule, whereas chronic hemophilic joint disease is characterized by irregular narrowing or total loss of the joint space, marginal spurring, and sclerosis of subchondral bone that often contains one or more areas of cystic translucency (Fig 38–2). The periarticular soft tissues are often thickened and increased in density. Enlargement of the head of the radius is a frequent finding in patients with elbow involvement.

Flattening of the inferior portion of the patella (squared off patella) is often noted in advanced disease of the knee and has been considered highly diagnostic of hemophilic arthropathy. In younger patients there is accelerated maturation and hypertrophy of adjacent epiphyses.

The recent availability of potent cryoprecipitates and other concentrated preparations of plasma coagulation factors and

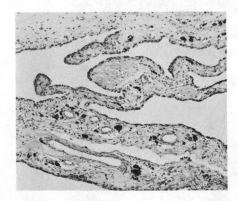

Fig 38–1. Photomicrograph of synovium obtained from the knee of a 76-year-old man with classic hemophilia (factor VIII deficiency) who had repeated episodes of hemarthrosis and developed severe osteoarthritis. Note heavy deposits of iron-containing pigment (hemosiderin) in lining cells and deeper portions of the synovium. (Reproduced from Arthritis and Allied Conditions. Ed 9, with permission of Dr Daniel J McCarty, Jr and the publishers, Lea & Febiger, Philadelphia)

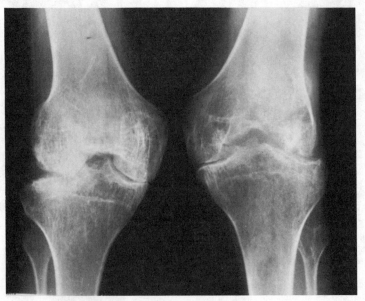

Fig 38–2. Roentgenogram of the knees of a 23-year-old man with classic hemophilia and repeated hemarthroses. Loss of articular cartilage and other changes indicative of degenerative joint disease are shown. (Reproduced from Arthritis and Allied Conditions)

the development of home treatment programs have made it much easier to attain effective hemostasis and have greatly improved, indeed revolutionized, the management of joint and muscle bleeding (3,6,7). Maintenance of low levels (3–5% of normal) of factor VIII activity by regular administration of relatively small amounts of concentrate sharply lowers the frequency of hemarthrosis and other serious hemorrhage. It has been noted, furthermore, that chronic joint changes are rare in hemophilic patients in whom the content of deficient coagulation factor is above 2–3% of normal.

Acute hemarthrosis. Every reasonable effort should be made to avoid trauma that may initiate joint hemorrhage. It is essential that the patient and his parents be instructed in the early recognition and immediate care of hemarthrosis. Home transfusion programs have proved highly successful in securing rapid relief of acute hemarthrosis. Prompt control of hemarthrosis is the key to the prevention of the chronic disability that results from repeated joint bleeding.

In acute hemarthrosis, the affected extremity should be elevated and the joint immobilized initially in a position of comfort. Ice packs lessen pain and inflammation. Aspirin should be avoided since this prolongs bleeding time by interfering with platelet aggregation. Acetaminophen and propoxyphane do not have this effect.

When hemarthrosis is severe, efforts should be made to correct the underlying defect in coagulation with the appropriate concentrate, or plasma if necessary, and thus prevent further bleeding. Joint aspiration can be accomplished safely during or after replacement therapy and often provides prompt relief of pain resulting from the joint tension caused by the effusion.

After pain and swelling subside, active exercise is encouraged and should be gradually increased until full motion is restored.

Chronic hemophilic joint disease. Chronic joint deformity, such as flexion contracture of the knee, can often be corrected by means of traction, wedging casts, and active resistive exercises.

In recent years, the ability to prevent or control postoperative hemorrhage by use of potent concentrates has made it possible to perform synovectomies and arthroplasties (including total hip and knee replacements) and a variety of other surgical procedures on the joints and has greatly improved the prospects for orthopedic rehabilitation.

1. Duthie RB, Rizza CR: Rheumatological manifestations of the haemophilias. Clin Rheum Dis 1:53–93, 1975

2. Rodnan GP: Arthropathies associated with hematologic disorders, storage disease, and dysproteinemias; Arthritis and Allied Conditions, ed 9. DJ McCarty, Jr, ed. Philadelphia, Lea & Febiger, 1979, pp 925–952

3. Mainardi CL, Levine PH, Werb Z, Harris ED: Proliferative synovitis in hemophilia. Biochemical and morphologic observations. Arthritis Rheum 21:137–144, 1978

4. Stein H, Duthie RB: The pathogenesis of chronic hemophilic arthropathy. J Bone Joint Surg 63B:601–609, 1981

5. Arnold WD, Hilgartner MW: Hemophilic arthropathy: current concepts of pathogenesis and management. J Bone Joint Surg 59A:287–305, 1977

6. Biggs R, ed: The Treatment of Haemophilia A and B and von Willebrand's Disease. Oxford, Blackwell Scientific Publications, 1978

7. Ingram GIC, Dykes SR, Creese AL, et al: Home treatment in haemophilia: clinical, social and economic advantages. Clin Lab Haemat 1:13–27, 1979

39. Infectious arthritis

An infectious agent may cause arthritis by a number of mechanisms. The microorganisms can directly invade the synovial membrane and the synovial fluid during a bloodborne infection or after direct penetration. The infectious agent then replicates in the synovium and can be recovered from the synovial fluid.

Also, a microorganism may cause an acute or chronic arthritis without necessarily being continuously present in the joint. For example, a hypersensitivity or an immunologic process may be triggered by an infection within or distant to the involved joint. Such "sterile synovitis" is present in the arthritis associated with acute rheumatic fever and Reiter's disease.

It is also possible that nonviable components of a microorganism may persist within the joint and potentiate a chronic inflammatory response. Such a mechanism has been postulated to play a role in the pathogenesis of chronic rheumatic conditions such as rheumatoid arthritis (1).

This section will cover those infectious diseases that cause arthritis by the direct invasion of the microorganism into the joint. The infectious agent may be a bacterium, a virus, or a fungus and these agents can usually be recovered from the synovial fluid or the synovial membrane. Thus they satisfy all the requirements for an infectious disease and generally can be quite specifically treated.

Pathogenesis. Most of these infectious agents arrive at the joint via the bloodstream. The synovial membrane is extremely vascular and the joint is susceptible to trapping of circulating foreign particles. As the infectious agents replicate in the synovium, they are phagocytosed by the synovial lining cells and inflammatory cells. During this phagocytosis, proteolytic enzymes are continuously released, causing further inflammation. Eventually, synovial lining cell regeneration and hyperplasia with chronic inflammation and granulation tissue will ensue. If the infection is untreated, cartilage erosions and finally articular destruction with fibrous or bony ankylosis will develop.

The rapidity of destructive joint changes depends on a number of factors, most prominently the specific infecting agent. For example, certain bacteria such as *Staphylococcus aureus* and Gram-negative bacilli will quickly destroy joint tissue. Other bacteria such as *Neisseria gonorrhoeae* and most viruses do not generally cause irreversible joint damage.

Host defense mechanisms are also intimately related to the development of infectious arthritis. If the host is immunocompromised by chronic illness or medications, an infectious arthritis is more likely to develop during septicemia. A previously damaged joint will be more likely to develop superimposed septic arthritis during an infectious process. This is especially important in patients with rheumatoid arthritis or with severe joint destruction due to a neuropathic arthropathy. Other factors that may influence the susceptibility of the host to infectious arthritis include: previous articular trauma, recent joint surgery, or intraarticular steroid injections.

Diagnosis. In any type of infectious arthritis, the diagnosis is definitive only if the infectious agent is recovered from the synovial fluid or synovial membrane. Thus an arthrocentesis is always required for the diagnosis of infectious arthritis. Whenever an infection is suspected, the joint should be drained under sterile conditions, a portion of the synovial fluid cultured, and a Gram stain smear immediately performed. In cases of suspected gonococcal arthritis, the synovial fluid should be plated on chocolate agar as well as on routine blood agar. Anaerobic infections are being seen more frequently, so anaerobic cultures should be included. If tuberculous or fungal arthritis is suspected, the laboratory should be alerted and appropriate culture media should be secured.

The yield of positive cultures or Gram stains varies on the basis of the specific infecting agent. For example, it is unusual to recover a virus from the infected joint, and *Neisseria gonorrhoeae* can be recovered in less than 50% of suspected individuals. Most other bacteria can almost always be recovered from the infected synovial fluid. Mycobacteria and fungi can be recovered in well over half of the patients simply by a synovial fluid culture. However the diagnostic yield can be increased further by a synovial membrane biopsy with appropriate tissue culture and histology.

Treatment. The principles of treatment of infectious arthritis are similar in most patients, although the response to the treatment will vary greatly depending on the infecting agent. Effective treatment requires the suspicion of an infected joint followed by an immediate arthrocentesis. Initially, all available synovial fluid should be drained for appropriate culture and analysis. Other helpful diagnostic clues obtained from the synovial fluid analysis include a marked leukocytosis, with greater than 50,000 cells/mm^3 and greater than 80% polymorphonuclear leukocytes and a synovial fluid glucose depressed in relation to the blood glucose.

A peripheral blood leukocytosis and an elevated erythrocyte sedimentation rate are usually present, but are not specific. Serial synovial fluid analyses will reveal a decrease in the leukocyte count and an increase in the synovial fluid glucose as parameters to determine an appropriate response to treatment. The synovial fluid should become sterile within a few days.

Once adequate cultures are obtained, an antibiotic is chosen on the basis of the most likely organism infecting the joint. Most often an accurate diagnosis can be made on the basis of the Gram stain smear or the clinical course including the presence of other obvious sites of infection even before the culture results are available. Any suspected infected body fluid including the blood must always be cultured.

Generally, antibiotics are initiated parenterally, often in large doses, when bacterial arthritis is suspected. Although no adequate data exist regarding the amount of antibiotics to give or the duration of therapy, most investigators tend to treat bacterial arthritis, other than that due to *Neisseria gonorrhoeae*, for 2–4 weeks depending on the clinical response. However, the arthritis due to *Neisseria gonorrhoeae* generally requires a much shorter treatment.

In addition to appropriate antibiotic therapy, the infected joint must be mechanically drained as often as fluid reaccumulates. This can generally be accomplished by closed needle joint aspiration although certain circumstances will necessitate open surgical drainage. These include hip and shoulder infections which often cannot be adequately drained by closed aspiration and any situation where a trial of closed needle aspiration has failed to sterilize the joint, or purulent accumulations or loculations cannot be adequately drained.

Even with appropriate mechanical drainage and antibiotics, the results of therapy vary greatly depending on the host, the infecting agent, and the rapidity of initiation of treatment. In the early stages of the infection, immobilization with splints or occasionally with traction may be needed to help control pain, but exercises should be begun quickly to prevent severe muscle atrophy. Joint drainage should be continued until there is no further accumulation of purulent synovial fluid. This may require daily or more frequent needle aspirations.

Although irrigation of the joint cavity with sterile saline and a large-bore needle may be helpful in removing clots and purulent exudate, antibiotics should not be directly instilled into the joint cavity. The systemic administration of the antibiotics provides adequate synovial fluid bactericidal activity, and a local inflammation may ensue from direct joint instillation of antibiotics.

Types of infectious arthritis

Nongonococcal bacterial arthritis. *Staphylococcus aureus*, various streptococcal species, and Gram-negative bacilli are common causes of nongonococcal bacterial arthritis in adults (2–4). In neonates who have not acquired maternal antibody, *Hemophilus influenzae* is the most common organism infecting the joint.

Often in adults a presumptive diagnosis of the specific infecting agent can be made when the suspected site of the initial bacteremia is identified. For example, when pneumonia is the site of infection, the bacteria recovered from the infected joint may be *Diplococcus pneumoniae*. Gram-negative bacilli will usually be cultured from infected joints in patients with an associated urinary tract infection and sepsis.

Nongonococcal bacterial arthritis generally affects a single joint, most commonly the weight-bearing joints and especially the knee. Most patients experience an abrupt onset of an extremely tender red warm swollen joint. The patients are usually febrile although shaking chills or a significant peripheral blood leukocytosis is present in only about 50%. Radiographs of the affected joint usually reveal only soft tissue swelling unless the infection has already been present for a few weeks or a contiguous osteomyelitis is present.

Patients with this type of joint infection are often either very young or very old and frequently have compromised defense mechanisms such as serious illness or prior treatment with corticosteroids or immunosuppressive agents. It is especially important to be aware of this type of infection superimposed on rheumatoid arthritis or another chronic rheumatic disease, since the joint effusion may otherwise be considered part of the underlying rheumatic illness and appropriate diagnosis and therapy delayed.

Gonococcal arthritis. The clinical manifestations, microbiology, and immunology of gonococcal arthritis are markedly different from other types of bacterial arthritis (5–7). Disseminated gonococcal infection (DGI) generally occurs in young, healthy, sexually active patients and is now the most common type of bacterial arthritis in urban populations. It has been estimated that it will occur in approximately 0.1–0.5% of patients who develop gonorrhea. Women are more likely to develop the infection than men.

Unlike nongonococcal bacterial arthritis, the typical musculoskeletal manifestations of gonococcal arthritis include migratory polyarthralgias, tenosynovitis, and polyarthritis. A skin rash occurs in about two-thirds of patients and can be maculopapular, pustular, vesicular, or bullous. Most patients have fever and other signs of bacteremia, especially when seen early in the course of the disease.

Purulent joint effusions are present in 30–50% of patients, but *Neisseria gonorrhoeae* can be recovered in less than 50% of those effusions. In most other patients scant transient sterile joint effusions can be detected or tenosynovitis will be the only articular manifestation of disseminated gonococcal infection. When the joint effusions can be aspirated, the synovial fluid analysis is similar to that of nongonococcal bacterial arthritis, although the average leukocyte count may not be quite as elevated.

The arthritis and tenosynovitis are seen more commonly in the upper extremities than in nongonococcal bacterial arthritis, and the wrist and small joints of the fingers are often affected.

The therapeutic response is also much more rapid than in other types of bacterial arthritis. Penicillin or other appropriate antibiotics generally reverse the symptoms within 24–48 hours. Mechanical joint drainage is usually not a major problem, even in gonococcal arthritis affecting the hip or shoulder.

Since the organisms are infrequently recovered from the blood or infected joint, the diagnosis is generally ascertained from the clinical observations, isolation of the organisms from a local site of infection such as the genitourinary tract, and rapid therapeutic response to antibiotics. A diagnosis is often made and treatment successfully given without the specific organism being isolated from any primary or disseminated site.

Many of the manifestations of disseminated gonococcal infection simulate a serum sickness–like picture and so are distinct from other types of bacterial arthritis. Because of this distinction and the difficulty in recovering *Neisseria gonorrhoeae* from the joints or the blood, it has been postulated that some of the musculoskeletal and other manifestations of DGI are due to immune-mediated or hypersensitivity mechanisms. Circulating immune complexes have been identified in the blood and synovial fluid of patients with gonococcal infection.

There is evidence that both host and bacterial factors are involved in the pathogenesis and specific clinical manifestations of this disease. For example, patients who are genetically deficient in complement will be predisposed to develop *Neisseria* infections and recurrent DGI. Women are more prone to develop DGI during menses and pregnancy.

The absence of a local inflammatory response to the initial gonococcal infection is characteristic in DGI. For example, women who develop DGI rarely have symptoms of pelvic inflammatory disease.

Important microbial virulent factors include certain phenotypic characteristics of the strain of *Neisseria gonorrhoeae*. For example, colony types 1 and 2 which have pili are isolated from patients with DGI. Transparent colonies are more virulent than opaque colonies.

The strains of *Neisseria gonorrhoeae* associated with DGI have specific nutritional requirements and are generally resistant to the bactericidal activity of normal human serum, unlike strains isolated from patients with local gonococcal infections. These same phenotypic characteristics may also be important in determining whether a patient develops purulent arthritis or bacteremic manifestations of disseminated gonococcal infection.

Arthritis associated with bacterial endocarditis. Bacterial endocarditis may be associated with purulent septic arthritis (rare) or with a sterile, moderately severe inflammatory synovitis (8). The latter, like many other extracardiac features of endocarditis, may be due to hypersensitivity or immune-mediated mechanisms. Musculoskeletal symptoms may precede the diagnosis of endocarditis by weeks or sometimes even months. Polyarthritis or polyarthralgias, monarthritis, myalgias, hypertrophic osteoarthropathy, disc infections, and low back pain are some of the more frequent findings.

Tuberculous arthritis. The frequency of tuberculosis of bones and joints has decreased in the past 3 decades, paralleling the decline in pulmonary tuberculosis. Tuberculous arthritis is relatively rare compared to other forms of extrapulmonary tuberculosis, occurring in less than 1% of these patients. At one large hospital, the incidence fell from more than 30 patients per year in 1953 to less than 2 per year from 1955–1970 (9).

The age incidence has also changed. Formerly a disease limited largely to children and young adults, tuberculous arthritis is now seen in all ages, including the elderly.

The joint infection usually results from hematogenous dissemination to bone. Synovial involvement occurs through invasion from a juxtaarticular osteomyelitic focus, although direct hematogenous spread to the synovium is possible.

Tuberculous arthritis characteristically presents as a chronic, insidious monarticular disease. The most common sites are the vertebral column and large weight-bearing joints, such as hips and knees, but elbows and wrists can also be infected. Tenosynovitis is common; the flexor tendon sheaths at the wrist may be involved, leading to the development of carpal tunnel syndrome.

Predisposing factors such as trauma, alcoholism, drug addiction, intraarticular corticosteroid injections, or systemic illnesses are found in a large proportion of patients. Only a small number have active pulmonary tuberculosis and less than half have a positive history of tuberculosis or radiologic evidence of inactive disease. However, almost all have a positive skin test to intermediate strength purified protein derivative, so that a negative skin reaction militates strongly against the diagnosis of tuberculous arthritis.

The most common clinical manifestation is pain, particularly on motion. The affected joint usually shows evidence of marked synovial proliferation and effusion with progressive limitation of motion. The adjacent muscles may be spastic and often there is rapidly progressive wasting.

Tuberculosis of the spine (*Pott's disease*) tends to involve the lower thoracic and lumbar vertebrae and is characterized by chronic back pain and the eventual appearance of sharp-angle kyphosis due to collapse of the affected vertebrae.

Neurologic disease may result from cord compression or meningitis. As the disease progresses, cold abscesses develop which dissect through the soft tissues anteriorly and may cause nerve compression symptoms or emerge to the exterior in areas distant from the vertebral focus.

Nonspecific systemic manifestations, such as low-grade fever and weight loss, frequently occur. More severe constitutional reactions such as high fever, night sweats, malaise, and anorexia are seen in the minority of patients with concomitant active pulmonary or miliary tuberculosis.

Roentgenographic examination may show soft tissue swelling and early diffuse osteoporosis of the adjacent bone, followed by the appearance of cystic lesions in the metaphysis and erosive destructive changes in the cartilage and subchondral bone. In tuberculosis of the spine, the destructive process usually involves 2 adjacent vertebrae and the intervertebral disc, with eventual collapse resulting in kyphosis. The cold abscess may appear as a paraspinal mass of variable size; in the late stages the abscess walls may calcify.

The synovial fluid findings vary: as a rule the protein concentration is greater than 3.5 gm/dl. The glucose concentration tends to be low. In more than half the patients, the level is below 50 mg/dl and the difference in the concentration between blood and synovial fluid is greater than 40 mg/dl. The synovial fluid leukocyte counts range from 1,000 to more than 100,000 cells/mm³, with an average of 10,000–20,000 cells/mm³, predominantly polymorphonuclear leukocytes (10). The proportion of polymorphonuclear leukocytes is seldom greater than 85%, a valuable finding that contrasts with that in pyogenic arthritis.

The diagnosis of tuberculous arthritis is usually not possible on clinical grounds alone; atypical mycobacterial and fungal infections have a similar clinical presentation, and occasionally rheumatoid arthritis with monarticular or oligarticular onset or bacterial arthritis may mimic granulomatous arthritis (11). An etiologic diagnosis of tuberculous arthritis is made by identifying the organism by cultures of synovial fluid or synovial tissue biopsy and culture. Synovial fluid cultures are positive in 80% of cases. Examination of the synovium reveals caseating granulomata and/or the presence of acid fast bacilli in over 90% of patients (Fig 39–1). Mycobacteria are cultured from biopsy material with the same frequency (10).

Because of the occurrence of granulomatous arthritis or tenosynovitis produced

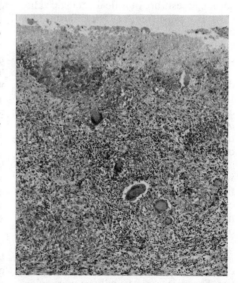

Figure 39–1. Photomicrograph of synovium from knee of a 79-year-old man with tuberculous arthritis. Note presence of numerous Langhans' giant cells.

by atypical mycobacteria resistant to the usual antituberculous drugs, it is important to determine the sensitivities of these organisms to the various chemotherapeutic agents available.

Treatment of tuberculous arthritis requires long-term administration of isoniazid and ethambutol or rifampin. A third drug may be added if pulmonary tuberculosis is active. Surgical excision of the affected synovium has been recommended to prevent destructive changes of the joint cartilage and tendons, but is seldom necessary.

Fungal arthritis. A significant proportion of chronic granulomatous arthritis is due to mycotic infection. Bone involvement usually develops after hematogenous dissemination from a primary focus, followed by secondary involvement of adjacent joints. In sporotrichosis, the joints may be involved by direct extension from infected skin or subcutaneous tissue. A majority of patients have some predisposing factor such as chronic debilitating or hematologic disease, alcoholism, drug addiction, indwelling intravenous catheters, prolonged antibiotic or corticosteroid administration, intravenous hyperalimentation, and prematurity.

Untreated, fungal arthritis usually follows a chronic indolent course with progressive destruction of bone and joints. Radiologically, the disease cannot be distinguished from other forms of granulomatous arthritis.

Diagnosis requires identification of the infective agent by histologic examination of suitable biopsy material and/or culture of synovial tissues and fluids. For these reasons, in patients with chronic mono- or oligarticular arthritis of unknown etiology, it is mandatory to obtain material for microbiologic studies.

Skin testing with fungal antigens and serologic tests are of little diagnostic value (11). The most frequent fungal arthritides in the United States are: coccidioidomycosis, sporotrichosis, blastomycosis, and candidiasis.

Coccidioidomycosis. This disease is endemic in the southwestern portion of the United States and Mexico. During the acute primary infection with *Coccidioides immitis,* as many as one-third of the patients experience episodes of transient recurring arthralgias which may last as long as a month. Erythema nodosum, with or without arthritis, may also develop during the course of the acute infection. In an estimated 0.1–0.2% of patients, the organism disseminates and approximately 20% of these will have bone and joint involvement.

The clinical manifestations are no different from any other granulomatous arthritis. The disease is usually monarticular, involving primarily large joints, such as the ankles, knees, elbows, or wrists. Destructive bone changes develop slowly over the course of months or years. If the disease is untreated, permanent joint destruction occurs.

The diagnosis is made by identification of the organisms in the synovial tissues and by recovery of the fungus from cultures of synovial tissue or fluid. Patients with desseminated disease are found to have rising serum titers of complement-fixing antibodies and may not react to intradermal injection of the antigen.

Treatment consists of systemic and/or intraarticular administration of amphotericin B. Surgical synovectomy may be an important adjunct procedure in the management of this condition (12).

Sporotrichosis. Joint infection with *Sporotrichum schenckii* may result from systemic sporotrichosis or from penetrating cutaneous inoculation of plant material, e.g., rose thorns. Alcoholism and outdoor activities such as gardening are predisposing factors. The large joints in both upper and lower extremities are the articulations most frequently involved, although any joint or tendon sheath may be infected.

Two clinical forms of sporotrichotic arthritis have been recognized: a unifocal form involving one or a few joints and a multifocal type occurring in compromised hosts, with involvement of multiple joints, skin, and viscera. The arthropathy is usually subacute or chronic, and skin lesions or fistuale overlying the affected joints develop frequently.

The diagnosis is made by recovery of sporotrichum from cultures of synovial fluid and tissue. Histologic examination reveals a granulomatous synovitis with central necrotic areas and multinucleated giant cells. The cigar-shaped organism is rarely found on histologic examination. Positive serologic tests suggest but do not establish conclusively the presence of sporotrichosis infection.

Systemic administration of amphotericin B and appropriate surgical debridement appear to be the treatment of choice. Because of limited experience with intraarticular injection of amphotericin B or with the concomitant administration of iodides, no conclusions about their effectiveness can yet be drawn (13).

Blastomycosis. Joint infection with *Blastomyces dermatitidis* results from dissemination of a primary skin or lung infection. Bone involvement occurs in 30–50% of patients with disseminated disease and the joints are often infected by direct spread. Isolated arthritis without bone involvement is seen occasionally.

Blastomycotic arthritis is difficult to distinguish from tuberculosis since concomitant lung and skin involvement always accompanies the arthritis. The diagnosis is made on the basis of positive cultures and microscopic examination of synovial fluid which often demonstrates numerous yeast-like organisms. Treatment with systemic amphotericin B has been highly successful (14).

Candidiasis. The frequency of candidial arthritis has increased in recent years, reflecting the increasing number of patients with systemic candidiasis. Almost all reported patients have underlying predisposing factors that interfere with normal host defense mechanisms against various species of *Candida.* Fifty percent of the affected patients are neonates or infants with prematurity, congenital defects, or respiratory distress syndrome. Among adults, narcotic addiction, parenteral hyperalimentation, increased antibiotic or corticosteroid administration, indwelling intravenous catheters, chronic debilitating disease, and carcinoma have been reported in association with candidiasis.

The arthritis occurs chiefly in patients with disseminated disease. It usually involves the knees, although a significant proportion of patients have polyarticular disease. In two-thirds of the patients, an adjacent osteomyelitic focus is found on roentgenographic examination.

The diagnosis is made by culture of organisms from the synovial fluid. Microscopic examination is usually unrewarding since the yeast-like organisms are only rarely detected. Treatment with parenteral amphotericin B and surgical debridement have been effective in most cases. Intraarticular injection of amphotericin B has been used in a few patients with good results. The compound, 5-fluorocytosine, was successful in a patient with recurrent disease (15).

Syphilitic arthritis. Congenital and acquired syphilitic infections are uncommon causes of joint disease. In congenital syphilis, osteochondritis or epiphysitis appears in infants 3 weeks to 4 months old and may lead to complete separation of the epiphysis, resulting in paraarticular swelling and pseudoparalysis of the affected limb. In children between the ages of 8 and 16, congenital syphilis may produce painless knee effusions which can be confused with pyogenic or rheumatoid arthritis (Clutton's joints) (16).

The most common rheumatic manifestation of acquired infection is arthralgias and/or arthritis associated with secondary syphilis (17). The patients present classic stigmata of secondary lues: rash, mucous plaques, alopecia, or lymphadenopathy. Back pain and knee, ankle, or occasionally other peripheral joint or tendon sheath involvement associated with small mildly inflammatory effusions are common complaints. Periostitis may also occur.

Serologic tests for syphilis are strongly positive in all patients (18). In tertiary syphilis, gummatous arthritis or periostitis involving tibia or clavicles is common. Neuropathic joint disease associated with tabes dorsalis (Charcot joints) is discussed in Section 37.

Mycoplasmal arthritis. Since the work

of Sabin with mice in 1938 (19), mycoplasmas have been found to cause arthritis in a number of animals, including rodents, cattle, swine, and birds. In many species, arthritis becomes chronic and in some ways resembles rheumatoid arthritis. Despite numerous attempts to relate mycoplasmas to rheumatoid arthritis, however, the accumulated evidence militates against such a relationship.

Although arthralgias and myalgias associated with mycoplasma infection (*Mycoplasma pneumoniae*) are rather common in humans, true arthritis has been observed in only a small number of individuals (20). These individuals have had serologic evidence of mycoplasmal infection and most have also had a history of upper or lower respiratory tract disease. Arthritis has been acute in onset, either mon- or polyarticular, and most often has occurred in the large joints of the lower extremities. In a few patients, elbows, shoulders, and the small joints of the hands have also been involved.

Respiratory symptoms have usually preceded arthritis by 1–4 weeks. In most patients, arthritis has been mild, and synovial fluid obtained from 2 patients has been considered class I (noninflammatory) in character. The duration of joint involvement has usually been brief (1–10 weeks), but in 3 the arthritis lasted 10–18 months. In 2 of these 3, the illness resembled rheumatoid arthritis.

Mycoplasma were cultured from the joints of 2 patients with congenital hypogammaglobulinemia and polyarthritis. *Ureaplasma urealyticum* was recovered from a synovial biopsy in the first patient (21) and *M pneumoniae* from synovial fluid of the second. The first responded to tetracycline.

Three neonates with monarticular arthritis due to *M hominis* have also been reported (22). *M hominis* is a common commensal in the female genital tract and has been implicated as a pathogen in cases of puerperal sepsis.

Viral arthritis. Since discovery of the hepatitis B surface antigen (HBsAg) in 1965, *hepatitis-associated arthritis* has been widely recognized and studied (23,24). The prevalence of articular involvement in patients with hepatitis B infection is approximately 20% (range 9–30%). Arthritis occurs as a prodrome, typically precedes the onset of clinically apparent liver disease, and is commonly associated with cutaneous disease and fever. Women are affected slightly more often than men.

Articular disease begins suddenly and is usually polyarticular and symmetrical, with the small joints of the hands most commonly involved, followed in decreasing frequency by the knees, ankles, shoulders, wrists, feet, elbows, and cervical spine. Patients may experience arthralgias alone, or the joints may be markedly in-

flamed. Bursitis and tendinitis also occur. Occasionally joint involvement is pauciarticular and asymmetrical.

Arthritis usually lasts about 3 weeks (range several days–six months) and in most cases resolves with the onset of jaundice. Synovial fluid leukocyte counts have varied from 500–90,000 cells/mm^3.

Many patients develop urticaria; less often there is a macular, papular, petechial rash or angioneuritic edema. Cutaneous disease without arthritis may occur in the prodromal phase. Low grade fever occurs in as many as half of those with arthritis. There may be renal involvement (glomerulitis). During the prodrome, HBsAg is usually present in blood, C3 and C4 are depressed, and immune complexes containing HBsAg and anti-HB are present. Cryoprecipitates are also present in many patients and contain HBsAg, anti-HB immunoglobulins, and complement components.

As the arthritis resolves, HBsAg disappears, complement components normalize, and anti-HB increases. These findings suggest that immune complexes play a pathogenetic role. Hepatitis B has not been propagated from the synovial fluid in tissue culture, but the antigen is demonstrable in synovium by immunofluorescence and Dane particles have been seen with electron microscopy.

Arthritis complicating naturally occurring *rubella* has been recognized for many years. The frequency in infected individuals varies from 15–61%; it is most common in young adult women and rare in men and children (25).

Arthritis occurs with an abrupt onset at the time of the rash or shortly after its development. It most often involves small joints of the hands, wrists, and knees; less commonly affected are the ankles, elbows, and small joints of the feet. The duration of arthritis averages approximately 9 days (range 1 day–7 weeks). Transient carpal tunnel syndrome occurs frequently. Synovial fluid is class II (inflammatory).

Arthritis also occurs after inoculation with live attenuated rubella virus vaccines and again is more common in adult women (26). Its distribution is similar to that of natural rubella, but is somewhat less inflammatory. Most children have knee disease, followed in frequency by the carpal tunnel syndrome and polyarthritis. Several children have been reported with persistent arthritis for months to years.

In both naturally occurring and vaccine-induced arthritis, virus has been recovered from synovial aspirates. Tests for rheumatoid factor are occasionally positive in naturally occurring, but not in vaccine-induced disease. Hypocomplementemia with the natural infection suggests a role for immune factors in the pathogenesis; this has not been consistently observed in children.

Articular disease is a common manifes-

tation of many other viral infections (27). These include the mosquito-borne group A arboviral diseases, Chickungunya (a dengue-like illness first observed in Tanganyika, 1952), O'nyong-nyong (meaning joint-breaker, Northern Uganda, 1959), sinbis (Africa and Asia), mayaro (Trinidad and Brazil), bunyamwera (Africa), and epidemic polyarthritis of south Australian adults presumably due to the Ross River virus.

Arthritis is also a rare complication of *mumps*, may precede the parotitis by several days, and can last 1–2 weeks. Articular disease has also been seen with type-6 echo virus, type-7 adenovirus, herpes viruses, and infectious mononucleosis.

1. Bennett JC: The infectious etiology of rheumatoid arthritis. Arthritis Rheum 21:531–538, 1978
2. Goldenberg DL, Cohen AS: Acute infectious arthritis: a review of patients with non-gonococcal joint infections (with emphasis on therapy and prognosis). Am J Med 60:369–376, 1976
3. Rosenthal J, Bole G, Robinson WB: Acute non-gonococcal infectious arthritis. Arthritis Rheum 23:889–897, 1980
4. Schmid FR, ed: Infectious arthritis. Clin Rheum Dis 4:1–241, 1978
5. Eisenstein BJ, Masi AT: Disseminated gonococcal infection (DGI) and gonococcal arthritis (GCA). I. Bacteriology, epidemiology, host factors, pathogen factors and pathology. Semin Arthritis Rheum 10:155–172, 1982
6. Handsfield HH, Weisner PJ, Holmes KK: Treatment of the gonococcal arthritis-dermatitis syndrome. Ann Intern Med 84:661–667, 1976
7. Rice PA, Goldenberg DL: Clinical manifestations of disseminated infection caused by Neisseria gonorrhoeae are linked to differences in bactericidal reactivity of infecting strains. Ann Intern Med 96:175–178, 1981
8. Churchill MA, Geraci JE, Hunder GG: Musculoskeletal manifestations of bacterial endocarditis. Ann Intern Med 87:754–759, 1977
9. Berney S, Goldstein M, Bishko F: Clinical and diagnostic features of tuberculous arthritis. Am J Med 53:36–42, 1972
10. Wallace R, Cohen AS: Tuberculous arthritis. A report of two cases with review of biopsy and synovial fluid findings. Am J Med 61:277–282, 1976
11. Goldenberg DL, Cohen AS: Arthritis due to tuberculous and fungal microorganisms. Clin Rheum Dis 4:211–223, 1978
12. Greenman R, Becker J, Campbell G, Remington J: Coccidioidal synovitis of the knee. Arch Intern Med 135:526–530, 1975
13. Crout JE, Brewer NS, Tompkins RB: Sporotrichosis arthritis: clinical features in 7 patients. Ann Intern Med 86:294–297, 1977
14. Fountain FF: Acute blastomycotic arthritis. Arch Intern Med 132:684–688, 1973
15. Bayer AS, Guze LB: Fungal arthritis. I. Candida arthritis: diagnostic and prognostic implications and therapeutic considerations. Semin Arthritis Rheum 8:142–150, 1978
16. Gray M, Philp T: Syphilitic arthritis: diagnostic problems with special reference to congenital syphilis. Ann Rheum Dis 22:19–25, 1963
17. Reginato AJ, Schumacher HR, Jimenez S, Maurer K: Synovitis in secondary syphilis: clinical, light, and electron microscopic studies. Arthritis Rheum 22:170–176, 1979
18. Gerster JC, Weintraub A, Vischer TL, Fallet GH: Secondary syphilis revealed by rheumatic complaints. J Rheumatol 4:197–200, 1977
19. Sabin AB: Identification of the filtrable transmissible neurolytic agent isolated from toxoplasma-infected tissue as a new pleuro-pneumonia-like microbe. Science 8:575–576, 1938

20. Ponka A: Arthritis associated with mycoplasma pneumoniae infection. Scand J Rheumatol 8:27–32, 1979

21. Stuckey M, Wuinn PA, Gelfand EW: Identification of Ureaplasma urealyticum (T-strain mycoplasma) in a patient with polyarthritis. Lancet 2:917–920, 1978

22. Verinder DGR: Septic arthritis due to muco-plasma hominis. J Bone Joint Surg 60B:224, 1978

23. Alpert E, Isselbacher KJ, Schur PH: The pathogenesis of arthritis associated with viral hepatitis. N Engl J Med 285:185–189, 1971

24. Alpert E, Schur PH, Isselbacher KJ: Sequential changes of serum complement in HAA related arthritis. N Engl J Med 287:103, 1972

25. Yanez JR, Thompson GR, Mikkelsen WM, Bar-tholomew LE: Rubella arthritis. Ann Intern Med 64:772–776, 1966

26. Thompson GR, Weiss JJ, Shillis JL, Brackett RG: Intermittent arthritis following rubella vaccination. Am J Dis Child 125:526–530, 1973

27. Hyer FH, Gottlieb NL: Rheumatic disorders associated with viral infection. Semin Arthritis Rheum 8:17–31, 1978

40. Lyme disease

Lyme disease, named after the Connecticut town where it was discovered in 1975, is an epidemic, systemic inflammatory disorder. It is recognized clinically by an early expanding skin lesion, *erythema chronicum migrans* (ECM) (Fig 40–1), which may be followed weeks to months later by neurologic, cardiac, or joint abnormalities (1–3).

The onset of Lyme disease occurs in summer or early fall. The illness may develop at any age in either sex. Foci of Lyme disease have been found elsewhere along the northeastern coast of the United States, in several other states, in western Europe, and in Australia (1 case).

Strong circumstantial evidence favors transmission of the penicillin-sensitive causative agent by the minute tick *Ixodes dammini* (4). A spirochete has recently been isolated from such ticks and is under study as a potential etiologic agent (5). ECM appears 3 days to 3 weeks after a tick bite and is often accompanied by chills and fever, malaise and fatigue, and headache or stiff neck.

Most patients with ECM have circulating immune complexes (6). Those who also have elevated levels of serum IgM and cryoglobulins containing IgM are at high risk for subsequent organ involvement. This high-risk group tends to have histocompatibility antigen DR2, which in turn correlates with the development of severe disease (but not with ECM alone).

Articular, neurologic, and cardiac abnormalities, alone or in combination, develop in approximately 50%, 20%, and 8% of patients, respectively. Early rheumatic complaints include migratory polyarthritis (without morning stiffness) and tendinitis. Later, patients experience longer attacks in a few large joints, especially the knees. These attacks typically recur for years. Chronic disease of the joints, with erosion

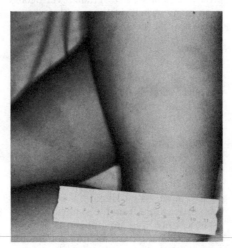

Fig 40–1. Thigh of child with Lyme disease shows erythema chronicum migrans. This first manifestation of Lyme disease begins as a red macule or papule that expands to form a large annular lesion. The outer border is intensely red and usually flat, the middle portion may be partially or completely clear, and the center is sometimes indurated in initial lesions. In some patients, the entire lesion is intensely red; in others, it may develop a bluish hue. (From Annals of Internal Medicine) (2)

of cartilage and bone, is much less common.

Changes in the synovium and synovial fluid are similar to those in rheumatoid arthritis. Immune complexes are present, even when absent from the blood. Rheumatoid factor and antinuclear antibodies are lacking.

Neurologic abnormalities often begin within a few weeks after ECM, last for months, and usually resolve completely. These include lymphocytic meningitis or meningoencephalitis, chorea, cerebellar ataxia, cranial neuritis (including bilateral Bell's palsy), motor and sensory radiculoneuritis, mononeuritis multiplex, and myelitis (7). Cardiac abnormalities, which also usually arise within a few weeks after ECM, include fluctuating degrees of A-V block and myopericarditis (8).

Oral penicillin G (or tetracycline) eradicates ECM and may prevent or attenuate subsequent arthritis (9). It is not yet clear whether neurologic, cardiac, or joint disease will respond to antibiotics. Symptomatic therapy for arthritis includes aspirin, other nonsteroidal antiinflammatory agents, intraarticular injection of corticosteroids, and occasionally synovectomy. Severe meningoencephalitis and complete heart block often respond to large doses of prednisone.

1. Steere AC, Malawista SE, Snydman DR, Shope RE, Andiman WA, Ross MR, Steele FM: Lyme arthritis: an epidemic of oligoarticular arthritis in children and adults in three Connecticut communities. Arthritis Rheum 20:7–17, 1977

2. Steere AC, Malawista SE, Hardin JA, Ruddy S, Askenase PW, Andiman WA: Erythema chronicum migrans and Lyme arthritis. Ann Intern Med 86:685–698, 1977

3. Steere AC, Gibofsky A, Patarroyo ME, Winchester RJ, Hardin JA, Malawista SE: Chronic Lyme arthritis. Ann Intern Med 90:896–901, 1979

4. Steere AC, Malawista SE: Cases of Lyme disease in the United States: locations correlated with distribution of *Ixodes dammini.* Ann Intern Med 91:730–733, 1979

5. Burgdorfer W, Barbour AG, Hayes SF, Benache JL, Grunwaldt E, Davis J: Lyme disease—a tick borne spirochetosis. Science 216:1317–1319, 1982

6. Hardin JA, Steere AC, Malawista SE: Immune complexes and the evolution of Lyme arthritis. N Engl J Med 301:1358–1363, 1979

7. Reik L, Steere AC, Bartenhagen NH, Shope RE, Malawista SE: Neurologic abnormalities of Lyme disease. Medicine 58:281–294, 1979

8. Steere AC, Batsford WP, Weinberg M, Alexander J, Berger HJ, Wolfson S, Malawista SE: Lyme carditis: cardiac abnormalities of Lyme disease. Ann Intern Med 93:8-16, 1980

9. Steere AC, Malawista SE, Newman JH, Spieler PN, Bartenhagen NH: Antibiotic therapy in Lyme disease. Ann Intern Med 93:1–8, 1980

41. Sarcoidosis

Sarcoidosis is a puzzling multisystemic disorder of unknown origin characterized by noncaseating granulomas in many organs (1). The disease predominantly affects young adults of either sex and begins most frequently with bilateral hilar lymphadenopathy, pulmonary infiltration, and skin and eye lesions.

Histologic examination of various tissues reveals granulomas composed primarily of epithelioid cells with occasional giant cells but without caseation necrosis.

Hyperglobulinemia and lymphopenia are the most common immunologic abnormalities, while a diminution in cutaneous delayed hypersensitivity and lymphocyte response to mitogenic stimulation, suggesting impaired T-cell function, may be present at certain stages of the disease (2).

The lung appears to be the site of increased antibody production in patients with pulmonary sarcoidosis (3). Elevations of serum angiotensin converting enzyme and lysozyme have been reported (4,5). Serial determinations of angiotensin converting enzyme may be useful in monitoring the dose and duration of corticosteroid therapy in pulmonary sarcoidosis (6).

The rheumatic manifestations of sarcoidosis include arthritis, osseous lesions, and muscle involvement. Arthritis, either acute or chronic, occurs in approximately 15% of patients (7). An acute symmetric, migratory, additive polyarthritis or periarthritis most frequently involving the ankles, and less often the wrists, proximal interphalangeal joints, and elbows is most common.

Acute arthritis is frequently the initial manifestation of sarcoidosis and is often associated with erythema nodosum. The arthritis may persist for weeks to months but usually resolves spontaneously without producing deformity or joint destruction.

Recent studies suggest the participation of circulating immune complexes in the pathogenesis of acute sarcoid arthritis (8) and an increased frequency of the HLA–B8 antigen has been observed (9).

Chronic sarcoid arthritis is characterized by recurrent or persistent oligarthritis frequently involving the knees and ankles. Joint destruction occasionally occurs. Synovial biopsy reveals characteristic noncaseating granulomas, which are generally absent in acute sarcoid arthritis or periarthritis. Bilateral hilar adenopathy is found in more than 90% of patients with either form of sarcoid arthritis. Diagnostic confusion with rheumatic fever, rheumatoid arthritis, or gout may occur because of the pattern of the arthritis or the presence of rheumatoid factor (14%) and hyperuricemia (20%). Therapy with salicylates, colchicine, or steroids has been effective in some cases.

Osseous sarcoidosis occurs in 3–9% of patients and most commonly involves the bones of the hands and feet (10). A striking association of bone lesions and chronic skin lesions (lupus pernio) has been noted. When osseous sarcoid involves the hands, a diffuse spongy thickening of the fingers and thumbs may be noted.

The most common radiographic abnormality consists of cortical defects or cysts in phalangeal or metatarsal heads. Bone disease treated with corticosteroids has healed.

From 50–80% of adequate muscle biopsy specimens from patients with sarcoidosis of less than 2 years contain typical noncaseating granulomas (11).

Patients with muscular involvement are usually asymptomatic but may have pain, weakness, or muscle wasting. Acute sarcoidal myopathy is occasionally indistinguishable from idiopathic polymyositis. Rarely, in acute sarcoidosis of muscle there may be tender, palpable muscle nodules or pseudohypertrophy. Patients with chronic disease may have palpably hard muscles. Although isolated muscular sarcoidosis may occur, multisystem involvement is usually evident.

1. Silzbach LE, James DG, Neville E, et al: Course and prognosis of sarcoidosis around the world. Am J Med 57:847–852, 1974
2. Tannenbaum H, Rocklin RE, Schur PH, Sheffer AL: Immune function in sarcoidosis. Clin Exp Immunol 26:511–519, 1976
3. Hunninghake GW, Crystal RG: Mechanisms of hypergamma-globulinemia in pulmonary sarcoidosis. J Clin Invest 67:86–92, 1981
4. Lieberman J: Elevation of serum angiotensin-converting enzyme level in sarcoidosis. Am J Med 59:365–372, 1975
5. Pascual RS, Gee JB, Finch SC: Usefulness of serum lysozyme measurement in diagnosis and evaluation of sarcoidosis. N Engl J Med 289:1074–1076, 1973
6. Rohatgi PK, Ryan JW, Lindeman P: Value of serial measurement of serum angiotensin-converting enzyme in the management of sarcoidosis. Am J Med 70:44–50, 1981
7. Spilberg I, Siltzbach LE, McEwen CE: The arthritis of sarcoidosis. Arthritis Rheum 12:126–137, 1969
8. Hedfors E, Norberg R: Evidence for circulating immune complexes in sarcoidosis. Clin Exp Immunol 16:493–496, 1974
9. Brewerton DA, Cockburn C, James DC, James DG, Neville E: HLA antigens in sarcoidosis. Clin Exp Immunol 27:227–229, 1977
10. Neville E, Carstairs LS, James DG: Bone sarcoidosis. Ann NY Acad Sci 278:475–487, 1976
11. Silverstein A, Siltzbach LE: Muscle involvement in sarcoidosis. Arch Neurol 21:235–241, 1969

42. Behçet's syndrome

In 1937 Behçet described a syndrome of recurrent oral ulceration, genital ulceration, and uveitis often leading to blindness (1). Additional features now recognized as part of the syndrome include cutaneous vasculitis resembling erythema nodosum, synovitis, aneurysms in large arteries, phlebitis, and meningoencephalitis. The disease affects mainly young adults; the mean age at onset is 30 years, and women are twice as commonly affected as men in the United States.

Criteria for the diagnosis of Behçet's disease are recurrent oral aphthous ulcerations in the presence of any 2 of the following: recurrent genital aphthous ulcerations, uveitis, cutaneous vasculitis, synovitis, and meningoencephalitis.

Incomplete forms of the syndrome may be suspected if recurrent aphthous ulceration coexists with one other finding. The diagnosis is clinical because there are no pathognomonic laboratory features. The approximate frequency of the major features is shown in Table 42–1.

Clinical features. Occurring as the initial manifestation, the oral ulcers are round or oval with a yellow or white exudate and a red rim. They resemble common canker sores, but are usually multiple and vary from 3–10 mm in diameter. They occur in painful crops that heal in weeks, leaving no scars.

Painful genital aphthous ulcers occur on the vulva or penis, recur less frequently than oral ulcers, and can cause dyspareunia, psychologic trauma, and rarely persistent vulvar perforations.

Bilateral nongranulomatous uveitis, present in two-thirds of patients, typically affects both anterior and posterior chambers of the eye (2). The resulting vasculitis infarcts the retina, often leading to blindness. Usually some years elapse between the onset of mucosal inflammation and uveitis. Patients present with blurred vision but seldom have much ocular pain or redness. Slit-lamp biomicroscopy may show cellular exudates in the anterior and posterior chambers. Hypopyon is rare nowadays.

A patient with ocular disease is best treated conjointly by an ophthalmologist and internist.

Mild synovitis, present at peaks of inflammation, generally affects the hands, knees, or ankles. It is almost never erosive or deforming. Synovial fluid cell counts

Table 42–1. Prevalence of major clinical features of Behçet's disease

Clinical feature	%
Recurrent oral ulcers	100
Recurrent genital ulcers	80
Uveitis	66
Cutaneous vasculitis	66
Synovitis	55
Meningoencephalitis	22

are inflammatory, e.g., 5,000–10,000 WBC/mm^3, with mostly polymorphonuclear leukocytes (6).

The HLA–B27 antigen is not usually implicated and spondylarthritis is rare.

Numerous types of cutaneous inflammation may be observed. Extremity nodules resemble erythema nodosum, but pustules, papules, and lesions due to phlebitis of small cutaneous veins are seen. A vasculitis affecting small veins and arteries is common. Patients seldom have extensive nodules or ulcerations. Their occurrence should lead the physician to suspect the condition with which Behçet's is most readily confused, i.e., Crohn's disease.

Some patients show a peculiar hyperreactivity of skin to minor trauma, i.e., pustules developing at sites of skin puncture or intradermal sterile saline injections.

About 20% of patients develop central nervous system disease (3). These patients usually present with findings of an aseptic meningitis, i.e., fever, headache, stiff neck, and cells in the cerebrospinal fluid (CSF). Most such patients eventually develop encephalitic episodes resembling stroke. Delay in diagnosis is frequent, while infective agents are sought in vain, unless the mucosal lesions are noticed. Typically lymphocytes predominate in the CSF during episodes of meningitis/meningoencephalitis except at onset when polymorphonuclear leukocytes predominate.

As in all other manifestations of Behçet's disease, asymptomatic intervals occur. There can be focal neurologic deficits from brain stem involvement; irreversible damage can result in hemiparesis, cerebel-

lar incoordination, and pathologic emotional states.

Deaths from Behçet's disease may result not only from central nervous system involvement but also from arteritis with aneurysm and rupture of pulmonary and systemic arteries and from perforation of discrete ulcerations in the ileum and ascending colon (4).

Pathogenesis. A viral etiology has long been considered but is not proved. Several immunologic abnormalities are seen. Serum antibodies to human mucosal cells are common, circulating immune complexes are present in half the patients, and lymphocytes from patients are cytotoxic to human oral epithelial cells in vitro. The neutrophils of patients have increased target-directed chemotaxis as compared with those of controls (5). Abnormalities in fibrinolysis and the secretory component of IgG have also been reported (6). The presence of lymphocytes in many of the pathologic sites, e.g., perivascular, CSF, and skin lesions, suggests a disorder of cellular immunity.

The disease is more prevalent in Eastern Mediterranean countries and Japan where there appears to be a linkage to HLA–B5. This association is not found in Western Europeans or Americans.

Differential diagnosis and treatment. Because Crohn's disease shares many features with Behçet's disease, a proctoscopic examination and colon x-ray are required to exclude this diagnosis. Other pitfalls in diagnosis are herpes simplex infections especially with recurrent aseptic meningitis, cicatricial pemphigoid, Cogan's syndrome (having a keratitis, rarely

uveitis), and such other rare causes of aseptic meningitis as Harada's syndrome or Mollaret's meningitis (3).

Although no treatment is curative, corticosteroids palliate the skin and joint lesions. Oral ulcerations usually continue despite moderate doses of prednisone. Systemic and topical corticosteroids reduce the ocular inflammation and prolong the duration before blindness.

For the 2 most serious consequences of Behçet's disease, i.e., uveitis and meningoencephalitis, immunosuppressive therapy is usually effective. One approach is to use chlorambucil 0.1 mg/kg/day until inflammation subsides, then tapering and withdrawal may be tried.

Because prevention of relapses may require years of low dosage, monitoring of blood counts to prevent dangerous leukopenia and thrombocytopenia is mandatory.

1. Behçet H: Uber Rezidivierende, Aphthose, Durch ein Virus verursachte Geschwure am Mund, am Auge und an den Genitalien. Derm Wschr 105:1152, 1937
2. Colvard DM, Robertson DM, O'Duffy JD: The ocular manifestations of Behçet's disease. Arch Ophthalmol 95:1813, 1977
3. O'Duffy JD, Goldstein NP: Neurologic involvement in 7 patients with Behçet's disease. Am J Med 61:170, 1976
4. Shimizu T, Ehrlich GE, Inaba G, Hayashi K: Behçet's disease (Behçet's syndrome). Semin Arthritis Rheum 8:223–260, 1979
5. Fordham JN, Davies PG, Kirk A, Currey HLF: Polymorphonuclear function in Behçet's syndrome. Ann Rheum Dis 41:421–425, 1982
6. Abdou NI, Schumacher HR, Colman RW, et al: Behçet's disease: possible role of secretory component deficiency, synovial inclusions and fibrinolytic abnormality in the various manifestations of the disease. J Lab Clin Med 91:409–422, 1978

43. Familial Mediterranean fever

Familial Mediterranean fever (FMF), also known as recurrent polyserositis and periodic disease, is a dramatic hereditary autosomal recessive disorder virtually restricted to Sephardic and Ashkenazi Jews, Armenians, and Arabs of the Middle East.

It is characterized by brief but disabling febrile attacks of peritonitis, synovitis, pleuritis, or an erysipelas-like erythema affecting the leg or foot. These episodes first appear during childhood or adolescence and recur at irregular intervals thereafter. Systemic amyloidosis develops and causes death from renal failure, usually at an early age. The febrile attacks and the amyloidosis are independent phenotypic expressions of a pleiotropic recessive gene (1).

Peritonitis is the most frequent manifestation of the disease, occurring in 95% of the patients. This is characterized by sudden onset with fever and pain spreading

over the entire abdomen from a variable point of origin. The physical signs of abdominal distention, rebound tenderness, board-like rigidity, and absence of peristalsis combine to suggest acute abdominal catastrophe. Surprisingly, after 6–12 hours, signs and symptoms recede and within 24–48 hours the attack is over (1).

Articular involvement is a cardinal feature of this disease. It is present in more than 70% of patients and appears as an acute monarthritis involving a large joint, most often in the lower extremity. Commonly, the attack subsides in 3–7 days, lasting somewhat longer than the peritoneal reaction (2).

In 5–7% of the patients, some of the joint attacks last for weeks to months; afterward functional and anatomic integrity is regained in most joints except the hip. Once affected by prolonged attacks, this joint may recover incompletely and its

function become moderately or severely restricted (3).

Amyloidosis, a major manifestation of familial Mediterranean fever, is extremely common in Sephardic Jews of North African extraction with the disease. Most of these people die from renal failure before they reach the age of 40. Systemic amyloidosis is infrequent in Armenians and Ashkenazi patients and moderately frequent in the Iraqui Jews.

The amyloid fibrils of familial Mediterranean fever consist of AA protein, structurally related to the serum acute phase reactant, serum amyloid A protein (SAA) (4) (see Section 21).

Daily colchicine administration markedly decreases the frequency and severity of all types of febrile attacks in FMF patients. Half the patients require 1 mg daily, whereas 10% fail to respond to a daily dose of 2–3 mg. Long-term colchicine treatment also seems to protect from or delay the development of amyloidosis in these patients (5–7).

1. Sohar E, Gafni J, Pras M, Heller H: Familial Mediterranean fever: a survey of 470 cases and review of the literature. Am J Med 43:227–253, 1967
2. Heller H, Gafni J, Michaeli D, Shahin N, Sohar E, Ehrlich G, Karten I, Sokoloff L: The arthritis of familial Mediterranean fever (FMF). Arthritis Rheum 9:1–17, 1966
3. Sneh E, Pras M, Michaeli D, Shahin N, Gafni J: Protracted arthritis in familial Mediterranean fever. Rheumatol Rehab 16:102–106, 1977
4. Pras M, Gafni J: The nature of amyloid, Immunochemistry. LE Glynn, MW Steward, eds. Chichester, John Wiley & Sons, 1977, pp 509–533
5. Zemer D, Revach M, Pras M, Modan B, Schor S, Sohar E, Gafni J: A controlled trial of colchicine in preventing attacks of familial Mediterranean fever. N Engl J Med 291:932–934, 1974
6. Zemer D, Pras M, Sohar E, Gafni J: Colchicine in familial Mediterranean fever. N Engl J Med 294:170–171, 1976
7. Wright DG, Wolff SM, Fauci AS, Alling DW: Efficacy of intermittent colchicine therapy in familial Mediterranean fever. Ann Intern Med 86:162–165, 1977

44. Intermittent hydrarthrosis

Intermittent hydrarthrosis is a rare problem of unknown cause in which a brief episode of joint effusion recurs fairly regularly (1). It is more common in women and usually develops in adolescents and young adults.

In most cases only one knee is involved at first, but bilateral effusions, during either the same or different episodes, are common. Rarely, other joints such as the ankle, hip, and elbow may be affected.

The effusion usually lasts 3–5 days. Fluid accumulates rapidly and is resorbed more slowly. Pain is seldom severe and warmth and tenderness are minimal or absent. The range of motion may be limited when a large effusion is present.

Attacks occur at intervals of 10 days to 4 weeks and are sometimes synchronized with the menstrual cycle. The joints appear quite normal between attacks. Although some patients have regular episodes throughout life, others experience temporary remissions for months or years, sometimes associated with a pregnancy. In some instances, the remission may be permanent.

Laboratory studies, including the levels of acute phase reactants, are normal and rheumatoid factor is absent. The joint fluid shows a small number of inflammatory cells and a good mucin clot, but no crystals. There are mild nonspecific changes in the synovium with scattered infiltrations of lymphocytes.

Radiographs demonstrate soft-tissue swelling during attacks but no other diagnostic findings.

Intermittent hydrarthrosis must be distinguished from similar episodes—usually occurring at more irregular intervals—during the early phase of rheumatoid arthritis (palindromic rheumatism) and familial Mediterranean fever, in which there may be similar recurrent effusions.

No treatment consistently aborts or prevents the attacks.

1. Ehrlich GE: Intermittent and periodic arthritic syndromes, Arthritis and Allied Conditions. Ed 9. DJ McCarty, Jr, ed. Philadelphia, Lea & Febiger, 1979, pp 663–680

45. Palindromic rheumatism

PS Hench and EF Rosenberg introduced the term *palindromic rheumatism* to describe an uncommon type of recurring acute arthritis and periarthritis with symptom-free intervals of days to months between attacks (1). Both sexes are affected equally, with the onset usually between the third and sixth decades.

Although originally described as a distinct condition, it is now evident that more than 30% of patients with palindromic rheumatism later develop rheumatoid arthritis (2), or much less commonly, systemic lupus erythematosus or some other connective tissue disease (3).

Each attack begins suddenly in 1 or 2 joints, often in the late afternoon or evening, with pain that may be intense and reaches a peak within a few hours. Swelling, warmth, and redness over or near the affected joint are noted shortly after the onset of pain. The evidence of inflammation usually disappears in 1–3 days, but may remain for as long as a week.

Constitutional symptoms are uncommon, but some patients have low-grade fever during the attack. Although objective signs of inflammation may not accompany every attack, a history of recurrent arthralgia is insufficient to justify this diagnosis. The episodes occur irregularly and attacks in individual joints may overlap. Any appendicular joint may be affected, but the knees, wrists, and shoulders are most commonly involved. Occasionally attacks are experienced in the vertebral column and temporomandibular joint. Periarticular attacks are marked by painful swelling of the fingerpads, heels, and other soft tissues. Poorly circumscribed subcutaneous nodes may also be present transiently.

Examination of the synovium and joint fluid reveals a nonspecific subacute inflammatory reaction with no crystals (2). Microvascular injury is prominent in synovial biopsies. Elevations of the erythrocyte sedimentation rate and various acute phase reactants may be found during an attack. Serum and synovial fluid complement levels are not depressed (4,5).

The extended clinical course is variable. A few patients enjoy a spontaneous remission, but many continue to have attacks without developing persistent synovitis or permanent joint damage. In patients who develop rheumatoid arthritis, rheumatoid factor may be detected either during the late palindromic phase or after chronic rheumatoid arthritis is established (2,3).

Antiinflammatory drugs do not prevent or mitigate the acute attacks, but chrysotherapy has been helpful in about half the patients treated (3). Penicillamine (6) or prophylactic colchicine (7) may also be effective.

1. Hench PS, Rosenberg EF: Palindromic rheumatism: a "new," oft recurring disease of joints (arthritis, periarthritis, para-arthritis) apparently producing no articular residues: report of 34 cases; its relation to "angioneural arthrosis," "allergic rheumatism," and rheumatoid arthritis. Arch Intern Med 73:292–321, 1944
2. Schumacher HR: Palindromic onset of rheumatoid arthritis: clinical, synovial fluid, and biopsy studies. Arthritis Rheum 25:361–369, 1982
3. Mattingly S: Palindromic rheumatism. Ann Rheum Dis 25:307–317, 1966
4. Williams MH, Sheldon PJHS, Torrigiani G, Elsen V, Mattingly S: Palindromic rheumatism: clinical and immunological studies. Ann Rheum Dis 30:375–380, 1971
5. Wajed MA, Brown DL, Currey HLF: Palindromic rheumatism: clinical and serum complement study. Ann Rheum Dis 36:56–61, 1977
6. Huskisson EC: Treatment of palindromic rheumatism with D-penicillamine. Br Med J 2:6042, 1976
7. Schwartzberg M: Prophylactic colchine therapy in palindromic rheumatism. J Rheumatol 9:341–342, 1982

46. Gout

Gout, a disease of long and distinguished lineage, is characterized by 1) recurrent paroxysms of violent articular inflammation provoked by the release of microcrystals of monosodium urate monohydrate in the joint cavity, and 2) the development of gross deposits of sodium urate (tophi) in and around the joints and in the kidneys (1–6). Approximately 20% of the patients have urinary calculi, consisting of uric acid (7).

The term *gout* is derived from the Latin *gutta*, "a drop," and reflects the ancient belief that the disease was caused by a malevolent humour dropping into the weakened joints (8).

Gouty arthritis represents a complication of prolonged hyperuricemia. In humans, who, unlike most other mammals, lack the enzyme uricase, uric acid constitutes the major end product of the catabolism of purines. Uric acid is only slightly miscible in body fluids; its solubility in plasma is approximately 8.0 mg/dl. Higher concentrations are the result of supersaturation, a state marked by a tendency toward precipitation of sodium urate in articular cartilage, synovium, and other tissues.

The deposition of sodium urate (the chief compound of uric acid existing at body pH) takes place not only in gouty humans but also in those species of animals in which uric acid represents the major end product in the breakdown of amino acid and purine nitrogen. Thus, *Homo sapiens* finds himself in the company of members of the uricotelic phyla, Insecta, Aves, and Reptilia, which are also subject to the development of tophaceous disease.

Gouty arthritis can now be treated so effectively that it may be difficult to appreciate the dread once inspired by this malady. The classic case of far advanced disease has become increasingly uncommon and it is unusual now to see examples of the massive tophaceous deposits which gouty English clubmen once boasted could be used to mark their game scores. Every so often, however, one encounters individuals in whom a failure to diagnose and/or treat properly has permitted full expression of the disease, and one understands why in ages past the gout was known as *opprobrium medicorum*.

Normouricemia. The normal values for serum urate concentration in adults are 5.1 ± 1.0 mg/dl in men and 4.0 ± 1.0 mg/dl in women (enzymatic uricase spectrophotometric method) (3). The concentration is lower in children (3.5–4.0 mg/dl). In boys it rises to the adult level during puberty. There is little or no change in the concentration of serum urate in girls at puberty.

The slightly lower value normally in women compared with that in men is attributable, at least in part, to the promotion of renal uric acid excretion by estrogenic hormones (9). After cessation of the menses the serum urate level tends to rise and approaches that found in the male.

Hyperuricemia. In the population at large, serum urate levels fall on a bell-shaped distribution curve, with skewing toward the higher values (3). Serum urate concentration constitutes a continuous variable, similar to blood pressure, and represents the result of a complex multifactorial inheritance modified by numerous other factors, including diet, body weight, and hemoglobin level, as well as social class and life style.

The interplay of genetic and environmental factors in the determination of hyperuricemia is illustrated by the observation of significantly higher mean serum urate level in Filipinos in the United States compared to racially identical individuals living in the Philippines. The basis for this difference appears to be a limited ability to excrete uric acid which cannot compensate for the increased purine content in the usual US diet (10).

In large-scale investigations of the serum urate concentrations in adult populations, approximately 5% of those surveyed have been found to have hyperuricemia (most often of mild degree) at some time or other during the study (11). Only a small minority of these individuals, however, have developed or are likely to develop gouty arthritis.

A direct relationship has been demonstrated between the level of serum urate and both the likelihood of subsequent development of gouty arthritis and age at time of the initial attack. In many instances the absence of gout in hyperuricemic individuals can be explained by a lack of sufficient severity and persistence in the hyperuricemia (various drugs and dietary factors may account for transient hyperuricemia).

All patients with gout, unless treated, have an increased quantity of dissolved urate in their extracellular fluid. Characteristically, this is manifested by an elevated serum urate level—first detected by AB Garrod in 1848. The mean average level in untreated patients is 9–10 mg/dl (1). Individuals with chronic joint disease and those in whom the gout is secondary to a blood dyscrasia have significantly higher concentrations of serum urate than others.

Biochemistry and purine metabolism

Classification of hyperuricemia. The biochemical hallmark and prerequisite of gout is hyperuricemia. The concentration of uric acid in body fluids is determined by the balance between rates of production and elimination of urate. Uric acid is formed by oxidation of purine bases, which may originate exogenously or endogenously.

About two-thirds of the uric acid produced each day is excreted into the urine (300–600 mg/day), while approximately one-third of that produced in excreted into the gastrointestinal tract where it is ultimately destroyed by colonic bacteria. The development of hyperuricemia may be due to an excessive rate of uric acid production, a decrease in the renal excretion of uric acid, or a combination of both events.

Hyperuricemia and gout may be classified as primary, secondary, or idiopathic (Table 46–1).

Primary hyperuricemia or gout refers to those cases that appear to be innate, neither secondary to another acquired disorder nor a subordinate manifestation of an inborn error that leads initially to a major disease unlike gout. Although some cases of primary gout have a genetic basis, others do not.

Secondary hyperuricemia or gout refers to cases that develop in the course of another disease or as a consequence of drugs.

Finally, *idiopathic hyperuricemia* refers to cases where there is elevated serum uric acid (but not gout) and a more precise classification cannot be assigned.

Further subdivisions within each major category are based on the identification of overproduction, underexcretion, or both as responsible for the hyperuricemia.

Primary hyperuricemia. Patients classified as exhibiting an overproduction of uric acid by definition excrete more than 600 mg of uric acid per 24 hours after 5 days of dietary purine restriction. Such patients probably represent less than 10% of the gouty population. In these patients with primary gout due to an overproduction of uric acid, the rate of purine biosynthesis de novo accelerates.

Purine metabolism. Several important elements related to the metabolism of purines deserve comment before considering those abnormalities related specifically to the overproduction of uric acid (Fig 46–1).

First, uric acid is the ultimate degradative product of purine catabolism in human beings. Second, although the purine pathway is regulated in a complex manner, the intracellular concentration of 5-phosphoribosyl-1-pyrophosphate (PRPP) appears to be a major determinant of the rate of synthesis of uric acid in humans. Generally, when the concentration of PRPP in the cell is elevated, uric acid synthesis is elevated; when the concentration of PRPP in the cell is reduced, the synthesis of uric acid is reduced. Although exceptions to this generalization exist, this concept is applicable to most clinical situations.

Two inborn errors of purine metabolism—hypoxanthine-guanine phosphoribosyltransferase (HGPRT) deficiency and PRPP synthetase overactivity—have now

Table 46–1. Classification of hyperuricemia and gout

Type	Metabolic disturbance	Inheritance
Primary		
Associated with specific enzyme defects		
Hypoxanthine-guanine phosphoribosyltransferase deficiency, partial	Overproduction of uric acid; increased purine biosynthesis de novo driven by surplus PRPP	X-linked
PRPP* synthetase variants; increased activity	Overproduction of PRPP and uric acid	X-linked
Molecular defects undefined		
Overproduction	Not established	Polygenic
Underexcretion	Not established	Polygenic
Secondary		
Associated with increased purine biosynthesis de novo		
Hypoxanthine-guanine phosphoribosyltransferase deficiency "virtually complete"	Overproduction of uric acid; Lesch-Nyhan syndrome	X-linked
Glucose 6-phosphatase deficiency or absence	Overproduction plus underexcretion of uric acid; glycogen storage disease, type I (von Gierke)	Autosomal recessive
Associated with increased nucleic acid turnover	Overproduction of uric acid	
Associated with decreased renal excretion of uric acid	Decreased filtration of uric acid, inhibited tubular secretion of uric acid, or enhanced tubular reabsorption of uric acid	
Idiopathic		Unknown

* PRPP = 5-phosphoribosyl-1-pyrophosphate.

been defined within the group of patients with primary hyperuricemia associated with an overproduction of uric acid.

HGRPT deficiency. Patients with a partial deficiency of HGPRT, the enzyme that catalyzes the conversion of hypoxanthine to inosinic acid and guanine to guanylic acid (reaction 2, Fig 46–1), typically have the onset of gouty arthritis at a young age (15–30 years) and a high incidence of uric acid nephrolithiasis (75%). A few of these patients may have mild neurologic dysfunction characterized by dysarthria, hyperreflexia, uncoordination, and/or mental retardation.

This disease is inherited in an X-linked manner so that males are affected through carrier females.

A more severe deficiency of the same enzyme leads to the development of the *Lesch-Nyhan syndrome*, a disease characterized by X-linked inheritance, selfmutilation, choreoathetosis, and mental retardation as well as a profound overproduction of uric acid, which leads to hyperuricemia and uric acid stone formation. The Lesch-Nyhan syndrome is considered a form of secondary hyperuricemia since the major clinical manifestations relate to the behavioral and neurologic disorder.

Overactive PRPP synthetase. PRPP, a normal substrate for HGPRT, accumulates intracellularly in each of these 2 syndromes related to a deficiency of the enzyme. This increased concentration of PRPP is thought to be primarily responsible for the accelerated rate of purine biosynthesis and the overproduction of uric acid characteristic of both disorders.

Several families are described who have an increased activity of the enzyme PRPP synthetase (reaction 3, Fig 46–1. At least 3 different types of mutant enzymes have now been described; all exhibit markedly increased activity in vivo, resulting in an increased intracellular concentration of PRPP, accelerated purine biosynthesis, and an exceptionally high daily excretion rate of uric acid.

The inheritance pattern in this disease is also X-linked. These patients, like those with partial hypoxanthine-guanine phosphoribosyltransferase deficiency, generally develop gout in the second or third decade and have a high incidence of uric acid stones.

The cause of the overproduction of uric acid in the majority of patients with a primary type of overproduction of uric acid who do not have 1 of these 2 enzymatic errors remains obscure.

Renal defect. A defect in the renal excretion of uric acid can be demonstrated in as many as 90% of gouty subjects. These patients require a plasma urate value of 1–2 mg/100 ml greater than nongouty subjects in order to achieve a given rate of uric acid excretion. This abnormality is most prominent in the gouty subject with a normal production of uric acid.

Although an abnormality in uric acid excretion does not appear to exist in most subjects with a profound overproduction of uric acid, a renal defect can be shown by careful study of some gouty subjects with modest uric acid overproduction.

The renal excretion of urate is dependent on glomerular filtration, tubular reabsorption, and tubular secretion. Uric acid appears to be completely filtered at the

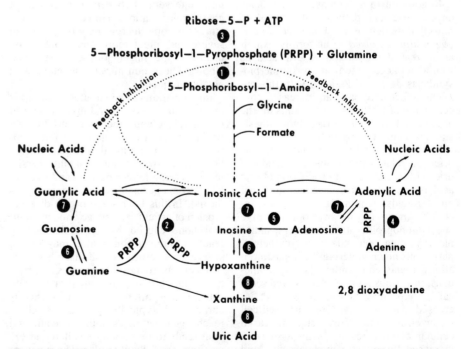

Fig 46–1. Outline of purine metabolism: 1) amidophosphoribosyltransferase; 2) hypoxanthine-guanine phosphoribosyltransferase; 3) PRPP synthetase; 4) adenine phosphoribosyltransferase; 5) adenosine deaminase; 6) purine nucleoside phosphorylase; 7) 5′-nucleotidase; 8) xanthine oxidase. (Adapted from Seegmiller, Rosenbloom, and Kelley: Science 155:1682–1684, 1967)

glomerulus and resorbed in the proximal tubule at a site proximal to secretion (i.e., presecretory reabsorption). Uric acid secretion then occurs in the proximal tubule, with a subsequent second reabsorptive site (i.e., postsecretory reabsorption) in the proximal tubule.

Although some uric acid reabsorption may also occur in the ascending limb of the loop of Henle as well as in the collecting duct, these latter 2 sites are thought to be quantitatively unimportant. Attempts to further define the location and nature of these putative sites or to quantify their contribution to uric acid transport in normal people or in those with various diseases have been largely unrewarding.

Theoretically, the altered renal excretion of uric acid exhibited by most patients with gout could be due to: 1) reduced filtration of uric acid, 2) enhanced reabsorption, or 3) decreased secretion. Although no unequivocal data establish any of these 3 mechanisms as the basic defect in a gouty patient at the present time, it seems likely that eventually any or all of the 3 types of abnormalities will be found within the gouty population.

Secondary hyperuricemia. Secondary hyperuricemia like primary hyperuricemia may be due to an overproduction of uric acid, a reduced clearance of uric acid, or a combination of both abnormalities. In some patients with secondary hyperuricemia due to an overproduction of uric acid, the predominant abnormality appears to be an accelerated rate of purine biosynthesis as it is in primary hyperuricemia. This is the case in patients with the Lesch-Nyhan syndrome.

In addition to a decreased renal clearance of uric acid, patients with glucose-6-phosphatase deficiency (*Von Gierke's glycogen storage disease*) uniformly exhibit an increased production of uric acid as well as an accelerated rate of purine biosynthesis de novo. Patients with this enzyme defect may have an increased concentration of PRPP which accounts for the accelerated rate of purine biosynthesis and uric acid overproduction.

In most patients with secondary hyperuricemia related to an overproduction of uric acid, the increased production of uric acid is due to an increased turnover of nucleic acids. A number of diseases, including many of the myeloproliferative and lymphoproliferative disorders, multiple myeloma, secondary polycythemia, pernicious anemia, certain hemoglobinopathies, thalassemia, other hemolytic anemias, infectious mononucleosis, and some carcinomas, may be associated with increased marrow activity or increased cell turnover at other sites. This increased cellular activity results in an associated increased turnover of nucleic acids, and thus hyperuricemia, hyperuricaciduria, and a compensatory increase in the rate of purine biosynthesis de novo.

Important renal causes of secondary hyperuricemia include renal insufficiency, most diuretic agents, chronic lead intoxication, low doses of aspirin, pyrazinamide, nicotinic acid, ethambutol, ethanol, and various types of organic acidosis.

Clinical features

In the majority of patients with gout, recurring bouts of acute joint inflammation constitute the first manifestation of the disease. In approximately 10–15% of the patients, arthritis is preceded by nephrolithiasis. A family history of the disease is found in approximately one-fourth of the patients (12). Gouty arthritis is a disorder chiefly of middle-aged and older men (who constitute 85–90% of patients) and postmenopausal women and is the most common form of inflammatory joint disease in men past 40 years of age.

Although gouty arthritis may commence as early as the second decade of life in rare individuals with a heritable deficiency in hypoxanthine-guanine phosphoribosyltransferase or some other enzymatic disturbance leading to congenital hyperuricemia, the peak period of onset is in the fourth and fifth decades (1)

Acute gouty arthritis. The inaugural attacks are typically monarticular (uncommonly oligarticular) and tend to affect the lower extremities, particularly the first metatarsophalangeal (MTP) and tarsal joints, ankles, and knees (5). The great toe is the most common site of initial involvement, and inflammation of the first MTP joint occurs in 75% or more of all patients.

In the beginning many months or years may intervene between paroxysms of gouty inflammation. However, in time, attacks become increasingly frequent and severe and affect more and more parts, including the finger joints, wrists, and elbows. Olecranon bursitis develops with notable frequency.

Inflammation of the shoulder and hip is uncommon, however, and involvement of the sacroiliac and other intervertebral articulations is rare. At first, the joints appear to return to normal between attacks, but in time, swelling and disability persist for longer and longer periods and eventually become permanent (chronic gouty arthritis). In this later stage of the disease, erosion of articular cartilage and subchondral bone caused by the inflammatory reaction to tophaceous matter may lead to severe joint deformity and disability.

In contrast to most other types of arthritis, the onset of joint inflammation in acute gout (which often occurs at night) is abrupt, and, typically, pain and swelling reach a peak within 24 hours. The affected joint tends to be notably swollen and exquisitely painful and tender. There is generally a considerable degree of periarticular swelling and erythema (dusky redness in the great toe). This feature, combined

with the low-grade fever and leukocytosis that often accompany the attack, frequently gives rise to the mistaken impression of cellulitis or thrombophlebitis. Thomas Sydenham, himself a victim of the disease, described (1683) the attack as follows:

The victim goes to bed and sleeps in good health. About two o'clock in the morning he is awakened by a severe pain in the great toe; more rarely in the heel, ankle, or instep. This pain is like that of a dislocation, and yet the parts feel as if cold water were poured over them. Then follow chills and shivers, and a little fever. The pain, which was at first moderate, becomes more intense. With its intensity the chills and shivers increase. After a time this comes to its height, accommodating itself to the bones and ligaments of the tarsus and metatarsus. Now it is a violent stretching and tearing of the ligaments—now it is a gnawing pain, and now a pressure and tightening. So exquisite and lively meanwhile is the feeling of the part affected, that it cannot bear the weight of the bedclothes nor the jar of a person walking in the room. The night is passed in torture, sleeplessness, turning of the part affected, and perpetual change of posture.

Mild attacks of the gout usually last for several days if untreated, while more severe seizures may persist for several weeks. Desquamation of the overlying skin may occur as the inflammation resolves, after which the joint returns to its previous state. Many patients experience numerous minor fits of joint inflammation in addition to the classically florid attacks.

Intercritical gout. During the interval between attacks the patient with early gout is usually entirely asymptomatic and no abnormalities may be found on examination of the joints.

Chronic tophaceous gout. Before the introduction of effective drugs for the control of hyperuricemia, approximately 50–60% of gouty patients developed clinically or radiographically detectable deposits of monosodium urate monohydrate in their tissues (Fig 46–2).

The ancients referred to these concretions or "articulation badges" of the gout as *tophi* (from the Greek, "chalk stone") in the belief that they represented an inspissated earthy humour. In 1797 WH Wollaston announced that the principal constituent of tophi was "a neutral compound, consisting of lithic [uric] acid and mineral alkali [sodium]." This epochal discovery provided the first direct evidence linking uric acid to the gout.

Sites. Tophi are rarely apparent at the time of the initial attack of gouty arthritis. They are generally first noted some time after onset, on an average of 10 years later. They occur most commonly in the synovium, subchondral bone, olecranon bursa, infrapatellar and achilles tendons, and subcutaneous tissue on the extensor surface of the forearm and overlying the

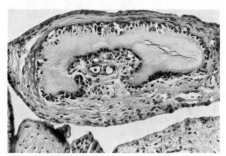

Fig 46–2. Photomicrograph of synovium (knee) of a 46-year-old man who had sustained repeated attacks of gouty arthritis for 15 years. Note large tophaceous deposit in synovial villus with surrounding histiocytic reaction.

joints. The cartilage of the helix of the ear, often cited as a location for tophi, is a relatively infrequent site for these deposits.

Composition. The tophus consists of a nodular core of monosodium urate with a surrounding inflammatory reaction that includes foreign body type giant cells. It may be difficult to clinically distinguish tophi from rheumatoid nodules. The former tend to be harder and may grow to be large and more irregular in shape; occasionally, the whitish contents of the tophus are apparent. The skin overlying bulky, more superficial tophi may ulcerate, with prolonged drainage of uratic matter.

When there is any doubt about the tophaceous nature of a given subcutaneous nodule, it should be aspirated and examined for the typical needle-shaped crystals of monosodium urate monohydrate (first describeα by Leeuwenhoek in 1684), or removed in its entirety and examined in frozen sections, or fixed in absolute alcohol to prevent dissolution of the deposit and scrutinized microscopically and chemically.

Association with chronic gout. The presence of tophaceous deposits is associated with a tendency toward more frequent and severe episodes of acute gouty arthritis. Chronic gouty arthritis, with joint deformity, develops as a result of the erosion of cartilage and subchondral bone caused by the inflammatory reaction to articular tophaceous matter. Tophaceous deposits may also be responsible for carpal tunnel syndrome and trigger finger deformity as a result of infiltration of the flexor tendons and their sheaths.

In exceptional instances tophi have been observed in the nasal cartilage, tongue, vocal cords, aorta, heart valves, and myocardium. The destruction of joint cartilage in chronic gout may lead to severe secondary osteoarthritis with or without chondrocalcinosis.

Tophus formation is related to the serum concentration of urate, as well as to the local tissue factors. In general, the higher the serum urate level, the earlier the appearance and more extensive the development of tophi (2). These deposits are relatively uncommon in those individuals with gout whose serum urate concentration (untreated) is less than 8.5 mg/dl (enzymatic method).

Secondary gout. The gout that occurs in the wake of various myeloproliferative disorders is clinically similar to primary gout, although the average age of onset and relative frequency with which women are affected are both greater in the secondary form of the disease (13). In further contrast, a history of familial involvement is unusual in secondary gout and there is a tendency toward higher serum urate levels and greater urinary uric acid excretion. Accordingly, a higher frequency of tophus and uric acid stone formation is found.

Gouty nephropathy. Individuals with longstanding gout may have kidney disease marked by proteinuria, diminution in concentrating capacity, and ultimately a decrease in creatinine clearance and azotemia (14,15). Uncommonly, severe renal insufficiency may develop. However, even before highly effective serum urate-lowering treatment, only a minority of gouty patients died of renal failure; most died of cardiovascular or cerebrovascular disease after a life span similar to that of nongouty individuals.

Histologic examination of the gouty kidney reveals a variety of abnormalities; tophaceous masses in the interstitium of the renal medulla are the most distinct and consistent abnormalities found (16). Other pathologic changes, including pyelonephritis, are believed to be secondary to these deposits. In addition, nephrosclerosis and other evidence of hypertensive disease are common. Tubular damage can result from intratubular deposition of uric acid.

Striking increases in serum urate levels (as high as 40–60 mg/dl) may occur in patients with leukemia or lymphoma as a result of the rapid breakdown of cellular nucleic acid after aggressive treatment with corticosteroids, x-irradiation, and alkylating agents. The precipitation of uric acid in the renal tubules of such patients may lead to severe urinary obstruction with prolonged oliguria. This hazard can be prevented or reversed by allopurinol treatment.

Uric acid stones. In the United States uric acid stones represent about 10% of all urinary calculi. Such stones occur in approximately 20% of all patients with gout (and 40% of those with secondary gout) (7).

Uric acid stones are usually relatively small, smooth, and rounded, and range from pale yellow through dark red to black. They are characteristically radiolucent, but some, particularly the larger ones, may contain calcium salts and hence are radiopaque.

At normal urinary pH, uric acid is large-ly or completely nondissociated. Nonionized uric acid is less soluble than sodium urate and markedly less soluble the lower the pH. Normally the urine is most acid at night and early morning; the pH rises sharply in the morning and remains at only mildly acid levels for most of the day.

In many patients with gout and uric acid nephrolithiasis, the urine pH remains persistently low throughout the day. This abnormality is related to a deficiency in ammonia buffer production by the kidney. Other factors that contribute to uric acid stone formation are hyperuricosuria and contraction of urine volume.

Complications and associated diseases. Patients with gout have a higher frequency of arterial hypertension and renal malfunction than do nongouty individuals, and they often have nephrosclerosis (1). The development of hyperuricemia in arterial hypertension appears to be related to an abnormality in uric acid transport by the renal tubules.

Diabetes mellitus, cardiac and cerebral atherosclerosis, and hypertriglyceridemia (3,17) all occur more frequently among those with gout. The precise explanation for these associations is not known, although a common connection with obesity has been suggested.

Avascular necrosis of bone, involving particularly the head of the femur, occurs with increased frequency in gouty individuals (18). In some instances this association is related to chronic alcoholism. The presence of lipoprotein abnormalities (hyperlipoproteinemia types II and IV) in a number of these cases has led to the suggestion that the bone necrosis may be caused by fat emboli.

Roentgenographic findings. At the time of the initial attack of gouty arthritis in younger individuals, roentgenographic examination of the affected joint (most often the first MTP joint) is usually normal. In older individuals signs of preexisting osteoarthritis are frequently found in this area. Later there is evidence of progressive damage of the articular cartilage and subchondral bone (19). Sharply defined marginal erosions of the subchondral bone have a thin shell-like overhanging edge of bone at the periphery. Such erosions occur most commonly in the first MTP joint (particularly in the base of the proximal phalanx) but are also found in the finger joints and other articulations affected by the disease.

Pathogenesis of acute gouty arthritis

Monosodium urate crystals. Monosodium urate is only sparingly soluble in body fluids and tends to precipitate in the tissues when the concentration in the plasma exceeds 8–9 mg/dl. These deposits form on the surface and within the substance of the articular cartilage as well as in the synovium (Fig 46–2) and related paraarticular structures, including bursae, tendons, and tendon sheaths. The basis for this affinity, which may be related to a preferential binding of urate to proteoglycans and other components of connective tissue, remains to be determined.

Inflammatory response. Acute gouty arthritis represents the inflammatory response induced by microcrystals of monosodium urate monohydrate which form within the joint cavity or, probably more commonly, are discharged into this space from preexisting intraarticular urate deposits ("crystal shedding") (20). Such crystals are invariably present (usually in abundance) in the synovial fluid of acutely inflamed joints, either contained within the cytoplasm of neutrophilic leukocytes or floating free.

The volume of synovia in the swollen joint tends to be large (often 50 ml or more in the knee) with a characteristically high white cell count (often 15,000/mm^3 or greater), containing a striking predominance of polymorphonuclear leukocytes (5). The crystals of monosodium urate monohydrate, which are rodlike or acerose (needle-shaped), average about 10μ in length. They are best seen by means of polarized light and are negatively birefringent (Fig 46–3). Experimental intrasynovial injection of these crystals has produced inflammation closely similar to natural gout (21).

Phagocytosis. Microcrystals of monosodium urate monohydrate (as well as other substances involved in the production of crystal-induced synovitis) are coated with plasma proteins, including immunoglobulins (22). IgG on these crystals may enhance their phagocytosis by neutrophilic leukocytes which carry Fc receptor sites on their surface. It has been postulated that once the microcrystals have been incorporated into phagolysosomes within the neutrophil, the surface proteins are removed, restoring the microcrystals' membrane-disrupting capacity.

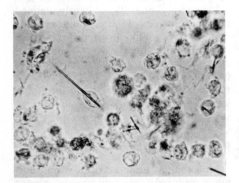

Fig 46–3. Photomicrograph of fresh preparation of synovial fluid obtained from the inflamed knee of a 45-year-old man with acute gouty arthritis. Note numerous small and large needle-shaped crystals of monosodium urate monohydrate which have been engulfed by neutrophilic leukocytes.

The phagocytosis of these microcrystals by polymorphonuclear leukocytes (and probably by phagocytic synovial lining cells as well) leads to the formation of a chemotactic factor that recruits additional leukocytes (23–25). Ingestion of urate crystals is followed by rapid degranulation and disintegration of these cells, with release of both cytoplasmic and lysosomal enzymes that may be responsible for dissolution of articular cartilage as well as injury to the soft tissue. Macrophages and synovial fibroblasts exposed to monosodium urate crystals are stimulated to produce prostaglandins and, in the case of fibroblasts, collagenase. Both prostaglandins and collagenase are believed to contribute to acute and chronic gouty inflammation and joint damage (26,27).

Note that urate crystals are not chemotactic per se but increase random motility of leukocytes. Phagocytosis is necessary for the production of chemotactic factors, one of which has been found to be a heat labile glycoprotein with a molecular weight of 8400 daltons (23).

The immediate mechanism of the initial crystallization is not fully known. In some instances gouty attacks take place after local trauma, which may rupture tophaceous deposits in the synovium and articular cartilage. Joint inflammation often develops in the wake of rapid fluctuations in serum urate levels (28,29). A sudden increase in serum urate concentration may lead to crystal precipitation in the already supersaturated synovial fluid, while a drop in serum urate concentration may give rise to the dissolution of the surface of intraarticular tophi and the release of undissolved crystals.

Gouty patients are also prone to develop acute arthritis after surgical procedures (postoperative gout), usually within 72 hours.

Eating, drinking, and the gout. The connection of gout with gluttony and the belief that attacks of articular inflammation followed sacrifice at the altar of Bacchus and Venus—that is to say, intemperance and venery—date to ancient times and serve as the basis for the extensive use of the gouty foot as a symbol of overindulgence and ill-gotten gain in satirical works throughout the centuries (Fig 46–4).

The association of primary gout with overeating and alcoholism is well documented. Approximately one-half of gouty individuals weigh 15% or more than ideal weight, and three-fourths or more exhibit hypertriglyceridemia, which appears to be correlated with the presence of obesity (17). It has been aptly noted that "the associates of a high [serum] uric acid are the associates of plenty" (30).

The observation that uric acid synthesis (as measured by the incorporation of glycine into urinary uric acid) is accelerated when the diet is fortified with protein, and

reports of the occasional correction of hyperuricemia in obese individuals by severe weight reduction (31) suggest that chronically excessive food intake may be import in persistent elevation in serum urate level. In general, however, adherence to a strict low-purine diet is followed by only a modest reduction in the concentration of serum urate, usually no more than 2 mg/dl (29).

The effects of heavy drinking, on the other hand, can be much more striking (28,29). The metabolism of ethanol gives rise to an increase in the concentration of blood lactate. Like a number of other small organic acids, lactic acid blocks the renal excretion of uric acid (presumably through inhibition of tubular secretion), and if the blood lactate level rises and remains above 20–25 mg/dl for a sufficient time, uric acid output by the kidney is sharply reduced. Recent studies suggest that alcohol also can increase urate production by activation of adenine nucleotide turnover (32).

The consumption of moonshine whiskey presents the additional hazard of lead poisoning (the lead derived from automobile radiators used in the distillation of this brew) and subsequent saturnine gout (33). The hyperuricemia that follows fasting is traceable to an increase in the plasma level of acetoacetic and β-hydroxybutyric acids (28).

When a large purine- and protein-rich meal is accompanied by the imbibition of copious amounts of ethanol, the lactic acid produced in the metabolism of the ethanol temporarily blocks the disposal of uric acid by the kidneys and leads to a greater rise in serum urate concentration than that produced by the same meal taken without spirituous fluids (29).

The rapid fluctuations in serum urate concentration induced by fasting, by the consumption of large amounts of ethanolic beverages, or especially by the combination of heavy drinking and a protein- and purine-rich meal are often followed by flares in gouty arthritis (aldermanic gout).

Similar swings in the level of serum urate precede the crises of gouty arthritis which often occur early in the course of treatment with uricosuric drugs or allopurinol or after the administration of various other drugs that affect the renal handling of uric acid, e.g., thiazides, furosemide, and ethacrynic acid.

Diagnosis

The diagnosis of gout should be considered in all patients who present the history and/or physical findings of characteristic inflammation described here. Individuals who have experienced monarticular arthritis involving the great toe and other joints of the feet are particularly suspect. Gouty inflammation is often mistaken for cellulitis because of the marked periarticular erythema and swelling. In wrist gout, for example, the entire hand may be swollen, as if severely injured, and it may be difficult to realize that there is underlying articular inflammation. By careful palpation, however, one can identify points of maximal tenderness over specific joints.

A record of uric acid stone, the presence of the disease in other members of the family, and the demonstration of hyperuricemia serve to strengthen the likelihood of gout. None of these features, however, is pathognomonic of gout. Each may exist coincidentally with other rheumatic diseases, a number of which may produce joint inflammation clinically indistinguishable from gout, e.g., calcium pyrophosphate dihydrate–induced synovitis (pseudogout) and calcific tendinitis.

It is improper to equate the finding of hyperuricemia with gout. Hyperuricemia is a necessary but not sufficient condition in the diagnosis of gout. Many individuals with hyperuricemia enjoy lifelong freedom from gout and show no evidence of urate deposits in their tissues (asymptomatic hyperuricemia) (34).

However, it is equally erroneous to dismiss the possibility of gout if the initial determination of serum urate concentration proves to be normal, since this may have been reduced from a naturally elevated value by antiinflammatory medication, e.g., large doses of salicylates, phenylbutazone, or corticosteroids.

Once considered, the diagnosis of gout can be established definitively and with little difficulty by 1) demonstration of the characteristic crystals of monosodium urate monohydrate in synovial fluid obtained from a joint either acutely inflamed (Fig 46–3) or asymptomatic (35) and/or 2) the demonstration of monosodium urate monohydrate in aspirates or tissue sections of tophaceous deposits (Fig 46–2) (5).

Only a single drop of fluid is necessary for detection of the tell-tale crystals, and even the small amount of synovia obtainable from the first metatarsophalangeal joint suffices.

The *needle-shaped crystals* of *sodium urate* usually range from 2μ–10μ in length, but may be much longer. Large numbers of crystals are generally present in the leukocytes of synovial fluid obtained during an acute attack.

The *strongly birefringent crystals* display *negative elongation (birefringence)* when viewed with a compensated polarized light microscope and a first-order red compensator is used (36). On occasion, repeated search of the synovial fluid may be required for detection of the monosodium urate crystals in gouty arthritis (37).

For histologic examination, care should be taken that the suspected tophus be fixed in absolute alcohol lest there be dissolution of the urate. The finding of

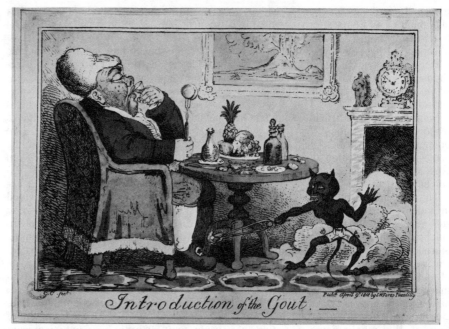

Fig 46–4. *Introduction of the Gout.* Copper-plate engraving by George Cruikshank, published by SW Fores, London, 1818. Note the decanter of wine on the table of the pinguid/gastronome and the illustration of a volcanic (gouty) eruption in the picture on the dining-room wall. (Reproduced by permission of the Trustees of the British Museum)

characteristic sharply defined erosions of subchondral bone on radiographic examination is also helpful in distinguishing gout from other forms of arthritis.

Course

The severity and rate of progression of untreated gouty arthritis are extremely variable. Some individuals experience no more than a few attacks in a lifetime. However, without treatment, these paroxysms can recur with increasing frequency and intensity and are associated with the gradual development of slowly progressive disability as a result of loss of articular cartilage, erosion of the subchondral bone, and infiltration of paraarticular structures. In extreme cases highly destructive joint disease and massive tophaceous deposits arise within a few years.

Treatment

The management of a patient with gout requires that 2 aspects be considered independently: 1) the immediate control of the acute attack of gouty arthritis; 2) the long-term treatment of hyperuricemia to prevent complications such as tophaceous deposits, joint destruction, renal calculi, or renal insufficiency. The approach to each is entirely different, the drugs used are dissimilar, and therapy aimed at one phase may in fact exacerbate the other.

However, current understanding of the pathophysiology of gout and the medications available make it possible to achieve both of these objectives successfully. The maintenance of normouricemia in most patients requires lifetime treatment, and it is important that the patient and his physician understand the rationale for treatment in this disease.

Management of acute gouty arthritis. Although *colchicine* was first used for "rheumatism" in the sixth century AD, it remains a valuable drug for treatment of an acute attack of gout. For the patient with a fully developed acute attack, 1 tablet (0.6 mg) of colchicine should be given every hour until the patient experiences relief of pain or develops side effects such as nausea or diarrhea. No more than 12 tablets should be given for any single acute attack in a 24-hour period.

Colchicine may also be administered intravenously (2 mg colchicine diluted with normal saline to a total volume of 20 cc and injected slowly over 5 minutes). Intravenous administration of colchicine produces a more prompt and effective response with fewer gastrointestinal side effects. No more than 4 mg of colchicine should be given intravenously during a 24-hour period.

Patients with renal insufficiency should be given even smaller doses, since they tend to excrete colchicine very slowly. About 75% of patients with acute gouty arthritis respond to colchicine. The best response occurs when colchicine is administered early in the acute attack and failure to respond is frequently the result of significant delay in therapy.

Colchicine has diagnostic as well as therapeutic value since a response to colchicine treatment in acute gouty arthritis is usually striking and occurs within a maximum of 48 hours after oral administration and within 12 hours of intravenous injection. In no other type of arthritis is there such a consistent and intense response to colchicine, and it thus may serve as a therapeutic trial, although it is not infallible.

Some patients with acute gout fail to respond, and occasionally patients with other types of arthritis, such as pseudogout, apatite deposition disease, or sarcoid arthritis, may show a response to colchicine.

The mechanisms of action of colchicine in patients with acute gouty arthritis are still not entirely clear. It is thought that colchicine acts by interfering with polymorphonuclear leukocyte function. Colchicine does interfere with the chemotaxis of leukocytes (38), but it is unlikely that this chemotactic effect is the major explanation for the impressive effects of colchicine in gouty arthritis. Further investigation of the mechanism of action of colchicine is still under way.

All the nonsteroidal antiinflammatory drugs are at least as effective as colchicine in the relief of acute gouty arthritis. These other agents, however, do not have the relative specificity for the gouty attack that colchicine has. However, because of the toxicity associated with colchicine, many patients prefer to use one of the nonsteroidal antiinflammatory agents.

Phenylbutazone and its analog, *oxyphenbutazone,* were the first of the nonsteroidal antiinflammatory drugs used in the treatment of gout and they proved effective. A dosage of 100 mg 4 times daily of phenylbutazone given for 2–3 days, with gradual tapering over the next few days, or oxyphenbutazone administered in an initial dose of 400 mg, with maintenance dosage of 100 mg 4 times daily, has been quite effective.

Although the toxic effects of phenylbutazone were minimal in the short-term use, potentially serious toxicity, such as bone marrow suppression, forces even the staunchest advocates to advise caution in its long-term use. Since other nonsteroidal agents have become available, they tend to be used more frequently for the treatment of gouty arthritis.

Indomethacin, in doses of 50 mg 3–4 times daily for 4–7 days, has been found very effective (39) and free from major toxicity. Some patients, however, do develop gastrointestinal intolerance, headaches, and other manifestations of toxicity from indomethacin and, therefore, must use one of the other agents.

Other nonsteroidal antiinflammatory drugs, such as ibuprofen, fenoprofen, naproxen, tolmetin sodium, sulindac, and piroxicam, have all been shown to be effective in the treatment of acute gouty arthritis. These should all be used in maximal recommended dosage as early as pos-

sible during an acute attack of gout and as soon as the symptoms have abated the drugs should gradually be tapered.

There is rarely any need for systemic corticosteroids or ACTH in the management of gout, since the previously mentioned drugs are all effective (40).

The rare exception is a patient who is having very severe recurrent acute attacks of gout, and either all other agents have failed or the patient is intolerant of the other drugs. In these instances some form of *corticosteroid* may be required. Although corticosteroids are effective, approximately one-third of patients treated with steroids have a flare of the disease after discontinuation of therapy; colchicine prophylaxis is of value in preventing this type of recurrence. Intraarticular depot corticosteroids can be used in patients with single joint involvement who are unable to take oral medications.

With the exception of phenylbutazone, none of the drugs used for the treatment of acute gouty arthritis have any significant effect on the serum uric acid concentration.

Treatment of hyperuricemia in patients with gout. Despite the fact that the hyperuricemia associated with gout might arise from a variety of causes, it seems quite clear that hyperuricemia still provides an acceptable explanation for the development of tophaceous deposits. Hyperuricemic body fluids are also a source from which crystals may precipitate to bring about an acute attack of gouty arthritis. The elimination of hyperuricemic body pools is the rationale for the treatment of hyperuricemia in patients with gout.

Since adequate means are now available for diagnosing hyperuricemia in patients with gout and effective drugs can decrease the serum urate concentration, there should no longer be any excuse for gouty patients developing progressive tophaceous complications. Therapy aimed at lowering the serum urate concentration is indicated in any patient with documented gout (either by demonstration of microcrystalline sodium urate in synovial fluid or documentation of uric acid deposition in the form of tophi) who continues to be hyperuricemic (serum urate persistently about 7 μg/dl).

Two types of treatment are available to decrease the serum urate concentration: 1) uricosuric therapy, 2) the use of a xanthine oxidase inhibitor to inhibit uric acid production.

Uricosuric acid therapy. The objective of uricosuric therapy is to increase the renal excretion of uric acid and thereby reduce the serum urate concentration. Uricosuric drugs act in the kidney by blocking the tubular reabsorption of urate. When uric acid lowering agents are used, frequent determination of the serum urate concentration is essential since this is the only guide to effective management.

To avoid the sudden exposure of the kidney to large quantities of uric acid and to prevent precipitation of an acute attack of gouty arthritis, uricosuric drugs should be started at low doses and gradually increased over 7–10 days.

Probenecid has proved to be an effective uricosuric agent for gout (41). One-gram daily dosage results in a mean increase of approximately 50% in the renal excretion of uric acid in gouty subjects and a mean fall of one-third of the serum urate concentration. Because the biological half-life of probenecid is 6–12 hours, it is advisable to administer this drug in divided doses. Maximum recommended daily dosage is 3 grams.

If toxicity occurs with probenecid or if this drug fails to be effective, administration of *sulfinpyrazone* is recommended. This phenylbutazone derivative has potent uricosuric but no antiinflammatory properties. The dosage should be increased until the desired serum urate concentration is achieved; the maximum dosage is 800 mg/day in divided doses.

Both probenecid and sulfinpyrazone have relatively few side effects and are usually well tolerated. The most common adverse reaction is gastric intolerance, although fever and drug rashes have been encountered.

Concomitant administration of salicylates in any dosage nullifies the uricosuric effect in both these agents. Acetaminophen, which has no effect on the serum urate concentration, may be used as an analgesic or antipyretic in patients with hyperuricemia when they are taking uricosuric drugs.

Inhibition of uric acid production. Another approach to the therapy of hyperuricemia is to inhibit uric acid production rather than to increase uric acid excretion. *Allopurinol,* a potent inhibitor of xanthine oxidase, has been very effective for this purpose (42). This compound is structurally similar to hypoxanthine. As a xanthine oxidase inhibitor, it prevents the conversion of hypoxanthine to xanthine and of xanthine to uric acid. Thus, these other oxypurines accumulate in the blood and are subsequently excreted.

Allopurinol, administered in doses of 300–800 mg/day is well tolerated by most patients. Some patients have shown drug rash, transient leukopenia, and transient aberations of liver function, but these side effects have rarely been serious and overall the drug has been well tolerated.

An acute attack of gouty arthritis may be precipitated during the early stages of allopurinol administration in a manner similar to the effect of institution of uricosuric therapy. This may be prevented by starting with small doses of allopurinol and gradually increasing the dose.

Since it has been shown that the renal clearance of oxypurines is much greater than that of uric acid and the solubility of xanthine and hypoxanthine exceeds that of uric acid, the inhibition of xanthine oxidase appears to be advantageous. Despite some of the apparent advantages of allopurinol, some theoretic concerns remain about the ultimate development of xanthine kidney stones in patients who received allopurinol for many years. A few instances of xanthine kidney stone formation in hyperexcretors of uric acid taking allopurinol for many years have been reported. Thus, it is generally believed that the conventional uricosuric therapy is sufficient for most patients with gout and hyperuricemia and that allopurinol should be reserved for specific indications.

The primary indications for the use of allopurinol in patients with hyperuricemia in gout include:

1. Patients who respond poorly to maximal uricosuric therapy, i.e., patients with renal impairment who cannot excrete an increased uric acid load. Allopurinol administration may afford the only means by which such patients may achieve normal serum urate concentrations.

2. Patients who have allergic reactions, or intolerance to uricosuric drugs

3. Patients with uric acid renal calculi. Uric acid calculi are a manifestation of the urinary uric acid concentration and only a xanthine oxidase inhibitor can lower urinary uric acid excretion while still causing a decrease in the serum urate concentration.

4. Patients with massive tophaceous involvement who may require treatment with both agents to block uric acid production and increase uric acid excretion

5. Patients with hyperuricemia secondary to myeloproliferative disorders, especially before treatment with cytotoxic agents. In some patients acute uric acid tubular blockade might otherwise develop.

It should be remembered that allopurinol is a potentiator of the purine antagonist agents frequently used as cytotoxic drugs (for example, 6-mercaptopurine and azathioprine). Therefore, the dosage of these drugs must be decreased if allopurinol is also administered.

Interval treatment. The interval or intercritical period in gout is between acute gouty attacks. Treatment during this time is concerned primarily with maintaining the serum urate concentration in the normal range and preventing subsequent acute gouty attacks. This therapy usually consists of a uric acid lowering agent (either a uricosuric drug or allopurinol) and prophylactic colchicine usually in doses of 2 or 3 tablets daily.

To be effective, the uric acid lowering agent must be given in a dosage sufficient to lower the serum uric acid concentration to the normal range. This aspect of therapy should help decrease the incidence of gouty nephropathy as well as prevent the development of tophaceous complications.

The uric acid concentration must be maintained in the normal range for the duration of the patient's lifetime. The prophylactic use of colchicine is helpful in preventing recurrent acute attacks. If the patient has had only one attack of gout, it is reasonable to discontinue colchicine or antiinflammatory agents after the uric acid has been returned to the normal range. However, if the patient continues to have recurrent attacks (more than 2 per year), prophylactic colchicine is useful in preventing these recurrences.

The only consideration currently given to diet is the avoidance of foods known to be of very high purine content (e.g., kidneys, liver, sweetbreads, sardines, anchovies, etc.). There is no therapeutic use for a purine-free diet. If significant hyperuricemia is a problem, it is better controlled with uricosuric drugs, than by dietary means alone.

For diagnostic purposes, a patient should be on a purine-free diet for 2–3 days before collection of 24-hour urinary samples for uric acid determinations used to establish whether the patient is an overproducer or underexcretor of uric acid.

Medications known to produce hyperuricemia and circumstances known to provoke acute attacks of gout should be avoided if possible in patients with gout. These include drugs such as thiazides and salicylates, alcohol, fasting or severe dieting, and physical or emotional stress.

Treatment of asymptomatic hyperuricemia. With the increased use of multiphasic screening programs in hospitals and clinics, the unanticipated or asymptomatic hyperuricemia is being recognized with increasing frequency. In patients with hyperuricemia associated with gout in whom deposition of urate in joints or other tissues has been demonstrated, it is quite clear that lowering the serum uric acid concentration in the blood is a rational basis for treatment.

However, no definitive data show the fate of untreated patients with asymptomatic hyperuricemia. Therefore, no firm guidelines exist for which of these patients should be treated. There is, however, some concern that asymptomatic hyperuricemia could result in renal dysfunction for some patients, even before they have gouty attacks. Studies have shown that some patients with asymptomatic hyperuricemia may have specific types of renal tubular dysfunction (43).

At the present time, it is clear that the likelihood of acute gouty arthritis increases proportionately to the serum urate concentration and that patients with serum urate concentrations greater than 9 μg/dl have a great chance of developing clinical gout.

It is probably, however, adequate to treat the clinical gout when it occurs.

There seems to be no rationale to treating asymptomatic hyperuricemia—either that occurring de novo or that related to ingestion of certain medications.

However, patients with persistent hyperuricemia should have their 24-hour urinary uric acid measured. If they are found to be significant hyperexcretors of uric acid (urinary uric acid excretions greater than 1,200 mg/24 hours), they are at greater risk for the development of uric acid renal calculi and should be treated with allopurinol to lower both the serum and urinary uric acid.

Surgical excision of tophi is rarely indicated, but if the tophus is very large and bulky, if there is external drainage, or if it is located in an area that bears weight or excessive pressure, then its removal might benefit the patient. However, excision of tophi or arthroplasties to repair severely deformed gouty joints should not be undertaken until the serum uric acid is brought into the normal range with appropriate medication and any evidence of acute gouty attacks are brought under control.

1. Grahame R, Scott JT: Clinical survey of 354 patients with gout. Ann Rheum Dis 20:895–900, 1977

2. Gutman AB: The past 4 decades of progress in the knowledge of gout, with an assessment of the present status. Arthritis Rheum 16:431–445, 1973

3. Wyngaarden JB, Kelley WN: Gout and Hyperuricemia. New York, Grune & Stratton, 1976

4. Talbott JH, Yü T-F: Gout and Uric Acid Metabolism. New York, Stratton Intercontinental Medical Book Corporation, 1976

5. Wallace SL, Robinson H, Masi AT, Decker JL, McCarty DJ, Yü T-F: Preliminary criteria for the classification of the acute arthritis of primary gout. Arthritis Rheum 20:895–900, 1977

6. Boss GR, Seegmiller JE: Hyperuricemia and gout: classification, complications and management. N Engl J Med 300:1459–1468, 1979

7. Yü T-F: Urolithiasis in hyperuricemia and gout. J Urol 126:424–430, 1981

8. Rodnan GP: Early theories concerning etiology and pathogenesis of the gout. Arthritis Rheum 8:599–609, 1965

9. Nicholls A, Snaith ML, Scott JT: Effect of oestrogen therapy on plasma and urinary levels of uric acid. Br Med J 1:449–451, 1973

10. Healey LA, Bayani-Sioson PS: A defect in the renal excretion of uric acid in Filipinos. Arthritis Rheum 14:721–726, 1971

11. Hall AP, Barry PE, Dawber TR, McNamara PM: Epidemiology of gout and hyperuricemia: a longterm population study. Am J Med 42:27–37, 1967

12. Becker MA, Seegmiller JE: Genetic aspects of gout. Ann Rev Med 25:15–28, 1974

13. Yü T-F, Weinreb N, Wittman R, Wasserman LR: Secondary gout associated with chronic myeloproliferative disorders. Semin Arthritis Rheum 6:247–256, 1976

14. Yü T-F, Berger L: Renal disease in primary gout: a study of 253 gout patients with proteinuria. Semin Arthritis Rheum 4:293–305, 1975

15. Yü T-F, Berger L: Impaired renal function in gout: its association with hypertensive vascular disease and intrinsic renal disease. Am J Med 72:95–100, 1982

16. Bluestone R, Waisman J, Klinenberg JR: The gouty kidney. Semin Arthritis Rheum 7:97–113, 1977

17. Yü T-F, Dorph DJ, Smith H: Hyperlipidemia in primary gout. Semin Arthritis Rheum 7:233–244, 1978

18. Mielants H, Veys EM, DeBussere A, Van Der Jeught J: Avascular necrosis and its relation to lipid

and purine metabolism. J Rheumatol 2:430–436, 1975

19. Resnick D: The radiographic manifestations of gouty arthritis. Crit Rev Diag Imag 9:265–335, 1977

20. Ginsberg M, Kozin F: Mechanisms of cellular interaction with monosodium urate crystals. Arthritis Rheum 21:896–903, 1978

21. McCarty DJ Jr: Crystal deposition joint disease. Ann Rev Med 25:279–288, 1974

22. Hasselbacher P, Schumacher HR: Immunoglobulin in tophi and on the surface of monosodium urate crystals. Arthritis Rheum 21:353–361, 1978

23. Spilberg I, Gallacher A, Mehta JM, Mandell B: Urate crystal-induced chemotactic factor: isolation and partial characterization. J Clin Invest 58:815–819, 1976

24. Phelps P, Andrews R, Rosenbloom J: Demonstration of chemotactic factor in human gout: further characterization of occurrence and structure. J Rheumatol 8:889–894, 1981

25. Spilberg I, Mehta J, Simchowitz L: Induction of a chemotactic factor from human neutrophils by diverse crystals. J Lab Clin Med 100:399–404, 1982

26. McMillan RM, Hasselbacher P, Hahn JL, Harris ED Jr: Interaction of murine macrophages with monosodium urate crystals: stimulation of lysosomal enzyme release and prostaglandin synthesis. J Rheumatol 8:555–562, 1981

27. McMillan RM, Vater CA, Hasselbacher P,

Hahn J, Harris ED Jr: Induction of collagenase and prostaglandin synthesis in synovial fibroblasts treated with monosodium urate crystals. J Pharm Pharmacol 33:382–383, 1981

28. Maclachlan MJ, Rodnan GP: Effects of food, fast and alcohol on serum uric acid and acute attacks of gout. Am J Med 42:38–57, 1967

29. Rodnan GP: The pathogenesis of aldermanic gout: procatarctic role of fluctuations in serum urate concentration in gouty arthritis produced by feast and alcohol (abstract). Arthritis Rheum 23:737, 1980

30. Acheson RM, Chan Y-K: New Haven Survey of Joint Diseases: the prediction of serum uric acid in a general population. J Chron Dis 21:543–553, 1969

31. Scott JT, Sturge RA: The effect of weight loss on plasma and urinary uric acid and lipid levels. Adv Exp Med Biol 76B:274–277, 1977

32. Feller J, Fox IH: Ethanol induced hyperuricemia. N Engl J Med 307:1598–1602, 1982

33. Halls JT, Ball GV: Saturnine gout: a review of 42 patients. Semin Arthritis Rheum 11:307–314, 1982

34. Rakic MT, Valkenburg HA, Davidson RT, Engels JP, Mikkelsen WM, Neel JV, Duff IF, Himes S: Observations on the natural history of hyperuricemia and gout. I. An 18 year follow-up 19 gouty families. Am J Med 37:862–871, 1964

35. Agudelo CA, Weinberger A, Schumacher HR, et al: Definitive diagnosis of gout by identification of

urate crystals in asymptomatic metatarsophalangeal joints. Arthritis Rheum 22:559–560, 1979

36. Gatter RA: The compensated polarized light microscope in clinical rheumatology. Arthritis Rheum 17:253–255, 1974

37. Schumacher HR, Jimenez SA, Gibson T, Pascual E, Traycoff R, Dorwart BB, Reginato AJ: Acute gouty arthritis without urate crystals identified on initial examination of synovial fluid: report on 9 patients. Arthritis Rheum 18:603–612, 1975

38. Caner JEZ: Cochicine inhibition of chemotactic migration of human polymorphonuclear leukocytes. Arthritis Rheum 7:297–298, 1964

39. Elder TD, Plotz CM: Discussion, Proceedings of Conference on Gout and Purine Metabolism. Arthritis Rheum 8:881–882, 1965

40. Klinenberg JR: Current concepts of hyperuricemia and gout. California Medicine 110:231–243, 1969

41. Yü TF, Gutman AB: Principles of current management of primary gout. Am J Med Sci 254:893–900, 1967

42. Klinenberg JR. Goldfinger S, Seegmiller JE: The effectiveness of the xanthine oxidase inhibitor allopurinol in the treatment of gout. Ann Intern Med 62:639–647, 1965

43. Klinenberg JR, Gonick H, Dornfeld L: Renal function abnormalities in patients with asymptomatic hyperuricemia. Arthritis Rheum 18:725–730, 1975

47. Calcium pyrophosphate deposition disease

Identification of the slightly soluble crystals of calcium pyrophosphate dihydrate (CPPD) ($Ca_2P_2O_7 \cdot 2H_2O$) in synovial fluid permits isolation of this condition from other inflammatory and degenerative arthropathies (Fig 47–1) (1). Thus, the preferred name for the disease incorporates its only specific feature.

The term **chondrocalcinosis** (2) is often used to describe the radiologic appearance of calcified joint cartilage, although it is now clear that CPPD crystals are also deposited in tendons, ligaments, articular capsules, and synovium as well as in cartilage. Moreover, it is clear that cartilaginous calcification can also be due to dicalcium phosphate dihydrate ($CaHPO_4 \cdot 2H_2O$), a much more soluble orthophosphate, or to hydroxyapatite ($Ca_5OH(PO_4)_3 \cdot H_2O$), a relatively insoluble orthophosphate (3), or to calcium oxalate. The term **pseudogout** was originally used to describe the acute inflammatory gout-like attacks that occur in patients with CPPD deposits (1).

Pathologic surveys of those who died at or near 72 years of age indicate that about 6% of the elderly population have articular CPPD crystal deposits (3). Radiologic surveys support this estimate and show a steadily increasing prevalence with advancing age, so that nearly 25% of individuals show evidence of chondrocalcinosis by the ninth decade of life (4,5). The incidence of symptomatic disease is about half that of classic gouty arthritis (6,7). Men are affected somewhat more often than women (1.4:1).

Clinical features. The acute pseudogout syndrome is only one of a number of clinical patterns exhibited by symptomatic patients (6). Joint inflammation and degeneration may occur independently or overlap, thus simulating many other arthritic diseases and leading to diagnostic confusion.

Acute pseudogout is marked by inflammation in 1 or more joints lasting for several days or longer. Although these episodes are generally less painful, these self-limited attacks may be as abrupt in

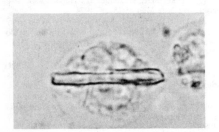

Fig 47–1. Neutrophilic leukocyte in fresh preparation of synovial fluid from an 84-year-old woman with acute inflammation of the knee (pseudogout). Note rod-shaped crystal of calcium pyrophosphate dihydrate.

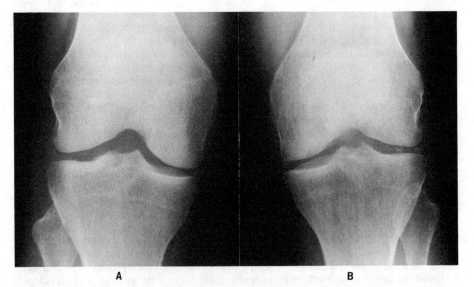

A   B

Fig 47–2. Anteroposterior radiographs of the knees of a 40-year-old woman showing greater cartilaginous calcification in the left knee (**B**) in which fracture of the patella had occurred than in the nontraumatized right knee (**A**). (Illustration provided by Dr DJ McCarty Jr)

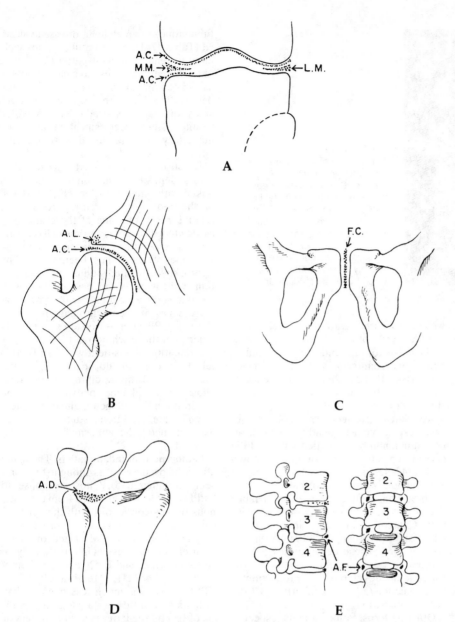

Fig 47–3. Diagrammatic representation of characteristic sites of CPPD crystal deposition. **A,** A.C. = articular cartilage; L.M. and M.M. = lateral and medial meniscus in knee joint shown in anteroposterior projection. **B,** A.L. = acetabular labrum in anteroposterior projection of hip joint. **C,** F.C. = fibrocartilaginous symphysis pubis in anteroposterior projection of pelvis. **D,** A.D. = articular disc of the wrist in anteroposterior projection. **E,** A.F. = anulus fibrosus of intervertebral discs in anteroposterior and lateral views. (From Bulletin on the Rheumatic Diseases)

onset and as severe as true gouty arthritis. "Petite" attacks occur, as in gout. The knee is the site of nearly half of all these paroxysms, although involvement of nearly all other synovial joints, including the first metatarsophalangeal joint, has been noted.

Provocation of acute attacks by surgery is common in both gout and pseudogout (8.3% of 168 gouty patients versus 9.4% of 106 patients with pseudogout). Severe medical illness (e.g., cerebrovascular accident or myocardial infarction) provoked attacks in 20.3% of 167 gouty subjects and in 24% of 104 patients with pseudogout (8). About 25% of patients show this pattern. Men predominate. Patients are typi-

cally asymptomatic between acute attacks.

About 5% of patients have multiple joint involvement, usually symmetrical, with low grade inflammation lasting for weeks or months. Morning stiffness, fatigue, synovial thickening, localized pitting edema, flexion contractures, and elevated sedimentation rate often lead to a mistaken impression of rheumatoid arthritis (RA). Prominent involvement of knees, wrists, and metatarsophalangeal joints further simulates rheumatoid arthritis in some patients.

Nearly half of all patients experience progressive degeneration of multiple joints. The knees are most commonly af-

fected, followed by the wrists, metacarpophalangeal (MCP) joints, hips, shoulders, elbows, and ankles. Although there is some overlap with the patterns of involvement in primary osteoarthritis (e.g., hip and knee), the joint degeneration associated with CPPD crystal deposits is unique.

Distal interphalangeal and proximal interphalangeal finger joint involvement (manifested by Heberden's and Bouchard's nodes) and first carpometacarpal joint involvement are no more common than would be expected by chance alone in an elderly population. Symmetrical involvement is the rule, although degeneration may be more advanced on one side, especially when severe trauma or fracture has occurred (Fig 47–2). Flexion contractures of the above-mentioned joints and varus deformities of the knees are common.

As in gouty arthritis, about 10% of patients with CPPD deposits are positive for rheumatoid factor (8), although patients with the "pseudorheumatoid" picture are no more likely to have positive tests than those with other clinical patterns. The negative association of RA and gouty arthritis does not hold for CPPD deposition, and about 1% of patients with these crystals have definite RA (6).

Crystals are sometimes not seen in fluid from joints in which there is no radiographic evidence of chondrocalcinosis, especially in those showing extensive joint space narrowing. Fine detail magnification may be helpful in detection of small deposits.

Changes in metacarpophalangeal joints, such as squaring of the bone ends, subchondral cysts, or hooklike osteophytes that are characteristic features of the arthropathy associated with hemochromatosis, are also found in patients with CPPD crystal deposition alone (9,10). These changes do occur more frequently in patients with CPPD crystal deposits and hemochromatosis than in those with crystal deposits only (11).

Another controlled study of the radiographic appearance of joint degeneration associated with CPPD crystal deposits disclosed certain differences from uncomplicated primary osteoarthritis (12). One of these is the occurrence in CPPD crystal deposition disease of isolated, patellofemoral joint space narrowing. Such differences may provide helpful clinical clues for diagnosis.

Most joints with radiologically evident CPPD calcification are not symptomatic, even in patients with symptoms in other articulations. Many (or even most) patients with CPPD crystal deposits do not have joint symptoms at all. A recent study of volunteer subjects in a home for the elderly revealed radiographic evidence of putative CPPD crystal deposits in 27.6% of knee joints. Wrist complaints and genu varus deformities, not acute attacks of

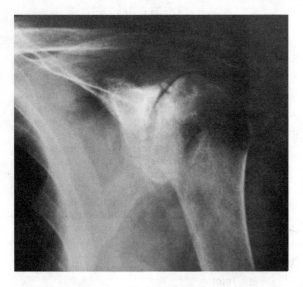

Fig 47–4. Anteroposterior view of left shoulder of a 70-year-old woman with radiographically demonstrable CPPD crystal deposits. There is nearly complete loss of joint space and severe destructive changes are present in the humeral head resembling those found in neuropathic arthropathy. The neurologic examination, however, was entirely normal. (Illustration provided by Dr DJ McCarty Jr)

joint inflammation, were more common in those with CPPD deposits as compared with subjects without CPPD deposits in the same population.

Radiologic features. The characteristic appearance of punctate and linear densities in articular hyaline or fibrocartilage is of diagnostic value. Trauma often accentuates the calcific process, as shown in Fig 47–2. The most characteristic sites of crystal deposition are presented diagrammatically in Fig 47–3. When the deposits are typical and unequivocal, the radiographic appearance is quite specific. Interpretation of atypical or faint deposits is often difficult. Fine detail radiographs of thin parts (such as hands) and focal-spot magnification views of thick parts (such as knees) may be helpful.

Calcific deposits may also occur in articular capsules, ligaments, and tendons. Synovial deposits have been so massive as to be mistaken for chondromatosis (13). Although the earliest calcific deposits occur in radiographically normal cartilage, degenerative changes often supervene with the passage of time (14).

For clinical purposes, a patient may be screened for CPPD crystal deposits with 4

Table 47–1. Classification of CPPD crystal deposition disease

Hereditary
    Slovakian
    Chilean
    Dutch
    French
    LaCrosse
Sporadic (idiopathic)
Probable metabolic disease associations
    Hyperparathyroidism
    Hemochromatosis
    Hypothyroidism
    Gout
    Hypomagnesemia
    Hypophosphatasia
    Aging

well-exposed radiographs, an anteroposterior (AP) view of both knees, an AP view of the pelvis for hips and symphysis pubis, and a posteroanterior view of the hands and wrists. If these show no evidence of CPPD deposition, it is unlikely that further study will prove fruitful.

Associated disorders. An associated severe destructive arthropathy has been reported in a number of patients with CPPD crystal deposition. An example is shown in Fig 47–4. In most cases, neurologic examination is entirely normal (14).

Three consecutive cases of mild tabes dorsalis were reported, however, with both Charcot arthropathy involving the knees and polyarticular CPPD crystal deposition (16). These observations led the authors to postulate that tabetic neuropathic joints develop in that proportion of the population (5%) with underlying CPPD crystal deposition.

Other patterns. Some patients, especially in familial series, have exhibited straightening and stiffening of the spine, simulating ankylosing spondylitis (17). True bony ankylosis of joints has been reported. Other patients have been thought to have rheumatic fever because of short-lived acute attacks of arthritis in multiple joints. Still others with mild attacks have been thought to have psychogenic joint complaints. Attacks induced by trauma are often called traumatic arthritis.

Thus, it is clear that articular complaints associated with CPPD crystal deposition can mimic not only gout, but rheumatoid arthritis, osteoarthritis, neuropathic arthropathy, and rarely, ankylosing spondylitis, rheumatic fever, psychogenic rheumatism, and traumatic arthritis. A patient may show 1 disease pattern (usually inflammatory) early in the disease course and later manifest another pattern (usually degenerative).

Etiologic classification. Cases of arthritis associated with CPPD crystal deposition can be classified as **hereditary, sporadic**

(idiopathic), or **metabolic disease-associated** (Table 47–1). Most familial series yield an autosomal dominant pattern and none of the hereditary cases have had any of the associated metabolic diseases discussed below. It is likely that a more thorough study of many "sporadic" cases would result in their reclassification as either hereditary or metabolic disease-associated.

Because of the high prevalence of CPPD crystal deposition, the condition has been linked with other disorders (18,19). Based on the frequency of such reports and the relative rarity of some of these allegedly associated disorders, the most likely significant associations are listed in Table 47–1. None of these has been proved by rigorously controlled studies. The association with aging is the best documented. Even in series of patients with hyperparathyroidism or hemochromatosis, those showing CPPD deposition are significantly older than those who do not (6).

Evaluation of a patient with CPPD crystal deposition should include measurements of serum calcium, magnesium, phosphorus, alkaline phosphatase, iron and iron-binding capacity, glucose, T_4 level, and urate. Additional studies should be made if metabolic abnormalities are uncovered.

Pathogenesis of inflammation. The acute attack of pseudogout is thought to represent an inflammatory host response to CPPD crystals that are shed from cartilaginous tissues contiguous with the synovial cavity (20). Phagocytosis of crystals by polymorphonuclear (PMN) and mononuclear phagocytes results in release of lysosomal enzymes and PMN-derived chemotactic factor (21). Membranolysis by CPPD crystals is much less marked than with sodium urate crystals (22) and binding of IgG by the latter is several orders of magnitude greater (23).

Inorganic pyrophosphate metabolism. Plasma and urinary inorganic pyrophosphate (PPi) levels are not altered in patients with CPPD crystal deposition (24,25). The concentration of synovial fluid PPi is elevated in most joints afflicted with CPPD crystal deposition (26), but this is not specific for this disease, since similar elevations are found in joint fluids from patients with osteoarthritis or other forms of joint diseases (27,28). Levels of PPi in synovial fluid correlate with the degree of osteoarthritis as estimated radiologically, irrespective of the clinical diagnosis (28) and the estimated turnover of PPi in joint fluid is similarly related (29). Joint fluid PPi levels have been found to be consistently lower during an acute attack than after subsidence of inflammation, probably because of fuller equilibration with plasma during the acute phase (28).

Articular chondrocytes are the most likely source of the excess synovial fluid PPi, as it has been shown that cartilage slices in organ culture liberate PPi into the surrounding medium (30). Such release occurs from both adult and immature hyaline and fibrocartilage from several species of animals, including humans (31). Release of PPi closely parallels release of alkaline phosphatase (30) and of proteoglycan (31). Again, this does not appear to be a specific phenomenon.

Crystal clearance. Radiolabeled synthetic CPPD crystals injected into human and rabbit joints were removed in inverse proportion to crystal size over a period of several weeks (rabbit) to several months (human) (32). Endocytosis and intracellular dissolution by fixed synovial macrophages appear to be the predominant routes of removal. There may be a "circulation" of crystals in some patients with the joint fluid crystal concentration representing the net effect of shedding from cartilage and synovial endocytosis and dissolution.

Treatment. Unlike uratic gout, there is no means available at present to remove CPPD crystals from joints. Treatment of the "associated" diseases such as hyperparathyroidism, hemochromatosis, or myxedema does not result in resorption of CPPD crystal deposits. In fact, thyroid hormone replacement is reported to lead to emergence of symptomatic disease (33).

Acute attacks in large joints can be treated by thorough aspiration or by aspiration combined with injection of microcrystalline corticosteroid esters. Phenylbutazone, indomethacin, other nonsteroidal antiinflammatory agents, or salicylates seem effective. Colchicine in usual therapeutic doses given intravenously appears to be effective in pseudogout (34). Oral administration of colchicine is less predictably effective in pseudogout than in gout (6). Whether crystal removal would prevent or slow the evolution of degenerative cartilaginous and bony changes is an important but still unanswered question.

1. McCarty DJ, Kohn NN, Faires JS: The significance of calcium phosphate crystals in the synovial fluid of arthritic patients: the "pseudogout syndrome". I. Clinical aspects. Ann Intern Med 56:711–737, 1962

2. Zitan D, Sitaj S: Articular chondrocalcinosis. Ann Rheum Dis 22:142–170, 1963

3. McCarty DJ, Hogan JM, Gatter RA, Grossman M: Studies on pathological calcifications in human cartilage. I. Prevalence and types of crystal deposits in the menisci of 215 cadavera. J Bone Joint Surg 48A:309–325, 1966

4. Ellman MH, Levin B: Chondrocalcinosis in elderly persons. Arthritis Rheum 18:43–47, 1975

5. Menin Y, Monville C, Ryckewaert A: Chondrocalcinosis over eighty (abstract #438). Proceedings XIVth International Congress of Rheumatology, San Francisco, California, June 1977

6. McCarty DJ: Calcium pyrosphate crystal deposition disease: pseudogout, articular chondrocalcinosis, Arthritis and Allied Conditions. Ed 9. DJ McCarty, ed. Philadelphia, Lea & Febiger, 1979, pp 1276–1299

7. O'Duffy JD: Clinical studies of acute pseudogout attacks: comments on prevalence, predispositions and treatment. Arthritis Rheum (suppl) 19:349–352, 1976

8. Wallace SL, Robinson H, Masi AT, Decker JL, McCarty DJ, Yu T-F: Preliminary criteria for the classification of the acute arthritis of primary gout. Arthritis Rheum 20:895–900, 1977

9. Martel W, Champion CK, Thompson GR, Carter TL: A roentgenographically distinctive arthropathy in some patients with pseudogout syndrome. Am J Roentgenol 109:587–605, 1970

10. Hamilton EBD, Williams R, Barlow K, Smith PM: The arthropathy of idiopathic haemochromatosis. Q J Med 37:171–182, 1968

11. Atkins CJ, McIvor J, Smith PM, Hamilton E, Williams R: Chondrocalcinosis and arthropathy: studies in haemochromatosis and in idiopathic chondrocalcinosis. Q J Med 39:71–82, 1970

12. Resnick D, Niwaygama G, Goergen TG, Utsinger DD, Shapiro RF, Haselwood DH, Weisner KB: Clinical, radiographic, and pathologic abnormalities in calcium pyrophosphate dihydrate deposition disease. Radiology 122:1–15, 1977

13. Ellman MH, Krieger MI, Brown N: Pseudogout mimicking synovial chondromatosis. J Bone Joint Surg 57A:863–865, 1975

14. Zitnan D, Sitaj S: Natural cause of articular chondrocalcinosis. Arthritis Rheum (suppl) 19:363–390, 1976

15. Menkes CJ, Simon F, Delrieu F, Forest M, Delbarre F: Destructive arthropathy in chondrocalcinosis articularis. Arthritis Rheum (suppl) 19:329–348, 1976

16. Jacobelli S, McCarty DJ, Silcox DC, Mall JC: Calcium pyrophosphate dihydrate crystal deposition disease in neuropathic joints: four cases of polyarticular involvement. Ann Intern Med 79:340–347, 1973

17. Reginato A, Valenzuela F, Martinez V, Passano G, Daza S: Polyarticular and familial chondrocalcinosis. Arthritis Rheum 13:197–213, 1970

18. McCarty DJ, Silcox DC, Coe F, Jacobelli S, Reiss E, Genan TH, Ellman M: Diseases associated with calcium pyrophosphate dihydrate crystal deposition—a controlled study. Am J Med 56:704–714, 1974

19. Hamilton EBD: Diseases associated with CPPD deposition disease. Arthritis Rheum (suppl) 19:353–357, 1967

20. Bennett RM, Lehr JR, McCarty DJ: Crystal shedding and acute pseudogout: an hypothesis based on a therapeutic failure. Arthritis Rheum 19:93–97, 1976

21. Tse RL, Phelps P: Polymorphonuclear leukocyte motility in vitro. V. Release of chemotactic activity following phagocytosis of calcium pyrophosphate crystals, diamond dust and urate crystals. J Lab Clin Med 76:403–415, 1970

22. Wallingford WR, McCarty DJ: Differential membranolytic effects of microcrystalline sodium urate and calcium pyrophosphate dihydrate. J Exp Med 133:100–112, 1971

23. Kozin F, McCarty DJ: Protein binding to monosodium urate monohydrate, calcium pyrophosphate dihydrate and silicon dioxide crystals. I. Physical characteristics. J Lab Clin Med 89:1314–1325, 1977

24. Pflug M, McCarty DJ, Kawahara F: Basal urinary pyrophosphate excretion in pseudogout. Arthritis Rheum 12:228–231, 1969

25. Ryan LM, Kozin F, McCarty DJ: Quantification of human inorganic pyrophosphate 1: normal volumes in osteoarthritis and calcium pyrophosphate crystal deposition disease. Arthritis Rheum 22:886–891, 1979

26. Russell RGG, Bisaz S, Donath A, Morgan DB, Fleish H: Inorganic pyrophosphate in plasma in normal persons and in patients with hypophosphatasia, osteogenesis imperfecta, and other disorders of bone. J Clin Invest 50:961–969, 1971

27. Altman R, Muniz O, Pita JC, Howell D: Microanalysis of inorganic pyrophosphate (PPi) in synovial fluid and plasma. Arthritis Rheum 16:171–178, 1973

28. Silcox DC, McCarty DJ: Elevated inorganic pyrophosphate concentrations in synovial fluids in osteoarthritis and pseudogout. J Lab Clin Med 83:518–531, 1974

29. Camerlain M, McCarty DJ, Silcox DC, Jung A: Inorganic pyrophosphate pool size and turnover rate in arthritic joints. J Clin Invest 55:1373–1381, 1975

30. Howell DS, Muniz O, Pita JC, Enis JE: Extrusion of pyrophosphate into extracellular media by osteoarthritic cartilage incubates. J Clin Invest 56:1473–1480, 1975

31. Ryan LM, Cheung HS, McCarty DJ: Extrusion of inorganic pyrophosphate (PPi) by mature lapine and canine hyaline and fibrocartilage (abstract). Arthritis Rheum 22:653–654, 1979

32. McCarty DJ, Palmer D, Halverson PB: Clearance of calcium pyrophosphate dihydrate (CPPD) crystals in vivo I. Studies using ^{169}Yb labelled triclinic crystals. Arthritis Rheum 22:718–727, 1979

33. Dorwart BB, Schumacher HR: Joint effusions, chondrocalcinosis and other rheumatic manifestations in hypothyroidism: a clinicopathologic study. Am J Med 59:780–790, 1975

34. Spilberg I, Berney S: Colchicine and pseudogout. Arthritis Rheum 22:427–428, 1979

48. Apatite and other calcium crystal deposition diseases

Apatite, $Ca_5(PO_4)_3OH$, is the normal form of calcium in bone and in most pathologic calcifications in the body. Evolving studies suggest a role for apatite crystals in clinical syndromes of calcific periarthritis (1–3) and acute or erosive arthritis (4–6). In addition, apatite crystals are demonstrable in osteoarthritic articular cartilage (7) and in a high percentage of osteoarthritic effusions (8,9).

Individual apatite crystals are visible only with the electron microscope. They are rod or needle shaped with diameters from 70–250 A. Crystals aggregate into masses and can be seen in joint or bursal effusions as glossy nonbirefringent clumps up to 10μ in diameter (Fig 48–1). The frequency of apatite deposition is not yet known. In an autopsy study using on x-rays, gross examination, and then x-ray diffraction, detectable deposits of apatite were found in only 1.4% of knee menisci (10).

Apatite deposition syndromes can be associated with acute recurrent or chronic periarthritis. Some patients have been described with similar attacks at many sites, most commonly at shoulders, greater trochanters of hips, elbows, wrists, digits, and medial aspect of the knee. Frequently,

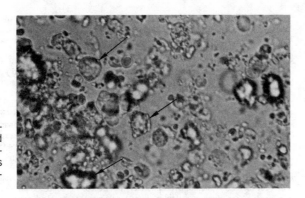

Fig 48–1. Clumps of apatite crystals **(arrows)** from synovial fluid appear glossy with irregular outlines in contrast to the leukocytes and erythrocytes. (Illustration provided by Dr HR Schumacher)

patients experience severe throbbing pain, often with swelling and erythema over inflamed superficial deposits. Usually 1 site is involved at a time.

Similarly, arthritis is usually present in 1 or a few joints, often with acutely painful gout-like episodes. Commonly involved joints are those of the fingers, toes, wrists, knees, and hips (5, 11). Polyarthritis with erosions has been reported (6), as has destructive shoulder arthritis in patients with rotator cuff tears (12) or those undergoing chronic dialysis (13).

As is the case with urate and CPPD deposition diseases, crystals can also be identified in tissues and fluids of asymptomatic subjects. In such asymptomatic situations, indolent damage to cartilage via mechanical effects and low-grade inflammation are under study as possible causative factors in osteoarthritis.

Radiologic studies may show soft tissue calcifications in or around joints. Typical deposits are distinguishable from the linear calcifications in cartilage that are characteristic of CPPD deposition disease.

Apatite can be tentatively identified in joint effusions by shiny (but nonbirefringent) globules and can be confirmed with x-ray diffraction. The diagnosis is readily made by using the white pasty material that can occasionally be aspirated from tendon sheaths or joints. Since most patients have many fewer crystals, other techniques must be used. Scanning electron microscopy (EM) can identify the clumps of apatite crystals, while transmission EM can detect the individual crystals (4,5). Electron probe elemental analysis can then add further support if the Ca:P ratio is in the range of 1.6:1, as would be expected with apatite. Alizarin red is used as a screening technique since it stains all calcium-containing crystals (or clumps) for light microscopic examination (14). ^{14}C EHDP binding is also being studied as a screening technique (15).

Synovial fluid leukocyte counts from symptomatic joints have ranged up to 49,000/mm^3, but generally tend to be lower and the fluid contains more monocytes than that in gout and CPPD disease. Occasionally, clumps of crystals are counted as leukocytes. This error causes confusion with septic arthritis.

Diseases associated with apatite-deposition arthritis and periarthritis include scleroderma, dermatomyositis, and undifferentiated syndromes (16–19), and renal failure in patients on dialysis (6,20). CPPD and apatite crystals can often coexist as they do in osteoarthritis (8). Apatite deposition has occurred in chronic gout and rheumatoid arthritis (21). In the latter, it may be a possible cause for some unexplained acute exacerbations.

Other syndromes involving apatite deposition include the acute periarticular calcification and ossifications of acute central neurologic injury (22,23), tumoral calcinosis (24), and vitamin D intoxication (25). Gouty tophi may calcify with apatite.

In most situations, the origin of apatite deposition is unknown. However, underlying systemic metabolic factors may be involved, at least in patients with multiple sites of intermittent calcification. Abnormal calcium or phosphorus serum levels are generally found only in patients with renal failure and tumoral calcinosis. Local cartilage or synovial connective tissue alterations (26,27) may also be a factor. Only occasionally, in advanced arthritis, does joint fluid apatite appear to be a result of actual bone fragments. Studies on the sequence of inflammation induced with apatite indicate involvement of phagocytosis, complement activation, prostaglandin, collagenase, and superoxide generation (28–32).

Patients with acute periarthritis or arthritis generally respond well to high doses of indomethacin or other nonsteroidal antiinflammatory drugs (5). Colchicine can also be effective (3,19). As yet, no method is known to deplete or mobilize abnormal apatite deposits in most idiopathic cases. Improved dialysis may help patients with renal failure. Phosphate restriction has good results for some patients with hyperphosphatemic tumoral calcinosis (24).

The joints are also the site of other calcium-containing crystals. Calcium oxalate has been described in joints of 3 patients undergoing hemodialysis for chronic renal failure (33). These crystals are large, bipyramidal, and birefringent. Deposits in cartilage produce chondrocalcinosis. Calcium hydrogen phosphate dihydrate (or brushlite) crystals have also

been reported in articular cartilage, synovium, and synovial fluid of patients who also have calcium pyrophosphate crystals (10,34,35). Crystals are brightly, positively birefringent. Their possible significance has not yet been explored.

1. Pinals RS, Short CL: Calcific periarthritis involving multiple sites. Arthritis Rheum 9:566–574, 1966
2. McCarty DJ, Gatter RA: Recurrent acute inflammation associated with focal apatite crystal deposition. Arthritis Rheum 9:804–819, 1966
3. Thompson GR, Ting YM, Riggs GA, et al: Calcific tendinitis and soft tissue calcification resembling gout. JAMA 203:464–472, 1963
4. Dieppe PA, Crocker P, Huskisson EC, et al: Apatite deposition disease: a new arthropathy. Lancet 1:266–269, 1976
5. Schumacher HR, Somlyo AP, Tse RL, et al: Arthritis associated with apatite crystals. Ann Intern Med 87:411–416, 1977
6. Schumacher HR, Miller JL, Ludivico C, et al: Erosive arthritis associated with apatite crystal deposition. Arthritis Rheum 24:31–37, 1981
7. Ali SY: Matrix vesicles and apatite nodules in arthritic cartilage, Perspectives in inflammation. DA Willoughby et al, eds. DA Willoughby. Baltimore, University Park Press, 1977, pp 211–223
8. Schumacher HR, Gordon G, Paul H, et al: Osteoarthritis, crystal deposition and inflammation. Sem Arthritis Rheum 11:116–119, 1981
9. Huskisson EC, Dieppe PA, Tucker AK, et al: Another look at osteoarthritis. Ann Rheum Dis 38:423–428, 1979
10. McCarty DJ, Hogan JM, Gatter RA, et al: Studies on pathological calcification in human cartilage. J Bone Joint Surg 48A:209–235, 1966
11. Fam AG, Pritzker KPH, Stein JL, et al: Apatite-associated arthropathy: a clinical study of 14 cases and of 2 patients with calcific bursitis. J Rheumatol 6:461–471, 1979
12. McCarty DJ, Halverson PB, Carrera GF, et al: "Milwaukee shoulder"—association of microspheroids containing hydroxyapatite crystals, active collagenase, and neutral protease with rotator cuff tears. Arthritis Rheum 24:464–473, 1981
13. Good AE, Rozboril MB, Port FK, et al: The dialysis shoulder (abstract) Arthritis Rheum 25:S34, 1982
14. Paul H, Reginato AJ, Schumacher HR: Alizarin red S staining as a screening test to detect calcium compounds in synovial fluid. Arthritis Rheum 26:191–200, 1983
15. Halverson PB, McCarty DJ: Identification of hydroxyapatite crystals in synovial fluid. Arthritis Rheum 22:389-395, 1979
16. Brandt KD, Krey PR: Chalky joint effusion. The result of massive synovial deposition of calcium apatite in progressive systemic sclerosis. Arthritis Rheum 20:792–796, 1977
17. Reginato A, Schumacher HR: Synovial calcification in a patient with collagen vascular disease: light and electron microscopic studies. J Rheumatol 4:261–271, 1977
18. Schumacher HR, Schimmer B, Gordon GV, et al: Articular manifestations of polymyositis and dermatomyositis. Am J Med 67:287–292, 1979
19. Taborn J, Bole GG, Thompson GR: Colchicine suppression of local and systemic inflammation due to calcinosis universalis in chronic dermatomyositis. Ann Intern Med 89:648–649, 1978
20. Mirahmadi KS, Coburn JW, Bluestone R: Calcific periarthritis and hemodialysis. JAMA 223:548–549, 1973
21. Reginato AJ, Paul H, Schumacher HR: Hydroxyapatite crystals in rheumatoid arthritis synovial fluid (abstract). Clin Res 30:662A, 1982
22. Rosin AJ: Ectopic calcification around joints of paralyzed limbs in hemiplegia, diffuse brain damage and other neurological diseases. Ann Rheum Dis 34:499–505, 1975
23. Goldberg MA, Schumacher HR: Heterotopic ossification mimicking acute arthritis after neurologic catastrophies. Arch Intern Med 137:619–621, 1977
24. Mozaffarian G, Lafferty F, Pearson OH: Treatment of tumoral calcinosis with phosphorus deprivation. Ann Intern Med 77:741–745, 1972

25. Kieff ED, McCarty DJ: Hypertrophic pulmonary osteoarthropathy with arthritis and synovial calcification in a patient with alcoholic cirrhosis. Arthritis Rheum 12:261–271, 1969

26. Steigerwald JC, Hardington TE, Muir H: The effect of proteoglycans on hydroxyapatite formation—possible relationship to joint calcifications (abstract). Arthritis Rheum 24:S69, 1981

27. Uhthoff HK, Sakkar K, Maynardi JA: Calcifying tendinitis: a new concept in pathogenesis. Clin Orthop 118:164–168, 1976

28. Maurer K, Schumacher HR: Hydroxyapatite phagocytosis by human polymorphonuclear leukocytes. Ann Rheum Dis 38:84–88, 1979

29. Hasselbacher P: C3 activation by monosodium urate monohydrate and other crystalline material. Arthritis Rheum 22:571–578, 1979

30. Denko CW, Petricevic M: Hydroxyapatite crystal-induced inflammation and prostaglandin E1. J Rheumatol 6:117-123, 1979

31. Cheung HS, Halverson RB, McCarty DJ: Release of collagenase, neutral protease and prostaglandins from cultured mammalian synovial cells by hydroxyapatite and CPPD crystals. Arthritis Rheum 24:1338-1344, 1981

32. Simchowitz L, Atkinson JP, Spilberg I: Stimulation of the respiratory burst in human neutrophils by crystal phagocytosis. Arthritis Rheum 25:181–188, 1982

33. Hoffman G, Schumacher HR, Paul H, et al: Calcium oxalate microcrystalline-associated arthritis in end stage renal disease. Ann Int Med 97:36–42, 1982

34. Moskowitz RW, Harris BK, Schwartz A, et al: Chronic synovitis as a manifestation of calcium crystal deposition disease. Arthritis Rheum 14:109–116, 1971

35. Gaucher A, Faure G, Netter, P, et al: Identification des cristaux observes dans les arthropathies destructrices de la chondrocalcinose. Rev Rhum 44:407-414, 1977

49. Hemochromatosis

Idiopathic hemochromatosis is a chronic disorder in which excessive deposition of iron in the parenchymal tissues is associated with hepatic cirrhosis, myocardial disease, diabetes mellitus, and other endocrine dysfunction. Increased skin pigmentation results largely from melanin.

Hemochromatosis affects men more often than women and is rarely recognized before age 40 (unless familial). Hereditary increased iron absorption (1) or prolonged excessive iron ingestion are etiologic factors. Repeated blood transfusions more often result in "hemosiderosis" with iron deposition occurring predominantly in macrophages and with less tissue damage and fibrosis.

The diagnosis of hemochromatosis is supported by the finding of an elevation in plasma iron concentration and saturation of the iron binding protein, transferrin. Liver biopsy showing hemosiderin in parenchymal cells usually provides histologic confirmation. Hemosiderin is also found in other tissues, including the synovial membrane and articular cartilage (2–5).

Iron can also be demonstrated in synovial membrane in rheumatoid arthritis, other inflammatory joint diseases, pigmented villonodular synovitis, hemophilia, and other causes of hemarthrosis. In these situations the hemosiderin tends to lie predominantly in deep synovial perivascular macrophages.

In hemochromatosis the iron deposits occur chiefly in the synovial lining cells and can be identified by electron microscopy as prominently involving the type B or synthetic cells (4). Synovial proliferation or inflammation is usually slight.

A characteristic arthropathy involving the hands occurs in approximately 40% of patients with hemochromatosis (2–3). The onset is most often coincident with other manifestations of hemochromatosis, but arthropathy has been seen in individuals as young as age 26 before any other detectable clinical manifestations of the disease. On occasion arthropathy becomes apparent only after initiation of phlebotomy therapy.

The proximal and distal interphalangeal joints and the second and third metacarpophalangeal joints show firm or bony enlargement. These joints are mildly tender, stiff, or painful on use without intense morning accentuation, and have limited motion. The larger joints including the wrists, knees, and hips may also be affected.

Bouts of acute joint inflammation have occasionally been described. Some of these may be due to associated chondrocalcinosis and crystal-induced synovitis. Radiographs most frequently reveal de-

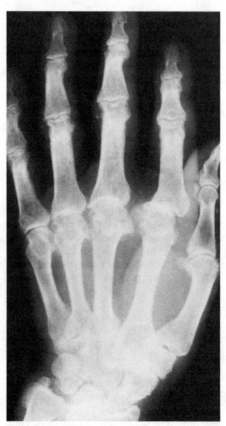

Fig 49–1. Radiograph of hand with hemochromatosis. Note the joint space narrowing, cystic subchondral lesions, joint space irregularity, mild subluxation, bony sclerosis, and small osteophytes in the metacarpophalangeal joints. Chondrocalcinosis is in the ulnar carpal joint and soft tissue has calcified around the interphalangeal joint of the thumb. (Illustration provided by Dr HR Schumacher)

generative changes in the metacarpophalangeal and interphalangeal joints (Fig 49–1). Similar changes may be present in the larger joints. Chondrocalcinosis is visible on radiographs in approximately 50% of patients with this arthropathy (3).

Synovial fluid tends to have good viscosity and leukocyte counts generally number less than 1,000/mm³. During acute exacerbations in which calcium pyrophosphate or apatite crystals are found in the synovia, the cell count may be much higher. Synovial fluid iron levels reflect the serum values. Rheumatoid factor is generally absent, serum urate levels are usually normal or low, and erythrocyte sedimentation rates rarely elevated. The pathogenesis of the arthropathy is not established, although iron damage to chondrocytes, cartilage matrix, or enzymes has been considered.

In Kashin-Beck disease, which occurs in certain parts of Asiatic Russia, an arthropathy with some similarity to hemochromatosis has been attributed to iron salts in the drinking water.

Phlebotomy therapy to deplete iron stores does not appear to improve established arthropathy but is indicated for the other systemic manifestations of hemochromatosis. Whether phlebotomy of asymptomatic relatives with early iron overload can prevent arthropathy is not known. Joint pain may be helped by analgesics, salicylates, or other nonsteroidal antiinflammatory agents.

Prosthetic hip and knee arthroplasties have been performed with some success in advanced disease.

1. Simon M, Bourel M, Genetet B, Fauchet R: Idiopathic hemochromatosis: demonstration of recessive transmission and early detection by family HLA typing. N Engl J Med 297:1017–1021, 1977

2. Schumacher HR: Hemochromatosis and arthritis. Arthritis Rheum 7:41–50, 1964

3. Dymock IW, Hamilton EBP, Laws JW, Williams R: Arthropathy of hemochromatsis. Ann Rheum Dis 29:469–476, 1970

4. Schumacher HR: Ultrastructure of the synovial membrane in idiopathic hemochromatosis. Ann Rheum Dis 31:465–473, 1972

5. Schumacher HR: Articular cartilage in the degenerative arthropathy of hemochromatosis. Arthritis Rheum 25:1460–1468, 1982

50. Wilson's disease (hepatolenticular degeneration)

Wilson's disease is an uncommon familial disorder characterized by marginal pigmentation of the cornea (Kayser-Fleischer ring), basal ganglion degeneration, and hepatic cirrhosis. The onset of symptoms may take place from age 4 to 50. Tremor, rigidity, athetosis, dysarthria, incoordination, or personality changes are generally the first manifestations.

Laboratory studies reveal a decrease in serum copper and the copper binding protein, ceruloplasmin. Copper concentration is increased in liver, brain, and other tissues. Copper levels have not been studied in articular structures or joint fluid. Renal tubular acidosis can produce uricosuria and hypouricemia.

An arthropathy frequently involving the wrists, knees, and hips, with joint effusions, is seen in as many as half of adults but is rare in children (1). Synovial effusions are clear and viscous with few cells; calcium pyrophosphate crystals have not been found.

Radiographic findings (1,2) include subchondral bone fragmentation, cortical irregularity, and sclerosis with or without narrowed joint spaces, chondromalacia patellae, osteochondritis dissecans, chondrocalcinosis, and periarticular calcifications.

The pathogenesis of the arthropathy is not understood. Joint manifestations do not correlate with neurologic, renal, or hepatic disease. Copper (like iron) inhibits pyrophosphatase in vitro, suggesting a mechanism for production of chondrocalcinosis.

Osteopenia is seen in as many as half the patients. Osteomalacia can result from the renal tubular disease. Early treatment with penicillamine and copper restriction can improve neurologic and possibly other manifestations. The effect of this treatment on the arthropathy is not known. Mild analgesics and nonsteroidal antiinflammatory agents may prove helpful.

Patients with Wilson's disease taking penicillamine have developed a lupus-like syndrome, polymyositis, and acute polyarthritis (3).

1. Finby N, Bearn AG: Roentgenographic abnormalities of the skeletal system in Wilson's disease (hepatolenticular degeneration). Am J Roentgenol 79:603–611, 1958
2. Feller EF, Schumacher HR: Osteoarticular changes in Wilson's disease. Arthritis Rheum 15:259–266, 1972
3. Golding DN, Walshe JM: Arthropathy of Wilson's disease. Ann Rheum Dis 36:99–111, 1977

51. Alkaptonuria (ochronosis)

Alkaptonuria is a rare, inherited (recessive) disorder resulting from a complete deficiency of the enzyme homogentisic acid oxidase (1,2). This deletion causes accumulation of homogentisic acid (a normal intermediate in the metabolism of phenylalanine and tyrosine) (Fig 51–1), which is excreted in the urine. Alkalinization and oxidation of this acid cause the urine to turn black. Some acid is retained in the body and deposited as a pigmented polymer in the cartilage, and to a lesser degree, in skin and sclerae. The darkening of these parts by this pigment is designated *ochronosis*.

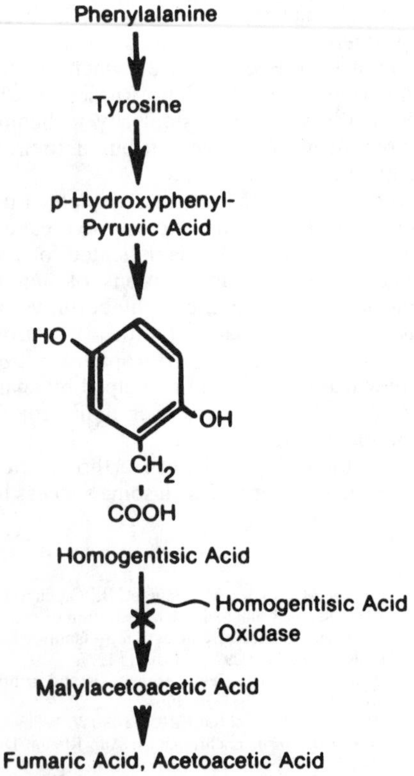

The pigment, which is found in the deeper layers of the articular cartilage, is bound to collagen fibers and causes this tissue to lose its normal resiliency and become brittle and fibrillated. The erosion of this abnormal cartilage leads to a denudation of subchondral bone and the penetration of tiny needle-like shards of pigmented cartilage into the synovium and bone.

A progressive degenerative arthropathy develops, with symptoms usually beginning in the fourth decade of life. This initially involves the vertebral column, where pigment is found in the annulus fibrosus and nucleus pulposus of the intervertebral discs (*ochronotic spondylitis*) (Fig 51–2), and later the knees, shoulders, and hips. The small joints of the hands and feet are rarely, if ever, affected, in contrast to osteoarthritis.

Stiffness and loss of joint mobility are the predominant complaints, with pain less prominent. Knee effusions are common, but other signs of articular inflammation are ordinarily lacking. Fragments of

Phenylalanine

↓

Tyrosine

↓

p-Hydroxyphenyl-
Pyruvic Acid

↓

Homogentisic Acid

─X─ Homogentisic Acid
Oxidase

Malylacetoacetic Acid

↓

Fumaric Acid, Acetoacetic Acid

Fig 51–1. Scheme of pathways involved in the normal metabolism of phenylalanine and tyrosine, indicating the block in the oxidation of homogentisic acid in alkaptonuria.

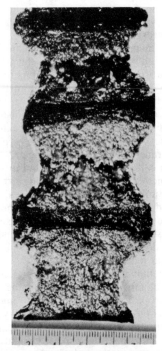

Fig 51–2. Part of lumbar vertebral column of 49-year-old woman with alkaptonuria who died of renal failure (ochronotic nephrosis). Blackened intervertebral discs are thin and focally calcified. This patient had incapacitating pain since age 36, with progressive limitation of back motion. Microscopic examination of the discs, which splintered easily, revealed nonrefractile granular pigment. (Illustration provided by Dr J Cooper and reproduced with permission of Cooper J, Moran TJ: Studies on ochronosis. I. Report of case with death from ochronotic nephrosis. Arch Pathol 61:46–53, 1957)

darkly pigmented cartilage can occasionally be found floating in the joint fluid. Osteochondral bodies which form in response to the deposition of cartilaginous fragments in the synovium are often palpable in and around the knee joint and may reach several centimeters in diameter.

In patients with severe, long-standing disease, the loss of lumbar lordosis and rigidity of the spine may resemble ankylosing spondylitis. Radiographs reveal calcification of the intervertebral discs (first apparent in the lumbar spine) and narrowing of the intervertebral spaces. The sacroiliac joints are spared.

The changes observed in the peripheral joints are similar to those in osteoarthritis: loss of cartilage space, marginal osteophytes, and eburnation of the subchondral bone.

No effective treatment is available for the underlying metabolic disorder. Surgical removal of osteochondral loose bodies from the knee joint is warranted when these interfere with motion.

1. Schumacher HR, Holdsmith DE: Ochronotic arthropathy. I. Clinicopathologic studies. Semin Arthritis Rheum 6:207–246, 1977
2. O'Brien WM, LaDu BN, Bunim JJ: Biochemical, pathologic, and clinical aspects of alcaptonuria, ochronosis, and ochronotic arthropathy: review of the world literature 1584-1962. Am J Med 34:813–838, 1963

52. Acromegaly

Acromegaly is associated with a distinct arthropathy resulting from the effects of excess growth hormone on cartilage, bone, and periarticular soft tissues, leading to a combination of hypertrophy, degeneration, and regenerative remodeling (1).

The characteristic early changes include generalized cartilaginous hypertrophy, apparent radiographically as widened joint spaces. The hypercellular and thickened cartilage appears to be unduly friable and prone to the development of superficial undercut ulceration at weight-bearing surfaces. Deeper fragmentation becomes filled in by healing fibrocartilaginous plugs. Eventually, the joint space narrows, as in osteoarthritis.

There is also capsular calcinosis, prolific marginal new bone formation appearing as large osteophytes or symmetrical bony rims, and remodeling of the adjacent shafts of long bones or vertebral bodies. The remodeling of metatarsal and metacarpal bones is most notable at insertions of the interosseous muscles and leads to cessation of the normal wasting. The vertebral bodies may become greatly hypertrophied anterocaudally with an increased posterior scalloping. A paradoxic radiographic picture may therefore evolve with greatly widened disc spaces despite bridging osteophytosis. Part of the new spinal bone formation may be a response to the axial hypermobility brought on by the thickened intervertebral cartilages. This spinal hypermobility is often evident as a remarkable degree of straight-leg forward flexion motion despite the frequent complaint of severe and chronic backache.

Other common rheumatic symptoms consist of widespread arthralgias and the paresthesias of the carpal tunnel syndrome. Osteoarticular findings include hypertrophy of articular and periarticular tissues, palpable bony lipping of small joints, and an occasional small effusion. Aside from the generalized increase of joint mobility, pronounced but painless crepitus may be felt and heard on movement of the shoulders and knees.

The carpal tunnel syndrome is immediately reversible after successful pituitary ablation, but once the other articular changes have developed, they are inevitably progressive, leading to secondary osteoarthritis. Thus, the patient with acromegalic arthropathy may require appropriate management for degenerative joint disease even after the endocrine disorder is arrested.

1. Bluestone R, Bywaters EGL, Hartog M, Holt PJL, Hyde S: Acromegalic arthropathy. Ann Rheum Dis 30:243–258, 1971

53. Arthropathies associated with other endocrine diseases

Musculoskeletal complaints may be the first clue in the detection of certain endocrine diseases and are often curable by treatment of the underlying disorder (1).

Hyperparathyroidism causes osteitis fibrosa cystica (Fig 53–1), subperiosteal bone resorption, generalized muscular aching and stiffness, joint laxity, osteoarthritis, spontaneous tendon avulsion and rupture, erosive arthritis of the hands (2), and back pain and vertebral fractures mimicking osteoporosis senilis (3). When renal failure supervenes, ischemic skin necrosis and periarticular calcification (hydroxyapatite) are also seen.

The typical neuromyopathy consists of proximal lower extremity weakness and atrophy, muscle aching after use, intact deep tendon reflexes, and normal creatine phosphokinase (CPK) levels (4). Thirty-five percent of hyperparathyroid patients have chondrocalcinosis (5).

Acute postoperative arthritis may be due to pseudogout (see Section 47) or gout (see Section 46) since both can coexist with hyperparathyroidism. Acute pseudogout continues to occur and may even be increased after parathyroidectomy.

With *hypoparathyroidism*, an ankylosing spondylitis–like disease with normal sacroiliac joints has been reported (6). The patient may have hypocalcemic muscular cramps, subcutaneous calcification (nodules), and carpopedal spasm with tingling. Vitamin D and calcium replacement alleviate the neuromuscular complaints. Pseudohypoparathyroidism (hypocalcemia resistant to parathormone) is associated with shortened metacarpals and metatarsals.

Hyperthyroid patients may complain of bone pain caused by osteopenia, muscle weakness (thyrotoxic myopathy, periodic paralysis, or myasthenia gravis), or shoulder periarthritis (see Section 72). Diffusely swollen hands and feet associated with periostitis (thyroid acropachy) (Fig 53–2) occur in Graves' disease but are generally unaffected by treatment of the hyperthyroidism. In prophylthiouracil-induced lupus, mild arthritis may be evident.

Musculoskeletal symptoms may occur in connection with Hashimoto's thyroiditis. This disorder occurs with increased frequency in association with rheumatoid arthritis and possibly with eosinophilic fasciitis (7), mixed connective tissue dis-

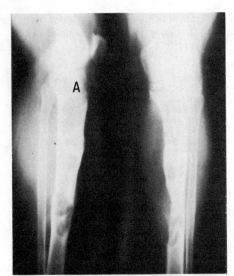

Fig 53–1. Roentgenogram of legs of patient with hyperparathyroidism. Subchondral bone absorption may lead to microfractures and premature osteoarthritis. (Illustration provided by Dr JJ Blizzard)

ease, and progressive systemic sclerosis (scleroderma) (8).

Primary *hypothyroidism* may be heralded by myalgias and other fibrositis-like complaints (see Section 56). Peripheral joints in myxedema are affected by symmetrical joint swelling mimicking rheumatoid arthritis (9). Unlike that in rheumatoid arthritis, the joint fluid in hypothyroidism is usually highly viscous and has low white cell counts (less than 1,000 cells/mm³). Calcium pyrophosphate deposition disease (pseudogout) coexists in many myxedematous patients. Crystals may be found in synovial fluids without any evidence of joint inflammation until thyroid replacement is begun; acute pseudogout often develops after replacement. Muscle weakness may be associated with very high levels of creatine phosphokinase activity (CPK), causing confusion with polymyositis.

The presence of otherwise unexplained carpal tunnel syndrome or flexor tendon thickening should also suggest the possi-

bility of hypothyroidism. Thyroid replacement results in striking resolution of all these rheumatic complaints.

Cortisol excess (*Cushing's syndrome*), whether idiopathic or from treatment with glucocorticoids, may cause severe osteoporosis with compression fractures of spine and ribs, osteonecrosis (especially of the femoral head), and proximal muscle wasting. CPK levels are normal in steroid myopathy.

In *adrenocortical insufficiency* muscle cramps are often severe. Pseudorheumatism (diffuse muscle, joint, and bony aching) occurs when exogenous corticosteroids are withdrawn.

Diabetes mellitus may be associated with several rheumatic problems (10). Charcot joints occur as a complication of neuropathy, predominantly in the tarsometatarsal area (11). These may not be completely painless and can be confused

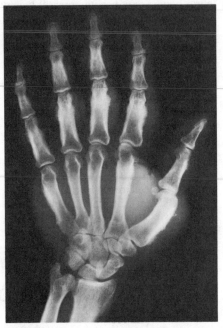

Fig 53–2. Thyroid acropachy showing an extreme example of the characteristic periosteal reaction in the hand.

with osteomyelitis, to which diabetics are also susceptible. Periarthritis of the shoulder (12), carpal tunnel syndrome, and flexor tendinitis in the palms also occur (13), as well as a peculiar form of digital sclerosis (in juvenile onset diabetes mellitus), and an increased frequency of scleredema.

In congenital vasopressin-resistant diabetes insipidus, an elevation in serum urate concentration may be as high as 15 mg/dl caused by decreased renal clearance of urate (14).

Acromegaly is discussed in the previous section.

1. Bland JH, Frymoyer JW, Newberg AH, Revers R, Norman RJ: Rheumatic syndromes in endocrine disease. Semin Arthritis Rheum 9:23–65, 1979
2. Resnick DL: Erosive osteoarthritis of the hand and wrist in hyperparathyroidism. Radiology 110:263–269, 1974
3. Dauphine RT, Riggs BL, Scholz DA: Back pain and vertebral crush fractures: an unemphasized mode of presentation for primary hyperparathyroidism. Ann Intern Med 83:365–367, 1975
4. Patten BM, Gilezikian JP, Mallette LE, Prince A, Engel WK, Aurbach GD: Neuromuscular disease in primary hyperparathyroidism. Ann Intern Med 80:182–193, 1974
5. Pritchard MH, Jessop JD: Chondrocalcinosis in first degree hyperparathyroidism. Ann Rheum Dis 36:146–151, 1977
6. Chaykin LB, Frame B, Sigler JW: Spondylitis: a clue to hypoparathyroidism. Ann Intern Med 70:995–1000, 1969
7. Smiley AM, Husain M, Indenbaum S: Eosinophilic fasciitis in association with thyroid disease: a report of 3 cases. J Rheumatol 7:871, 1980
8. Gordon MB, et al: Thyroid disease in progressive systemic sclerosis: increased frequency of glandular fibrosis and hypothyroidism. Ann Intern Med 95:431–435, 1981
9. Dorwart BB, Schumacher HR: Joint effusions, chondrocalcinosis and other rheumatic manifestations in hypothyroidism. Am J Med 59:780–790, 1975
10. Gray RB, Gottlieb NL: Rheumatic disorders associated with diabetes mellitus: literature review. Semin Arthritis Rheum 6:19–34, 1976
11. Sinha S, Munichoodappa CS, Kozak GP: Neuro-arthropathy (Chartcot joints) in diabetes mellitus. Medicine 51:191–210, 1972
12. Bridgman JF: Periarthritis of the shoulder and diabetes mellitus. Ann Rheum Dis 31:69–71, 1972
13. Jung Y, Hohmann TC, Gerneth JA, Novak J, Wasserman RC, D'Andrea BJ, Newton RH, Danowski TS: Diabetic hand syndrome. Metabolism 20:1008–1015, 1971
14. Gordon P, Robertson GL, Seegmiller JE: Hyperuricemia, a concomitant of congenital vasopressin-resistant diabetes insipidus in the adult. N Engl J Med 284:1057–1060, 1971

54. Arthropathies associated with hematologic diseases and storage disorders

Sickle cell anemia. The crises of sickle cell anemia are often associated with severe polyarthralgia (1). Occasionally the pain is accompanied by hydrarthrosis and other evidence of inflammation. The synovial fluid in such cases is generally clear and the cell count <1,000 cells/mm³; in some cases, however, the number of cells is large.

Synovial biopsy specimens have revealed microvascular thrombosis. This is consistent with the belief that joint effusion results from infarction of the synovium (1). Bone scans have provided evidence of vascular obstruction in the marrow adjacent to painful joints, indicative of localized reduction or absence of blood flow (infarction).

The skeletal lesions, so characteristic of this hemoglobinopathy, may be separated into those related to hyperplasia of the marrow and those that are the result of local sickle cell thrombosis and infarction. The expanded bone marrow with its sluggish circulation and high oxygen demand is especially vulnerable in the latter condition (2). Results of hyperplasia of the

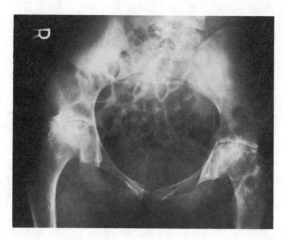

Fig 54–1. Roentgenogram of the pelvis of a 24-year-old woman with sickle cell anemia illustrates osteonecrosis of both femoral heads.

marrow include widening of medullary cavities, thinning of cortices, coarsening and irregularity of trabecular markings, and cupping of vertebral bodies. Most notable among the bony changes caused by sickle cell thrombosis (or, as has been suggested, possibly from fat emboli originating in necrotic marrow) is osteonecrosis of the head of the femur (Fig 54–1) and, less commonly, the head of the humerus (Fig 54–2), patella, and vertebral bodies (3).

This complication has been encountered in the variant forms of the hemoglobinopathy (S-C, S-thalassemia, S-F) as well as in S-S disease and rarely in sickle cell trait. Total hip replacement has been carried out successfully in a number of these patients.

Young children with sickle cell disease may experience transient swelling and ten-

derness of the hands and feet as a result of periostitis of the metacarpal, metatarsal, and proximal phalangeal bones (**sickle cell dactylitis**) (Fig 54–3).

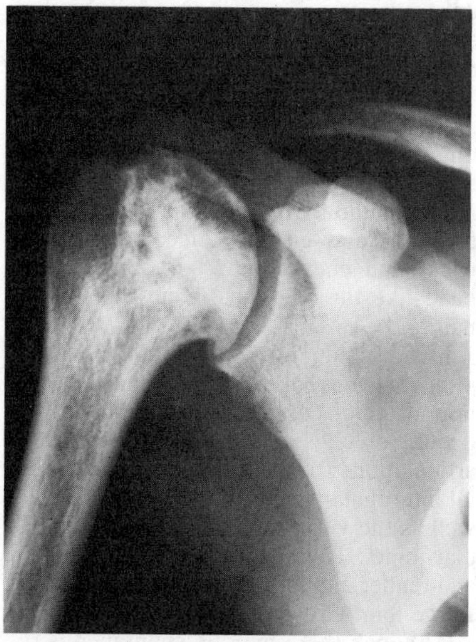

Individuals with sickle cell disease are particularly susceptible to salmonella osteomyelitis. This may be attributed to a defect in the alternative complement pathway which interferes with the normal phagocytosis and lysis of salmonellae and certain other microorganisms (4).

The occurrence of hyperuricemia in patients with sickle cell disease appears to result from a combination of over-production of uric acid (as a result of greatly increased rate of erythropoiesis) and its diminished excretion due to impaired renal function (**sickle cell kidney**) (5). Children and younger adults with this disorder exhibit evidence of an increased tubular secretion of urate that permits them to remain normouricemic despite overproduction of uric acid and may account for the relatively low frequency of secondary gout in this condition.

A specific osteoarthropathy associated with beta thalassemia has been recognized. It is marked by pain and swelling of the ankles and by hyperplasia and hemosiderosis of the synovium (6). This joint disease develops as patients approach the second and third decades of life and ap-

pears to be related to underlying bone changes found in this hemoglobinopathy, although the role of iron overload in pathogenesis remains to be determined. A similar form of pauciarticular nonerosive arthropathy has also been observed in thalassemia minor and avascular necrosis of the femoral heads has been reported in a patient with this condition.

1. Schumacher HR: Rheumatological manifestations of sickle cell disease and other hereditary hemoglobinopathies. Clin Rheum Dis 1:37–53, 1975
2. Moseley JE: Skeletal changes in the anemias. Semin Roentgenol 9:169–184, 1974
3. Chung SM, Alvai A, Russell MD: Management of osteonecrosis in sickle cell anemia and its genetic variants. Clin Orthop 130:158–174, 1978
4. Hand WL, Kind NL: Serum opsonization of salmonella in sickle cell anemia. Am J Med 64:388–394, 1978
5. Diamond HS, Meisel AD, Holden D: The natural history of urate overproduction in sickle cell anemia. Ann Intern Med 90:752–757, 1979
6. Gratwick GM, Bullough PG, Bohne WHO, Markenson AL, Peterson CM: Thalassemic osteoarthropathy. Ann Intern Med 88:494–501, 1978

Myelomatosis and Waldenström's macroglobulinemia. In most cases, the pain that occurs in the back of the extremities and that is so frequently the initial manifestation of myelomatosis is attributable to disease of the bone, and roentgenograms often reveal osteolytic defects. Some patients with myelomatosis, however, develop pain and swelling of the joints and have extensive deposits of amyloid in the synovium and paraarticular tissues including muscle (1).

Amyloidosis is found in all forms of myelomatosis but occurs most frequently in light chain disease and IgA myeloma. The hands, wrists (carpal tunnel syndrome), antecubital fossae, shoulders, and clavicles are most often affected. There may be striking enlargement of the shoulders (*shoulder pad sign*), and they may dislocate as a result of the deposition of large masses of amyloid in the glenoid fossa (Fig 54–4).

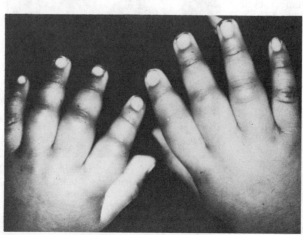

Fig 54–2. Roentgenogram of right shoulder of a 35-year-old woman with hemoglobin S-C disease illustrates avascular necrosis of the head of the humerus. This patient also had bilateral osteonecrosis of the femoral heads. (From Arthritis and Allied Conditions, Ed 9, with permission of Daniel J McCarty, Jr, editor, and Lea & Febiger, Philadelphia)

Fig 54–3. Sickle cell dactylitis

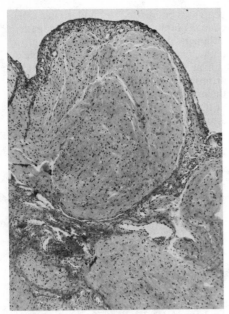

Fig 54—4. Photomicrograph of synovium from right shoulder of a 56-year-old woman with myelomatosis who dislocated her right humerus following a fall. At the time of open reduction of this dislocation, large deposits of amyloid were found in the glenoid fossa. Note large mass of amyloid covered by thin rim of synovium. The material in this nodule stained metachromatically with crystal violet. (From Arthritis and Allied Conditions)

Polyarticular involvement, sometimes mistaken for rheumatoid arthritis, may be associated with nodular periosteal deposits of amyloid. Typically, the highly viscous synovial fluid of such patients contains a relatively small number of cells ($200–4,500/mm^3$), chiefly mononuclear forms. Fragments of villi containing amyloid material may be detected in the sediment. Primary amyloidosis is also marked by a high frequency of carpal tunnel syndrome and by the occasional deposition of amyloid in and around the joints (2,3).

The bones of the patient with myelomatosis may appear normal on roentgenographic examination. More often, however, generalized rarefaction of bone, circumscribed lytic areas, or expansile lesions are present. In some instances, complete lysis of bone or ill-defined wide areas of bone destruction ("motheaten" bone) is apparent. Generalized osteoporosis, with or without discrete oteolytic defects, is a common finding in patients with amyloidosis. It may be difficult to differentiate lytic bone lesions due to amyloid from those due to myeloma.

Myelomatosis may serve as a basis for the development of secondary gout in some patients. Low levels of normal serum immunoglobulins leading to an impairment in humoral immune responses explain the vulnerability of these patients to infection (particularly by pneumococci), including septic arthritis.

The osseous changes found in Waldenström's macroglobulinemia are similar to those of myelomatosis (4). Although articular involvement is rare in Waldenström's macroglobulinemia, there have been isolated reports of amyloid arthropathy and of neuropathic joint disease secondary to amyloid neuropathy.

1. Gordon DA, Pruzanski W, Ogryzlo MA, Little HA: Amyloid arthritis simulating rheumatoid disease in five patients with multiple myeloma. Am J Med 55:142–154, 1973
2. Wiernik PH: Amyloid joint disease. Medicine 51:465–479, 1972
3. Cohen AS, Canoso JJ: Rheumatological aspects of amyloid disease. Clin Rheum Dis 1:149–161, 1975
4. Vermess M, Pearson KD, Einstein AB, Fahey JL: Osseous manifestations of Waldenström's macroglobulinemia. Radiology 102:497–504, 1972

Gaucher's disease. This is a heritable lysosomal sphingolipid storage disease resulting from a deficiency in the enzyme glucocerebroside, β-glucosidase. Gaucher's disease is characterized by an accumulation of the glycolipid glucocerebroside (or glucosylceramide) in reticuloendothelial cells in the bone marrow, spleen, liver, lymph nodes, and other internal organs (1,2).

Three clinical forms of Gaucher's disease are now recognized: type 1 (by far the most common)—the chronic non-neuropathic adult form; type 2—infantile or active neuronopathic form; type 3—juvenile or subacute neuronopathic form. Osteoarticular complaints are an important feature in both type 1 and type 3 Gaucher's disease. These are often the earliest manifestation of the disease and result from infiltration of the marrow of subchondral bone.

Polyarthralgia affecting the larger peripheral joints is a common complaint. Pathologic fracture of a long bone or compression of vertebrae giving rise to low back pain may occur. There are numerous reports of severe degenerative hip disease, a result of avascular necrosis and collapse of the head of the femur (Fig 54–5). Changes in the femoral neck may lead to pathologic fracture or coxa vara deformity. Patients with long-standing disease may have an elevation of levels of serum immunoglobulins, which increase, often monoclonally.

One of the most frequent roentgenographic features in Gaucher's disease is widening of the distal portion of the femur, just above the medial condyles ("Erlenmeyer flask" deformity). Similar flaring may be present in the tibia and humerus, together with changes in the other long bones, pelvis, skull, vertebrae, and mandible. Characteristically, areas of rarefaction are mingled with patchy sclerosis and cortical thickening which is the result of new bone formation.

The role of enzyme replacement with purified glucocerebrosidase is under study. In some patients, bone pain has been relieved following x-irradiation or treatment with corticosteroids.

1. Peters SP, Lee RE, Glew RH: Gaucher's disease, a review. Medicine 56:425–442, 1977
2. Brady RO: Glucosyl ceramide lipidosis: Gaucher's disease, The Metabolic Basis of Inherited Disease, Ed 4. JB Stanbury, JB Wyngaarden, DS Fredrickson, eds. New York, McGraw-Hill, 1978, pp 731–746

Multicentric reticulohistiocytosis (lipoid dermatoarthritis). This rare disorder of unknown origin occurs in adults and is characterized by a profusion of histiocytic nodules in the skin and mucous membranes and by severe, often mutilating polyarthritis (1). Women are affected 3 times as often as men. The firm reddish-brown or yellow papulonodules appear most commonly on the fingers and hands, forearms and elbows, face, scalp, ears, neck, and chest (Fig 54–6). Small coral bead–like tumefactions occur around the nail fold.

In approximately two-thirds of cases, joint changes represent the first manifestation of the disease. Symmetric polyarthritis may involve virtually all the peripheral articulations (frequently including the distal interphalangeal joints of the fingers) as well as the vertebral and temporomandibular joints. The affected parts are swollen and tender and may be intensely inflamed. Large joint effusions occur.

Although there may be spontaneous remission, chronically active disease leading to severe joint deformity is the rule. Radiographs of the joints reveal extensive destruction with loss of cartilage and striking resorption of subchondral bone (2). Early erosion of the odontoid process leading to atlantoaxial subluxation has

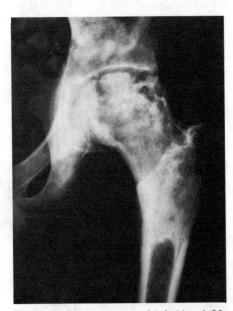

Fig 54—5. Roentgenogram of left hip of 22-year-old man with Gaucher's disease illustrates osteonecrosis of the head of the femur. This roentgenogram was obtained 2 years after the onset of pain in the hip. (From Arthritis and Allied Conditions)

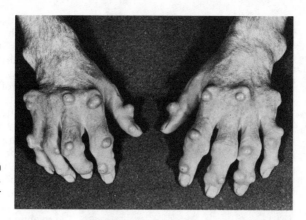

Fig 54-6. Hands of a man with multicentric reticulohistiocytosis. (Illustration provided by Dr Stephania Jablonska)

been described. The skin and synovium are infiltrated by histiocytes and multinucleated giant cells with homogeneous cytoplasm. The latter contain large amounts of a PAS-positive material which appears to be a mixture of lipids, including triglycerides, cholesterol esters, and several phospholipids (Fig 54-7). Similar cells are found in the bone marrow, lymph nodes, bone and periosteum, muscle, larynx, and endocardium.

The exact origin of multicentric reticulohistiocytosis remains unknown, although present evidence suggests that it is a lipid storage disease, involving glycolipid or phospholipid. Often this rarely fatal disease is spontaneously quiescent. Although the mucocutaneous nodules may diminish in size or disappear completely, patients are often left with serious joint damage.

There is no treatment that is regularly beneficial. Cyclophosphamide or other cytotoxic agents have been reported to be helpful in a few cases, but confirmation is difficult since the disease course is highly unpredictable.

1. Barrow MV, Holubar K: Multicentric reticulohistiocytosis: a review of 33 patients. Medicine 48:287–305, 1969
2. Gold RH, Metzger AL, Mirra JM, Weinberger HJ, Killebrew K: Multicentric reticulohistiocytosis (lipoid dermatoarthritis): an erosive polyarthritis with distinctive clinical, roentgenographic and pathologic features. Am J Roentgenol 124:610–624, 1975

Fabry's disease. Fabry's disease or glycolipid lipidosis, a hereditary sex-linked disorder of glycosphingolipid metabolism, is characterized by accumulation of triglycosylceramide, and to a lesser extent a diglycosylceramide, in the cells of the blood vessels, autonomic nervous system, kidney, bone marrow, synovium, and many other tissues (1). This pathologic storage is the result of a defect in the activity or the absence of the lysosomal enzyme α-galactosidase A.

In addition to the characteristic rash (angiokeratoma corporis diffusum universale), the disease is marked by recurrent bouts of fever and severe pain in the extremities. The latter is often induced by changes in environmental temperature. Painful swelling of the fingers, elbows, and knees as well as deformity and limitation in extension of the distal interphalangeal joints of the fingers are the most common rheumatic complaints (2). In addition, avascular necrosis of the head of the femur or talus as well as other bones sometimes occurs.

1. Desnick RJ, Klionsky B, Sweeley CC: Fabry's disease (α-galactosidase A deficiency), The Metabolic Basis of Inherited Disease. Ed 4. JB Stanbury, JB Wyngaarden, DS Fredrickson, eds. New York, McGraw-Hill, 1978, pp 810–840
2. Sheth KJ, Bernhard GC: The arthropathy of Fabry disease. Arthritis Rheum 22:781–783, 1979

Farber's disease. Farber's disease or disseminated lipogranulomatosis is a rare sphingolipidosis of early childhood. Farber's disease is characterized by painful swollen joints, periarticular, and subcutaneous nodules, dysphonia, pulmonary infiltrations, and retardation of mental and motor development (1,2). The pattern of familial occurrence is compatible with an autosomal recessive disorder.

Ceramide, a glycolipid, accumulates in the cytoplasm of neurons in the central nervous system and in granulomatous deposits in the larynx, lungs, synovium, and bone as well as a number of other organs.

The underlying defect probably results from a deficiency in the lysosomal enzyme, acid ceramidase. Articular manifestations usually appear between 2 weeks and 4 months of age and have been the dominant initial manifestation in the small number of reported cases. Few patients have survived beyond the age of 2 years, most succumbing to pulmonary disease.

1. Moser HW, Prensky AL, Wolfe JH, Rosman NP: Farber's lipogranulomatosis: report of a case and demonstration of an excess of free ceramide and ganglioside. Am J Med 47:869–890, 1969
2. Moser HW: Ceramidase deficiency: Farber's lipogranulomatosis, The Metabolic Basis of Inherited Disease, Ed 4. JB Stanbury, JB Wyngaarden, DS Fredrickson, ed. New York, McGraw-Hill, 1978, pp 707–717

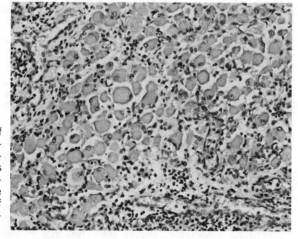

Fig 54-7. Photomicrograph of synovium (knee) from a 54-year-old woman with multicentric reticulohistiocytosis shows numerous histiocytes and multinucleated giant cells that contain large amounts of periodic-acid Schiff (PAS)-positive material. (From Arthritis and Allied Conditions)

55. Hyperlipoproteinemia

A variety of musculoskeletal problems complicate the hyperlipoproteinemias. In type II hyperlipoproteinemia tendinous and tuberous xanthomas are common features. Tendinous xanthomas occur in the achilles tendons, patellar tendons, and extensor tendons of the hands and feet, and tuberous xanthomas occur as subcutaneous masses over extensor surfaces of the elbows, knees, hands, and in the buttocks. Similar xanthomas are seen with type III hyperlipoproteinemia. Types I, IV, and V are more often characterized by eruptive xanthomas over the knees, buttocks, shoulders, and back (1).

Type II. Recurrent episodes of a migratory polyarthritis have been reported in about 50% of patients homozygous for type II hyperlipoproteinemia (2). Articular disease chiefly affects large peripheral joints, and inflammation varies from mild to severe. In many patients, the illness resembles rheumatic fever because of both the nature of the arthritis and the concurrence of aortic valvular disease, elevated erythrocyte sedimentation rate (ESR), and increased titer of anti-streptolysin-O. The valvular disease and elevated ESR also occur in individuals without arthritis and are presumably due to the hyperlipoproteinemia itself. Episodes of arthritis last several days to 2 weeks.

In patients with heterozygous type II hyperlipoproteinemia, arthritis may be limited to a single joint or changes in one or both achilles tendons, or a migratory polyarthritis may affect large peripheral joints as well as the small joints of the hands and feet (3). Attacks occur 4–12 times per year and have recurred over spans of up to 40 years without residual joint deformity. Tendinous xanthomas of the achilles tendons are frequently present in these cases, but in some instances do not become noticeable until many years after the initial episode of joint inflammation.

In a more recent series of 41 heterozygous type II hyperlipoproteinemia patients, 13 had inflammatory symptoms involving not only achilles tendons, great toes, and knees, but also proximal interphalangeal joints, ankles, wrists, shoulders, elbows, and hips (4). In all patients arthritis was sudden in onset, reached a peak in 24 hours, and resolved in each affected joint within 48 hours. However, the disorder was migratory in all cases, and the symptoms averaged 6 days (4).

Type IV. A number of patients have now been reported with arthritis associated with type IV hyperlipoproteinemia.

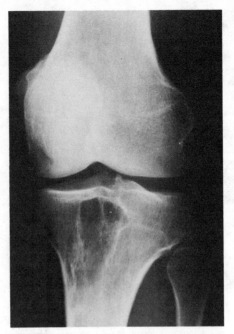

Fig 55–1. Roentgenogram of left knee of a patient with familial type IV hyperlipoproteinemia, illustrating large cystic lesion in tibia. (Illustration provided by Dr RB Buckingham)

Twelve individuals had predominantly asymmetric oligoarthritis involving small and large joints (5). Inflammatory joint disease was usually mild and persistent, but occasionally episodic and recurrent. Joint fluid in 1 patient was class I and in a second patient, class II. Of note, joint radiographs in 5 of these patients revealed prominent paraarticular bone cysts (Fig 55–1).

In another report on musculoskeletal complaints associated with type IV hyperlipoproteinemia, joint tenderness, morning stiffness, and paraarticular hyperesthesias were emphasized (6).

Associations. Some of the cases of articular disease described earlier with types II and IV hyperlipoproteinemia might have been associated instead with familial combined hyperlipidemia. It is now clear that this latter disorder is an additional form of familial hyperlipoproteinemia distinct from types II and IV. Individuals within a single kindred who suffer with this abnormality may have any of 3 apparent lipoprotein profiles including type IIa, type IIb, and type IV hyperlipoproteinemia. Patients often convert from one abnormal lipoprotein pattern to another.

There are other reports of skeletal lesions associated with hyperlipoproteinemic states. One patient with probable type V hyperlipoproteinemia had cystic lesions in both proximal femurs. Curettage yielded yellowish fragments that on microscopic examination showed foamy histiocytes and a granulomatous reaction around cholesterol clefts (7). Another report described a patient with lesions in the calvarium and femur with similar histologic characteristics. Neither of these reports mentioned objective or subjective joint involvement.

An increased frequency of hyperuricemia is seen in types III, IV, and V hyperlipoproteinemia.

1. Fredickson DS, Levy RI, Lees RS: Fat transport in lipoproteins: an integrated approach to mechanisms and disorders. N Engl J Med 276:34–44, 94–103, 148–156, 215–225, 273–281, 1967
2. Kachadurian AK: Mgratory polyarthritis in familial hypercholesterolemia (type II hyperlipoproteinemia). Arthritis Rheum 11:385–393, 1968
3. Glueck CJ, Levy RI, Fredrickson DS: Acute tendinitis and arthritis: a presenting symptom of familial type II hyperlipoproteinemia. JAMA 206:2895–2897, 1968
4. Rooney PJ, Third J, Madkour MM, Spencer D, Dick WC: Transient polyarthritis associated with familial hyperbetalipoproteinemia. Q J Med 187:249–259, 1978
5. Buckingham RB, Bole GG, Bassett DR: Polyarthritis associated with type IV hyperlipoproteinemia. Arch Intern Med 135:286–290, 1975
6. Goldman JA, Glueck CJ, Abrams NR, Steiner P, Herman JH: Musculoskeletal disorders associated with type IV hyperlipoproteinemia. Lancet 2:449–452, 1972
7. Siegelmann SS, Schlossberg I, Becker NH, Sachs BA: Hyperlipoproteinemia with skeletal lesions. Clin Orthop 87:228–232, 1972

56. The fibrositis syndrome

The term *fibrositis* has been used to describe trunk or limb pain, perhaps accompanied by tenderness, but without other local objective findings. There may be a subtle local abnormality, but sometimes the pain (and tenderness) seem to represent referred pain phenomena, postural pain, or unexplained amplified pain.

The essential feature for the diagnosis of fibrositis is the presence of a large number of tender points (Table 56–1).

Patients with *primary* fibrositis have no other underlying disease. In *secondary* fibrositis an associated disease state is identified. Two types of secondary fibrositis may exist: one in which an underlying disease produces pain and tenderness, and another where the pain is amplified by the same mechanisms operative in patients with primary fibrositis.

Clinical features. The symptoms are pain, stiffness, and exhaustion (1,2). The *pain* is widely distributed, aggravated by fatigue or chilling, and eased by heat or massage. The *stiffness* and *exhaustion* may be the most disabling and may discourage as well as punish activity. The patients wake unrefreshed, more exhausted than the night before.

Pain is not the only amplified sensation. Individuals may also be sensitive to weather, cold, bright lights, and loud noises. They may develop urinary frequency because of an enhanced sense of bladder fullness or may have intermittant bowel complaints.

Table 56–1. Tender points (14) in the fibrositis syndrome (see Fig 56–1)

Trapezius (right and left). Middle of upper fold
Second costochondral junctions (right and left)
Lateral epicondyles (right and left). 1–2 cm distal
Supraspinatus origin (right and left). Near medial portion of scapula
Low cervical spine. Front of intertransverse spaces
Low lumbar spine. Interspinous ligaments L4–S1
Gluteus medium (right and left). Upper outer portion of buttock
Medial fat pad (right and left). Over ligament

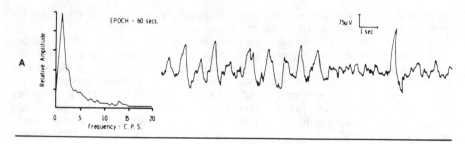

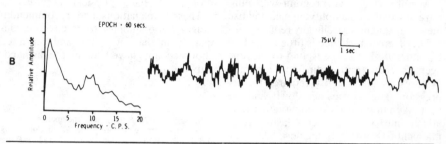

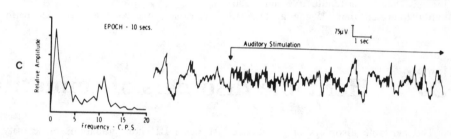

Fig 56–2. Frequency spectra and EEG from **A**, non-REM (delta) sleep in a healthy 25-year-old; **B**, non-REM sleep in a patient with fibrositis, amplitude at both 1 cycles per second (cps) (delta) and 8–10 cps (alpha); **C**, non-REM sleep of a healthy subject during delta sleep deprivation. Note association between arousal and alpha onset. (Reproduced with permission of the editor of Psychosomatic Medicine (3), the American Psychosomatic Society, and American Elsevier Publishing Company, Inc.)

Some patients are demanding of themselves and others. They can be trying, but are often very effective at work because of their dedication. They may dislike drugs, alcohol, or other crutches. The majority are females.

During examination they can give the impression that they are not making a full effort. Tenderness is often not simply reported; it may be demonstrated in sudden dramatic twisting leaps. Grip strength is reduced, inconsistent, and poorly sustained. Ill-defined and variable areas of partial numbness may also be described. The interview is often exhausting for the examiner as well as the patient, indicative of the stresses generated between the patient and others.

The cardinal clinical features are consistent, however, from patient to patient. The *tender points* (Fig 56–1) are largely unknown to the patient and often not even central to their areas of pain. There is marked skinfold tenderness, especially over the upper scapular region. *Reactive hyperemia* will often give visible evidence of the amplified responses to pain in this region.

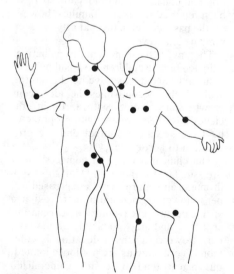

Fig 56–1. Location of 14 typical sites of deep tenderness in the fibrositis syndrome. (From the Bulletin on the Rheumatic Diseases)

Probable causes. A specific disturbance in sleep in many patients with the fibrositis syndrome may operate as a factor in producing or exaggerating the pain (3,4). Overnight increase in measures of muscle tenderness and a coincident disturbance in non-REM sleep (Fig 56–2) have been shown (3). Experimental reproduction of fibrositis symptoms was achieved in healthy university students who were disturbed during slow wave sleep by a buzzer. This produced alpha intrusion in the electroencephalographic pattern and an increase in tenderness as measured by dolorimeter scores.

Research has begun to clarify the mechanisms by which pain is eased. This progress has refreshed interest in disorders of pain modulation and the concept of pain amplification syndromes. The fibrositis syndrome appears to be such a disorder, as are reflex dystrophies, the pain of narcotic withdrawal, and others. The amplified pain is real pain, of deep origin.

A "body image" of the surface of the body is based on cerebral cortical representation and is required for normal function. No such detailed information is available about deeply lying structures, and

pain arising in deep structures must be referred. Experimental studies have established that deep pain is referred distally to deep structures within the segment of origin (the sclerotome) and may be markedly exaggerated by cold (5–7).

Referred deep tenderness deserves emphasis. Physicians find it difficult to accept that there may be no structural abnormality in a localized area of deep tenderness which disappears after an injection of an anesthesic. In the presence of referred pain, points of referred tenderness can be found, not necessarily central to the regions of spontaneous pain, but usually at the "fibrositic" sites within the affected region and side. Subtle local pathology has been sought in the tender muscles, but important points do not involve muscles.

Patients with rheumatoid arthritis may develop the fibrositis syndrome and present a sharp increase in pain and stiffness without objective evidence of incre___ inflammation (8). These patie___ recognized by their hig___ it is striking how___ their innoc___ cent s___ fla___

ing change in life situation and may respond to time and appropriate therapies.

Therapy. Patients with fibrositis often dislike medication and may improve with a clear explanation of the nature of their diagnosis and symptoms. A minimal program of salicylates, support for the neck during sleep, and short-term use of benzodiazepines such as diazepam, 5–20 mg at night, are also helpful.

A more aggressive program will minimize those factors amplifying pain and use measures that nonspecifically reduce pain.

The sleep disturbance is little helped by barbiturates, but may respond to tricyclic agents such as amitriptyline or imipramine in doses far below those required for depression. These drugs act slowly and are best taken in the early evening rather than at bedtime, to give effects lasting from midnight to 8 AM. A 10 mg dose taken at 8 PM may then be more effective and much better tolerated than 25 mg at 11 PM.

Occasionally, much larger doses are required.

Mechanical stresses in the neck and low back are commonly important primary deep pain sources and require specific therapy. Heat, massage, injections, electrical stimulation all give real if temporary relief, possibly through endorphin release. Instruction about proper posture while sitting and standing can be helpful as can a program of regular physical exercise.

These explanations and recommendations are too complex to be covered adequately in one interview, and reprinted short accounts have been helpful as handouts (9,10).

1. Smythe HA: Nonarticular rheumatism and the fibrositis syndrome, Arthritis and Allied Conditions. Ed 9. DJ McCarty, Jr, ed. Philadelphia, Lea & Febiger, 1979, pp 881–891
2. Yunus M, Masi AT, Calabro JJ, et al: Primary fibromyalgia (fibrositis): clinical study of 50 patients with matched normal controls. Semin Arthritis Rheum 11:151–171, 1981
3. Moldofsky H, Scarisbrick P, England R, Smythe HA: Musculoskeletal symptoms of nonREM sleep disturbance in patients with "fibrositis syndrome" and healthy subjects. Psychosom Med 37:341–351, 1975
4. Moldofsky H, Scarisbrick P: Induction of neurasthenic musculoskeletal pain syndrome by selective sleep stage deprivation. Psychosom Med 38:35–44, 1976
5. Kellgren JH: Observations on referred pain arising from muscle. Clin Sci 3:174–190, 1938
6. Kellgren JH: On distribution of pain arising from deep somatic structures, with charts of segmented pain areas. Clin Sci 4:35–46, 1939
7. Kellgren JH, McGowan AM, Hughes FSR: On deep hyperalgesia and cold pain. Clin Sci 7:13–27, 1948
8. Moldofsky H, Chester WJ: Pain and mood patterns in patients: a prospective study. Psychosom Med 32:309–318, 1970
9. Smythe HA: Fibrositis syndrome, Current Therapy. Ed 27, HF Conn, ed. Philadelphia, WB Saunders Company 1975, pp 706–708
10. Smythe HA, Moldofsky H: Two contributions to understanding of the "fibrositis" syndrome. Bull Rheum Dis 28:928–931, 1977

57. Heritable disorders of connective tissue

The heritable disorders of connective tissue are diseases in which there is a genetically determined defect in the biosynthesis or degradation of one or another of the structural components of the connective tissue (1). The underlying defects are transmitted by single gene, Mendelian inheritance and may be conveniently classified into 1) those in which biochemical abnormalities in the fibrous components—collagen and elastin—either have been demonstrated or are suspected, 2) disturbances in mucopolysaccharide metabolism, and 3) the skeletal dysplasias.

The heritable disorders of collagen and elastin metabolism include Marfan's syndrome, the Ehlers-Danlos syndrome, osteogenesis imperfecta, homocystinuria, cutis laxa, pseudoxanthoma elasticum, and alkaptonuria (see Section 51).

The **Ehlers-Danlos syndrome** is a group of disorders characterized by fragile, stretchable skin that heals with atrophic, paper-like scars and by joint hypermobility with frequent subluxations. Easy bruisability is commonplace. Many of these patients have a mitral click and murmur. Both inguinal and diaphragmatic hernias are frequent. Visceral rupture, most often of the large vessels or the gastrointestinal tract, also takes place and may prove fatal. Ocular difficulties, most often myopia and retinal detachment, are common. Surgery in these patients may be difficult because of the fragility of the tissues.

Subtypes. On the basis of clinical, genetic, and biochemical evidence, several ᵇtypes have been distinguished (2,3).

Types I–III show gradations of severity (Ehlers-Danlos type I—gravis; II—mitis; III—benign hypermobile). Electron microscopy of skin specimens from patients with types I and II Ehlers-Danlos syndrome has shown collagen fibrils 20–40% larger in diameter than normal, with irregular disordered aggregates (4,5).

Patients with Ehlers-Danlos type IV have thin, translucent, fragile skin and are prone to large vessel and gastrointestinal rupture. The tissues from these patients have a decreased amount of type III collagen. This is inherited in an autosomal recessive pattern.

Ehlers-Danlos type V is inherited in an X-linked recessive pattern and is clinically similar to Ehlers-Danlos type II. The biochemical defect is unknown.

In Ehlers-Danlos type VI, a deficiency of the enzyme lysyl hydroxylase results in a decrease in collagen hydroxylysine and decreased collagen crosslinking (6). This disease is inherited in an autosomal recessive pattern. Clinically, these patients have scoliosis at an early age and are prone to intraocular bleeding and aortic rupture.

In Ehlers-Danos type VII decreased conversion of the collagen precursor, procollagen, to collagen has been reported (6,7). These patients have excessively mobile joints and congenital hip subluxation.

Marfan's syndrome is characterized by abnormal growth and body habitus, ocular difficulties, and cardiac disease. These people are unusually tall, have a decreased upper to lower segment ratio, unusually long arm span, and long slender fingers (*arachnodactyly*). They are loose jointed and have frequent joint subluxations.

Scoliosis is common, usually during adolescence. Pectus excavatum or carinatum is also frequently present. Patients frequently have upward subluxation of the lens and myopia. They commonly have mitral prolapse and aortic insufficiency. Dissection of the aorta is a frequent cause of death. This disorder is inherited as an autosomal dominant trait; however, variable penetrance may obscure the clinical diagnosis.

Defects in hyaluronic acid overproduction and collagen chain biosynthesis have been reported in isolated families; however, the basic defect in the majority of cases remains unknown.

Therapy in these patients is palliative. Affected female children have had puberty induced to avoid excessive height and the scoliosis that accompanies the adolescent growth spurt. Adults with aortic insufficiency have been treated with propranolol to decrease cardiac output and the progression to aortic aneurysm.

The clinical features in **homocystinuria** are similar to those in Marfan's syndrome. Tall stature, with a decreased upper to lower segment ratio, increased arm span, pectus excavatum or carinatum, scoliosis, and arachnodactyly all may occur. Downward lens dislocation is common. These patients are not loose jointed, but instead tend to be stiff. Generalized osteoporosis is frequent, and pathologic fractures may occur. These patients are prone to arterial and venous thromboses, especially during surgery. The most severely affected patients are mentally retarded.

Homocystinuria is due to a defect in the enzyme cystathionine synthetase, with a resultant failure to convert homocysteine and serine to cystathionine. This disorder is inherited as an autosomal recessive trait.

Therapy in these patients has been directed toward improvement of enzyme activity with large doses of pyridoxine, a cofactor for cystathionine synthetase. The mildly affected patients usually improve symptomatically, but the most severely affected patients are resistant. Drugs that inhibit platelet aggregation, such as sulfinpyrazone and aspirin, have been used to prevent thromboses.

The hallmarks of **osteogenesis imperfecta** are osteopenia with fracture diathesis, blue sclerae, and deafness due to osteosclerosis. In the most severe form, *osteogenesis imperfecta congenita*, the neonate has multiple fractures from trauma in utero. Stillbirths resulting from cerebral hemorrhage during birth are common. Osteogenesis imperfecta congenita is most often due to a mutation, but autosomal dominant inheritance has been documented and autosomal recessive inheritance suggested in certain cases.

A milder form of the disease, *osteogenesis imperfecta tarda*, results in a fracture diathesis during childhood. This disorder is inherited in an autosomal dominant pattern.

No medical therapy has proved efficacious. Orthopedic procedures are often required. Patients with osteogenesis imperfecta have the peak incidence of fractures during childhood and adolescence, experience fewer fractures after puberty, and again become prone to fracture after menopause.

An alteration in the ratio of type I to type III collagen biosynthesis has been detected in cultured skin fibroblasts and skin biopsies from certain patients with osteogenesis imperfecta.

Cutis laxa is a rare disorder in which the skin hangs loosely in redundant folds. Unlike the Ehlers-Danlos syndrome with which it is often confused, the skin is neither elastic nor fragile and the joints are not hypermobile. Cutis laxa may occur in an acquired or a hereditary form. Autosomal dominant and recessive forms of cutis laxa have been described. Patients with hereditary cutis laxa frequently develop emphysema and hernias.

Histologic and biochemical evidence suggests that cutis laxa results from impaired elastin metabolism. In a family with an X-linked variety of the disease, an impairment of lysyl oxidase, the enzyme that facilitates crosslinking in elastin, has been described.

Pseudoxanthoma elasticum, also known as the Grönblad-Strandberg syndrome,

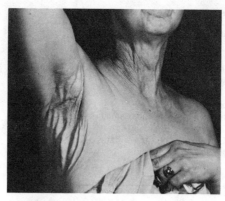

Fig 57-1. Pseudoxanthoma elasticum. This patient compared her skin to "turkey skin." The wrinkled skin was inelastic. Similar changes were noted in other flexural folds.

begins with cutaneous, ocular, cardiovascular, and gastrointestinal abnormalities. The elastic fibers in the corium undergo degeneration and give rise to yellowish papules in the flexural folds and mucous membranes (Fig 57-1). Elastic degeneration in the inner membrane of the choroid (Bruch's membrane) is perceived clinically as angioid streaks (Fig 57-2). Ultimately, retinal hemorrhage and macular degeneration may lead to severe impairment of vision.

The elastin in the large and small arteries degenerates and becomes calcified and the small arteries become occluded. These patients are prone to vascular accidents such as cerebral thrombosis and myocardial infarcts. Gastrointestinal bleeding may result from the vascular disease and is a frequent presenting complaint.

Pseudoxanthoma elasticum is most commonly inherited as an autosomal recessive disorder. The basic defect is that of an increased degradation of elastin,

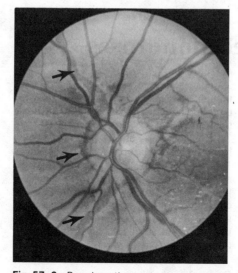

Fig 57-2. Pseudoxanthoma elasticum: angioid streaks (**arrows**) in the left retina of a sister of the patient whose axilla is shown in the previous figure. This woman had no visual complaints.

which may result from increased protease activity in pseudoxanthoma elasticum fibroblasts (8).

Alkaptonuria, a rare inborn error of metabolism due to a deficiency of homogentisic oxidase, is discussed in Section 51.

The **mucopolysaccharidoses and mucolipidoses** are lysosomal storage diseases in which there is defective degradation of glycoproteins and glycolipids (9). The abnormal cellular storage results in a skeletal dysplasia (*dysostosis multiplex*) manifested by stiffness, limitation of motion, and skeletal malformations. These disorders are inherited as autosomal recessive diseases, except for the Hunter syndrome, which is inherited in an X-linked recessive pattern (9,10).

Biochemical defects have been characterized in cultured skin fibroblasts from patients with mucopolysaccharidoses and have corroborated the heterogeneity in these disorders, initially detected by clinical and genetic studies. The classification of these diseases is shown in Table 57-1 (10).

The *Hurler syndrome* (mucopolysaccharidosis I) serves as the prototype of these disorders. Symptoms begin shortly after birth and include coarsening of the facial features, hirsutism, indurated skin, claw hands, stiff joints, kyphosis, corneal clouding, hepatosplenomegaly, and growth and mental retardation. Most of these patients die in their teens from intractable congestive heart failure.

Although the *Scheie syndrome* is due to a defect in the same enzyme as in the Hurler syndrome, symptoms are much milder. Patients have normal intelligence, and most notable manifestations are claw hands, stiff joints, and corneal clouding.

The *Hunter syndrome* (mucopolysaccharidosis II) is similar to the Hurler syndrome, but with milder symptoms. The *Sanfilippo syndrome* (mucopolysaccharidosis III) is characterized by severe mental retardation, with only mild skeletal, ocular, and visceral changes.

The *Morquio syndrome* (mucopolysaccharidosis IV) is characterized by severe short stature due to platyspondyly and by corneal clouding. The patients have lax, rather than stiff joints and excrete large amounts of keratan sulfate in the urine.

The *Maroteaux-Lamy syndrome* (mucopolysaccharidosis type VI) has a phenotype similar to that found in the Hurler syndrome, except that intelligence is preserved despite severe somatic abnormalities.

Mucopolysaccharidose type VII is clinically similar to the Hurler syndrome. The mucopolysaccharidoses are characterized by excessive mucopolysacchariduria-dermatan sulfate, heparan sulfate, and/or keratan sulfate.

The **mucolipidoses** have a phenotype similar to the mucopolysaccharidoses but

Table 57–1. Classification of the mucopolysaccharidoses and mucolipidoses (10)

I. Mucopolysaccharidosis type 1 (alpha-L-iduronidase deficiency)
    A. Hurler form
    B. Scheie form (formerly mucopolysaccharidosis type V)
II. Mucopolysaccharidosis type II—Hunter syndrome (sulfoiduronate sulfatase deficiency)
III. Mucopolysaccharidosis type III—Sanfilippo syndrome
    A. Type A (heparin sulfamidase deficiency
    B. Type B (N-acetyl-glucosaminidase deficiency)
IV. Mucopolysaccharidosis type IV—Morquio syndrome (N-acetylgalactosamine-6-sulfate sulfatase deficiency)
V. Mucopolysaccharidosis type VI—Maroteaux-Lamy syndrome (aryl sulfatase-B deficiency)
VI. Mucopolysaccharidosis type VII—(beta-glucoronidase deficiency)
VII. Mucolipidoses II (I-cell disease)
VIII. Mucolipidosis III (pseudo-Hurler polydystrophy)

do not have mucopolysaccharidura (9,10). These patients have a lysosomal storage disease due to a deficiency of multiple lysosomal hydrolases in connective tissue despite marked elevations of lysosomal enzymes in plasma.

Mucolipidosis II is the clinically more severe condition, with death usually in the first decade, while *mucolipidosis III* (*pseudo-Hurler polydystrophy*) is a milder disease, manifest primarily by skeletal dysplasia and mental retardation.

The **skeletal dysplasias** are a large group of diseases with abnormal chondrogenesis and osteogenesis. A complete listing of these disorders is presented in the 1976 revision of the International Nomenclature of Constitutional Diseases of Bone (over 150 entries are listed) (11). These disorders are characterized clinically by abnormalities of growth and skeletal malformations. Most of these disorders result in short stature, abnormal body proportions (such as rhizomelia in achondroplasia), and skeletal malformations (such as the polydactyly in chondroectodermal dysplasia).

Many skeletal dysplasias are marked by the development of premature osteoarthritis due to the joint abnormalities resulting from the underlying chondrodystrophy.

Patients with degenerative hip diseases and back pain in the first or second decade should be suspected of skeletal dysplasia. *Achondroplasia* and *vitamin D–resistant* rickets are two of the more common examples of these disorders.

Achondroplastic patients have a large skull, with a characteristic facies, rhizomelia, brachydactyly with a trident hand, and increased lumbar lordosis (1). They are particularly prone to disc disease with frequent nerve root compression. This disorder is inherited in an autosomal dominant pattern.

Vitamin D–resistant rickets (familial hypophosphatemic rickets) is inherited in a X-linked dominant pattern. Males are more severely affected than females (12). Most of these patients are short. Patients are prone to stiffening of the back due to progressive calcification in the paraspinous ligaments. Neurologic symptoms may result from nerve root compression by

syndesmophytes. Ankylosis of other joints such as the carpals, radioulnar, and tibiofibular joints also occurs with periarticular calcium deposits. Laboratory studies show hypophosphatemia and hypophosphaturia. Treatment consists of lifelong supplementation with vitamin D and phosphate.

1. MuKusick VA: Heritable Disorders of Connective Tissue. Ed 4. St. Louis, CV Mosby, 1972
2. Uitto J, Lichtenstein JR: Defects in the biochemistry of collagen in diseases of connective tissue. J Invest Dermatol 66:59–79, 1976
3. Bornstein P, Byers PH: Collagen metabolism, Current Concepts, Scope Publication, 1980
4. Vogel A, Holbrook KA, Steinman B, Gitzelmann R, Byers PH: Abnormal collagen fibril structure in the gravis form of the Ehlers-Danlos syndrome. Lab Invest 40:201–206, 1979
5. Holbrook KA, Byers PH: Ultrastructural characterization of several varieties of the Ehlers-Danlos syndrome. Clin Res 26:570A, 1978
6. Pinnell SR, Krane SM, Kenzora JE, Glimcher MJ: An heritable disorder of connective tissue: hydroxylysine deficient collagen disease. N Engl J Med 286:1013–1020, 1972
7. Lichtenstein JR, Martin OR, Kohn L, Byers PH, McKusick VA: Defect in conversion of procollagen to collagen in a form of Ehlers-Danlos syndrome. Science 182:298–300, 1973
8. Gordon SG, Overland M, Foley J: Evidence for increased protease activity secreted from fibroblasts from patients with pseudoxanthoma elasticum. Connec Tissue Res 6:61–68, 1978
9. Neufeld EF, Lim TW, Shaprio LJ: Inherited disorders of lysosomal metabolism. Ann Rev Biochem 44:357–376, 1975
10. McKusick VA, Neufeld EF: The mucopolysaccharide storage diseases, The Metabolic Basis of Inherited Disease. Ed 5. JB Stanbury, JB Wyngaarden, DS Fredrickson, et al, eds. New York, McGraw-Hill, 1983, pp 751–802
11. International Nomenclature of Constitutional Disease of Bone. Revision May, 1977. J Pediatr 93:614–616, 1978
12. Rasmussen H, Anast C: Familial hypophosphatemic rickets and vitamin D–dependent rickets, The Metabolic Basis of Inherited Disease. Ed 5. JB Stanbury, JB Wyngaarden, DS Fredrickson, et al eds. New York, McGraw-Hill, 1983, pp 1743–1773

58. Juvenile osteochondroses

The term *juvenile osteochondroses* (or osteochondritides) embraces a series of regional clinical entities, each designated by its own eponym. These conditions have been united in one group chiefly because of the prevailing, albeit erroneous, belief that they share a common pathogenesis (1,2).

These conditions, occurring primarily in children, have somewhat similar roentgenographic characteristics. Historically, the characteristic lesions are interesting in that most were described in the early days of roentgenography and were differentiated from tuberculosis of bone, and hence considered to represent "aseptic" necrosis (as opposed to septic). The lesions for the most part affect the epiphyseal or

apophyseal centers of the child and were thought to cause a disturbance of growth that ultimately led to structural malformations.

Critical analysis of these conditions has led to their separation into 2 basic groups: 1) those due to localized osteonecrosis of an apophyseal or an epiphyseal center, 2) those related to abnormalities of endochondral ossification, either because of a genetically determined "normal variation" or as a result of chronic or sometimes acute trauma.

Group 1

The true osteonecrotic osteochondroses include those following.

Legg-Calvé-Perthes disease. Idiopathic osteonecrosis of the proximal femoral (capital) epiphysis occurs principally in boys between 3 and 12 years and is much more common in whites than in blacks (3). The disease is bilateral in approximately 10% of patients. The principal clinical finding is a slowly evolving painless limp, often in association with limitation of abduction and internal rotation and a flexion contracture of the affected hip.

Generally, affected children have no other complaints or findings, although many have delayed skeletal maturation. Thyroid function has been shown to be normal. The cause of this disease is obscure.

Biopsy specimens show osteonecrosis.

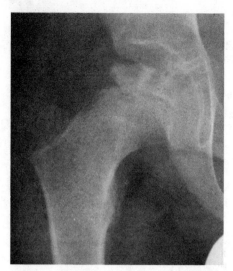

Fig 58–1. Right hip of patient with Legg-Calvé-Perthes disease in early healing phase. (Illustration provided by Dr HJ Mankin)

Roentgenographic monitoring shows progression through phases, indicating gradual revascularization often associated with loss of the normal contour and the development of a large, flat femoral head with a wide, short neck (coxa magna et plana) (Fig 58–1). Revascularization and restoration of bone usually takes 3–5 years (sometimes longer).

Treatment consists principally of various techniques to prevent deformity during this period by limitation of weight bearing on the weakened femoral head. In recent years, osteotomy of the femur or innominate osteotomy has been advocated to improve "coverage" of the femoral head and thus diminish the likelihood of deformity, particularly of the vulnerable lateral portion of the head.

Freiberg's disease is an osteonecrosis of the epiphyseal center of the second metatarsal bone arising in children between 12 and 15, presumably as a result of trauma. There is localized tenderness. The radiograph discloses areas of increased density and rarefaction with flattening of the ossification center of the metatarsal head. The condition is self-limited, but may require protective inserts in the shoe during the revascularization and may leave a permanent minor deformity in the foot.

Panner's disease is an osteonecrosis of the capitellum of the humerus that occurs in children in the early teenage years, principally in association with trauma. Revascularization, as followed by roentgenographic studies, occurs relatively rapidly. Significant disability rarely results.

Kienbock's disease, or idiopathic osteonecrosis of the carpal lunate, occurs in adults rather than in children and in some cases is more clearly related to trauma than many of the others. It may occur as a result of dislocation of the carpus, but congenital variations in ulnar length have been implicated in pathogenesis (4). The

condition is troublesome and sometimes requires corrective surgery, paticularly if significant collapse occurs. The analogous lesion in the carpal navicular is known as *Preiser's disease* and is much less common.

Osteochondritis dissecans, discussed in detail in Section 65, also represents a form of localized osteonecrosis, probably due to trauma.

Group 2

The second group of juvenile osteochondroses are either normal variants of ossification or related to derangements of endochondral ossification.

Osgood-Schlatter disease is a self-limited disorder, occurring most frequently in boys between 10 and 16 years (5). It is associated with pain and tenderness over the tibial tubercle and with some inflammation and thickening at the insertion of the patellar tendon. The condition is bilateral in approximately half the patients.

Roentgenographic examination discloses irregularity and fragmentation of the apophysis of the tibial tubercle similar to that seen in the true osteochondroses (Fig 58–2). Histologic study and followup evaluation have suggested that this is more likely to be a mechanical tendinitis with partial avulsion of the tibial tubercle by extraordinary stress during a critical phase of growth, resulting in a disturbance of endochondral ossification and in new bone formation.

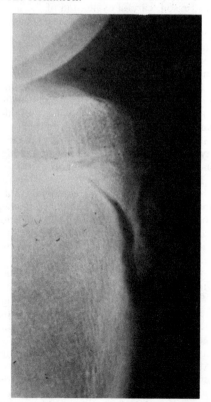

Fig 58–2. Tibia of a young patient with Osgood-Schlatter disease. (Illustration provided by Dr HJ Mankin)

The disease usually remits spontaneously in 1–2 years. However, patients occasionally have considerable distress, and limited activity and braces or even plaster casts may be required to relieve symptoms. Increased prominence of the tibial tubercle, often a late sequel, is not a cause of symptoms in adults.

Blount's disease, or tibia vara, results from an abnormality of endochondral ossification in the medial portion of the proximal tibial epiphyseal plate (6). With continued growth, structural changes are noted in this part of the epiphysis and in the shaft of the tibia. The disease may occur very early in life (infantile form) or later (adolescent form) and is characterized by a progressive, often severe, bowleg deformity, usually bilateral.

On roentgenographic examination the abnormality is rather striking. Irregularity of the epiphyseal line, abnormal sloping of the medial side of the proximal tibial epiphysis, and an irregular "break" on the metaphyseal side of the epiphyseal plate are prominent features.

Ligamentous laxity frequently occurs, so that the bowing deformity is much more severe when the patient is standing than when he is in the recumbent position. Bracing is sometimes successful in preventing progression of the deformity, and if instituted early enough, may reverse the growth abnormality. Most frequently, however, tibial osteotomies or stapling procedures of the lateral side are necessary to prevent progressive genu varum.

In very severe cases the anatomic change is so great that repeated osteotomies are unsuccessful in correcting the deformity and the child enters adulthood with a short malaligned extremity that renders the knee prone to early osteoarthritis.

Sever's disease is a lesion similar to Osgood-Schlatter disease, occurring in the achilles tendon at its insertion into the posterior apophysis of the os calcis. Increased density and partial fragmentation of the calcaneal apophysis may be found but true bone death does not occur. It is much more likely that this condition represents a tendinitis with partial avulsion of the insertion resulting in growth irregularities.

The condition is most common in the 6–10-year-old group and is characterized by pain, tenderness, and swelling along the tendon. Treatment is symptomatic and complete relief is often obtained by elevation of the heel of the shoe.

Scheuermann's disease is a condition of unknown origin, characterized by multiple deformities of the thoracic and upper lumbar vertebrae, presumably caused by an irregularity of ossification and endochondral growth of the ring apophyses. The condition arises in preteen or early adolescent years and results in a slowly progressing, usually painless roundback deformity. Occasionally, however, patients experience a dull aching pain in the thoracic spine.

Roentgenographic studies reveal irregularities of ossification at the margins of the vertebral bodies and the eventual development of anterior wedging, producing a kyphotic deformity.

In many patients the condition is self-limited and the degree of curvature will cause no problem other than a cosmetic one. In some instances, however, the curve is progressive and will require bracing throughut the teen years and possibly corrective surgery including spinal instrumentation and fusion.

Calvé disease, otherwise known as vertebra plana, was thought to represent an isolated osteonecrosis of a vertebral body, with resultant compression and complete collapse. It has been shown, however, that many of these lesions result from a pathologic compression fracture through a focus of eosinophilic granuloma. The pattern may be simulated in Gaucher's disease and other infiltrative disorders.

Köhler's disease may on rare occasions represent a true osteonecrosis of the tarsal navicular. However, strong evidence now supports the view that most patients with a roentgenographic finding of increased density and fragmentation of the navicular have a normal variant of ossification, frequently present on the opposite side, and sometimes familial.

A number of other conditions are normal variants but may under some circumstances be responsible for complaints. These include Köhler's disease of the primary patellar center, Sinding Larsen's disease of the secondary patellar center, Van Neck's disease of the ischial pubic synchondrosis, Milch's disease of the apophysis, Buchman's disease of the iliac crest, Pierson's disease of the symphysis pubis, and Mandl's disease of the greater trochanter.

1. Pappas AM: The osteochondroses. Pediatr Clin N Am 14:549–570, 1967
2. Caffey J: Pediatric X-ray Diagnosis. Ed 5. Chicago, Yearbook Medical Publishers, 1967
3. Inoue A, Freeman MAR, Vernon-Roberts B, Mizuno S: The pathogenesis of Perthes' disease. J Bone Joint Surg 58B:453–461, 1976
4. Gelberman RH, Salamon PB, Jurist JM: Ulnar variance in Kienbach's disease. J Bone Joint Surg 57A:674–676, 1975
5. Ogden JA, Southwick WO: Osgood-Schlatter disease and tibial tuberosity development. Clin Orthop 116:180–189, 1976
6. Kessel L: Annotations on the etiology and treatment of tibia vara. J Bone Joint Surg 52B:93–99, 1970

59. Congenital dysplasia and dislocation of the hip

Congenital dislocation or dysplasia of the hip is one of the most common causes of hip problems in children and of subsequent osteoarthritis in later life. Although the cause of this condition is unknown, it is generally believed to be of genetic origin, based principally on the frequency with which the disorder occurs in families and on the sexual and racial distribution. Dysplasia or dislocation of the hip is approximately 6 times more common in women than men and over 30 times more common in whites than blacks. Individuals of northern Italian or Scandinavian stock run the highest risk.

The left side is affected 1.5 times more often than the right, and when bilateral disease is present, as it is in approximately 30% of cases, the left side is usually more severely involved. The anatomical abnormalities in children (and adults) with this disorder have been well defined and consist principally of an excessively oblique placement of a shallow, defective acetabulum and a small anteverted femoral head.

Ideally, the condition is recognized at birth by the finding of an abnormal click which may be palpated over the hip region as the infant's hip is abducted and adducted. Within a few weeks, this click can no longer be elicited and the diagnosis is then dependent on the findings of limitation of abduction, shortening of the femur, instability of the hip, abnormally placed thigh creases, and on widening of the perineum in bilateral cases. The diagnosis is readily confirmed by roentgenographic demonstration of an abnormal position of the ossified portions of the femur in relation to the pelvis (1–5).

If treatment can be started in the nursery or during the first few weeks of life, the prognosis is usually excellent, and for this reason, careful evaluation of the hips has become an essential part of the examination of the newborn. Splinting in abduction for several months may be all that is necessary to allow the child to develop a normal acetabulum and proximal femur.

If the problem is discovered later in life, it may be necessary to perform a closed or open reduction (usually following preliminary traction), an innominate or femoral varus and derotation osteotomy, or a variety of other procedures to relocate the hip and correct the anatomic abnormality.

Patients who have not been treated or who were inadequately treated in childhood may in later life exhibit manifestations ranging from a mild tilting of the acetabulum, excessive anteversion, and poor acetabular coverage of the femoral head (Fig 59–1) to complete dislocation, with the femoral head abutting on the iliac wing.

The complaints and physical signs in these patients will vary considerably with the degree of abnormality present, but pain is rarely a prominent feature. Generally, patients experience shortening of the extremity, altered range of motion, and a gait abnormality related to malfunction of the gluteus medius muscle. This is characterized by a lurch toward the side of the lesion during the stance phase of gait, known as a Trendelenburg gait.

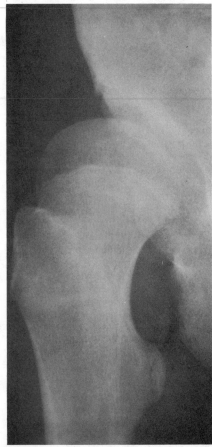

Fig 59–1. Roentgenogram of hip of a 12-year-old girl with acetabular dysplasia. Note the shallowness of the acetabulum and poorly covered femoral head. (Illustration provided by Dr HJ Mankin)

As the patient grows older, osteoarthritis is likely to occur. Over 10 or more years, an asymptomatic or slightly unstable hip will become painful and progressively more limited in motion. Treatment of the disorder differs considerably at this later stage. There are no conservative measures that will reverse or alter the pathologic state, but rest, exercises, nonsteroidal antiinflammatory drugs, and use of a cane may be successful in decreasing symptoms and perhaps delaying the progress of the osteoarthritic lesion. Operative procedures which may be of value in restoring function to these patients include a variety of osteotomies and arthroplastic procedures. Total hip replacement often provides an excellent result but is technically difficult because of the limited bone stock in acetabular area.

1. Stanisavljevic S: Diagnosis and Treatment of Congenital Hip Pathology in the Newborn. Baltimore, Williams & Wilkins, 1964
2. Hirsch C, Scheller S: Result of treatment from birth of unstable hips. Clin Orthop 62:162–166, 1969
3. Harris WH, Crothers O, Oh I: Total hip replacement and femoral head bone-grafting for severe acetabular deficiency in adults. J Bone Joint Surg 59A:752–759, 1977
4. Jones D: An assessment of the value of examination of the hip in the newborn. J Bone Joint Surg 59B:318–322, 1977
5. Paterson DC: The early diagnosis and treatment of congenital dislocation of the hip. Clin Orthop 119:28–38, 1976

60. Slipped capital femoral epiphysis

The proximal femoral epiphysis unites to the neck of the femur when a person is between the ages of 16 and 19. Before this, between the ages of 10 and 17 (with a peak incidence at 11–13 for girls and 13–16 for boys), the femoral head may "slip," displacing medially and posteriorly in relation to the shaft, producing an adduction, lateral rotation, and extension deformity (1,2). The condition is usually insidious in onset, but is occasionally associated with acute trauma.

The frequency of slipped capital femoral epiphysis (adolescent coxa vara, proximal femoral epiphysiolysis) in boys is considerably greater than in girls (2:1); approximately 30–50% of the cases are bilateral.

The child complains of pain in the hip, often referred to the medial side of the knee, and is found to have slight shortening of the extremity, an abnormal (Trendelenburg) gait, and limitation of abduction, medial rotation, and often, flexion.

The origin of the problem is obscure. Aside from the sex predilection, 2 somatotypes are more frequently affected: the short, obese male with poorly developed secondary sex characteristics and the extraordinarily tall and lean child. The oblique angle assumed by the femoral head in relation to the neck at this age suggests increased susceptibility to shearing stress. In addition, some inherent abnormality of the epiphyseal plate probably predisposes to the slip. This abnormality has been attributed to hormonal imbalance (3), genetic error, and an altered anatomic structure.

The diagnosis is established by roentgenographic examination of the hips and the degree of slip is obviously a factor in determining treatment and prognosis (Fig 60–1).

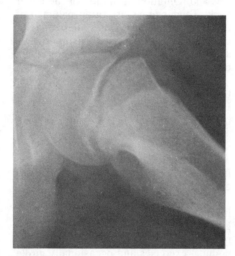

Fig 60—1. Left hip (lateral view) of a patient with slipped capital femoral epiphysis, illustrating posterior displacement of the femur. (Illustration provided by Dr HJ Mankin)

Minimal slips are best treated by fixation in situ with threaded pins (4), but more severe slips may require osteotomies (5) or osteoplastic procedures on the femoral neck. If the patient is seen early and treated effectively, the prognosis is generally good.

With a more advanced degree of slip, the possibility of anatomic restoration is diminished and the likelihood of early and late complications is increased. The principal late complication is osteoarthritis. If closely studied, large numbers of patients formerly thought to have "idiopathic" osteoarthritis show roentgenographic signs of an old mild slipped capital femoral epiphysis (6).

Chondrolysis is one of the early complications of the slipped capital femoral epiphysis. This condition usually occurs in blacks or Hispanics and is much more prevalent in females.

Pathologically, the cartilage shows a severe depletion of proteoglycan, structural derangement without evidence of repair or osteophyte formation, and occasionally pannus formation (7). The condition should be suspected in patients with moderate or severe slipped capital femoral epiphysis who have persistent pain and limitation of motion, especially after surgical correction.

Roentgenograms show progressive narrowing of the joint space and osteopenia of the femoral head and adjacent acetabulum. If treated by prolonged non-weight bearing, about 40% of the patients recover at least partially, but the remainder develop a severe limitation of hip function and eventually require further surgery.

The cause of the disorder is unknown, but some form of autoimmune process in susceptible populations has been suggested.

1. Wilson PD, Jacobs B, Schecter L: Slipped capital femoral epiphysis: an end result study. J Bone Joint Surg 47A:1128–1145, 1965
2. Ponseti IV, McClintock R: The pathology of slipping of the upper femoral epiphysis. J Bone Joint Surg 38A:71–83, 1956
3. Ogden JA, Southwick W: Endocrine dysfunction and slipped capital femoral epiphysis. Yale J Biol Med 50:1, 1977
4. Bianco AJ: Treatment of slipping of the capital femoral epiphysis. Clin Orthop 48:103–110, 1966
5. Southwick WO: Biplane osteotomy for very severe slipped capital femoral epiphysis, The Hip: Proceedings of the Third Open Meeting of the Hip Society. St. Louis, CV Mosby, 1975, pp 105–114
6. Solomon L: Patterns of osteoarthritis of the hip. J Bone Joint Surg 58B:176–183, 1976
7. Eisenstein A, Rothschild A: Biochemical abnormalities in patients with slipped capital femoral epiphysis and chondrolysis. J Bone Joint Surg 58A:459–467, 1976

61. Disorders of the lower back

Despite the low priority accorded, back pain is a major cause of rheumatic disability. In typical rheumatology practices in the United States, 20% of patients have back pain as their presenting complaint (1). In the United Kingdom, back pain is responsible for more than half of all loss of work due to rheumatic complaints (2).

Spinal problems are associated with heavy manual work, particularly that involving stooping, lifting, and twisting.

The causes of pain in the lower back are

Table 61–1. Causes of back pain

Structural
  Prolapsed intervertebral disc
  Spondylosis and apophyseal osteoarthritis
  Diffuse idiopathic skeletal hyperostosis
    (hyperostotic spondylosis)
  Lumbosacral strain
  Spondylolisthesis
  Spinal stenosis
  Other congenital anomalies
  Scheuermann's osteochondritis
  Fractures
  Nonspecific back pain
Inflammatory
  Ankylosing spondylitis and related
    seronegative spondylarthropathies
  Rheumatoid arthritis
  Infection
Neoplastic
  Primary and secondary neoplasms
  Myelomatosis and reticulosis
Metabolic
  Osteitis deformans (Paget's disease of bone)
  Alkaptonuria
  Other forms of bone disease
  Chondrocalcinosis
Referred pain

---

legion. They range from a wide variety of congenital disorders to traumatic states, inflammatory and osteoarthritic processes, infectious diseases, metabolic abnormalities, and primary and metastatic neoplastic diseases (Table 61–1) (3,4). In addition, in many patients with abdominal visceral disorders, pain in the lower back is the primary complaint.

The evaluation of patients with low back pain should always include a complete history and physical examination, appropriate roentgenograms, scans, and laboratory studies to rule out some of the more pernicious processes. Radiographic evidence of degenerative changes is common in the middle-aged and older population. It is essential to exclude other sources of back pain before attributing symptoms to degeneration since spondylitic changes frequently occur in symptomless individuals.

In addition to intervertebral disc syndromes (see Section 62) and diffuse idiopathic skeletal hyperostosis (see Section 63), several mechanical disorders are sufficiently common to warrant further description. These include low back derangement (lumbosacral strain), spondylolisthesis, and lumbar stenosis.

Although disc disease is fairly common, particularly in an industrial community, the largest number of patients with pain in the lower part of the back have insufficient findings to warrant such a diagnosis and are grouped into a category simply titled "low back derangement." The cause of this syndrome is unknown, but it is probably diverse and a number of relatively minor or reversible pathologic states may produce a similar clinical disturbance. These include facetal joint subluxation, transient disc prolapse, partial ligament tear, muscle insertion tear, and muscle hemorrhage.

The patient usually has a history of injury, often significant but sometimes minor, followed by immediate or delayed onset of pain in the lower part of the back. Occasionally pain radiates to the buttocks or, in rare cases, to the leg. Motion of the spine causes pain, but there is usually no increase with cough or strain. Some patients assume an abnormal posture which can be bizarre.

Physical examination discloses tenderness and spasm of the paravertebral muscles and limitation of motion of the lower back. Tender areas are often palpated at the posterior superior iliac spines. Characteristically, a straight leg raising sign is absent, and no sensory, motor, or reflex changes are noted in the legs.

The syndrome of low back derangement tends to be self-limited in most cases. Patients are often severely incapacitated, however, and seek help because of pain and inability to walk or to carry on normal activities.

Treatment consists of rest, usually in bed, analgesics and muscle relaxants, local application of heat, and flexion exercises to relieve the spasm. Occasionally injections of trigger areas or facetal regions with xylocaine and depot corticosteroids are helpful (5). In later phases, abdominal exercises and occasionally girdle support are useful in preventing recurrences.

Spondylolysis and spondylolisthesis. The lesion in spondylolysis is a defect in the pars intraarticularis of the pedicle of one or, rarely, several lumbar segments (6–9). The process is most frequent in males and usually begins in late childhood or early adult life. L5 is most frequently affected, and the defect may be unilateral or bilateral. The basic abnormality in the bone is probably congenital, although a traumatic episode may be involved in its pathogenesis.

Familial cases are common and the abnormality is prevalent in certain racial groups such as the Eskimos. The process is often associated with a spina bifida of L5 or even more frequently of S1.

Patients with spondylolysis are often asymptomatic, but occasionally the syndrome appears to be causally related to chronic or recurrent acute low back pain.

The diagnosis can be best made by oblique roentgenograms of the lumbar spine, in which the defect is clearly demonstrable.

Of considerably greater importance clinically is spondylolisthesis, the sequel of spondylolysis. In this disorder, the affected vertebral body and the entire column cephalad to it slip anteriorly, leaving the posterior elements firmly attached to the caudad segments. The degree of slip ranges from minimal (less than one-third of width of the vertebral body) to complete (a rarely seen circumstance in which the entire body is displaced anterior to the caudad segments), but with any degree the lower lumbar segments are considered unstable and may produce significant symptoms in some individuals.

Patients with symptomatic spondylolisthesis and spondylolysis complain of low back pain, often with radiation into the buttocks or into both lower extremities. The pain is aggravated by forward bending, a motion often severely limited by tight hamstrings. The physical findings, aside from bilateral pain on straight leg raising and occasionally bilaterally depressed ankle jerks, will depend on the degree of spondylolisthesis. With moderate or greater slips, the trunk may be foreshortened, the pelvis tilted, and a sometimes tender palpable "step" is noted posteriorly in the midline at the level above the segment that has slipped forward.

Therapy for patients with symptomatic spondylolysis and spondylolisthesis may include an exercise program, bracing, and restriction of activities, but often these measures are insufficient to control symptoms and an arthrodesis with or without resection of the loose posterior element is indicated. In recent years, bilateral posterolateral fusion has been advocated and is often successful in reducing the pain and disability of this disorder.

Lumbar stenosis. This disorder has recently gained wide recognition as a major cause of lumbar spinal and lower extremity disability in 2 groups of patients: 1) young adults in whom the lumbar spinal canal is congenitally narrowed and assumes a trefoil configuration instead of the usually ovoid one, and 2) older people, in whom posterior osteoarthritic spurring, chronic disc degeneration, facetal joint arthritis and, on occasion, osteitis deformans, conspire to produce a narrowing of not only the lumbar canal but the foramina through which the roots exit to form the lumbosacral plexus (10,11).

Patients with this disorder complain of mild to moderate backache, but more frequently of weakness and numbness of the lower extremities in association with pain, often quite severe, which is intensified by ambulation. This latter complaint is often so prominent as to suggest vascular insufficiency, particularly in older individuals, and hence is known as "lumbar claudication." The symptoms almost always disappear with rest but patients may be severely disabled by the problem, often being required to stop and rest after walking only short distances.

Physical examination usually shows little or no abnormality of the spine with a good range of motion and no limitation of straight leg raising. Absent or depressed ankle jerks and patchy sensory and motor deficits are commonly seen but no well defined pattern has been reported.

The diagnosis can be suspected on routine roentgenograms, which show a narrow disc space, posterior osteophytes, facetal hypertrophic osteoarthritis, and retro- or pseudospondylolisthesis (both without pars intraarticularis, spondylolytic defects) (12). Either myelogram or computerized axial tomography is required to confirm the diagnosis and quantitate the degree of stenosis or the congenital trefoid configuration of the canal (13,14).

The treatment of this disorder in young people is usually a wide decompression with a lateral bilateral arthrodesis, a technique that relieves the symptoms in most patients. In older individuals with the acquired disorder, such surgery is less likely to be successful, possibly because the disorder may be associated with a chronic myelopathy.

Because the surgery is fairly extensive, conservative measures (bracing, exercise, limitation of activities, nonsteroidal antiinflammatory drugs) are preferred for the elderly.

Spondylosis and apophyseal osteoarthrosis. The term *spondylosis* refers strictly to degenerative changes in the intervertebral disc and is distinct from osteoarthrosis of the apophyseal joints. However, because the 2 commonly coexist they are usually considered together. Pathologic evidence of spondylosis is common, and indeed, virtually universal in older subjects. However, many deny back symptoms despite gross radiologic changes.

Pathologic examination shows disorganization of the intervertebral disc with drying up and cleft formation in the nucleus and loss of the clear distinction from the anulus. The disc space becomes narrowed so that if several are involved, the spine may become shorter. Osteophytes develop around the vertebral rims and the apophyseal joints and may compress nerve roots by encroachment into the intervertebal foramina.

Congenital anomalies. Other anomalies of the spine such as failure of separation of vertebral bodies, lumbarization of the first sacral vertebra, sacralization of the fifth lumbar vertebra, and other defects are common. They do not lead directly to back pain but may be responsible for premature disc degeneration.

Fractures. After gross trauma, fractures of the vertebral bodies lead to acute episodes of pain and are easily recognized. However, fractures may also occur after repeated minor stresses. They have been identified in the trabeculae of the vertebral bodies and in the apophyseal processes and pars interarticularis and appear to develop in areas of stress concentration. These small fractures are difficult if not impossible to detect in life, but, nevertheless, may well be responsible for many episodes of acute back pain.

Investigation of back pain. Investigation should regularly include a full blood count, measurement of the erythrocyte sedimentation rate, a biochemical profile including measurements of the serum calcium, phosphate, and alkaline phosphatase, serum proteins and electrophoresis, and in men, acid phosphatase.

Radiographs of the lumbar spine generally reveal no abnormality in acute disc prolapse other than a possible reduction in disc height. Later the changes of lumbar spondylosis may appear with disc space narrowing, endplate sclerosis, osteophytes, and osteoarthritic changes in the apophyseal joints. Oblique radiographs may show encroachment on the intervertebral foramina by osteophytes.

The routine use of radiographs for back pain is probably unnecessary. Their use can be restricted to patients whose clinical evaluation and laboratory tests indicate special back problems (15). However, medicolegal pressures often dictate the need for roentgenographic examination even though the findings may not influence clinical management.

Myelography using oily medium has largely been replaced by radiculography using a water-soluble medium such as metrizamide. This allows the nerve roots to be seen in considerably greater detail and laterally placed lesions which would be missed by myelography may be recognized. Radiculography is indicated only if spinal surgery is being considered. Discography not only demonstrates the ap-pearance of disc degeneration but also reproduces the symptoms when the responsible disc is injected.

Computerized axial tomography provides detailed information about the spine and with high resolution instruments, it is now possible to identify prolapse of an intervertebral disc without need to inject radiopaque dye into the vertebral canal (15).

All patients who have suffered from lumbar pain should be instructed on the correct ways to bend and lift. Prophylactic advice given to manual workers can significantly reduce the incidence of episodes of back pain.

1. American Rheumatism Association: A description of rheumatology practice. Arthritis Rheum 20:1278–1281, 1977

2. Anderson JAD: Back pain and occupation, Lumbar Spine and Back Pain. MIV Jayson, ed. Kent, England, Pitman Medical, 1980, pp 57–82

3. Mankin HJ, Admans RD: Pain in the back and neck, Harrison's Principles of Internal Medicine, ed 8. New York, McGraw-Hill, 1977, pp 37–48

4. Brown MD: Diagnosis of pain syndromes of the spine. Orthop Clin N Am 6:233–248, 1975

5. Mooney V: The facet syndrome. Clin Orthop 115:149–156, 1976

6. Wiltse LL, Widell EH Jr, Jackson DW: Fatigue fracture: the basic lesion in isthmic spondylolisthesis. J Bone Joint Surg 57A:17–22, 1975

7. Rosenberg NJ: Degenerative spondylolisthesis. Predisposing factors. J Bone Joint Surg 57A:467–474, 1975

8. Wiltse LL, Newman PH, McNab I: Classification of spondylosis and spondylolisthesis. Clin Orthop 117:23–29, 1976

9. Taillard WF: Etiology of spondylolisthesis. Clin Orthop 117:30–39, 1976

10. Kirkaldy-Willis WH, Paine KW, Couchoix J, McIvor G: Lumbar spinal stenosis. Clin Orthop 99:30–50, 1974

11. Verbiest H: Pathomorphologic aspects of developmental lumbar stenosis. Orthop Clin N Am 6:177–196, 1975

12. Baddeley H: Radiology of lumbar spinal stenosis, The Lumbar Spine and Back Pain, MIV Jayson, ed. New York, Grune & Stratton, 1976, pp 151–171

13. Jacoby RK, Sims-Williams H, Jayson MIV, Baddeley H: Radiographic stereoplotting: a new technique and its application to the study of the spine. Ann Rheum Dis 35:168–170, 1976

14. Porter RW: Measurement of the spinal canal by diagnostic ultrasound, The Lumbar Spine and Back Pain. MIV Jayson, ed. Kent, 1980, pp 231–245

15. Meyer GA, Haughton VM, Williams AL: Diagnosis of herniated lumbar disc with computed tomography. N Engl J Med 22:1166–1167, 1979

62. Intervertebral disc disease

The joints between the human vertebrae have 2 types of articulations. The posterior facetal joints are diarthrodial (synovial). In the anterior synchondrosis, the cartilage endplates of the bodies of the vertebrae are connected by a fibrocartilaginous intervertebral disc. (A third variety, the uncovertebral joints, is found in the cervical vertebrae.)

The components of the intervertebral discs are the **anulus fibrosus**, densely fibrous rings which surround the **nucleus pulposus**, an internal mass of gelatinous material (1). The anulus consists of circumferential sheets of collagen with fibers that run obliquely. This structure ensures great strength but allows little range of motion.

Water content of normal pulposus is approximately 80%. The remaining mass is collagen and proteoglycan. The macromolecular material of proteoglycan has a protein core linked to polyanionic glycosaminoglycans. The principal glycosaminoglycan is chondroitin sulfate. Low concentrations of keratan sulfate are also present. Hyaluronic acid serves as the filament on which the individual proteoglycan subunits are linked to form large aggregates.

Aging or degeneration related to chronic trauma distorts the arrangement of fibers in the anulus. In the nucleus pulposus, water content and proteoglycan decrease. Chrondroitin 4-sulfate diminishes and the concentration of keratan sulfate increases. The disc develops abnormal structural changes: clefts, scarring, neovascularization, and resiliency, a property that lets the disc act as a shock absorber, decreases.

With advancing age or traumatic insults to the anulus, the intervertebral discs become increasingly prone to posterior prolapse, protrusion, or extrusion into the spinal canal. The weakest site appears to lie posterolaterally, and most protrusions occur in this area, adjacent to the nerve roots as they enter the foramina to exit from the canal.

The clinical syndromes associated with lumbar disc prolapse, protrusion, or extrusion are characterized by low back pain (2). The usual pattern is sciatica associated with specific neurologic deficits, depending on the anatomic site of the lesion and the nerve root which is irritated or compressed.

Lumbar disc disease most commonly involves the L5 and S1 roots (protrusions of discs between L4–5 and L5–S1, respectively). Protrusions above this level are uncommon. Double lesions (both L5 and S1 roots) occur in about 10% of patients.

This condition is somewhat more common in men than in women and generally occurs between the third and sixth decade, with the peak incidence in the 35–45 year age group. Symptoms may appear following a single episode of trauma, but more commonly there is a history of chronic intermittent low back distress, perhaps indicating prolapse or an intermittent bulging phase.

The back pain in disc disease is usually located in the lumbar area, in the midline, or to one side or the other. It is frequently described as dull and aching and is aggravated by movement and relieved by rest. Characteristically, the pain is accentuated by bending forward, coughing, or straining.

Sciatica is distinguished by dull pain in the posterior aspect of the thigh and lateral aspect of the calf that occasionally extends to the foot. This referred component is intensely aggravated by straight leg raising, forward bending, or any other maneuver that places the sciatic nerve, and hence the lumbosacral root, on a stretch. The patient may complain of numbness, particularly of the foot and toes, or weakness, especially of the foot. Bladder symptoms are rarely encountered.

Physical examination may demonstrate limitation of lumbar motion, localized tenderness, spasm of the musculature, and reversal of the normal lumbar lordosis.

Some patients, particularly during an acute episode, manifest extraordinary spasm of the low back, causing the assumption of bizarre postures, tilts, or curves.

If the L4 root (L3–4 disc herniation) is involved, sensory loss over the anterolateral aspect of the thigh, medial aspect of the leg, and posterior portion of the foot may occur. Quadriceps weakness may be present in association with diminution or absence of the knee jerk.

With L5 root irritation (L4–5 disc herniation), there may be atrophy and weakness of the glutei and dorsiflexors of the foot, but knee and ankle reflexes are generally intact. A sensory defect may be noted over the anterolateral aspect of the leg and dorsum of the foot, including the great toe and 1 or 2 adjacent ones. Generally, there is weakness of the extensor hallucis longus.

In patients with S1 involvement (L5–S1 disc herniation), there may be atrophy of the glutei, hamstrings, and calf. The area of hyperesthesia may include the lateral aspect of the foot, especially on the plantar surface. The ankle jerk is frequently diminished or absent.

In patients with L5 or S1 root irritation, maneuvers which stretch the sciatic nerve cause increase of pain. This is the physiologic basis for the straight leg raising test and its variations. In addition, the sciatic nerve, in its course through the sciatic notch or in the posterior thigh, is often very tender to palpation.

Roentgenographic evaluation of patients with lumbar disc disease may fail to reveal any abnormality, particularly in patients in whom the symptoms are of recent origin. In long-standing cases, there may be significant narrowing of the disc space, but this is often very difficult to interpret. Myelography, discography, and electromyography may be valuable in localizing the lesion, but usually the diagnosis can be made without these aids on the basis of history and physical findings. Myelography should probably be reserved for those patients in whom there is to be surgical intervention, and discography, considered hazardous by some, remains controversial.

Disc protrusions occasionally occur in the thoracic region, where they are the cause of either symptoms of cord compression (central discs) or peculiar radicular-type pains (peripheral placement). These syndromes are fortunately rare. The other major location for disc protrusions is in the cervical region, where the syndrome generally affects the C6 and C7 roots (C5–6 and C6–7 interspaces, respectively) (3).

Patients with cervical disc disease (or its late counterpart, bony spur formation, also known as cervical spondylosis) generally complain of chronic aching pain in the neck that radiates to the shoulder or some-

times into the head. The pain may extend into the arm and hand and the patient may experience numbness of the hand or digits. The pain is usually increased by extension of the neck or extremes of other motions. Motion is limited and occasionally the head will be held in a tilted position, presumably due to protective muscle spasm. However, a fairly large number of patients, particularly in a late stage of this disease, have little or no neck pain but only the symptoms of root compression.

Patients with a C6 radiculopathy may experience pain and sensory deficit over the radial aspects of the forearm, thumb, and index finger. These symptoms are associated with weakness and atrophy of the biceps muscle and diminution of the biceps reflex.

Involvement of the C7 root is characterized by pain and sensory defect over the dorsum of the forearm, wrist, and the index and middle fingers. There is usually weakness and atrophy of the triceps muscle and diminution of the triceps reflex.

Unlike the lumbar syndrome, it is possible to have a significant midline protrusion in the cervical area that causes a myelopathy with long tract signs and urinary bladder problems. Roentgenographic studies, particularly oblique views of the cervical spine, may show significant foraminal encroachment by bony spurs or narrowing of disc spaces. Patients with cervical radiculopathy frequently have a reversal of the normal cervical lordosis, probably due to muscle spasm. Myelography may be very helpful in cervical spine disease to demonstrate the site of a significant encroachment on the canal or root, particularly in the accurate delineation of the level of involvement prior to surgical intervention.

In diagnosing patients with the disc syndromes, it is important to first rule out, as far as possible, other causes of local or radicular pain that may simulate the pattern of herniated intervertebral disc. All patients with back or neck distress should have a thorough physical examination, appropriate radiographic scanning, and laboratory studies to exclude the possibility of metastatic cancer, myeloma, other mechanical derangements, or neuropathy from other causes. If the patient fails to respond to conservative treatment, the physician should consider the possibility that the root irritation or local symptoms may be due to some cause other than mechanical derangement.

Treatment of the cervical and lumbar syndromes will vary according to the age and occupation of the patient, the severity and duration of symptoms, the degree and extent of clinical impairment, and many other factors. In general, conservative management, consisting of a soft collar, traction, physical therapy, analgesics, and exercises for the cervical areas, or bed rest, physical therapy, exercises, analgesics, and corset support for the lumbar area will be successful in alleviating symptoms in most patients.

For those who do not respond or who have acute episodes at frequent intervals, nerve root, epidural, or intrathecal injections of corticosteroids are sometimes useful (4). In the small portion of patients refractory to prolonged conservative therapy, myelography and surgical intervention (5), a laminectomy at the involved segment and removal of the disc (6), may be necessary. Local arthrodesis may be indicated for instability or posterior facet arthritic changes at the involved site. In the cervical area, posterior laminectomy, with or without fusion, may be necessary (7), but in recent years anterior approaches with disc removal and fusion by bone plug have gained favor in selected cases.

1. Coventry MB: Anatomy of the intervertebral disc. Clin Orthop 67:9–15, 1969
2. Armstrong JR: Lumbar Disc Lesions, Ed 3. Baltimore, Williams & Wilkins Company, 1965
3. Friedenberg AB, Miller WT: Degenerative disc disease of the cervical spine. J Bone Joint Surg 45A:1171–1183, 1963
4. Brown FW: Management of diskogenic pain using epidural and intrathecal steroids. Clin Orthop 129:72–78, 1977
5. Wiltse LL: Surgery for intravertebral disk disease of the lumbar spine. Clin Orthop 129:22–45, 1977
6. Naylor A: Late results of laminectomy for lumbar disk prolapse. J Bone Joint Surg 56B:17–29, 1974
7. Robinson RA, Walker AE, Ferlic DC, Wiecking DK: The results of anterior interbody fusion of the cervical spine. J Bone Joint Surg 44A:1569–1587, 1962

63. Diffuse idiopathic skeletal hyperostosis

Diffuse idiopathic skeletal hyperostosis (DISH), also called ankylosing hyperostosis of Forestier and Rotes-Querol, is a common skeletal disorder associated with distinct alterations in both spinal and extraspinal structures (1–3).

Radiographic criteria for establishing the diagnosis of this disease are based on characteristic alterations in the spine. These include: the presence of flowing calcification and ossification along the anterolateral aspect of at least 4 contiguous vertebral bodies, relative preservation of intervertebral disc height, and absence of intraarticular bony ankylosis of the sacroiliac and apophyseal joints.

Diffuse idiopathic skeletal hyperostosis is a disorder of middle-aged and elderly individuals and is more frequent in men. Its frequency in patients over 65 years is approximately 5–10%. The patient may be asymptomatic or may have clinical manifestations that relate to the spinal sites (stiffness, restricted range of motion, dysphagia), extraspinal sites (restricted motion, tendinitis), or both.

Laboratory analysis is generally unrewarding although the disorder is more common in individuals with diabetes mellitus.

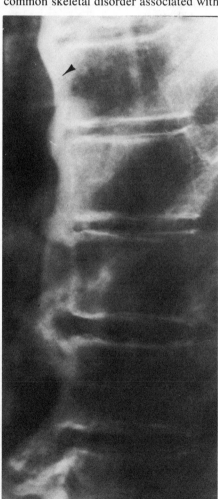

Fig 63–1. Spinal abnormalities in DISH. A lateral radiograph of the thoracic spine reveals ossification along the anterior aspect of the vertebral bodies (**arrowhead**). Observe the bumpy spinal contour, radiolucent extensions at the level of the intervertebral disc, and a linear radiolucency between the deposited bone and the anterior surface of the vertebra. The intervertebral discs are mildly narrowed. (Illustration provided by Dr D Resnick).

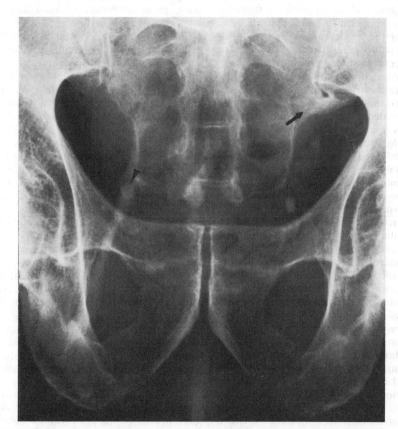

Fig 63–2. Pelvic abnormalities in DISH. Findings include a well defined osteophyte along the inferior aspect of the sacroiliac joint (**arrow**) and sacrotuberous ligament ossification (**arrowhead**). (Illustration provided by Dr D Resnick).

The distinct radiographic findings in the vertebral column include bony deposition which has a predilection for the anterolateral aspect of the vertebrae, particularly in the mid- and lower thoracic region, although cervical and lumbar spine abnormalities may also be apparent. Apposition of bone creates a bumpy spinal contour with large irregular excrescences and a diagnostic radiolucency between the deposited bone and the anterior margin of the vertebral body (Fig 63–1). Deposition of bone on the posterior margin of the vertebrae is less common and less severe, although occasionally calcification and ossification of the posterior longitudinal ligament is found, which may lead to neurologic symptoms and signs (4). The intervertebral discs are generally normal in height.

Radiographic changes in extraspinal locations are most often apparent in the pelvis, heel, foot, and elbow. These changes are characterized by proliferation at sites of tendon and ligament attachment to bone, ligament calcification and ossification, and paraarticular osteophytes. Particularly characteristic are sacrotuberous and iliolumbar ligament calcifications in the pelvis (Fig 63–2), paraacetabular bony outgrowths, olecranon and calcaneal spurs, patellar hyperostosis, and bony proliferation in the tarsal and metatarsal areas. Some of these outgrowths, such as those involving the calcaneus and olecranon, may produce local symptoms and signs sufficient to warrant surgical intervention.

Recurrent osseous proliferation may take place after removal of osteophytes. Heterotopic bone formation after arthroplasty is another apparent complication of the disease (5).

The etiology of DISH is unknown. Although hyperostosis of the spine may be seen in several other disorders such as fluorosis, hypervitaminosis A, ankylosing spondylitis, psoriasis, Reiter's syndrome, acromegaly, and hypoparathyroidism, no convincing evidence exists that links hyperostosis in DISH to any of these disorders.

Although occasional reports emphasize a possible association of DISH with HLA–B27, this has not been verified by others.

1. Forestier J, Rotes-Querol J: Senile ankylosing hyperostosis of the spine. Ann Rheum Dis 9:321–330, 1950
2. Resnick D, Shaul SR, Robins JM: Diffuse idiopathic skeletal ostosis: Forestier's disease with extraspinal manifestations. Radiology 115:513–524, 1975
3. Resnick D, Niwayama G: Radiographic and pathologic features of spinal involvement to diffuse idiopathic skeletal hyperostosis. Radiology 119:559–568, 1976
4. Resnick D, Guerra J, Robinson CA, Vint V: The association of diffuse idiopathic skeletal hyperostosis and calcification and ossification of the posterior longitudinal ligament. Am J Roentgenol 131:1049–1053, 1978
5. Resnick D, Linovitz RF, Feingold ML: Postoperative heterotopic ossification as a manifestation of ankylosing hyperostosis of the spine (Forestier's disease). J Rheumatol 3:313–320, 1976

64. Neoplasms of the joints, including villonodular synovitis and osteochondromatosis

Despite the many types of tissue found in the joint and its supporting structures, primary neoplasms of the joint are rare. Most of the lesions considered to be tumors are actually localized swellings or deformities resulting from inflammatory, mechanical, or degenerative disease. Most true neoplasms arise from the synovium and are benign (1,2).

Pigmented villonodular synovitis is one of the more common synovial lesions which is considered by some to be neoplastic (1–5). The tumor consists of a mass of matted reddish-brown villous projections and nodules densely adherent to the capsule and synovium of the joint and occasionally encroaching on the cartilage surfaces or burrowing into the subchondral bone. Histologic examination shows monotonous deep synovial cell proliferation, increased vascularity and fibrosis with infiltration by lymphocytes, multinucleated giant cells, iron deposition, and lipid laden macrophages interspersed with areas of hemorrhage (1–3).

The condition occurs most frequently in the knee, but occasionally involves the hip, elbow, ankle, or foot, and produces a swollen, warm tender joint with a limited range of motion. Roentgenographic examination may show only widening of the soft tissue shadows with rounded, whorled masses. In long-standing cases, the roentgenogram occasionally shows rarefaction of the adjacent bones and sometimes erosions and joint destruction

(4–6). Aspiration of the joint often reveals dark serosanguineous synovial fluid, an important diagnostic feature.

The diagnosis can be made by arthography which shows nodular masses encroaching on the joint space or by arthroscopy which reveals the abnormal tissue and allows a biopsy under direct vision. A meticulous excision of the synovium, often through both anterior and posterior approaches, is necessary for adequate treatment, but at times the disease progresses to a point where joint destruction is necessary. If the synovectomy is incomplete, the lesion may recur (2,4).

Localized pigmented villonodular synovitis has a histologic appearance essentially identical to the diffuse form (Fig 64–1), but usually presents as a solitary nodule in either the medial or lateral compartment of the knee joint. This is often mistaken for a meniscal tear or a parameniscal cyst (5). The serosanguineous effusion seen in the diffuse form is rarely present with this lesion, and simple excision results in cure. The localized form of the disease is more common in tendon sheaths, especially in the hands and feet, where it is sometimes known as giant cell tumor of tendon sheath (1,3,5).

Synovial chondromatosis is an uncommon disorder characterized by the presence of multiple foci of cartilage metaplasia within the synovium (2,7,8). As these masses grow, they first form nodules within the synovial tissue and then become

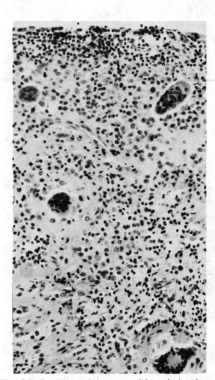

Fig 64–1. Villonodular synovitis: photomicrograph of synovium from nodule removed from the knee joint of a 13-year-old boy who had had recurrent knee effusions for 8 months. Note multinucleated giant cells amidst dense infiltrate of small lymphocytes and large cells with pale, spindle-shaped nuclei. (Reproduced from Arthritis and Allied Conditions. Ed 9, with permission of the editor, Dr Daniel J. McCarty, Jr, and the publishers, Lea & Febiger, Philadelphia)

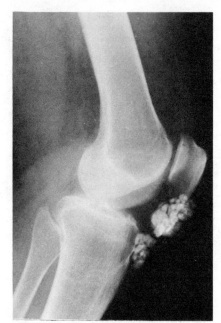

Fig 64–2. Synovial osteochondromatosis: knee of a 58-year-old woman who had painless swelling of the infrapatella bursa. (Reproduced from Arthritis and Allied Conditions)

excrescences, either sessile or pedunculated. The nodules may calcify, or if the blood supply from the synovium remains intact, ossification may take place within their central portions. A characteristic roentgenographic appearance results (Fig 64–2).

The disease is almost always monarticular, affecting principally the knee but occasionally the hip, ankle, elbow, or other joints. The diagnosis may be suspected in adults in whom limitation of motion, crepitation, and locking episodes gradually appear without antecedent trauma. Roentgenographic examination is helpful, but findings in milder cases may be confused with calcium crystal deposition diseases. The diagnosis is best made by arthroscopic examination and surgical biopsy.

The process appears to be self-limited, but extensive joint destruction can occur unless a complete synovectomy is performed. An aggressive form of the disorder has been described, which tends to recur and, in rare cases, may have distant metastases. In these instances the lesion must be regarded as a form of synovial chondrosarcoma (9).

Benign lesions. Other, less common, benign lesions that affect the joints include: *lipoma*, which may be intracapsular or intrasynovial and may demonstrate a bizarre configuration (*lipoma arborescens*); *chondroma*, a solitary firm mass usually located anteriorly in the knee joint with characteristics typical of benign cartilage tumors; *hemangioma*, either localized or diffuse, usually synovial in origin and an occasional cause of recurrent hemarthrosis; and *xanthoma*, probably a variant of

the localized pigmented nodular synovitis, in which there are extensive deposits of neutral lipids (1,2).

The paraarticular and paratendinous tissues also demonstrate a variety of benign lesions, which include: *ganglion*, a thin-walled sac filled with a viscous fluid, often in continuity with a joint or tendon sheath, and possibly resulting from a rupture or hernia of the membranes of these fluid-filled cavities; *localized pigmented villonodular tenosynovitis*, identical with that found within the knee, but sometimes called xanthoma or giant cell tumor of tendon sheath (Fig 64–3); *chondromatosis* of tendon sheath, more common in the upper extremity and difficult to excise locally; and *lipoma* (1,2).

Malignant tumors. Fortunately, primary malignant tumors of joints are rare. The principal lesion that may arise within or adjacent to a joint is the *synovioma*, also called *synovial sarcoma* or malignant synovioma (1,2,10–12). This highly malignant fibroblastic neoplasm usually occurs in late childhood or early adult life and arises most often in the lower extremity within the fascial planes of the thigh or leg, adjacent to, and occasionally within, the knee or, uncommonly, in other joints.

The mass may be present in a quiescent state for a number of years, and calcifications may occur within its substance, producing a characteristic roentgenographic appearance. Synovial sarcomas are made up of two types of malignant cells: one epithelioid in appearance, the other resembling fibroblasts (Fig 64–4).

Occasionally, one encounters a *monophasic synovioma*, which raises considerable difficulty in distinguishing the lesion

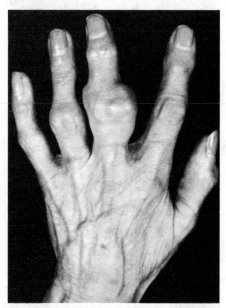

Fig 64–3. Localized pigmented villonodular tenosynovitis ("fingeroma") of middle finger in a 67-year-old woman. Note also Heberden's and Bouchard's nodes.

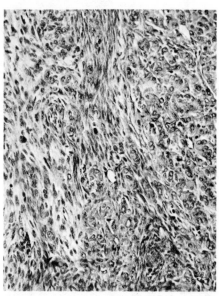

Fig 64–4. Photomicrograph of synovial sarcoma (synovioma) removed from the leg of a 65-year-old man. There is an inextricable admixture of 2 types of malignant cells: one is present in clumps and cords of polyhedral and ovoid cells that are epithelioid in appearance; the other consists of fibroblast-like elements with large fusiform nuclei.

from other spindle cell sarcomas. After local excision, the tumor rapidly recurs, and metastases appear in the lungs or lymph nodes in a high percentage of patients despite radical surgery, radiation therapy, or chemotherapy.

Several unusual malignant tumors may be associated with tendon sheaths, particularly in the upper extremities. These include *clear cell sarcoma*, the origin of which is obscure (2,13). The lesion is highly malignant with considerable propensity for local recurrence and distant metastasis.

Epithelioid sarcoma is occasionally found in the subcutaneous tissue of the hand and forearm but may appear in the tendon sheaths or adjacent to joints (2,14). Despite its small size at original observation and the disarmingly bland histologic picture, the tumor is highly malignant and long survival is unusual, despite treatment.

Synovial chondrosarcoma is a rare neoplasm that may arise either within a focus of, or closely simulating the appearance of, synovial chondromatosis (9). The lesion occurs most frequently in the knee joint and its growth is slow. Local recurrence is common, but distant metastasis is a late occurrence. The histologic pattern is indistinguishable from chondrosarcoma of bone or other soft parts, and the question of origin from the joint or invasion from without is as yet undecided.

Metastatic tumors from other sites may also be present in various joints, occasionally including even the digits (15,16).

Other lesions. As indicated, most of the "tumors" of joints are, in fact, not neoplasms, and represent a variety of lesions that produce a localized swelling in or around the joint. These include adventitious bursae, ganglions, Baker's cysts, parameniscal cysts, free bodies, loculated effusions, osteophytes, and traumatic deformities.

Roentgenographic evaluation is helpful in differential diagnosis, but frequently arthroscopy or exploration is necessary for definitive evaluation and treatment.

1. Jaffe HL: Tumors and Tumorous Conditions of the Bone and Joints. Philadelphia, Lea & Febiger, 1958

2. Schajowicz F: Tumors and Tumor-like Lesions of Bone and Joints. New York, Springer-Verlag, 1982, p 519

3. Schumacher HR, Lotke P, Athreya B, et al: Pigmented villondular synovitis: light and electron microscopic studies. Semin Arthritis Rheum 12:32–43, 1982

4. Chung SMK, Janes JM: Diffuse pigmented villonodular synovitis of the hip joints. J Bone Joint Surg 47A:293–303, 1965

5. Granowitz SP, D'Antonia J, Mankin HJ: The pathogenesis and long term end results of pigmented villonodular synovitis. Clin Orthop 114:335–351, 1976

6. Rosenthal DI, Coleman PK, Schiller AL: Pigmented villonodular synovitis: correlation of angiographic and histologic findings. Am J Roentgenol 135:581–585, 1980

7. Jeffreys TE: Synovial chondromatosis. J Bone Joint Surg 49B:530–534, 1967

8. Milgram JW: Synovial chondromatosis: a histopathologic study of 30 cases. J Bone Joint Surg 59:792–801, 1977

9. Goldman RL, Lichtenstein L: Synovial chondrosarcoma. Cancer 17:1233–1246, 1964

10. Cole S: Synovial sarcoma. J R Coll Surg Edinb 8:1–51, 1962

11. Cadman NL, Soule EH, Kelly PJ: Synovial sarcoma: an analysis of 134 tumors. Cancer 18:613–627, 1965

12. Murray JA: Synovial sarcoma. Orthop Clin N Am 8:963–972, 1977

13. Hayden SI, Shiu MH, Fortner JB: Tenosynovial sarcoma: a clinical-pathological study of 136 cases. Cancer 39:1201–1217

14. Enzinger FM: Epithelioid sarcoma: a sarcoma simulating a granuloma or carcinoma. Cancer 26:1029–1041, 1970

15. Fam AG, Kalin A, Lewis AJ: Metastatic carcinomatous arthritis and carcinoma of the lung. J Rheumatol 7:98–104, 1980

16. Vaczy A, Budson DC: Phalangeal metastases from bronchogenic carcinoma. JAMA 239:226–227, 1978

65. Osteochondritis dissecans

Osteochondritis dissecans, possibly a form of osteonecrosis, is localized to subchondral bone (1). The knee is the most common site, but it also can occur in the elbow, hip, ankle, or in almost any diarthrodial joint.

Onset usually follows a traumatic event, resulting in a shearing fracture of the subchondral cortex and medullary bone. Loss of blood supply ensues, with no initial injury to the overlying cartilage. Additional trauma may cause the fragment to loosen, separate further, and, in some cases, discharge into the joint, producing a "loose body."

The symptoms are vague before the fragment loosens and consist principally of mild aching pain and intermittent swelling. However, when loosely attached or free bodies are discharged into the joint, symptoms are accentuated and may result in mechanical locking, the clinical hallmark of osteochondritis dessicans. In the knee joint, where the favored site of osteo-

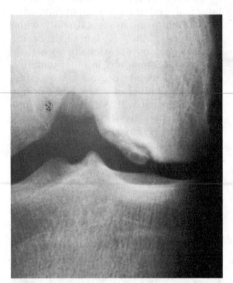

Fig 65–1. Right knee of patient with osteochondritis dissecans involving lateral portion of medial femoral condyle. (Illustration provided by Dr HJ Mankin)

chondritis dissecans is the lateral face of the medial femoral condyle, localized tenderness often develops.

The condition is most common in males in the second and third decades. The occurrence of the syndrome in families and of occasional bilateral involvement clouds the issue of a purely traumatic etiology.

The diagnosis is readily confirmed by roentgenographic examination (Fig 65–1). Arthrography or arthroscopy may occasionally be helpful.

The prognosis depends upon age; young children (under 15) frequently heal spontaneously in a year or more. In older individuals or those in whom the bone has separated, surgical intervention and replacement or removal of the segment may be necessary.

1. Green JP: Osteochondritis dissecans of the knee. J Bone Joint Surg 48B:82–91, 1966

66. Loose bodies

Loose bodies, or "joint mice," may occur in any diarthrodial joint. The bodies may be composed entirely of cartilage or have a central area of dead bone. The number of loose bodies in a joint may vary considerably. They may be entirely silent or cause pain, deformity, and significant interference with mechanical function.

Since articular cartilage is avascular and derives its nutrition from synovial fluid, a segment of cartilage (with or without underlying bone) that breaks off into the joint may not only retain its viability but, for

some unknown reason, may actually enlarge in size. Thus, over a period of years, many large bodies may accumulate in a joint without gross defect in the articular surface.

Free bodies may originate in the joints from many causes including osteoarthritis, synovial chondromatosis, osteochondral fractures, osteochondritis dissecans, neuroarthropathy, meniscal injuries, or joint infections. The complaints and physical findings depend on the joint involved and the number and location of bodies. Most

frequent physical manifestations are crepitation, intermittent locking, swelling, pain, and limitation of motion.

Roentgenographic evaluation reveals only those bodies that have a bony or calcified center. Free bodies should generally be removed unless they are firmly fixed in a recess, such as the suprapatellar pouch. In addition to the symptoms that loose bodies cause, the constant trauma of contact with the articular surface may lead to osteoarthritic change.

67. Osteitis pubis

Osteitis pubis is an uncommon, self-limited affliction of adults, characterized by pain and tenderness in the pubic rami adjacent to the symphysis. The pain is aggravated by walking or standing and is generally relieved by rest (1). The discomfort is accentuated by stretching of the adductor muscles and one of the common findings is spasm of these muscles and tenderness at their origins. This condition often occurs as a sequel to urologic surgery (retropubic prostatectomy) or gynecologic procedures (cystocele repair).

Osteitis pubis may be diagnosed by roentgenographic findings of patchy increased density of both pubic rami, often associated with mottled areas of rarefaction. Symptoms may be mild, subsiding spontaneously in a few weeks, or incapacitating. In the most severe cases, the patient may require complete bed rest for many months for relief of intense pain.

The pathogenesis of this disorder is obscure, and it is agreed that there may be several causes. Frankly purulent or indolent osteomyelitis of the parasymphyseal bone is sometimes responsible, but in most cases, tissue cultures are sterile (2).

Though many forms of treatment have been used, no single method has been satisfactory for all patients. Fortunately, the condition appears to be self-limited and may subside after a period of several weeks or months, although some cases persist for a much longer time.

1. Schute W: Osteitis pubis. Clin Orthop 20:187–192, 1961
2. Gilbert DN: The bacterial causation of postoperative osteitis pubis. Surg Gynecol Obstet 141:195–198, 1975

68. Regional osteoporosis

Regional osteoporosis is defined as osteoporosis confined to one region or segment to the body, almost always part of the appendicular skeleton (1). The classic example of such a disorder is osteoporosis associated with disuse or immobilization of a limb or portion of a limb. Other examples include reflex sympathetic dystrophy and transient regional osteoporosis.

As contrasted to the uniform increase in skeletal radiolucency typical of generalized osteoporosis, the radiographic patterns of regional osteoporosis are more variable. Uniform osteopenia (a decrease in radiographic density of the bone) may accompany regional osteoporosis of long duration, such as that associated with chronic disuse in patients who are paralyzed or have undergone amputation.

Band-like osteopenia (in the subchondral or metaphyseal regions) and patchy osteopenia (particularly in the epiphyses) may indicate a more acutely developing osteoporosis, such as that occurring in reflex sympathetic dystrophy. Acutely, both cortical and spongy bone may exhibit striking alterations. The cortical abnormalities, which include subperiosteal, intracortical, and endosteal erosion, may require high quality radiography for their detection.

In reflex sympathetic dystrophy, the radiographs may reveal rapid and severe osteopenia, particularly in periarticular regions, which simulates the appearance of primary articular disorders. The absences of significant intraarticular erosions and joint space narrowing usually allow accurate differentiation of reflex sympathetic dystrophy from these other disorders.

Transient regional osteoporosis is an appropriate term for conditions that share certain features: rapidly developing osteoporosis affecting periarticular bones; self-limited and reversible nature; and absence of clear-cut evidence of inciting factors such as trauma and immobilization.

Two important diseases (which are probably related) fall into this category: transient osteoporosis of the hip and regional migratory osteoporosis. The former is seen in young and middle-aged adults, particularly men. In men, either hip may be involved, whereas in women, the left hip is affected almost exclusively, and changes may begin during the third trimester of pregnancy. Progressive and marked osteoporosis of the femoral head is associated with less extensive involvement of the femoral neck and acetabulum. The joint space is not reduced and the few synovial biopsy specimens that have been obtained have been normal. The cause is unknown although various theories have been proposed, including neurogenic mechanisms (2).

Regional migratory osteoporosis migrates from one articulation to another. The hip is affected less frequently than other parts, such as the knee, ankle, and foot. This condition occurs more frequently in men than women and usually becomes evident in the fourth or fifth decade of life.

Radiographs reveal osteoporosis which becomes apparent within weeks or months after the onset of clinical findings. Radioisotopic joint imaging can sometimes suggest this syndrome at sites before the osteopenia is detectable (3). Radiographically the joint space is not narrowed, nor is intraarticular erosion evident.

1. Arnstein AR: Regional osteoporosis. Orthop Clin N Am 3:585–600, 1972
2. McCord WC, Nies KM, Campion DS: Regional migratory osteoporosis, a denervation disease. Arthritis Rheum 21:834–838, 1978
3. Tannenbaum H, Esdaile J, Rosenthall L: Joint imaging in regional migratory osteoporosis. J Rheumatol 7:237–244, 1980

69. Paget's disease of bone

Paget's disease of bone (osteitis deformans), is a "focal disorder of unknown etiology characterized initially by excessive resorption and subsequently by excessive formation of bone culminating in a 'mosaic' pattern of lamellar bone associated with extensive local vascularity and increased fibrous tissue in adjacent marrow" (1). Paget's disease of bone is a focal disorder since some bone is always spared no matter how widespread the pagetic process.

In the United States, it is estimated that Paget's disease occurs in approximately 1–3% of persons past age 45 and is usually polyostotic. Males tend to predominate and the disease is almost always first detected after the age of 40. Familial clustering may take place.

The cause of Paget's disease of bone is unknown, although it has been suggested that the disorder is a late manifestation of a viral infection. Osteoclasts from patients with Paget's disease of bone have been found to contain intranuclear and cytoplasmic inclusions that resemble most closely the nucleocapsids of viruses such as measles. Definitive identification of these inclusions, however, has not been accomplished.

The primary event in Paget's disease is probably a focal, intense resorption of bone (osteolytic phase) leading to the formation of typical resorption lacunae filled with osteoclasts. The osteoclasts may assume bizarre shapes and contain as many as 100 nuclei, a feature not seen normally or in other pathologic states.

Early in the disease, the osteolysis is accompanied by some element of repair, usually observed in focal regions near the excessive resorption. The newly deposited bone is abnormal, but usually lamellar, although woven bone may also be found. The local fatty or hematopoietic marrow is replaced by a loose, fibrous connective tissue stroma that frequently appears hypervascular.

The pagetic process occurs in both cancellous and cortical bone. The characteristic and diagnostic "mosaic" pattern of Paget's disease results from the abnormal deposition of lamellar bone. The so-called cement lines are formed at sites where these lamellae are joined.

In some patients the rate of resorption diminishes whereas bone formation continues, resulting in an increased mass of bone per unit volume (osteoblastic or sclerotic phase). In general, however, in this disease a close coupling between formation and resorption is observed, even though formation may appear excessive and involved bones may be larger than normal.

Overall, there may be enormous increases in rates of resorption and formation of bone which involve increased fluxes of mineral ions from resorbing bone into newly forming bone. In addition, bone matrix is resorbed, as reflected in the increased urinary excretion of hydroxyproline-containing peptides, which may exceed 1,000 mg/24 hr. The increased bone accretion and the increased local vascularity account for the increased uptake of bone-seeking isotopes by pagetic lesions as detected by scanning procedures.

Levels of alkaline phosphatase activity in the serum are characteristically elevated in patients with Paget's disease of bone. These increased levels reflect bone formation and generally correlate with the extent and activity of the pagetic process. In rare instances, radiographically typical Paget's disease of bone may be associated with a normal level of alkaline phosphatase activity, when only a small bone or portion of a bone is involved.

Levels of alkaline phosphatase activity tend to rise gradually often reaching a plateau characteristic for each individual, although in some cases wide fluctuations are seen, with decreases associated with immobilization or intercurrent infections. In the rare individuals who develop sarcoma at the site of pagetic involvement, an explosive rise in alkaline phosphatase levels is seen.

The radiographic appearance of pagetic bone reflects the predominant pathologic process and the stage of the disorder. The initial lesion is a focal area of radiolucency, particularly evident in the skull where the term "osteoporosis circumscripta" is used. In long bones, particularly the tibia and the femur, the resorption is marked by an advancing wedge of radiolucency.

Attempts at repair are observed as islands of increased density or as coarsened trabecula. In some instances, the dimensions of the involved bone may increase and thickening of the cortex results, progressing to a sclerotic appearance. Thickening of the pelvic brim or iliopectineal line ("brim sign") is a helpful finding in differentiating Paget's disease from metastatic carcinoma of bone.

The most common sites of involvement are the spine, pelvis, skull, femur, and tibia. In individuals with widespread disease, almost every bone may be involved, including the small ones. In most instances, Paget's disease of bone is asymptomatic. It becomes clinically apparent when the involvement results in pain, gross deformity, compression of neural structures, fracture of an involved bone, alteration of joint structure and function, or the consequences of increased vascularity. When bone of the appendicular skeleton is involved, the overlying skin may be abnormally warm. Occasionally the excessive circulation in the hypervascular bone contributes to the development of high output cardiac failure.

Specific features are associated with each site of involvement (2). Skull involvement may produce obvious enlargement of the head with increased frontal bossing, or occasionally involve the facial bones, resulting in a leonine appearance.

Deafness results from involvement of the ossicles or neural elements.

Symptomatic spinal involvement can produce pain directly or as a result of neural compression. Spinal cord compression is a rare complication. Pain in the limbs may be localized over the lesion or result from nerve root compression or associated joint disease. Degenerative disease of the hip secondary to involvement of the subchondral bone is common in Paget's disease of bone and may be associated with a striking degree of protrusio acetabulae (Fig 69–1). A similar arthropathy may occur in knees due to involvement of the distal femurs or the patellae.

The dread complication of Paget's disease of bone is osteosarcoma, which fortunately occurs in less than 1% of patients. Other associated neoplasms include giant cell tumors and non-neoplastic granulomas. Malignant tumors occasionally metastasize to pagetic bone.

Metabolic complications usually result from some interruption of the mechanism that controls the close bone formation-resorption coupling. Immobilization or fracture may lead to hypercalciuria, or rarely, hypercalcemia.

Since Paget's disease of bone is asymptomatic in most individuals and does not result in significant clinical disability, no therapy is indicated (2,3).

In symptomatic individuals, specific therapy is available but careful clinical evaluation is essential to determine the nature of the pain or disability. Antiinflammatory agents (e.g., aspirin, or indomethacin) may suppress pain, although in dosages commonly used these do not affect the biochemical abnormalities. Other agents can suppress pagetic bone resorption (decrease urinary hydroxyproline excretion) and subsequently produce a decrease in bone formation (decrease serum alkaline phosphatase levels) accompanied by lessening of pain and improvement in function. Synthetic salmon calcitonin administered subcutaneously usually results in clinical improvement within several weeks.

When therapy is discontinued, symp-

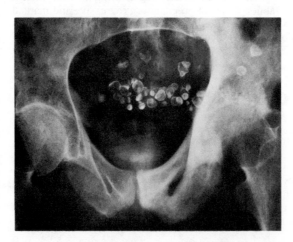

Fig 69–1. Pelvis of an 82-year-old man who had Paget's disease of bone for at least 10 years. The joint (cartilage) space of the left hip joint is severely narrowed and the iliopectineal line ("brim sign") is thickened, as evidenced by comparison with the opposite side.

toms usually return. Some patients may experience a plateau in the response or symptoms may return and alkaline phosphatase levels increase despite continued therapy. Antibodies to the salmon calcitonin are responsible for the refractory state in some patients.

Disodium etidronate, a diphosphonate compound administered orally in dosages of 5 mg/kg/day for no longer than 6 months, also decreases bone resorption. Clinical and biochemical improvement may first become evident after the drug has been discontinued; improvement may last longer than 6 months.

Mithramycin is also effective, although its use should probably be restricted to patients with severe disease who require a rapid therapeutic effect or who have not responded to other therapy. Patients with hip involvement who have not had a satisfactory response to medical treatment may be candidates for total hip replacement. It is worthwhile to administer calcitonin before surgery to reduce the activity of the disease and decrease local vascularity.

1. Singer FR, Schiller AL, Pyle EB, Krane SM: Paget's disease of bone, Metabolic Bone Disease. LV Avoli, SM Krane, eds. New York, Academic Press, 1977, pp 490–575
2. Altman RD, Singer F, eds: Proceedings of the Kroc Foundation Conference on Paget's Disease of Bone. Arthritis Rheum 23:1073–1240, 1980
3. Krane SM: Etidronate disodium in the treatment of Paget's disease of bone. Ann Intern Med 96:619–625, 1982

70. Osteonecrosis

Death of a bone or part of a bone, without evidence of an inflammatory process or sepsis, is usually regarded as secondary to loss of the blood supply (avascular necrosis of bone). Some argue that metabolic changes in the osteocytes are responsible for bone death in certain forms of the disease and recommend a more general term—osteonecrosis (1). An older synonym that emphasizes the lack of an inflammatory component is aseptic necrosis. Since the precise pathogenesis remains unknown and major vascular loss is not always evident, the term osteonecrosis seems preferable at this time.

The most simple classification divides osteonecrosis into traumatic and nontraumatic categories (2) (Table 70–1).

Traumatic osteonecrosis. Here the pathogenesis seems clear: a fracture involving the end of a bone interrupts the tenuous blood supply and osteocytes die. The proximal end of the femur is particularly vulnerable since the blood supply to the head is primarily intraosseous, with the major secondary source lying unprotected in a thin periosteum along the neck. Fractures or dislocations of the hip can severely damage these vessels and produce osteonecrosis.

Several features of the epidemiology suggest, however, that this simplistic explanation is incomplete and that even in the traumatic group, the etiology is multifactorial (3).

Treatment methods appear to exert some influence on the frequency of osteonecrosis after hip fracture since 30 years ago it was reported as 34% (4) and is now reported as approximately 15% (4–7).

Displaced fractures have twice the frequency of undisplaced fractures (12% versus 7%) (5). In undisplaced, "impacted," fractures, the incidence is virtually nil unless there is an excessive valgus position (8). Even with displaced fractures, perfect reduction is reported to reduce the likelihood of osteonecrosis to nearly zero, whereas excessive residual varus or valgus reduction increases the incidence to 54%, and a gross malreduction carries an 86% risk (6).

Because of the particularly vulnerable blood supply to the femoral head in children with open growth plates (and therefore no intraosseous blood supply to the head), the frequency of osteonecrosis is greatly increased after femoral neck fractures in this age group (9).

Dislocations of the hip are complicated by osteonecrosis in 15–40% of cases, depending on type, severity of the injury, and delay before treatment (10). The cause is considered to be rupture of the ligamentum teres and capsular vessels, leaving an inadequate intraosseous blood supply.

Osteonecrosis of the hip is rarely detected before 6 months after fracture or dislocation and may not be detected for 3 years or more, although 90% of cases are evident by 2 years with careful review of radiographs.

Several individuals have been reported who developed osteonecrosis after major impact to the femoral head without recognizable fracture or dislocation. Originally reported in sailors whose ships were torpedoed (11), it is seen in civilian practice after falls or jumps (12). The presumed cause is extensive trabecular microfracture with interruption of intraosseous blood supply to the femoral head or its segments.

Certain fractures of the shoulder, so-called 4-part fractures (13), render the proximal articular end of the humerus avascular and produce the same sequence of events seen in the hip.

In the knee, osteonecrosis of the femoral condyles is rarely due to trauma and is usually seen as a primary process, without recognizable antecedent causes or as a complication of corticosteroid therapy for rheumatoid arthritis or systemic lupus erythematosus (14,15).

Nontraumatic osteonecrosis. The multitude of diseases associated with this category suggests that no single etiology accounts for all examples. Proponents of the fat embolization theory (3) may be hard-pressed to explain osteonecrosis in a patient given a brief course of corticosteroids for an acute asthmatic attack. The one tenuous thread running through most of the lists of conditions associated with osteonecrosis is an abnormality of lipid metabolism and/or an abnormality of blood coagulation. It has been suggested that in predisposed individuals (emphasizing the multifactorial nature of the process), microemboli of lipids, aggregated platelets, or red cells block the terminal vessels supplying the subchondral area of susceptible bones. These microemboli produce infarcts that initiate changes similar to those seen in traumatic osteonecrosis. The osteonecrosis associated with certain hematologic diseses and storage disorders may be related to an increase in intraosseous (marrow) pressure.

Osteonecrosis is a major problem in patients with systemic lupus erythematosus who are treated with corticosteroids (16–21). The development of osteonecrosis, which often involves multiple bones (Figs 70–1 and 70–2), has been correlated with the use of high initial doses of corticosteroids (18). Osteonecrosis in most of

Table 70–1. Categories of osteonecrosis

Traumatic	Nontraumatic
Fracture of the hip, shoulder, carpal navicular, etc	Idiopathic (Chandler's disease)
	Alcohol abuse
	Corticosteroid treatment
	Rheumatoid arthritis
	Systemic lupus erythematosus
Dislocation of the hip	Caisson disease
Slipped femoral capital epiphysis	Hyperuricemia (? hyperlipoproteinemia)
	Sickle cell disease
	Sickle cell–hemoglobin C disease
	Gaucher's disease
	Fabry's disease
	Liver disease
	Pancreatitis
	Polycythemia
	Cushing's syndrome
	X-irradiation

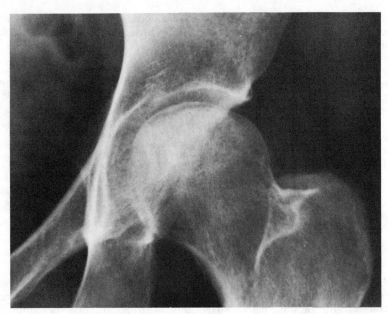

Fig 70–1. Osteonecrosis of head of left femur of a 20-year-old woman with systemic lupus erythematosus of 7 years duration. The patient had developed hip pain 5 months before this roentgenogram, while taking prednisone, 25 mg/day. Note zone of subchondral lucency (crescent sign).

these individuals is clinically silent and nonprogressive (19). Evidence of increased bone marrow pressure and altered venous drainage, as documented by venography, has been found in all stages of osteonecrosis in patients with SLE, including the period before radiographic changes appear, and may be the earliest detectable change in this disorder (21).

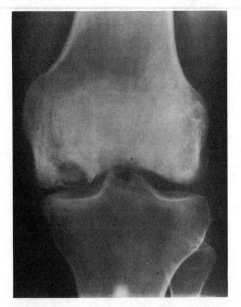

Fig 70–2. Osteonecrosis of medial condyle of left femur of another 20-year-old woman (November 1973) with systemic lupus erythematosus of 2 years duration. This patient also had osteonecrosis of both femoral heads and tali and subsequently (age 24) developed avascular necrosis of the heads of both humeri. She had taken large quantities of prednisone (60 mg/day) early in her illness, but had discontinued this medication 2 years earlier.

Osteonecrosis, believed to be related to corticosteroids, has been reported to occur in 1.4–16.9% of individuals with kidney transplants and is the most common cause of major long-term disability in patients surviving for more than a year who are otherwise well with stable renal function (22).

Dead bone has the same radiographic appearance as living bone and is just as strong. The radiographic appearances of increased density and focal collapse are therefore signs of repair and appear late in the disease course. A relative increase in density of the avascular segment may be seen early in the process if immobility or disuse leads to osteopenia of the adjacent bony structures. Since disuse osteopenia is dependent on an intact blood supply, the avascular segment remains dense. This appearance is common after fractures, but in nontraumatic osteonecrosis, the patient often remains mobile, active, and asymptomatic until late in the process so that these early radiographic signs fail to develop.

Revascularization of the necrotic segment first involves resorption of dead bone to provide new vascular channels, after which new bone is deposited along the walls of these channels. Often the earliest radiographic findings are these areas of patchy loss of bone substance, interspersed with focal areas of increased density secondary to new bone formation.

Two other processes may also produce radiographic changes. The first is microfracture of trabeculae. Although dead bone is just as strong as living, it cannot repair the microfractures that frequently take place in the trabeculae supporting the articular surface. As sequential microfrac-

tures occur, collapse of the subchondral plate may produce a radiographic picture of mottled density (due to compaction of old dead bone) with some flattening or collapse of the articular surface.

Second, with vascular resorption occurring around the periphery of an avascular segment, a weakened zone may result into which the entire necrotic segment collapses. In the femoral head these segments are often wedge-shaped (like an infarct) and the resulting segmental collapse produces an unmistakable radiographic sign of advanced osteonecrosis.

A fracture may be evident in the late stages of osteonecrosis of the hip, knee, or shoulder. The fracture originates at the junction of articular cartilage and periosteum where presumably a site of vascular invasion accompanies the repair process. The fracture propagates centrally through the trabecular bone supporting the subchondral plate; this produces in radiographs a "crescent sign" representing the segment of detached dense subchondral bone and cartilage (Fig 70–1). In osteonecrosis secondary to fractures, this stress fracture may extend deeply into the center of the head producing a somewhat different appearance.

In end-stage osteonecrosis, the mixture of resorption, collapse, spotty increased density, and fragmentation produces an unmistakable image.

Since the common pathogenetic feature of both traumatic and nontraumatic osteonecrosis is considered to be an infarct, radionuclide scanning should be of help in determining the presence of such an avascular infarcted area. Unfortunately, scanning has been of limited usefulness since symptoms often appear late in the disease course, at which time the avascularity of a segment of bone is concealed by the hypervascularity of the repair process surrounding it. Thus far the resolution of radionuclide scanning has not allowed a distinction between the hypervascularity of the repair process and the avascularity of the infarct.

Because of the frequency of bilateral involvement in nontraumatic osteonecrosis (23), radionuclide scanning has been useful in detecting early changes in the contralateral hip.

Treatment. Treatment has been largely unsatisfactory since it approaches the problem indirectly. In traumatic osteoarthritis, major intra- and extraosseous vessels are injured. Immediate primary repair before the death of osteocytes would be the appropriate direct treatment.

In nontraumatic osteonecrosis, emboli or metabolic changes damage the arborizing capillary network. Removal of fat embolism by "clearing agents" would be appropriate with this cause while decompression of the marrow cavity would be appropriate if extravascular compression were involved. Both approaches have been reported, but their effectiveness cannot yet be evaluated (24,25). Early core decompression has been advocated in the management of avascular necrosis in lupus patients (26).

Bone grafting has long been a controversial treatment with mixed reults. Critics point out that inserting a dead piece of bone (the graft) into the dead segment of osteonecrosis doesn't make biological sense. Advocates either invoke a stimulatory effect of the graft on bone repair or point out that since the deleterious effect of osteonecrosis is late collapse with disruption of the joint, the use of a strut to support the articular surface mechanically is rational. All agree such grafts are only of use early in the process, before collapse produces joint incongruity.

The use of vascularized bone grafts attached to a muscle pedicle has been reported (27), but the series are too small and the followup too brief to allow conclusions.

Most patients with osteonecrosis of the hip, whether secondary to fracture or idiopathic, eventually require prosthetic replacement to relieve symptoms and restore full activity. Since the congruity of the joint is usually lost by the time patients come to surgery, hemiarthroplasty is not satisfactory and total joint replacement is required. In the knee, osteotomy to relieve stress on the affected femoral condyle is often satisfactory (14). Osteonecrosis of the carpal navicular can be treated early by bone grafting, but patients with late diagnosis benefit by prosthetic replacement.

1. Glimcher MJ, Kenzora JE: The biology of osteonecrosis of the human femoral head and its clinical implications: an abridged communication. Clin Orthop 130:47–50, 1978
2. Herndon JH, Aufranc OE: Avascular necrosis of the femoral head: a review of its incidence in a variety of conditions. Clin Orthop 86:43–62, 1972
3. Jones JP, Jr: Osteonecrosis. Clin Orthop 130:2–4, 1978
4. Boyd HB, George IL: Complications of fractures of the neck of the femur. J Bone Joint Surg 29:13–18, 1947
5. Arnold WD, Lyden JP, Minkoff J: Treatment of intracapsular fractures of the femoral neck. J Bone Joint Surg 56A:254–262, 1974
6. Garden RS: Malreduction and avascular necrosis in subcapital fractures of the femur. J Bone Joint Surg 53B:183–197, 1971
7. Metz CW, et al: The displaced intracapsular fracture of the neck of the femur. J Bone Joint Surg 52A:113–127, 1970
8. Aufranc OE, Jones WN, Harris WH: Undisplaced femoral neck fracture. JAMA 189:314–317, 1964
9. McDougall A: Fractures of the neck of the femur in childhood. J Bone Joint Surg 43B:16–28, 1961
10. Epstein HC: Posterior fracture-dislocations of the hip: long term followup. J Bone Joint Surg 56A:1103–1127, 1974
11. Draeger RH, Barr JS, Sager WW: Blast injury. JAMA 132:762–767, 1946
12. Ficat RP, Arlet J: Ischemia and Necrosis of Bone. DS Hungerford, ed. Baltimore, Williams and Wilkins, 1980
13. Neer CS II: Fractures and dislocations of the shoulder. Part 1: Fractures about the shoulder, Fractures, vol 1. CA Rockwood, Jr and DP Green, eds, Philadelphia, JB Lippincott, 1975, pp 585–623
14. Bauer GCH: Osteonecrosis of the knee. Clin Orthop 130:210–217, 1978
15. Ahuda SC, Bullough PG: Osteonecrosis of the knee. A clinicopathological study in 28 patients. J Bone Joint Surg 60A:191–197, 1978
16. Leventhal GH, Dorfman HD: Aseptic necrosis of bone in systemic lupus erythematosus. Medicine 4:73–93, 1974
17. Klipper AR, Stevens MB, Zizic TM, Hungerford DS: Ischemic necrosis of bone in systemic lupus erythematosus. Medicine 55:251–257, 1976
18. Abeles M, Urman JD, Rothfield NF: Aseptic necrosis of bone in systemic lupus erythematosus: relationship to corticosteroid therapy. Arch Intern Med 138:750–754, 1978
19. Klippel JH, Gerber LH, Pollak L, Decker JL: Avascular necrosis in systemic lupus erythematosus: silent symmetric osteonecroses. Am J Med 67:83–87, 1979
20. Griffiths ID, Maini RN, Scott JT: Clinical and radiological features of osteonecrosis in systemic lupus erythematosus. Ann Rheum Dis 38:413–422, 1979
21. Zizic TM, Hungerford DS, Stevens MB: Ischemic bone necrosis in systemic lupus erythematosus. I. The early diagnosis of ischemic necrosis of bone. Medicine 59:134–142, 1980
22. Habermann ET, Cristofaro RL: Avascular necrosis of bone as a complication of renal transplantation. Semin Arthritis Rheum 6:189–206, 1976
23. Springfield DS, Enneking WJ: Surgery for aseptic necrosis of the femoral head. Clin Orthop 130:175–185, 1978
24. Wang GJ, Moga DB, Richemer WG, Sweet DE, Reger SI, Thompson RC: Cortisone induced bone changes and its response to lipid clearing agents. Clin Orthop 130:81–85, 1978
25. Hungerford DS, Zizic TM: Alcoholism associated ischemic necrosis of the femoral head: early diagnosis and treatment. Clin Orthop 130:144–153, 1978
26. Hungerford DS, Zizic TM: Ischemic bone necrosis in systemic lupus erythematosus. II. The treatment of ischemic necrosis of bone in systemic lupus erythematosus. Medicine 59:143–148, 1980
27. Meyers MH: The treatment of osteonecrosis of the hip with fresh osteochondral allografts and with the muscle pedicle graft technique. Clin Orthop 130:202–209, 1978

71. Carpal tunnel syndrome

The carpal tunnel syndrome represents one of the so-called entrapment neuropathies and is a common cause of paresthesias in the hands (1–3). At the wrist, the median nerve and flexor tendons pass through a common tunnel whose rigid walls are bounded dorsally and on the sides by the carpal bones. This tunnel is enclosed on the volar aspect by the transverse carpal ligament (Fig 71–1).

Any process that encroaches on this crowded tunnel results in compression of the most vulnerable structure, the median nerve. This nerve innervates the thenar muscles (flexion, opposition, abduction) the radial lumbricals, and the skin of the radial side of the palm, the thumb, second and third fingers, and the radial half of the fourth finger.

Clinical features. The symptoms that result from compression of the median nerve at this site are variable. Episodes of burning pain or tingling in the hands are common, often occurring during the night and relieved by vigorous shaking or exercising of the hand. Numbness (hypesthesia) is a common complaint, affecting the middle or 3 radial fingers and occasionally the thumb. The patient may feel a sensation of swelling of the affected parts, when in fact no swelling is visible.

In time, weakness of the muscles of the thenar eminence may appear, with difficulty in abducting the thumb or opposing the thumb to the index finger. Some patients merely complain of numbness, without much pain, in the distribution of the median nerve. In a smaller group of patients progressive wasting of the muscles of the thenar eminence is associated with weakness and numbness, but with little or no pain. Occasionally the pain may spread above the wrist into the forearm or, rarely, even to the upper arm. Bilateral involvement is common.

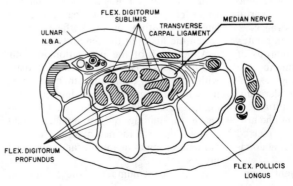

Fig 71–1. Cross-section of wrist illustrating the position of the transverse carpal ligament (flexor retinaculum) and the structures occupying the osseous-fibrous carpal tunnel.

The diagnosis should be suspected on the basis of the history, especially if the symptoms are aggravated by compressing the median nerve locally (Tinel's sign), using digital pressure, percussion hammer, tourniquet, sphygmomanometer cuff, or even by forced flexion of the wrist. Loss of sensation may be demonstrated in the index, middle, or radial side of the fourth finger. Weakness and wasting of the thenar muscles is usually a late sign.

Confirmation of median nerve involvement and loss of innervation can be obtained by measuring impulse conduction times during electromyography.

Other entrapment neuropathies that occur in the arm include compression of the median nerve by the pronator teres or a fibrous band near the origin of the deep flexor muscles, the so-called *pronator syndrome*. The ulnar nerve may be similarly compressed within the ulnar tunnel at the wrist or at the medial side of the elbow (4).

A variety of disorders may give rise to the syndrome. These include edema after trauma or associated with the fluid retention of pregnancy, overgrowths (osteophytes) of bone, ganglia related to tenosynovial sheaths, lipomata, and anomalous muscles, tendons, and blood vessels that compress the median nerve.

Carpal tunnel syndrome has been observed in a variety of systemic disorders and infections such as tuberculosis, histoplasmosis, sporotrichosis, coccidioidomycosis, and rubella. Thickening of the transverse carpal ligaments is a reported cause of primary familial carpal tunnel syndrome, and vitamin B6 deficiency has been said to culminate in this syndrome.

Enlargement of the median nerve as in leprosy or hypertrophic polyneuropathy rarely produces compression symptoms.

Perhaps the most common cause (after pregnancy) is thickening of the tendon sheaths by rheumatoid granulation tissue. Gout, pseudogout, and other inflammatory diseases of the wrist can cause median nerve compression. Deposits of amyloid of the primary type or in association with multiple myeloma have a predilection for this site, and the carpal tunnel syndrome may constitute the initial manifestation of the disease. Occurrence of the syndrome has also been reported in myxedema and acromegaly.

In many instances, however, no obvious cause can be demonstrated or there may be a nonspecific tenosynovitis. Patients with the carpal tunnel syndrome may have other forms of tenosynovitis such as deQuervain's disease, rotator cuff tendinitis at the shoulder, or trigger fingers. Many of the "idiopathic" cases are in reality due to occupational stress, while others are seen in menopausal women, suggesting a hormonal aberration.

Symptoms similar to those of the carpal tunnel syndrome may be from cervical nerve root compression, reflecting the origin of the median nerve from the sixth and seventh cervical roots. Unlike carpal tunnel syndrome, cervical root compression is apt to be symptomatic when the person assumes erect posture or moves the neck, and Tinel's sign is not detectable.

Treatment. In the milder cases where edema is a factor, splinting of the wrist or the administration of a diuretic may relieve symptoms. Local injections of corticosteroids are helpful for tenosynovitis, whether nonspecific or due to proliferation of rheumatoid granulation tissue. However, the benefit may be only temporary.

Decompression of the tunnel by surgical release of the transverse carpal ligament, with removal of any tissue compressing the median nerve, often provides gratifying results (3). It should be considered in all patients in whom conservative treatment has failed.

1. Phalen GS: The carpal-tunnel syndrome: 17 years' experience in diagnosis and treatment of 654 hands. J Bone Joint Surg 48A:211–228, 1966

2. LaBan MM, Zemenick GA, Meerschaert JR: Neck and shoulder pain: presenting symptoms of carpal tunnel syndrome. Michigan Med 74:549–550, 1975

3. Gainer JV, Nugent GR: Carpal tunnel syndrome: report of 430 operations. South Med J 70:325–328, 1977

4. Sedal L, McLeod JG, Walsh JC: Ulnar nerve lesions associated with the carpal tunnel syndrome. J Neurol Neurosurg Psychiat 36:118–123, 1973

72. The shoulder

The shoulder is not only the most movable of the body's joints but one of the most complicated, since motion occurs not only at the enarthrodial glenohumeral joint, but synchronously in varying degrees at the acromioclavicular, sternoclavicular, and scapulothoracic articulations. Numerous tight ligaments are required to hold the component parts of the less movable joints together, while in contrast, the most movable juncture, the glenohumeral, has only a loose capsule. The glenohumeral joint depends on muscles and tendons to provide stability and at the same time create force couples which allow powerful action throughout the enormous range.

This anatomic complexity contributes materially to the difficulty of analysis of patients with complaints referable to "the shoulder" (1–3). In differentiating the clinical syndromes that include shoulder pain, it is essential to remember the multiarticular structure of the shoulder joint and also that the region may be the site of referred pain from cervical, intrathoracic, abdominal, and diaphragmatic foci.

By careful analysis of a patient's complaints and findings, it is possible to delineate a series of shoulder syndromes which include those following.

Calcific tendinitis and bursitis. Because of some degenerative process, possibly related to chronic trauma, the tendons of the supra- and infraspinatus (the superior central and superior posterior portions of the rotator cuff) undergo an alteration in structure during the middle years. This change causes the normally orderly parallel bundles of collagen to become frayed and irregular and undergo calcification, with little or no inflammatory change. Large plaques of hydroxyapatite may be laid down within, on the surface, or between the fibers of the tendons.

Almost 3% of the population in their middle years have such calcific deposits with little or no complaint other than perhaps some limitation of abduction. This limitation is related to the decrease in space for gliding of the humeral head beneath the arch formed by the acromion, coracoarcromial ligament, and coracoid process.

A significant number of these patients, however, do develop symptoms as a result of irritation and inflammation of the parietal surface of the subdeltoid (subacromial) bursa or of frank rupture and discharge of the calcific contents into the bursal sac. The syndrome may be acute, subacute, or chronic, presumably dictated by the pathologic process and the body's responses to the foreign material (considered to be similar to crystal-induced inflammation seen in gout and chondrocalcinosis). See also Sections 46 and 47.

The syndromes occur in a peak incidence between the ages of 40 and 45 years, and women are affected slightly more often than men. The dominant arm is usually affected, and approximately 15% of cases are bilateral. A smaller percentage of patients also have involvement of the lower extremities with calcifications at sites such as the trochanteric bursae.

The acute syndrome, which may be associated with trauma, is characterized by the sudden onset of pain in the shoulder area, often with radiation into the base of the neck, the deltoid insertion, or occasionally extending even further down the arm. The pain is severe and accentuated by almost any motion of the shoulder girdle, particularly those of abduction, medial rotation, or forward flexion. Night pain is a prominent feature, and the patients complain bitterly about the difficulty of inserting their arms into a coat or shirtsleeve. Examination during this phase often reveals notable voluntary splinting of the shoulder, and commonly exquisite local tenderness is observed in the anterior and sometimes also the anterolateral or posterolateral portions of the shoulder joint.

Roentgenographic study frequently discloses a calcific mass in the subdeltoid area, usually paralleling the course of the tendon (Fig 72–1). The calcification may display discrete margins consistent with its intratendinous location, pseudopodic projections indicative of beginning "escape" into the bursa, or a diffuse, more lacy pattern indicative of a rupture into the cavity of the subdeltoid bursa.

The subacute and chronic forms of the disorder have virtually identical complaints and findings, but are usually much less pronounced. The range of motion may be limited by pain only at the extremes and tenderness may be minimal. The roentgenographic characteristics may be indistinguishable from the more acute form but more often the calcific deposit is small and difficult to see without multiple views.

Treatment. The treatment of this entity depends somewhat on the severity of symptoms. The natural history of the disorder is one of gradual improvement, corresponding to the disappearance of the calcific mass, but periodic recurrences are common. When acute, aspiration of the calcified material from the bursa or the region of the tendinous cuff may give prompt relief. Injections of a slightly soluble corticosteroid in combination with xylocaine into the bursa are sometimes successful in relieving the discomfort. Several antiinflammatory agents (such as phenylbutazone or indomethacin) or physical measures (such as ultrasound) are successful in varying degrees.

The treatment for subacute and chronic varieties is essentially the same as for the acute, but is often less successful in effecting the dramatic relief of symptoms.

An occasional patient is found to be completely refractory to these methods of treatment and, in such cases, surgical exploration, excision of the calcific deposit, and section of the coracoacromial ligament (and possibly subtotal acromionectomy) may become necessary.

Bicipital tendinitis. The long head of the biceps originates from the superior surface of the glenoid and travels intraarticularly to lie in a groove between the greater and lesser tuberosities along the anterolateral aspect of the head and neck of the humerus. In some patients with the shoulder

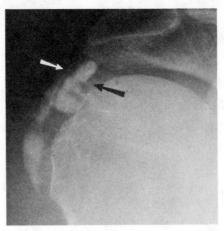

Fig 72–1. Right shoulder of a 44-year-old man, illustrating massive calcareous deposits in the supraspinatus tendon (**white arrow**) and subdeltoid bursa (**black arrow**)

pain syndrome who do not have calcific deposits on roentgenographic examination, there may be a tenosynovitis of the biceps tendon within its groove. This lesion is associated with tenderness localized to this anatomic region and an accentuation of the pain with resisted supination of the forearm, with the elbow flexed at 90 degrees.

The syndrome frequently responds to local injections of slightly soluble corticosteroid with xylocaine or other measures, as defined above, but occasionally requires surgical exploration, section and tenodesis of the bicipital tendon.

Rotator cuff tears. The supraspinatus, infraspinatus, and teres minor tendons undergo degenerative change with aging and, presumably, chronic stress. Under conditions of acute or, more commonly, minor repetitive trauma, this change may result in a rupture of the tendinous envelope (the rotator cuff) which ordinarily not only aids in rotation in the humeral head, but by approximating the humeral head to the glenoid allows the deltoid to abduct or forward flex the arm (4). The rupture may be minimal, with little functional deficit, or complete, resulting in inability to abduct the glenohumeral joint from the side, although it can be held in abduction once elevated to 90 degrees or more (by deltoid muscle action).

In incomplete lesions, the abnormality is much more subtle since the patient may have only mild pain, atrophy of muscles in the shoulder region, slight weakness of abduction, and a normal roentgenogram (rarely demonstrating calcification).

The diagnosis in these patients is aided materially by contrast arthrography which often demonstrates the abnormal communication between the joint and the subdeltoid bursa.

The treatment depends on the degree of the tear, the age of the patient, and the level of disability. Minor tears may be

treated symptomatically with gentle exercises, partial immobilization (in acute situations), or nonsteroidal antiinflammatory drugs. Major tears may require operative intervention and repair of the ruptured tendinous structures.

The "frozen shoulder," pericapsulitis, and the shoulder–hand syndrome. The group of syndromes discussed in this section may have a variety of causes and some differences in presentation. However, all are characterized by profound and eventually virtually complete limitation of glenohumeral motion together with obliteration of the normal capsular folds and fibrosis in the capsular and pericapsular tissues.

The condition principally affects patients in their middle years and is often "triggered" by an acute illness, such as coronary occlusion, angina pectoris, cerebral vascular accident, trauma to the distal part of the upper extremity, calcific tendinitis, or pulmonary problems, such as tuberculosis or postthoracotomy syndrome. Diabetes and some drugs, including phenobarbital and isoniazid, have been suggested etiologic factors.

Clinical features. The patient complains of a dull, aching pain in the shoulder and limitation of motion. In the patient with advanced disease, this limitation is obvious on physical examination, particularly when rotation is tested (since abduction, flexion, and extension can occur, in part, at one of the other joints that comprise the total shoulder articulation).

Occasionally, in more severe forms of this disorder, pain extends into the neck or down the arm, which may be associated with clinical and roentgenographic findings consistent with Sudeck's atrophy (osteoporosis) of bone. In these patients, the hand may become swollen and reddened, with changes characteristic of a sympathetic dystrophy, including loss of extension or full flexion of the fingers and irregular punctate rarefactions of the bony structures (see Section 75).

Treatment. The severity of the symptoms and dysfunction determines the type of treatment necessary. For milder cases, which are considered to be self-limited, exercises, local physical measures (heat), and injections of corticosteroids and xylocaine may be all that is necessary. Manipulation under anesthesia is sometimes successful in releasing the contracted shoulder but may be hazardous since the tendinous, capsular, or even bony structures may be damaged.

In more severe cases, systemic corticosteroids, stellate ganglion block, physiotherapy, and certain exercises may be required to bring about control of this extremely disabling syndrome.

In patients who have sustained a myocardial infarction, cerebral vascular accident, trauma to the distal part of the upper extremity, or in those with pulmonary tuberculosis or cervical radicular syndromes, it is advisable to begin exercises of the shoulder as soon as possible to prevent this complication.

Other syndromes. In any patient with persistent shoulder pain or in individuals with atypical syndromes not responsive to the customary measures, it is essential to consider other possible causes of the pain. Thoracic outlet syndrome, Pancoast tumor, a cervical spine lesion (spondylosis, disc, or tumor), metastatic carcinoma, referred pain, and other disorders should be considered and attempts made to rule them out by appropriate studies.

1. Booth RE Jr, Marvel JP Jr: Differential diagnosis of shoulder pain. Orthop Clin N Am 6:353–379, 1975
2. Kessel L, Watson M: The painful arc syndrome: clinical classification as a guide to management. J Bone Joint Surg 59B:166–172, 1977
3. Kozin F: Painful shoulder and the reflex sympathetic dystrophy syndrome, Arthritis and Allied Conditions. Ed 9. DJ McCarty, Jr, ed. Philadelphia, Lea & Febiger, 1979, pp 1091–1120
4. Nixon JE, DiStefano V: Ruptures of the rotating cuff. Orthop Clin N Am 6:423–447, 1975

73. The foot

The feet contain one-fourth of the body's joints and bones (Fig 73–1). As moving appendages, they are rivaled in lifetime work only by the heart and lungs. It has been estimated that in a lifetime the average person walks as many as 250,000 miles and that foot problems affect 9 of 10 people at some time during their lives.

Most of these problems are primarily static, the consequence of inborn structural defects or abusive shoes that produce faulty support and promote poor posture. Whether congenital or acquired, static foot afflictions are frequently multiple, since faulty mechanics from one disability often lead to another, thereby adding to the complexity of diagnosis and management. Other major causes of foot pain are injuries, vascular disorders, and arthritis (1–3).

Forefoot problems. Metatarsalgia, or pain at the ball of the foot, may be due to pes cavus (high longitudinal arch), a shortened achilles tendon, Morton's neuroma, or the inflammation of the metatarsophalangeal (MTP) joints frequently observed in rheumatoid arthritis (RA) and other forms of inflammatory joint disease.

Hammer and cockup toes may be congenital but are more often due to abnormal foot mechanics, tight shoes, or chronic rheumatic disorders. Foot pain may also result from hallux valgus, an outward turning of the great toe, or from hallux rigidus, a complete fixation of the first metatarsophalangeal joint. These, in turn, are often accompanied by a painful bunion from adjacent bursal inflammation. Corns and calluses are other painful soft tissue lesions that arise secondary to irritation from confining shoes in the presence of other deformities, particularly hammer or cockup toes and metatarsal subluxation.

Midfoot problems. The most common are foot strain and flat feet (pes planus) either congenital or resulting primarily from obesity or occupational stress. Overstretching muscles and ligaments leads to varying degrees of foot pronation and valgus of the heel, abnormalities seen only with weight bearing.

The major causes of flat feet are developmental (faulty posture, obesity), occupational, traumatic, neurologic, and rheu-

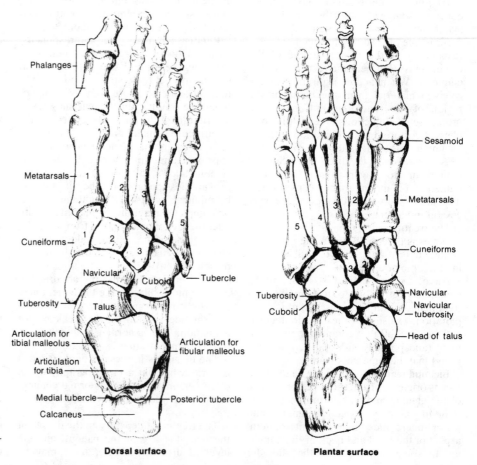

Fig 73–1. Bones of the feet. (Illustration provided by Dr JJ Calabro)

Dorsal surface

Plantar surface

matic (RA). Flat feet may be flaccid (static), spastic, or rigid. When they are flaccid, which is the most common variety, the longitudinal arch is depressed only on weight bearing. If untreated, peroneal muscle spasm may result in a spastic flat foot characterized by painful limitation of inversion. The end stage is a rigid flat foot fixed in abduction by contractures.

Heel pain. Heel pain is most frequently caused by bursitis, tendinitis, periostitis or spurs from trauma, or common rheumatic disorders such as acute gouty arthritis, RA, Reiter's syndrome, psoriatic arthritis, and ankylosing spondylitis. Heel pain may also result from infection, osteomyelitis, fracture, local lipodystrophy, Sudeck's atrophy, Paget's disease of bone, xanthoma of the achilles tendon, bone tumor, osteochondritis, callus, or pump bumps.

Pain in back of the heel may be due to achillotendinitis or bursitis or from a bony spur originating at the insertion of the achilles tendon. In children, it may also be due to calcaneal apophysitis (osteochondritis) and in young women, to shoe-induced achillotendinitis, callus, or pump bumps. The latter are painful soft tissue enlargements caused by irritation of prominent posterior calcanei from high-heel or pump shoes (4).

Pain at the base of the heel may be due to a subcalcaneal bursitis or plantar fasciitis. These may be idiopathic, traumatic, or secondary to rheumatic diseases, particularly Reiter's syndrome. Plantar fasciitis frequently leads to calcaneal periostitis or new bone and spur formation.

Diffuse foot pain. Diffuse foot pain, often severe, may be due to Sudeck's atrophy, synovitis, vasculitis, peripheral vascular disease, or nerve entrapment. The tarsal tunnel syndrome is a compression neuropathy of the posterior tibial nerve within the tarsal tunnel that causes intermittent burning pain and parasthesias of the toes and sole which worsen at night (5). Point tenderness occurs at the medial side of the ankle, especially with tapping or direct pressure (*Tinel's sign*).

Rheumatoid arthritis. In terms of frequency of initial joint symptoms in rheumatoid arthritis, foot problems outrank those of the hand and are second only to those of the knee (1,6). The feet eventually become affected in 90% of patients with rheumatoid arthritis, often constituting the major disability.

The metatarsophalangeal joints are usually the first to become involved. Tenderness is elicited by applying light pressure to each of the MTP joints or by compression of the forefoot. Heel pain may also

occur, occasionally as the initial complaint, from achillotendinitis or bursitis and plantar fasciitis (1).

Continued inflammation of the MTP joints can induce contractures of ligaments and supporting structures, leading to progressive hallux valgus, hammer or cockup toes, MTP subluxation, spreadfoot, and spastic flat foot. Secondary discomfort arises from shoe-induced microtrauma producing bunions, corns, and calluses.

All these afflictions require aggressive treatment (2,6), lest malalignment of the weight-bearing leg produces a valgus deformity of the knee. Modified inserts and padding in the shoes can help some problems. Other treatments are discussed in Section 74.

1. Calabro JJ: A critical evaluation of the diagnostic features of the feet in rheumatoid arthritis. Arthritis Rheum 5:19–29, 1962
2. Locke RK, Mennell JM, Sgarlato TE: Foot complaints. Patient Care 6:20–47, 1975
3. Hamilton EBD: Painful feet. Br Med J 3:343–344, 1969
4. Dickinson PH, Coutts MB, Woodward EP, Handler D: Tendoachilles bursitis. J Bone Joint Surg 48A:77–81, 1966
5. Goodgold J, Kopell HP, Spielholz NI: The tarsal-tunnel syndrome. N Engl J Med 273:742–745, 1965
6. Dixon AStJ: The rheumatoid foot, Modern Trends in Rheumatology–2. AGS Hill, ed. New York, Appleton-Century-Crofts, 1971, pp 158–173

74. Regional rheumatic pain syndromes

The rheumatic pain syndromes described in this section are often secondary to acute or chronic trauma, minor congenital defects, or structural disorders. They sometimes result from improper body mechanics during work or sports. They may also complicate another rheumatic disease. A careful history is essential with particular emphasis on sport or leisure activity, work habits, and personality.

The physical examination must include attention to the patient's body habitus, structural disorders such as short limb, dorsal kyphosis, scoliosis, joint laxity, and tests and maneuvers that reproduce or accentuate the pain.

Most of the regional rheumatic disorders cannot be defined radiographically or by laboratory tests. When a regional pain disorder is considered in muscle or fascia, the clinician must carefully palpate for soft tissue tender points that reproduce the pain that is located some distance away in a "target zone" (1,2). When pain overlies a joint, examination must exclude synovitis or internal joint derangement.

Some guidelines for management are shown in Table 74–1.

Drug therapy. Most regional disorders respond to rest, local protection, and counterirritants. Ice applied promptly may

prevent excessive bleeding or swelling of the soft tissues. Salicylates and safe analgesics such as diflunisal (250–1,000 mg immediately, 250–500 mg twice daily thereafter) may also be required. For selected conditions presenting with acute pain and swelling (bursitis or tenosynovitis), a short course of phenylbutazone (100 mg 4 times daily for not over 5 days) will often provide relief. Indomethacin (75–150 mg per day for up to 10 days) and other nonsteroidal antiinflammatory agents may be used depending on the acuteness and severity of the disorder.

The judicious use of tricyclic drugs at bedtime may be helpful when sleep disturbance is thought to contribute to symptoms. Meprobamate (400 mg at bedtime) may be helpful when anxiety, tension, or muscle cramp is a problem.

However, drug therapy should never be the only method of treatment for these disorders.

Aggravating factors. Most regional rheumatic pain disorders arise from specific injurious activities that can cause recurrences. For example, muscle contraction headache, myofascial neck pain, and occipital neuralgia may result from falling asleep in a chair and allowing the head to drop down, from lying on a sofa with the

head propped forward, or from working with the head too close to the work material.

Trigger finger, tenosynovitis, or tendinitis often result from prolonged repetitive tasks (needlepoint, potato peeling) and not from direct trauma. Gluteal pain is often precipitated by bending over with straight legs.

Plantar fasciitis and heel pain may result from moving to a home with a concrete slab foundation, a change to a job that requires more prolonged standing on concrete, or increased body weight. Failure to condition properly before a sport activity can lead to serious soft tissue injury for the older weekend athlete (3).

Intralesional injections. Use of local crystalline corticosteroid (triamcinolone acetonide or methylprednisolone acetate) combined with 1% procaine or xylocaine often quickly reduces pain and spasm. Not over 40 mg of the steroid agent should be administered and 1–6 ml of the anesthetic agent is adequate. If used judiciously and infrequently and if sepsis has been excluded, this therapy has proved useful, safe, and cost effective after nearly 30 years (see Section 93).

Physical therapy. Measures to relieve pain and spasm must be followed by mobilizing exercises and posture correction where needed. Individualized exercises are an integral part of long-term management and are often overlooked or underemphasized. Although the services of a physiatrist or physical therapist are useful, the clinician can direct the patient in the performance of simple exercises with adequate instructions. Frequently the exercise program must be modified as treatment progresses.

The patient should realize that pain relief may depend on a conscientious effort carried out daily for an adequate period of time. Routine work and chores are not the same as mobilizing or strengthening exercises (see Section 95).

Disorders of the arm

Tennis elbow. Subacute or chronic pain in the region of the lateral epicondyle has become known as *tennis elbow*. The pain is aggravated by grasping, extending the wrist, or supinating the arm. Usually considered a lesion of the extensor communis apparatus, the pain can arise from a bursa that overlies the radiohumeral joint. The disorder is often occupational in carpenters, plumbers, gardeners, dentists, sportsmen, and politicians—from excessive handshaking!

Examination reveals normal range of joint motion, no joint instability, and characteristically, point tenderness over the lateral epicondyle or over the head of the radius. Often careful palpation will reveal a firm, tender cord in one of the extensor tendons of the forearm located 2–4 cm distal from the epicondyle.

Treatment consists of elimination of the aggravating factors, rest, use of a tennis elbow band, intralesional injection of a local anesthetic and corticosteroid agent, and institution of an exercise program to stretch and strengthen the forearm extensor muscles. The patient sits with the forearm across a table, the wrist lying over the edge, at first palm down. A 3-pound weight is grasped and the wrist is alternatively flexed and extended. Then the wrist is rotated palm up and the motions repeated. Stretching is accomplished by having the patient press the back of the hand against a wall with the fingers pointed downward and the hand slowly raised upward starting at the level of the patient's waist. A pulling sensation in the area of the extensor tendons should occur and this position is then held for a minute and repeated several times a day.

Olecranon bursitis. The superficial olecranon bursa may become inflamed after trauma, gout, infection, rheumatoid arthritis, or other inflammatory arthritides. Visible distention of the bursa over the olecranon process occurs. The bursa is easily aspirated and the bursal fluid should be examined by Gram stain, culture, white blood cell count with differential, and crystal identification with polarizing microscopy. If the joint fluid is not septic, an intralesional injection of a corticosteroid is appropriate.

Avoidance of bearing weight on the elbow when arising or when sitting is essential to recovery. A protective elbow pad is often helpful.

Stenosing tenosynovitis. Also known as "DeQuervain's tendinitis" when tendons of the extensor pollicis brevis and abductor pollicis longus are involved, the disorder presents as a subacute or chronic and disabling pain at the radial aspect of the wrist. Careful examination often reveals swelling over the involved tendons bordering the radial styloid process.

The Finkelstein test distinguishes tendinitis from underlying osteoarthritis. With the patient's thumb folded into the palm, the remaining fingers flexed over the thumb, the examiner grasps the patient's fist and gently ulnar deviates the patient's wrist, thus putting the involved tendons on the stretch and resulting in acute exacerbation of pain. The usual aggravating factor is excessive repetitive hand work such as peeling vegetables, knitting, or working at needlepoint.

Injection of the tendon sheath with 1% local anesthetic and a corticosteroid agent is usually helpful. Surgical incision of the tendon sheath is sometimes necessary. Occasionally, rheumatoid arthritis can present with bilateral tendinitis.

Trigger finger and trigger thumb. Flexor tendon sheath inflammation in association with development of a tendon nodule can give rise to intermittent locking of a digit. The digit often locks in flexion when the patient arises from sleep. Although the sensation is perceived at the proximal interphalangeal joint, the nodule can be palpated in the palm just proximal to the metacarpophalangeal joint. Aggravating factors include excessive repetitive hand work or unconscious fist clenching, osteoarthritis of the underlying joint, tendon dislocation, and sesamoid bones. Injection of the tendon sheath with a corticosteroid agent (0.3–0.5 ml) relieves symptoms. Surgical incision of the sheath is occasionally necessary.

Ganglia. Most commonly these cystic lesions arise over tendons or joints of the wrist or hand. They can result from a defect in the joint capsule or tendon sheath with extravasation of synovial fluid forming the cyst. When the communication becomes obliterated, the fluid becomes gelatinous. The cyst may regress spontaneously. Treatment includes: 1) doing nothing, 2) aspiration with a large bore needle (#16) followed by instillation of a corticosteroid, or 3) surgical excision during which the communication must be traced to the defect in the joint or tendon sheath followed by repair of the defect.

The hypermobility syndrome. Joint laxity may result in symmetric upper or lower limb joint stiffness and pain. This benign syndrome may be mistaken for early rheumatoid arthritis. A sensation of joint pain, stiffness, and swelling that lasts for hours rather than for days may follow intense physical activity. Although joint laxity has been reported in 5% of the adult population, only a minority develop the syndrome (4). Features of joint laxity include:

1. Passive dorsiflexion of a finger until it is parallel to the forearm
2. Passive opposition of the thumb to the flexor aspect of the forearm
3. Extension of the elbow or knee 10 degrees beyond normal
4. Ability to bend forward and touch palms to floor with knees straight

Some patients have other familial orthopedic disorders including dislocations of the hip or shoulder, laterally displaced patellae, scoliosis, or flat feet. Other disorders associated with joint laxity include inherited connective tissue disorders (Marfan's syndrome, Ehlers-Danlos syndrome), neurologic diseases, rheumatic fever, and rare metabolic disorders.

By definition, the hypermobility syndrome is not associated with skin hyperelasticity or involvement of the eye. Patients may have a floppy mitral valve. Treatment includes establishing and maintaining good extensor muscle tone at the involved joint locations. Vigorous conditioning programs should be recommended for these patients if possible.

The leg

Trochanteric bursitis. A common rheumatic pain disorder, trochanteric bursitis presents with lateral hip pain, often acute, and usually more severe at night. Physical examination reveals point tenderness over the bursa in the region of the greater trochanter. The bursitis may arise from trauma to the overlying gluteal muscles or may occur in association with hip arthritis, back surgery, or improper work habits such as bending over while holding the knees straight.

Treatment includes injection of the superficial or deep trochanteric bursa with a local anesthetic and corticosteroid agent. Often a spinal needle will be needed to reach the deep trochanteric bursa. If tender points are detected in the overlying muscles (including the piriformis), they should be injected also.

Fascia lata fasciitis. The fascia lata, which is a fascial plane extending down the lateral aspect of the thigh may be the source of pain extending down the lateral leg to the upper foreleg. Tender points can be detected along this fascial band. Causes include inflammation from sport or running activities, or the disorder may occur in association with lumbar disc disease and sciatica. Snapping hip syndrome may also occur.

Treatment includes injecting the tender points with a local anesthetic and corticosteroid agent, stretching exercises, and conditioning exercises before engaging in sport activities. Lumbar disc disease with nerve root impingement should be excluded. Meralgia paresthetica, back pocket wallet syndrome, piriformis syndrome, spinal stenosis, and osteoarthritis of the hip are among the many other disorders that cause persistent hip pain.

Prepatellar busitis. Inflammation of the prepatellar bursa (located in the soft tissues in front of the patella) usually results from direct trauma that can occur during repeated kneeling. Foreign body penetration with resulting infection must be excluded. It can be seen nuns, carpet layers, plumbers, and carpenters. The bursa may be warm and tender; if an effusion is present, it should be aspirated and examined.

Anserine bursitis. This common cause for pain at the medial aspect of the knee often occurs in association with osteoarthritis. The pain is located in the area of the medial tibial collateral ligament and is troublesome at night. The patient often seeks comfort by sleeping with a pillow between the thighs. Point tenderness is

greater than that in uncomplicated osteoarthritis.

Local intralesional injection with a local anesthetic and corticosteroid agent provides immediate improvement, thus aiding in diagnosis. The bursa may be buried within a large panniculus; night pain should alert the clinician to examine the knee carefully for tenderness. The valgus stress test for collateral ligament involvement should be performed before injection. If the legs are weak, the patient should perform quadriceps resistance exercises for improved knee stability.

Popliteal (Baker's) cyst. Pain in the posterior (popliteal) knee region may result from knee joint synovitis, hamstring tenosynovitis, hamstring contracture, or a Baker's cyst (5). This lesion represents enlargement of one or more bursae that communicate with the knee joint. The enlargement results from increased synovial fluid arising in the knee, usually as a result of arthritis. Careful examination for a Baker's cyst includes palpation for a pulsating mass (aneurysm), knee joint synovitis, and other manifestations of arthritis. Examination for hamstring tightness by the straight leg raising maneuver is important.

If present, a tight hamstring should be stretched by twice a day mobilizing exercise. Treatment includes aspiration of the cyst and/or the knee joint, followed by injection of a corticosteroid agent. Surgical excision should be considered for recurrent cysts. Spontaneous rupture of a Baker's cyst can mimic acute deep vein thrombophlebitis or thrombophlebitis can result from venous obstruction by a large cyst. Prolonged sitting, squatting, and stair climbing should be avoided.

Leg cramp. This common disturbance may be familial and often results from prolonged squatting, kneeling, or standing on concrete floors. Metabolic derangement is seldom found.

Stretching exercises are performed by standing and facing a wall with the feet approximately 3 feet from the wall; hands are placed upon the wall and "walked" slowly up the wall until the posterior leg muscles begin to pull. Without allowing the heels to rise from the floor, the patient stretches the leg muscles maximally. Performed several times a day with several repetitions each time, the exercise often provides relief (6).

Use of quinine for 7–10 days has also been helpful.

Achilles tendinitis. Heel pain may result from many disorders. Achilles tendinitis presents with heel pain and tenderness over the insertion of the tendon. Usually the tendinitis results from the trauma of improperly fitting shoes with a stiff heel counter or from a new sport activity. The spondylarthropathies and calcific tendinitis must also be considered if inflammation is more acute.

The achilles tendon is vulnerable to rupture, and local injection of a corticosteroid is contraindicated in the vicinity of the tendon unless the ankle can be rested for at least a week thereafter.

Plantar fasciitis. This common cause for plantar heel or foot pain often results from foot strain. New sports activities, jogging, jumping, or a new job that requires prolonged standing are common causes. Obesity and flat feet may be associated with the disorder. Spondylarthritis occasionally causes similar irritation. The patient usually notes heel or foot pain with the onset of weight bearing after rest; each step is painful.

Examination reveals tautness to the plantar fascia when compared with normal. The examiner should dorsiflex the toes with one hand and palpate for tender points with the other hand. These points can be injected with a local anesthetic and a corticosteroid agent and the patient should be instructed to stretch the tight tissue with non-weight-bearing exercise.

Proper shoes or sandals, particulary with rubber soles for working on concrete, may be helpful. Excessive heel strike (as in jogging, rope skipping, or an improper gait) should be curtailed and obesity should be controlled.

1. Sheon RP, Moskowitz RW, Goldberg VM: Soft Tissue Rheumatic Pain: Recognition, Management, Prevention. Philadelphia, Lea & Febiger, 1982
2. Sheon RP: Soft tissue rheumatic pain. Comprehensive Therapy 8:19–28, 1982
3. James SL, Bates BT, Osternig LR: Injuries to runners. Am J Sports Med 6:40–50, 1978
4. Sheon RP, Kirsner AB, Farber SJ, Finkel RI: The hypermobility syndrome. Postgrad Med 71:199–209, 1982
5. Bywaters EGL: Tendinitis and bursitis. Clin Rheum Dis 5:883–927, 1979
6. Hench PK: Nonarticular rheumatism, Rheumatic Diseases: Diagnosis and Management. WA Katz, ed. Philadelphia, JB Lippincott, 1977

75. Reflex sympathetic dystrophy syndromes

The reflex sympathetic dystrophy syndromes (RSDS) are characterized by *causalgia*, a distinctive nonsegmental pain in 1 or more extremities combined with trophic skin changes, vasomotor instability,

increased local blood flow, and radiographic evidence of local osteopenia (Table 75–1). Trauma, spinal cord or peripheral nerve injuries, immobilization, certain drugs, and a particular personality type,

have all been implicated as inciting factors (1).

Early mobilization after myocardial infarction, stroke, and injury have reduced the frequency of, but not eliminated, re-

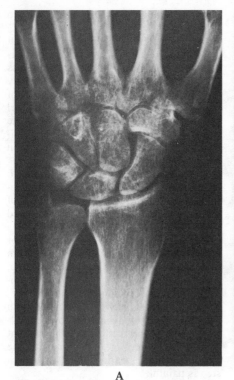
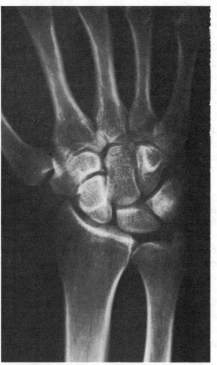

A   B

Fig 75–1. Roentgenograms of the hands of a 42-year-old woman with shoulder–hand syndrome involving the left hand (**A**) illustrates changes of patchy osteoporosis (Sudeck's atrophy). Compare with normal right hand (**B**). These roentgenograms were obtained 2 months after the onset of burning pain and swelling in the left hand and of pain and limitation of motion in the left shoulder.

Table 75–1. Features of reflex sympathetic dystrophy syndromes

Pain or burning in distal portion of extremity
Tenderness and swelling (often with pitting edema) over entire distal portion of extremity with periarticular accentuation
Cool, cyanotic, moist skin in distal portion of extremity, often associated with scaling, desquamation, and atrophy of skin and skin appendages (e.g., hair loss, dyskeratotic nails)
Shoulder pain and limitation of motion (in shoulder–hand variant of syndrome)
Condition often bilateral; may be subclinical on 1 side
Synovial cell proliferation with subsynovial fibrosis without inflammatory cell infiltrate
Blood flow to deep tissues of extremity greatly increased with nonspecific patchy osteopenia (Sudeck's atrophy) that is accentuated around joints. Resorption of subchondral bone may lead to cortical breaks mimicking the surface erosions of rheumatoid arthritis, and to peculiar "crumbling" erosions

flex sympathetic dystrophy syndromes. Trauma, often minor, is the most frequent antecedent factor, although in fully one-third of patients, no etiologic event can be identified.

Men and women are affected with equal frequency, and RSDS has been reported in both children and young adults. Although the entire hand (or foot) is usually afflicted, instances of involvement of only 1 or more rays of the hand or foot (radial form) or a segment of a long bone such as the femoral head (zonal form) have also been reported.

Tenderness and swelling are accentuated around joints, even when the entire hand or foot is affected. The motion of joints in the distal portion of the extremity is often limited, and in the common variant of RSDS known as the shoulder–hand syndrome, movement is both painful and restricted. Bilateral involvement occurs in 18–50% of patients with RSDS. Clinical and scintigraphic analysis of a small number of patients with the fully developed syndrome revealed all had bilateral abnormalities, although 1 side was sometimes asymptomatic. This observation reinforces the classic notion that the disease is mediated by a central neurogenic mechanism.

The appearance of a patchy osteoporosis in roentgenograms of the hands and sometimes the feet (Sudeck's atrophy) (Fig 75–1) is characteristic of, but not specific for, RSDS. Recent use of fine detail roentgenograms has shown that bone resorption is also accentuated around joints, sometimes leading to peculiar "crumbling" erosions (Fig 75–2) or to breaks in subchondral bone reminiscent of the surface erosions of rheumatoid arthritis (Fig 75–3). There is an average loss of

approximately one-third of the bone mineral in the affected extremity. Treatment appears to halt the progression of osteopenia but does not reverse the process except in children.

The usual clinical course in the fully expressed case can be separated into 3 overlapping stages. The first or acute stage lasts 3–6 months and has the features described in Table 75–1. The second or dystrophic stage persists for several months and is characterized by trophic skin changes with total or partial resolu-

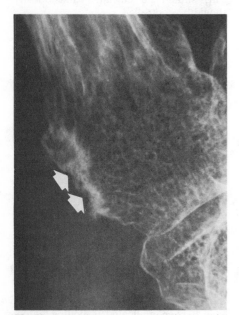

Fig 75–2. A paraarticular "crumbling" erosion (**arrows**), not specific for reflex sympathetic dystrophy, but seen in other conditions such as osteoarthritis and hyperparathyroidism. (Illustration provided by Dr Harry Genant)

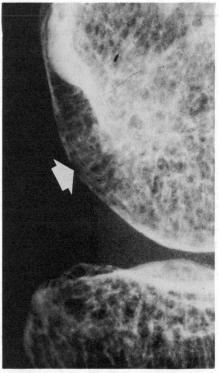

Fig 75–3. A surface erosion in subchondral bone (**arrow**), thought to result from the bony demineralization that is accentuated in the metaphyseal and paraarticular areas. (Illustration provided by Dr Harry Genant)

tion of the acute manifestations. In the third or atrophic stage, there is gradual thinning of skin, subcutaneous tissue, and muscle, and the development of contractures of tendons and joint capsules. The end result is a painless contracted functionless appendage with cool shiny skin. Radiographs then show a "ground glass" osteopenia.

Histologic examination of the synovium during the active stages of the disease reveals synovial cell hyperplasia, subsynovial fibrosis, and increased vascularity but almost no evidence of inflammation.

Treatment is most successful when begun early in the acute stage. Analgesic medications and range of motion exercises (especially shoulder) within the patient's pain tolerance should be prescribed. Nonsteroidal antiinflammtory drugs may be of value. If these measures fail to provide satisfactory relief, treatment with corticosteroids or sympathetic blockade may be pursued. After a brief course of prednisone, a mild exacerbation may occur. This usually subsides within 2 weeks. Some patients relapse and require a second course of treatment.

Sympathetic blockade with local anes-

thetic agents may provide transient relief from pain, especially if carried out on a daily or alternate-day schedule. Patients deriving *any* benefit from this treatment are candidates for surgical sympathectomy, which often produces excellent results in treatment of reflex dystrophy syndromes of either the upper or lower extremity.

1. Kozin F: Painful shoulder and the reflex dystrophy syndrome, Arthritis and Allied Conditions, Ed 9. DJ McCarty, Jr, ed. Philadelphia, Lea & Febiger, 1979, pp 1091–1120

76. Dupuytren's contracture

Dupuytren's contracture is caused by a thickening and shortening of the palmar fascia; the plantar fascia may also be affected. Occasionally fibrosis is more widespread and may include involvement of the penis, as in Peyronie's disease. Fibrous nodules are often the earliest abnormality, probably resulting from a contraction of proliferative fibroblasts in the superficial compartment of the palm (1). There does not appear to be any direct involvement of joints, tendons (and their sheaths), muscles, or nervous or vascular tissue, but the dermis is frequently invaded by fibroblastic cells resulting in fixation to the deeper structures (2).

In most instances, Dupuytren's contracture affects the ulnar side of both hands. In almost all patients, the fourth finger is involved with associated involvement of the fifth, third, and second fingers in decreasing order of frequency. The disease evolution is unpredictable. Some individuals show little change or incapacity over a period of many years. In others, fascial

contraction progresses rapidly with severe deformity and loss of hand function.

Although the cause of this condition is unknown, there appears to be an underlying hereditary predisposition (Mendelian dominant). The disorder is about 5 times more frequent in men than in women, predominates in whites, and is more common in Europe. There is a gradual increase in incidence of the disease with age.

Most authors agree that an association exists between Dupuytren's contracture and chronic alcoholism or epilepsy (3), but trauma, long thought to be a contributing factor, is now considered to be of minor, if any, relevance. Some researchers suggest that this condition may at times result from increased sympathetic tone and may be a part of the spectrum of reflex neurovascular dystrophy (shoulder–hand syndrome) following myocardial infarctions and a variety of other thoracic and skeletal disorders.

Treatment depends entirely on the se-

verity of the findings. Heat, stretching exercises, ultrasound, and intralesional injection of corticosteroids may be helpful in early stages. If there is evidence of shoulder–hand syndrome, more intensive physical and systemic therapy is warranted. When actual contractures are occurring, surgical intervention may be desirable. Limited fasciectomy is effective in most instances, but more radical procedures, including digital amputation, may be necessary. Palmar fasciotomy is a useful and more benign procedure, but if the disease remains active recurrence is likely.

1. Hineston JT, Hurley JV, Whittingham S: The contracting fibroblasts as a clue to Dupuytren's contracture. The Hand 8:10–12, 1976
2. Vijanto JA: Dupuytren's contracture: a review. Semin Arthritis Rheum 3:155–176, 1973
3. Pojer J, Radiwojevic M, Williams TF: Dupuytren's disease: its association with abnormal liver function in alcoholism and epilepsy. Arch Intern Med 129:561–566, 1977

77. Clubbing and hypertrophic osteoarthropathy

Clubbing is the term used to describe an abnormal appearance of the fingers and toes. It occurs chiefly in adults and is characterized by widening of the fingertips, loss of the normal angle between the nail and the cuticle, increased convexity of the nail, and enlargement of the distal finger pad (Fig 77–1). The adjacent skin and nail are usually shiny. Clubbing usually affects the fingers and toes symmetrically but is sometimes unilateral (1).

Hypertrophic osteoarthropathy (HO) refers to a syndrome of periositis of the long bones, joint effusion, and clubbing. Clubbing need not be associated with HO,

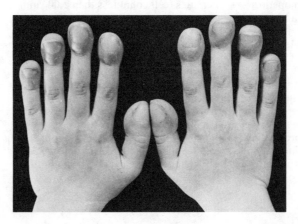

Fig 77–1. The hands of an 8-year-old girl with cystic fibrosis illustrate severe clubbing. (Illustration provided by Dr JB Rodnan)

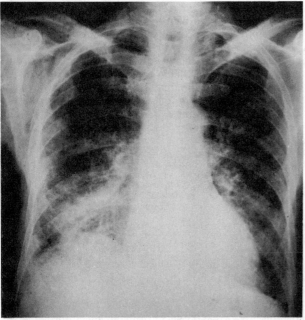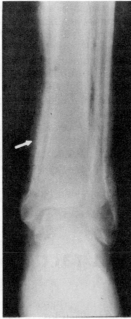

Fig 77–2. Chest and left leg of a 67-year-old man with bronchogenic carcinoma and associated hypertrophic osteoarthropathy. Extreme degree of periosteal new bone formation (**arrow**) involves both the tibia and fibula.

clarify the diagnosis because radionuclide deposits are pericortical in HO, whereas with bony metastases uptake is central. Radioscans may be used to document regression of HO after therapy.

Although endocrine (12), humoral (3), and neuronal (13) theories have been investigated and HO has been reported in animals (14), the mechanisms responsible for HO are not known. Moreover, because clubbing and HO can each occur independently, different mechanisms may be responsible. While familial clubbing is usually asymptomatic, the course of HO varies considerably. Regression may follow treatment of a pulmonary neoplasm by surgical resection, radiotherapy (15), chemotherapy (16), or less specific measures such as hilar denervation, surgical or chemical vagotomy, and sympathectomy. Symptomatic relief may be obtained by salicylates, indomethacin, or corticosteroids.

whereas HO is almost invariably associated with clubbing (2,3). Although clubbing may be hereditary, it is usually secondary to some other disorder (4). Bronchogenic carcinoma, chronic pulmonary sepsis, and cyanotic congenital heart disease account for most cases, but there are a variety of other causes including cystic fibrosis in children, mesothelioma, nasopharyngeal carcinoma, bacterial endocarditis, biliary cirrhosis, ulcerative colitis, regional enteritis, and pituitary and thyroid disease.

Compared with clubbing, HO is uncommon (1–3,5). Because most cases are associated with some form of pulmonary disease, HO is also known as hypertrophic pulmonary osteoarthropathy. Bronchogenic carcinoma accounts for most cases of HO, but in rare instances, it may be secondary to pleural tumors, pulmonary metastases, or one of the many other causes of clubbing (5). With arterial graft sepsis, HO occasionally may affect only the lower extremities (6).

In an unusual variety of idiopathic familial HO, known as pachydermoperiostitis, postpubertal clubbing and bone changes are accompanied by increased sweating of the palms and soles and a marked thickening of the skin of the face, forehead, and scalp (7,8).

Clubbing usually develops insidiously, years after the onset of a nonmalignant condition, whereas HO may appear suddenly, with pain and tenderness in the distal parts of the legs and forearms or with a polyarthritis affecting knees, ankles, elbows, wrists, or metacarpophalan-geal joints. Symptoms in the affected limbs may worsen with dependency and improve with elevation (1). Morning stiffness, raised sedimentation rate, and response to antiinflammatory medication may reinforce a mistaken impression of rheumatoid arthritis. The articular features may precede the clubbing and/or radiographic evidence of periostitis. Clubbing and HO sometimes constitute the first manifestation of an occult bronchogenic carcinoma. In rare cases, clubbing may be associated with acrolysis (9). This syndrome occasionally occurs in older patients with neoplasm (2).

Although the presence of clubbing and arthritis is suggestive of HO, the radiographic appearance of the long bones is usually diagnostic (Fig 77–2). Sometimes the condition is first discovered when roentgenograms of the painful joints reveal periosteal proliferation. Synovial fluid from patients with HO with polyarthritis tends to clot spontaneously, but otherwise displays noninflammatory characteristics (cell count less than 2,000/mm^3) in contrast to that of rheumatoid arthritis (3).

Although electron dense material may be found in vessel walls of patients with HO synovitis (3), evidence of circulating immune complexes (10) or synovial deposits of immunoglobulin and complement is lacking in those with HO. Radioscan of imaging with ^{99m}technetium phosphate complexes may be used to determine the presence and extent of HO before radiologic changes appear (11). Scanning may

1. Altman RD, Tenenbaum J: Hypertrophic osteoarthropathy, Textbook of Rheumatology. WN Kelley, ED Harris, S Ruddy, C Sledge, eds. Philadelphia, WB Saunders, 1981, pp 1647–1657
2. Calabro JJ: Cancer and arthritis. Arthritis Rheum 10:553–567, 1967
3. Schumacher HR: Articular manifestations of hypertrophic pulmonary osteoarthropathy in bronchogenic carcinoma. Arthritis Rheum 19:629–635, 1976
4. Fischer DS, Singer DH, Feldman SM: Clubbing, a review with emphasis on hereditary acropachy. Medicine 43:459–479, 1964
5. Coury C: Hippocratic fingers and hypertrophic osteoarthropathy: a study of 350 cases. Br J Dis Chest 54:202–209, 1960
6. Walter RD, Resnick D: Hypertrophic osteoarthropathy of a lower extremity in association with arterial graft sepsis. Am J Radiol 137:1059–1061, 1981
7. Rimoin DL: Pachydermoperiostosis (idiopathic clubbing and periostosis): genetic and physiologic considerations. N Engl J Med 272:923–931, 1965
8. Lauter SA, Vasey FB, Huttner I, Osterland CK: Pachydermoperiostosis: studies on the synovium. J Rheumatol 5:85–95, 1978
9. Hedayati H, Barmada R, Skosey JL: Acrolysis in pachydermoperiostosis—primary or idiopathic hypertrophic osteoarthropathy. Arch Intern Med 140:1087–1088, 1980
10. Auerbach MS, Brooks PM: Role of immune complexes in hypertrophic osteoarthropathy and nonmetastic polyarthritis. Ann Rheum Dis 40:470–472, 1981
11. Rosenthal L, Kirsh J: Observations on radionuclide imaging in hypertrophic pulmonary osteoarthropathy. Radiology 120:359–362, 1976
12. Ennis GC, Cameron DP, Burger HG: On the aetiology of hypertrophic pulmonary osteoarthropathy in bronchogenic carcinoma: lack of relationship to elevated growth hormone levels. Aust NZ J Med 3:157–161, 1973
13. Carroll KB, Doyle L: A common factor in hypertrophic osteoarthropathy. Thorax 29:262–264, 1974
14. Hancey JB, Pass MA: Hypertrophic pulmonary osteoarthropathy in a great dane. Can Vet J 13:118–120, 1972
15. Steinfeld AD, Munzenrider JE: The response of hypertrophic pulmonary osteoarthropathy to radiotherapy. Radiology 113:709–711, 1974
16. Evans WK: Reversal of hypertrophic osteoarthropathy after chemotherapy to bronchogenic carcinoma. J Rheumatol 7:93–97, 1980

78. Rheumatic syndromes of the anterior chest wall

Tietse's syndrome, costochondritis, the hypersensitive xiphoid, and the syndrome of the slipping rib (1–4) must be differentiated from problems involving the thoracic viscera, particularly those of the heart, great vessels, and mediastinum, as well as from illness originating in the head, neck, or abdomen.

The terms **Tietse's syndrome** and **costochondritis** are often used interchangeably. Although both disorders are characterized by inflammation of 1 or more costal cartilages, Tietse's syndrome is associated with notable local swelling, while costochondritis is not. Tietse's syndrome is far less common than costochondritis.

In most cases, the cause of Tietse's syndrome is unknown. The syndrome occurs in all age groups, including children, with a predilection for the second and third decades (2). The clinical manifestations are consistent: the sudden or gradual onset of upper anterior chest pain associated with fusiform or bulbous swelling of the involved costal cartilage. Chest pain is mild to severe and sometimes radiates to the shoulder and arm. It is often aggravated by sneezing, coughing, inspiration, bending, recumbency, or exertion. Approximately 80% of patients have only single sites of involvement, most commonly the second or third costal cartilage.

Table 78–1. Differences between Tietse's syndrome and costochondrosis

	Tietse's syndrome	Costo-chondritis
Female:male	1:1	3:1
Age at onset	Most < 40 yrs	Most > 40 yrs
No. sites involved	Single, 80%	Multiple, 90%
Most frequent site involved	2nd, 3rd	3rd, 4th, 5th
Local swelling	Present	Absent

When swellings are multiple, neighboring articulations are usually affected.

Costochondritis (costal chondritis), also known as the anterior chest wall syndrome, the costosternal syndrome, and parasternal chondrodynia, is characterized by pain of the anterior chest wall that may radiate widely, thereby simulating intrathoracic or intraabdominal disease (4).

Costochondritis may follow trauma or may be associated with systemic rheumatic disease.

Palpation of the affected portion of the thoracic cage elicits tenderness. Inflammation of upper costal cartilages may cause annoying chest pain (3), while inflammation of lower costal cartilages may cause abdominal discomfort. Differences between Tietse's syndrome and costochondritis are noted in Table 78–1.

Yet another cause of upper abdominal pain is the **hypersensitive xiphoid**, also known as the cartilage syndrome or xiphoidalgia. This syndrome is manifest as epigastric pain, nausea, and vomiting (1). The xiphoid is tender to palpation and local pressure may cause nausea and vomiting.

In the **syndrome of the slipping rib** (usually the tenth), the involved cartilage moves upwards overriding the one above it, thereby causing pain.

These disorders are usually benign and self-limiting. Most patients respond to reassurance and to 1 or more local injections of xylocaine and long-acting corticosteroids. Surgical intervention is rarely necessary.

1. Lipkin M, Fulton LA, Wolfson EA: The syndrome of the hypersensitive xiphoid. N Engl J Med 253:591–597, 1955
2. Calabro JJ, Marchesano JM: Tietze's syndrome: report of a case with juvenile onset. J Pediatrics 68:985–987, 1966
3. Wolf E, Stern S: Costosternal syndrome: its frequency and importance in differential diagnosis of coronary heart disease. Arch Intern Med 136:189–191, 1976
4. Calabro JJ: Costochondritis: N Engl J Med 296:946–947, 1977

79. Metabolic bone disease

Patients with metabolic bone disease complain of musculoskeletal pain and weakness, symptoms that may be confused with rheumatic diseases. Osteopenia is an additional complicating problem in many individuals with rheumatic diseases, especially those taking glucocorticoids (1).

Bone formation and resorption, normally in equilibrium, are controlled by 1) **mechanical stress** stimulating osteoblast formation and synthesis of ground substance and collagen (osteoid); 2) **levels of calcium and phosphate ions** in the extracellular fluid (ECF) regulating levels of parathyroid hormone (PTH) and calcitonin (CT); 3) **parathyroid hormone** maintaining normal ionized calcium levels in ECF by stimulating osteoclasts to resorb mineralized bone, increasing renal tubular calcium retention and excretion of phosphate, sodium and bicarbonate, and favoring the conversion of vitamin D to its most active metabolite; 4) **calcitonin** lowering ionized calcium levels by reducing bone resorption, enhancing renal excretion of calcium, phosphate, sodium, and chloride, and possibly by inhibiting conversion of vitamin D; and 5) **vitamin D** regulating intestinal absorption of calcium.

Vitamins D_2 and D_3 are ingested in foods; D_3 is synthesized in skin from 7-dehydrocholesterol, which is activated by ultraviolet light. These compounds are not hormonally active, but their conversion in the liver to 25-hydroxycholecalciferol (25-OH D) produces a metabolite which enhances intestinal absorption of calcium (2). Drugs that induce hepatic microsomal enzyme activity promote conversion of 25-OH D to inactive metabolites. Osteomalacia occasionally results from this process. In the renal tubule, 25-OH D is metabolized to 1,25-dihydroxycholecalciferol (1,25-$(OH)_2$D). This is the most active form of the vitamin and greatly increases intestinal absorption of calcium. High levels of PTH are favorable for the formation of 1,25-$(OH)_2$D.

Osteopenia is a reduction of bone mass greater than expected for a given age, race, and sex. Clinical manifestations include bone pain and/or multiple fractures. Evaluation includes roentgenograms of the bones (30–50% of mass must be lost before routine roentgenograms detect osteopenia); fasting blood levels of calcium, phosphate, alkaline phosphatase activity and PTH; 24-hour urine calcium excretion; and tests to rule out other disorders associated with osteopenia. Newer techniques for measurement of bone mass, such as single photon osteodensitometry or computerized tomography of the vertebra may be used, if available.

In adults, the differential diagnosis includes *osteoporosis, osteomalacia, osteitis fibrosa, hyperthyroidism, neoplasms* (especially *multiple myeloma*), and *inherited bone disorders* (Table 79–1).

In osteoporosis, serum levels of calcium, phosphate, alkaline phosphatase activity, and PTH are usually normal. In osteomalacia, serum phosphate level is low and calcium normal; alkaline phosphatase activity is normal or high; PTH levels are usually slightly elevated. In osteitis fibrosa, the PTH level is always high

Table 79–1. Differential diagnosis of generalized osteopenia in adults*

Osteoporosis: parallel loss of mineral and matrix
  aging—genetic, sex, race, dietary predispositions
  immobilization or reduced physical activity
  premature menopause
Osteomalacia: inadequate mineralization
  vitamin D deficiency
    inadequate intake and reduced exposure to sunlight
    drug-induced catabolism of vitamin D
    intestinal malabsorption
  phosphate-wasting syndromes
    acquired renal tubular defects with isolated phosphate loss
    combined tubular defects (Fanconi syndrome)
    renal tubular acidosis
    antacid abuse
Osteitis fibrosa: PTH-induced increase in mineral and matrix resorption
  primary hyperparathyroidism
  secondary hyperparathyroidism
    vitamin D-deficiency states
    primary decrease in intestinal calcium absorption with age
    reduced renal mass
Corticosteroid-induced osteopenia
  iatrogenic
  adrenal corticosteroid overproduction
Other disorders
  hyperthyroidism
  diffuse osteolytic malignancies (e.g., multiple myeloma)
  congenital disorders: osteogenesis imperfecta tarda, vitamin D-resistant rickets

* From Seminars in Arthritis and Rheumatism (1)

with elevated levels of serum calcium and alkaline phosphatase activity, low serum phosphate level, and normal or high urine calcium excretion.

Osteoporosis is defined as osteopenia associated with parallel loss of bone mineral and matrix; resorption rates are always greater than formation rates (3). Loss of bone mass is in part a consequence of aging. Both diaphyseal and metaphyseal mass decline after age 25, more rapidly in women than in men, with considerable individual variability. Acceleration of bone loss from the appendicular skeleton occurs at menopause (especially if menopause is premature) in some, but not all, women. In contrast, loss of vertebral mass may be constant after puberty and is less sensitive to sex hormones than the appendicular skeleton (4).

Average bone mass is greater in men than in women and greater in blacks than in whites or Asians. Therefore, females have less bone mass and lose it faster, and white and Asian women are at highest risk for the development of symptomatic osteopenia.

The multifactorial pathogenesis of osteoporosis includes age, race, sex, genetic predisposition, reduced physical activity, menopause, reduced dietary calcium intake, impairment of intestinal calcium absorption in some individuals over 50 years of age, and reduced exposure to sunlight.

Treatment of symptomatic osteoporosis often has disappointing results. Prevention is a more useful approach. Individuals at high risk should be identified before menopause. Preventive measures include regular exercise that moves bones against gravity (walking, running, tennis), adequate daily intake of Vitamin D (at least 400 IU per day), and supplemental calcium. The average American diet provides approximately 500 mg of calcium daily; 500–1,000 mg should be added (if serum and urine calcium levels are normal) to provide the minimal daily requirement of 1,000–1,500 mg.

Several studies have demonstrated a reduced rate of postmenopausal bone loss in women treated with estrogen, especially if such treatment is instituted within 3 years of menopause. Other studies have shown no benefit from this approach. Hazards of this therapy include increased risk of endometrial and breast carcinoma, thromboembolic disease, and arterial hypertension. Estrogen reduces bone resorption, but formation may also diminish after several months. Estrogen therapy is probably indicated in order to preserve bone mass in women with premature (before age 45) menopause (5,6).

Symptomatic osteoporosis may be treated with regular exercise and adequate intake of Vitamin D and calcium, especially if calcium malabsorption is present (1,7). Sodium fluoride, 20 mg twice a day, is sometimes prescribed as an experimental drug. Fluoride stimulates formation of osteoid, reduces bone resorption, and is incorporated in the hydroxyapatite crystal. This process confers greater density to bone. Bone mass has been found to increase and bone fractures to decrease in some osteoporotic patients treated for 12–18 months with sodium fluoride (7). Calcium and vitamin D should also be provided so that osteoid can mineralize. Unde-

sirable side effects of fluoride include gastrointestinal disturbances, joint pain, and osteomalacia.

Estrogens may also be given to symptomatic patients: 1.25 mg of conjugated estrogens or 0.5 mg of stilbesterol daily for 20 of 25 days may be effective in increasing mass and in decreasing fractures (5–7). Benefits are controversial. Androgenic hormones have been used to treat osteoporosis, but there is little evidence that they increase bone mass for long periods.

Osteomalacia is the pathologic loss of mineralized bone due to reduction of calcium–phosphate levels, with resultant accumulation of unmineralized matrix (osteoid) (8). The most common causes in adults are reduced vitamin D absorption due to biliary tract or intestinal disease, accelerated vitamin D catabolism due to drug-induced increase in hepatic oxidases (especially barbituates and diphenylhydantoins), and acquired renal tubular defects with phosphate wasting.

Patients with osteomalacia have rheumatic complaints: generalized aching, muscle weakness, periarticular tenderness, and sensory polyneuropathy. Treatment is directed toward the underlying problem. It is often necessary to give supplemental vitamin D, calcium, and/or phosphate. Correction of acidosis may be necessary if renal tubular acidosis is present, since acidosis per se impairs mineralization of bone.

Osteitis fibrosa represents a histologic diagnosis based on the finding of increased osteoclast numbers and resorption sites; bone is thus replaced by fibrous tissue. This condition occurs in primary or secondary hyperparathyroidism, the latter resulting from prolonged hypocalcemia. Associated symptoms include bone, muscle, and joint pain, weakness, fractures, morning stiffness, and occasionally calcium pyrophosphate dihydrate crystal–induced synovitis (pseudogout).

Primary hyperparathyroidism should be treated by surgical resection of 3½ parathyroid glands. Secondary hyperparathyroidism usually results from vitamin D malabsorption (this may be at least partially corrected), from chronic renal failure, or from PTH-producing malignancies of the lung, kidney, or urogenital tract.

Steroid-induced osteopenia occurs in more than 40% of individuals treated for 3 years or longer with daily supraphysiologic doses of glucocorticoids (>5 mg prednisone or equivalent). Severity is related to a number of factors, including status of bone mass when therapy is instituted—menopausal white and Asian women again are at high risk. Physical inactivity caused by the primary disease accelerates bone loss. Large cumulative doses of glucocorticoids, small body size, age over 50 years, and the postmenopausal state are also risk factors for symptomatic steroid-induced osteopenia.

Fractures of the vertebrae and ribs are the most frequent clinical manifestations of this disorder. This is probably a result of the high content of trabecular bone, which is metabolically more active than cortical bone, in these areas.

Mechanisms by which glucocorticoids produce osteopenia include reduced bone formation and increased bone resorption resulting from reduced intestinal absorption of calcium with subsequent secondary hyperparathyroidism. In addition, there is some controversial evidence for accelerated conversion of 25–OH D and 1,25–(OH)$_2$D to inactive metabolites in corticosteroid-treated individuals—a situation which results in relative vitamin D deficiency.

Prevention or reduction of corticosteroid-induced osteopenia may be possible. Regular administration of vitamin D, 25–OH D, or 1 α-OH–D (a synthetic analog of vitamin D) enhances intestinal absorption of calcium. In studies with 25–OH D, the restoration of normal calcium absorption was associated with a reduction in serum PTH from elevated to normal levels, increased bone mass assessed by photon absorption osteodensitomitry (a technique that is capable of detecting an 8% reduction in bone mass), and reduced numbers of osteoclasts in posttreatment bone biopsy specimens. These benefits were sustained during 18 months of treatment (9). It should be emphasized that this therapy reduces corticosteroid-induced bone resorption but may not alter reduced formation rates and that a change in fracture rate has not been documented.

The therapy currently recommended for controlling steroid-induced osteopenia is the reduction of glucocorticoid doses to as low as possible; the encouragement of physical activity; and for high risk patients, vitamin D supplements, 50,000 units 2 or 3 times a week, and calcium 500–1,000 mg daily (preferably calcium carbonate, which is absorbed well). Supplemental vitamin D and calcium therapy should not be instituted unless serum and urine calcium levels are normal. Hypercalcuria and even hypercalcemia can result from this therapy. Serum and urine calcium levels should be measured at 2–3 month intervals until stable, then every 6 months while supplementation is continued.

1. Hahn TJ, Hahn BH: Osteopenia in patients with rheumatic diseases: principles of diagnosis and therapy. Semin Arthritis Rheum 6:165–188, 1976
2. Raisz LG: Bone metabolism and calcium regulation, Metabolic Bone Disease. Vol 1. LV Avioli, SM Krane, eds. New York, Academic Press, 1977, pp 1–48
3. Avioli LV: Osteoporosis: pathogenesis and therapy, Metabolic Bone Disease. Vol 1. LV Avioli, SM Krane, eds. New York, Academic Press, 1977, pp 307–385
4. Riggs BL, Wahner HW, Dunn WL, Mazess RB, Offord KP, Melton LJ III: Differential changes in bone mineral density of the appendicular and axial skeleton with aging: relationship to spinal osteoporosis. J Clin Invest 67:328–335, 1981
5. Lindsay R, Hart DM, Forrest C, Baird C: Prevention of spinal osteoporosis in oophorectomized women. Lancet 2:1151–1154, 1980
6. Paganini-Hill A, Ross RK, Gerkins GR, Henderson BE, Arthur M, Mack TM: Menopausal estrogen therapy and hip fractures. Ann Intern Med 95:28–31, 1981
7. Riggs BL, Seeman E, Hodgson SF, Taves DR, O'Fallon WM: Effect of the fluoride/calcium regimen on vertebral fracture occurrence in postmenopausal osteoporosis. N Engl J Med 306:446–450, 1982
8. Dent CE, Stamp TCB: Vitamin D, Rickets and osteomalacia, Metabolic Bone Disease. Vol 1. LV Avioli, SM Krane, eds. New York, Academic Press, 1977, pp 237–305
9. Hahn TJ, Halstead LH, Teitelbaum SL, Hahn BH: Altered mineral metabolism in glucocorticoid-induced osteopenia: effect of 25-hydroxyvitamin D administration. J Clin Invest 64:655–665, 1979

80. Nodular panniculitis

As used here, the term nodular panniculitis encompasses idiopathic Weber-Christian disease (less a disease than a nonhomogeneous syndrome) and nodular panniculitis due to pancreatic disease (1–5). Various causes for inflammatory fat disorders include infection, trauma, drug reaction, neoplasia, and intestinal bypass. Only rarely do these syndromes encompass joint pain or arthritis and neither they nor panniculitis occurring in connective tissue disease will be discussed. Since alleged distinctions among the various types are often not observed and until further facts detailing mechanisms of disease are available, rigid systems of classification should be avoided. Erythema nodosum is also excluded from this discussion of nodular panniculitis, even though these nodules may exhibit infiltration of neutrophils and macrophages as well as the necrosis common to all panniculitis syndromes.

Of particular interest are reports of more than 40 patients in whom nodular panniculitis, arthritis, and rarely, lytic lesions of bone appear related to pancreatitis, pancreatic cancer, or less often, to ischemic necrosis of the pancreas (1,4,5). Pancreatic disease, even pancreatitis, has not been symptomatic in all cases. Thus, serum amylase or lipase levels may be elevated in the absence of symptoms. Skin and joint lesions may come and go despite persistence of hyperamylasemia or hyperlipasemia (6).

The subcutaneous nodules of nodular panniculitis resemble those of erythema nodosum, but differ in a tendency to liquefy and ulcerate and in their distribution over the trunk and buttocks as well as the legs. These nodules are sometimes painful, and are usually formed around joints and in other areas subject to pressure.

Arthritis or periarthritis may occur without skin lesions and resemble the arthritis of gout or sarcoidosis or joint infection. Synovial fluid has been infrequently examined and variously described as purulent, creamy, or watery; fat droplets are sometimes seen. Other systemic manifestations include eosinophilia, ascites, and pleural and pericardial effusions.

Panniculitis is most likely related to lipolysis in patients with increased serum lipase activity (7). This syndrome has not been clearly shown to be the cause of arthritis, which may be immune-mediated. Nodular panniculitis without demonstrable cause or association, previously designated as Weber-Christian disease, is perhaps more common than nodular pancreatitic panniculitis. Nodular panniculitis may be confined only to the skin, or through involvement of many organ systems, it may simulate diseases such as rheumatic fever and systemic lupus erythematosus.

1. Moore S: The relation of pancreatic disease to Weber-Christian disease. Can Med Assoc J 88:1238–1241, 1963
2. Förström L, Winkelmann RK: Acute panniculitis, a clinical and histopathologic study of 34 cases. Arch Dermatol 113:909–917, 1977
3. Niemi KM, Förström L, Hannuksela M, Mustakallio KK, Salo OP: Nodules on the legs: a clinical, histological and immunohistological study of 82 patients representing different types of nodular panniculitis. Acta Derm Venerol 57:145–154, 1977
4. Tannenbaum H, Anderson LG, Schur PH: Association of polyarthritis, subcutaneous nodules, and pancreatic disease. J Rheumatol 2:14–20, 1975
5. Smukler NM, Schumacher HR, Pascual E, Brown S, Ryan WE, Sadeghian MR: Synovial fat necrosis associated with ischemic pancreatic disease. Arthritis Rheum 22:547–553, 1979
6. Mori K, Hiratsuka I, Sakai H, Hiwatashi K, Takahashi T, Maruhama Y, Yamagata S: Hemorrhagic diathesis with Weber-Christian disease. Tohoku J Exp Med (suppl)118:227–243, 1976
7. Case Records of the Massachusetts General Hospital (Case 17–1982). N Engl J Med 306:1035–1043, 1982

81. Erythema nodosum

Erythema nodosum is characterized by crops of dusky-red, painful, tender, and indurated subcutaneous nodules of variable diameter (up to 15 cm). These nodules are most frequently encountered on the extensor surfaces of the legs but can also occur on the thighs and forearms.

Usually, the lesions are of all ages, with older ones resolving side by side with newer, redder nodules. The emergence of these nodules is sometimes accompanied by fever and arthralgias, and, less often, arthritis. Swelling of the knees or ankles is usually associated with overlying skin lesions. The nodular lesions usually resolve in 2–3 weeks, but they may become chronic and relapsing.

The pathologic features of erythema nodosum vary and may be evident only in sizeable excision biopsy specimens (1). The principal lesion occurs in the subdermal panniculus where an acute inflammation of the septum is most characteristic (2). The initial exudate consists of polymorphonuclear leukocytes, but most later infiltrates are lymphocytic. The inflammatory process may involve arterioles, arteries, or veins, resulting in perivascular cuffing and even hemorrhage. The inflammatory exudate occasionally extends throughout the panniculus and is accompanied by small foci of fat necrosis and reactive adipocyte hypertrophy. A more granulomatous response with giant cells and numerous histiocytes is detectable in rare cases.

Many patients suffer an attack of erythema nodosum with no obvious underlying cause. In some patients, the dermal lesions are associated with active tuberculosis, mycoses, sarcoidosis, a recent streptococcal infection, or as part of a drug sensitivity reaction. Erythema nodosum may occur in pregnancy or after use of oral contraceptive agents, in the course of gastrointestinal infection with *Yersinia enterocolitica*, and in chronic nonspecific inflammatory bowel disease. The presence of hilar lymphadenopathy suggests the diagnosis of sarcoidosis, although there are other processes that may lead to simultaneous nodose skin lesions and hilar lymph node enlargement, e.g., Hodgkin's disease.

Circulating immune complexes have been reported in the serum of certain patients with the syndrome. Local immunofluorescence studies, however, rarely reveal the presence of perivascular immunoglobulin deposits (3), although small quantities of cryoglobulins may be detected in the patient's serum.

The treatment is that of the underlying associated condition. Patients with very severe or relapsing attacks usually show an excellent response to salicylates or to a short course of corticosteroids in low doses.

1. Winkelmann RK, Förström L: New observations in the histopathology of erythema nodosum. J Invest Dermatol 65:441–446, 1975
2. Förström L, Winkelmann RK: Acute panniculitis: a clinical and histopathologic study of 34 cases. Arch Dermatol 113:909–917, 1977
3. Niemi KM, Förström L, Hannuksela M, Mustakallio KK, Salo OP: Nodules on the legs: a clinical, histological and immunohistological study of 82 patients representing different types of nodular panniculitis. Acta Dermatovener 57:145–154, 1977

82. Arthritis associated with intestinal bypass

Arthritis is one of several medical problems that may develop as a result of intestinal bypass surgery for morbid obesity. It has been reported after both jejunocolostomy (1,2) and jejunoileostomy (3–7), but less frequently after the latter. Both these operations have now been almost completely abandoned because of serious side effects.

The frequency of arthritis after bypass surgery remains to be determined, and varies from 0–40% in different series. Confusion arises because many of these patients have had a variety of rheumatic complaints before surgery as well as afterwards. In some patients these symptoms were attributed to other complications such as electrolyte disturbances, abnormalities in magnesium balance, or psychophysiologic factors.

Large and small joints can be affected symmetrically. Onset may occur from 1 month to as long as 9 years after surgery. Joint symptoms tend to be episodic and migratory, usually lasting a few days to several weeks. Symptoms are occasionally persistent, and the findings may mimic those of rheumatoid arthritis.

In 1 study, 9 patients have been described who apparently developed rheumatoid arthritis following bypass surgery (5). Sacroiliitis has also been described (2–4). Tenosynovitis, a rash, Raynaud's phenomenon, erythema nodosum, vasculitis, paresthesias, renal pathology, and pericarditis also have been reported (1–7). Cutaneous vasculitis has been observed in two-thirds of cases. Manifestations varied from macules, urticarial papules, and nodular plaques to typical vesiculopustular lesions (4).

Several investigators (2–7) have found circulating complement–fixing immune complexes and cryoprecipitates in sera of patients who had undergone 1 or the other of the bypass procedures. Incorporated in these complexes and cryoprecipitates were IgG, IgM, IgA, rheumatoid factor, complement components, C3, C4, and C5, and antibodies to *Escherichia coli* and *Bacteroides fragilis*. These findings, present at the time of the arthritis, disappeared when joint symptoms resolved. Synovial fluid immune complexes have also been reported (3). Immune deposits have been observed in biopsied skin lesions with immunoglobulins and complement present at the dermoepidermal junction (3,4).

The synovial fluid is usually mildly to moderately inflammatory, with a predominance of polymorphonuclear leukocytes. The erythrocyte sedimentation rate is elevated. Serum rheumatoid factor and antinuclear antibody are absent in almost all cases described. Serum C3 and C4 levels are normal or low. HLA–B27 was reported when sacroiliitis was present, but the relationship is not clear in these bypass patients.

Intestinal bacterial antigens, absorbed from the blind loop formed during the surgical procedures, have been implicated in the pathogenesis of the arthritis. It has been proposed that these antigens lead to the formation of circulating immune complexes that activate both the classical and alternate complement pathways, and thus initiate joint inflammation and other complications. This hypothesis is supported by the occasional improvement in joints of patients who have undergone reanastomosis of the bowel. In addition, improvement has resulted in some patients when the potential bacterial antigens in the blind loop were treated by administering antibiotics or when a sphincteroplasty was performed at the blind loop preventing bacterial reflux.

Treatment has varied. Spontaneous improvement has occurred most frequently. At times, nonsteroidal antiinflammatory drugs, corticosteroids, antibiotics, and corrective surgical measures have proved useful.

1. Shagrin JW, Frame B, Duncan H: Polyarthritis in obese patients with intestinal bypass. Ann Intern Med 75:377–380, 1971
2. Rose E, Espinoza LR, Osterland CK: Intestinal bypass arthritis: association with circulating immune complexes and HLA–B27. J Rheumatol 4:129–134, 1977
3. Utsinger PD: Systemic immune complex disease following intestinal bypass surgery: bypass disease. J Am Acad Dermatol 2:488, 1980
4. Stein HB, Schlappner OL, Boyko W, Gourlay RH, Reeve CA: The intestinal bypass arthritis–dermatitis syndrome. Arthritis Rheum 24:684–690, 1981
5. Utsinger PD, McLaughlin GE, Hicks JT, Moidel RA: Rheumatoid arthritis following the reactive arthritis of bypass disease (abstract). Arthritis Rheum 25:S24, 1982
6. Wands JP, LaMont JT, Mann E, Isselbacher KJ: Arthritis associated with intestinal bypass procedure for morbid obesity. New Engl J Med 294:121–124, 1976
7. Utsinger PD: Absorption and articular deposition of ingested I 131 E coli cell wall in reactive arthritis (abstract). Arthritis Rheum 24:S58, 1981

83. Arthritis associated with hypogammaglobulinemia

Both acquired and congenital (sex-linked recessive) hypogammaglobulinemia are associated with a rheumatoid arthritis–like illness, with a reported frequency as high as 30% (1). Progressive systemic sclerosis, systemic lupus erythematosus, and a particularly severe form of dermatomyositis have been reported in patients with hypogammaglobulinemia. The ever present possibility of septic arthritis must always be considered in the differential diagnosis. Since all these patients produce a small quantity of gammaglobulin, *hypogammaglobulinemia* is a more accurate designation than the term *agammaglobulinemia*.

The arthritis associated with hypogammaglobulinemia may be indistinguishable from rheumatoid arthritis but often differs in various ways. Symmetric polyarthritis involving small joints is often seen. It is rare, however, to find tenosynovitis, radiographic evidence of joint space narrowing indicative of cartilage loss, marginal erosions, extensive joint damage, and periarticular osteoporosis.

Histologic studies have revealed little or no proliferation of synovial lining cells or subsynovial blood vessels. The extensive cellular infiltrates of plasma cells, lymphocytes, and lymphoid follicles seen in rheumatoid synovium are not found. Although T cells are present in large numbers, B lymphocytes are virtually absent as are rheumatoid factors. Synovial fluid complement levels are usually normal (2). In some patients limited local immunoglobulin production has been demonstrated, but immune complexes have not been detected (3,4).

The arthritis occasionally responds dramatically to the administration of gammaglobulin (5), but such a reaction is exceptional (2). In some cases, thymectomy results in improvement.

Selective IgA deficiency is also associated with an increased incidence of arthritis, and conversely, the incidence of IgA deficiency in juvenile arthritis patients is 40 times that of the general population. The usual strong association between uveitis and pauciarticular juvenile arthritis is not seen in patients with hypogammaglobulinemia but is present in patients with IgA deficiency. Patients with IgA deficiency have a uniquely high incidence of both antinuclear antibodies and antibody to IgA (6).

The arthritis occurring in hypogammaglobulinemia may be a disease entirely unrelated to rheumatoid arthritis. Viral, bacterial, or other toxic substances could be responsible for articular inflammation in an individual with defective humoral immunity.

However, since the pathologic changes of this disease bear a resemblance to those of rheumatoid arthritis, it raises questions about the pathogenesis of rheumatoid arthritis. Is rheumatoid arthritis an "immune complex disease," or is it a "T cell disease" in which T cells account directly for joint disease, perhaps, in part, because of the absence of feedback inhibition by B cells?

1. Good RA, Rotstein J: Rheumatoid arthritis in agammaglobulinemia. Bull Rheum Dis 10:203–206, 1960
2. Grayzel AI, Marcus R, Stern R, Winchester RJ: Chronic polyarthritis associated with hypogammaglobulinemia. Arthritis Rheum 20:887–894, 1977
3. Rawson AJ, Hollander JL, Abelson NM, Reginato A, Torralba T: Immunoglobulins in the joint fluid and cells of arthritis with agammaglobulinemia (abstract). Arthritis Rheum 9:534, 1966
4. Barnett EV, Winkelstein A, Weinberger HJ: Agammaglobulinemia with polyarthritis and subcutaneous nodules. Am J Med 48:40–47, 1970
5. Webster ADB, Loewi G, Dourmashkin RD, Golding DN, Ward DJ, Asherson GL: Polyarthritis in adults with hypogammaglobulinemia and its rapid response to immunoglobulin treatment. Br Med J 1:1314–1316, 1976
6. Petty RE: Immunodeficiency and arthritis, Juvenile Rheumatoid Arthritis. JJ Miller, ed. Littleton, Mass, PSG Publishing Co, 1979, pp 51–59

84. Miscellaneous rheumatic syndromes involving skin and joints

Acne arthralgia. Severe acne, specifically febrile ulcerative conglobate acne, may be associated with myalgias, polyarthralgias, and otherwise unexplained nonseptic joint effusions (1,2). Large joints are most commonly involved. Most reported cases have been in young males. There is a tendency for improvement with resolution of the acne.

Sweet's syndrome (acute febrile neutrophilic dermatosis). The characteristic tender, red or purple, discrete 0.5–4 cm skin plaques (Fig 84–1) of Sweet's syndrome are associated with myalgias, arthralgias, or noninflammatory joint effusions in about 20% of patients (3). All manifestations usually resolve over 2–3 months, but recurrences have been observed in suspected cases (4). Sjögren's syndrome and episcleritis have been reported, as has facial rash and glomerulonephritis, causing confusion with systemic lupus erythematosus.

Systemic corticosteroids are effective if treatment is required.

Erythema elevatum diutinum. This syndrome is characterized by chronic, very painful, primarily acral erythematous to purple (hemorrhagic) plaques, bullae, and nodules located chiefly on extensor surfaces (Fig 84–2). Local irritation may worsen lesions, which result from leukocytoclastic inflammation of small vessels with prominent fibrin deposition. A variety of constitutional symptoms including fever, pleurisy, and abnormal results of liver function tests may occur (5,6).

Treatment has been difficult but some patients may respond to phenformin (possibly due to its fibrinolytic effect) or to dapsone.

Pyoderma gangrenosum. This painful,

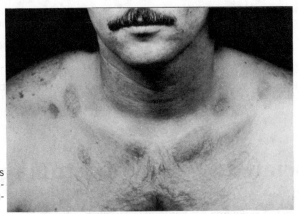

Fig 84-1. Typical cutaneous plaques of Sweet's syndrome. (Illustration provided by Dr HR Schumacher)

ulcerating, purplish-red elevated skin lesion is found on the legs and is typically associated with ulcerative colitis but can also be seen with rheumatoid arthritis and other systemic diseases or without any identifiable underlying disorder (7,8). Approximately 30% of patients have arthralgias or arthritis. In patients without colitis, an inflammatory polyarthritis resembling rheumatoid arthritis or seronegative spondylarthritis, with or without radiographic evidence of erosions has been described.

Rheumatoid factor is generally absent. Synovial fluid analyses have shown mildly increased leukocyte counts with predominantly mononuclear cells (7,8). Synovial biopsies have revealed infiltrations of lymphocytes and plasma cells plus lining cell hyperplasia. Various abnormalities of immune mechanisms have been described (7) but none are consistently found (8). Sulfones and sulfapyridine rarely help and corticosteroids may be needed for the skin lesions. The arthritis has been described as occasionally antedating the skin lesion and persisting after the skin has resolved.

Urticaria. Urticaria occurs with arthritis or arthralgia in viral hepatitis, in some patients with systemic lupus erythematosus, and also in some patients with an idiopathic syndrome of urticaria associated with vasculitis, frequent hypocomple-

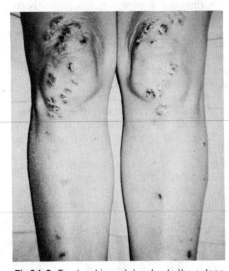

Fig 84-2. Tender skin nodules due to the cutaneous vasculitis of erythema elevatum diutinum. (Illustration provided by Dr HR Schumacher)

mentemia, and occasional multisystem manifestations such as myositis, pulmonary disease, and glomerulonephritis (9,10). Joint pain and swelling are episodic, involving most often the knees, ankles, wrists, and fingers. Radiographs reveal only soft tissue swelling. Antihistamines are often ineffective. A familial syndrome of urticaria, arthralgia or arthritis, and nerve deafness has also been described (9,11).

1. Kelley AP, Burnes RE: Acute febrile ulcerative conglobate acne with polyarthralgia. Arch Dermatol 104:182–187, 1971

2. Davis DE, Viozzi FJ, Miller OF, et al: The musculoskeletal manifestations of acne fulminans. J Rheumatol 8:317–321, 1981

3. Krauser RE, Schumacher HR: The arthritis of Sweet's syndrome. Arthritis Rheum 18:35–41, 1975

4. Trentham DE, Masi AT, Bole GG: Arthritis with an inflammatory dermatosis resembling Sweet's syndrome: report of a unique case and review of the literature on arthritis associated with inflammatory dermatoses. Am J Med 61:424–432, 1976

5. Schumacher HR, Carroll E, Taylor F, Shelley WB, Wood MG: Erythema elevatum diutinum: cutaneous vasculitis, impaired clot lysis, and response to phenformin. J Rheumatol 4:103–112, 1977

6. Katz SI, Gallin JI, Hertz KC: Erythema elevatum diutinum: skin and systemic manifestations, immunologic studies, and successful treatment with dapsone. Medicine 56:443–455, 1977

7. Lazarus GS, Goldsmith LA, Rocklin RE, Pinals RS, et al: Pyoderma gangrenosum, altered delayed hypersensitivity, and polyarthritis. Arch Dermatol 105:46–51,1972

8. Holt RTA, Davies MG, Saunders KG, Nuki G: Pyoderma gangrenosum: clinical and laboratory findings in 15 patients with special reference to polyarthritis. Medicine 59:114–133, 1980

9. Soter N: Chronic urticaria as a manifestation of necrotizing venulitis. N Engl J Med 296:1440–1442, 1977

10. Schwartz HR, McDuffie F, Black LF, et al: Hypocomplementemic urticarial vasculitis: association with chronic obstructive pulmonary disease. Mayo Clinic Proc 57:231–238, 1982

11. Prost A, Barrière H, Legent F: Rhumatisme intermittent révélateur d'un syndrome familial arthrites-éruption urticarienne-surdité: syndrome de Muckle et Wells sans amylosa rénale. Rev Rhum 43:201–208, 1976

85. Roentgenographic features of the rheumatic diseases

William Martel, MD

The skeletal system can react to disease in a limited number of ways, and it is, therefore, not surprising that different pathologic conditions may to some extent exhibit similar radiographic features. Nevertheless, certain combinations of changes are more likely to occur in a particular disease (1). One should consider the "predictive value" of radiologic features relative to the clinical conditions being considered (1).

Rheumatoid arthritis. Any synovial joint may be affected in rheumatoid arthritis (RA), but there is a predilection for the small joints of the hand, wrist, and foot with the exception of the distal interphalangeal joints (2–4). The arthritis may be asymmetric at first, but as the disease progresses, some degree of symmetry is evident in most cases. The cervical spine is frequently affected, but the sacroiliac joints are only occasionally involved.

Soft tissue swelling, due to joint effusion, synovitis, and periarticular edema is easily detected in the hands and feet, but may also be visualized in large joints by virtue of displacement of normal periarticular fat. This swelling characteristically involves all aspects of the affected joints and tends to be fusiform in the fingers, although it may be lobulated if synovial hypertrophy predominates. Atrophy of soft tissues develops late in the disease. Regional osteoporosis (bone atrophy) is an early finding and often appears in the juxtaarticular areas. Rarely, osteoporosis is absent in the early stages despite the presence of bone erosion. Generalized osteoporosis usually develops subsequently.

Loss of articular cartilage leads to a characteristically *uniform* narrowing of the interosseous joint (cartilage) space which represents an early irreversible alteration that usually precedes or coincides with bone erosion (Figs 85–1 and 85–2). Rarely, slight widening of the joint space is seen in the hands and feet; this probably reflects ligamentous laxity and joint effusion. Although subperiosteal bone apposition is common in children, it is only rarely seen in adults. Furthermore, it is invariably subtle in adults and tends to be found at capsule and tendon attachments. In some cases it results from subclinical trauma in the presence of osteoporosis. In fact, the *lack* of new bone formation is so characteristic of the rheumatoid arthritis in adults that the presence of exuberant bone apposition should suggest another diagnosis.

Joint malalignment and subluxation often follow a typical pattern and are a consequence of soft tissue involvement. Tenosynovitis and inflammation of the periarticular ligaments result in edema and joint laxity which alter the relationship of the tendons to the joints across which they act. These change the action of individual muscle groups so that normal muscular balance, for example, between flexors and extensors, is disturbed (5). Thus, ulnar deviation and volar subluxation may be seen at the metacarpophalangeal (MCP)

joints, and radial deviation of the radiocarpal joints is characteristic even in the early stages; individual carpal bones are often displaced. Hallux valgus and fibular deviation with plantar subluxation of the metatarsophalangeal (MTP) joints is common. Nontraumatic cervical subluxation is frequent, particularly at the atlantoaxial level.

Bone erosions. Bone erosion occurs near the attachments of the joint capsule, where the articular cartilage ends and the synovial reflection begins. The most conspicuous sites of erosion correspond to those parts of the bone within the joint that are not covered with articular cartilage, the so-called bare areas (3) (Fig 85–2). Thus, in the MCP joints the erosions tend to occur earliest and most extensively on the radiovolar aspect of the metacarpal heads and are larger on the proximal than on the distal side of the proximal interphalangeal joints of the hands.

An erosion often develops in the thumb at the ulnar side of the volarbasilar aspect of the distal phalanx. The ulnar styloid is commonly eroded and there is often a characteristic broad, notched erosion of the radius at the distal radioulnar joint.

Erosions in the feet are frequently detectable on the medial aspects of the metatarsal heads, although the earliest erosion of the fifth metatarsal is often on its lateral aspect (Fig 85–3). Calcaneal erosion adjacent to the retrocalcaneal bursa is common and a well-marginated spur may develop posteroinferiorly at the attachment

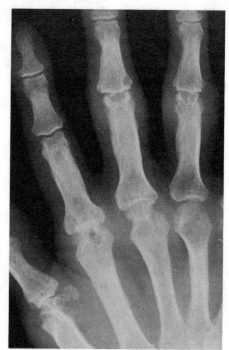

Fig 85–2. Rheumatoid arthritis. Fusiform soft tissue swelling of the interphalangeal joints is seen with characteristic marginal bone erosions at the "bare areas." Note uniform narrowing of the interosseous spaces and lack of subperiosteal bone apposition.

of the plantar aponeurosis. The lower cervical and odontoid processes are often eroded, as are the cervical apophyseal and intervertebral joints (6). The odontoid erosions are best shown by laminography (7). The margins of erosions are not sclerotic at the outset, but may become so after a time during which the bone reconstitutes (Fig 85–3).

Bone never returns to normal at the site of erosions. Large, sharply marginated, cyst-like erosions in the subchondral bone may appear to be unconnected to the joint. These "pseudocysts" are more common in large joints, such as the knee, but occasionally occur in the small joints of the hands and feet. If a pseudocyst is present, it is likely that additional ones will be found in relation to other joints.

Rarely, there is a superficial resorption of the subperiosteal surface of the bone at tendon attachments, probably due to tenosynovitis. A severe form of bone destruction characteristic of advanced disease is due in part to an attenuation of the articular cartilage resulting in its inability to withstand compressive forces. In such cases muscular activity causes compression of the essentially "unprotected" osteoporotic bones with subsequent dramatic resorption of their intraarticular portions.

Bony ankylosis may be observed in the tarsal and carpal joints and uncommonly in the interphalangeal joints but is extremely rare in the MCP and MTP groups.

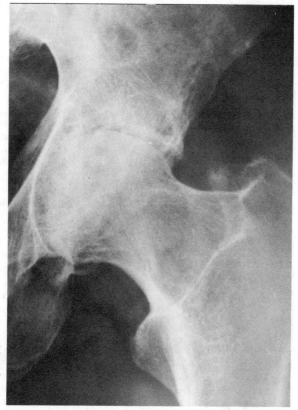

Fig 85–1. Rheumatoid arthritis. Note uniform narrowing of the interosseous joint space, small subchondral erosions, and secondary sclerosis. There is a characteristic absence of osteophytes.

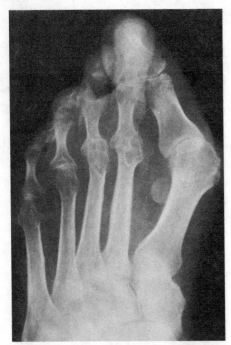

Fig 85–3. Rheumatoid arthritis. Metatarsophalangeal joints are affected with erosions of the metatarsal heads. Sclerosis (minimal) of the eroded margins of the second metatarsal indicates that this lesion has been present for some time. Note hallux valgus deformity. Plantar subluxation of the metatarsophalangeal joints was evident in lateral view.

Because any inflammatory joint disease, particularly a chronic disorder such as rheumatoid arthritis, may irreversibly alter a joint and interfere with its subsequent mechanical function, secondary osteoarthritis may supervene, particularly in weight-bearing joints. Hence, marginal osteophytes and minimal subchondral sclerosis may be observed in long-standing RA but the osteophytes tend to be small and poorly developed compared with those seen in primary osteoarthritis (Fig 85–1).

It generally takes at least 3 months for irreversible joint changes to appear (e.g., cartilage thinning or bone erosion). Occasionally, these changes may not be evident for 6 months or longer; it is unusual to see them within weeks after clinical onset.

Chronic arthritis in childhood. Chronic arthritis in children comprises a heterogeneous group of disorders (8). The radiologic manifestations are determined primarily by the type of disease and the age at onset. The types of such arthritis include juvenile rheumatoid arthritis, Still's disease, juvenile ankylosing spondylitis, psoriatic arthritis, and Reiter's disease. It is difficult to distinguish juvenile rheumatoid arthritis from Still's disease on radiologic grounds.

Juvenile rheumatoid arthritis commonly affects the wrists, knees, or ankles selectively and may spare the joints of the hands and feet in the early years (9). Monarticular inflammation is common and

tends to involve the knee most often. Cartilage destruction is characteristically minimal and bone erosion is rare in monarticular disease (10). Unlike adult rheumatoid arthritis, linear subperiosteal bone apposition adjacent to involved joints is an early and frequent finding (Fig 85–4). It probably reflects the ease with which new bone is stimulated in the young and is common in the metacarpals and metatarsals. Bony ankylosis is probably more common than in adults. Subluxation occurs not only in the small joints of the hands and feet but also in large joints, such as the hip.

As in adults, cervical spondylitis and atlantoaxial subluxation are common. There is a greater tendency toward cervical apophyseal joint ankylosis in children than in adults.

These cases should not be confused with ankylosing spondylitis. Skeletal growth disturbances are frequent but do not necessarily reflect the severity of joint destruction.

Gout. Although there is a predilection for involvement of the first metatarsophalangeal joint, arthritis of other joints occasionally occurs, sparing the toe. The lesions are not usually symmetric. The spinal column is generally unaffected, although tophi in the sacroiliac joints have been demonstrated on rare occasions. Joint effusion is common in both the acute attack and the chronic tophaceous stage of the disease.

Tophi appear as nodules or lobulated soft tissue masses which tend to arise near joints but may be adjacent to a diaphysis. They may calcify producing coarse irregular, opaque deposits or finely dispersed, homogeneous densities (Fig 85–5). Tophi

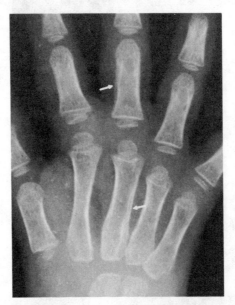

Fig 85–4. Juvenile arthritis illustrating characteristic linear subperiosteal bone apposition in the proximal phalanx and metacarpal of the middle finger (**arrows**).

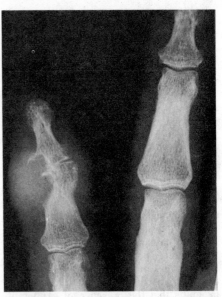

Fig 85–5. Gout. There is a tophus at the lateral aspect of the distal joint of the fifth finger with an adjacent bone erosion showing characteristic overhanging margin. Note remarkable density of the soft tissue mass.

may develop in virtually any location but show a particular affinity for certain sites such as the dorsum of the foot and ankle, extensor surface of the forearm, the achilles tendon, and certain bursae, particularly the olecranon and infrapatellar bursae. Paraarticular tophi are often eccentric with respect to the joint.

Bone erosions usually develop near tophi and may be paraarticular or intraarticular. Marginal erosions may develop in joints at the "bare areas," probably reflecting chronic synovitis. There may be surprisingly little interosseous space narrowing but in later stages this narrowing is common and typically uniform.

These features may be responsible for a mistaken radiologic diagnosis of rheumatoid arthritis. However, bone erosions in gout may exhibit a characteristic *overhanging margin*, a segment of eroded cortex extending over the tophus, elevated and displaced from the normal bone contour (11) (Figs 85–5 and 85–6). This displacement, which may be likened to a small blowout deformity, helps distinguish these lesions from the pocketed erosions of rheumatoid arthritis.

Subperiosteal bone apposition is not a conspicuous feature but is occasionally present, especially in the metacarpals or metatarsals; it is usually associated with an obvious tophus (Fig 85–6). Joint ankylosis occasionally occurs. Neither osteoporosis nor soft tissue atrophy occur in gout but regional osteoporosis may be observed in patients with chronic arthritis and severe bone destruction. There are no characteristic malalignments or subluxations in gout, but where there are large intraarticular tophi causing ligamentous

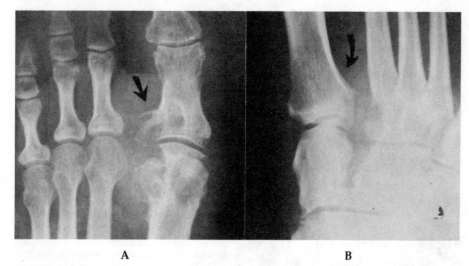

A   B

Fig 85–6. A, Gout. Left first metatarsophalangeal joint exhibits sharply marginated erosions with overhanging margins (**straight arrow**). **B,** There is a large destructive lesion in the right tarsus with minimal adjacent new bone formation (**curved arrow**); this was associated with a large soft tissue tophus on the dorsum that was apparent in the lateral projection.

and bone destruction, there may be gross deformity.

Minimal malalignment may be due to secondary osteoarthritis. It usually takes years of intermittent episodic arthritis before tophi and bone erosion become radiologically evident.

Calcium pyrophosphate dihydrate (CPPD) deposition disease. Although chondrocalcinosis is a hallmark of calcium pyrophosphate deposition disease, the cartilage calcification may not be detectable radiographically despite the presence of calcium pyrophosphate dihydrate crystals in the joint fluid (12–14).

Primarily the fibrocartilages are affected, particularly the menisci of the knee (Fig 85–7), triangular cartilage of the wrist, acetabular and glenoid labra, symphysis pubis, and intervertebral discs.

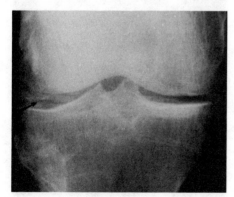

Fig 85–7. Chondrocalcinosis. Calcification is present in both menisci but more evident in the lateral meniscus (**arrow**). There is slight narrowing of the interosseous space medially with subchondral sclerosis, reflecting degenerative change in the cartilage. Hyaline cartilage calcification was evident in the lateral view but, as is common, was obscured by the fibrocartilaginous calcification in this projection.

Calcification may also involve hyaline articular cartilage, usually appearing finely linear; the calcium deposits in fibrocartilage are usually more coarse. Chondrocalcinosis is usually bilateral. It is not pathognomonic of CPPD deposition disease since it may occasionally represent dicalcium phosphate dihydrate or calcium hydroxyapatite.

Chondrocalcinosis has been observed in elderly persons who have had no significant joint symptoms (15). Some of these individuals may be at risk to develop crystal-induced joint inflammation.

Chondrocalcinosis has also been observed in a number of other rheumatic diseases including gout, rheumatoid arthritis, systemic lupus erythematosus, and neuropathic arthropathy. In these situations the chondrocalcinosis tends to be restricted to a few joints, particularly the knees and wrists and tends to involve mainly the fibrocartilages. Although chondrocalcinosis may be localized to a few joints in CPPD deposition disease, it is usually a more generalized phenomenon. CPPD deposition may be associated with a variety of underlying conditions.

Calcification in CPPD deposition disease is not limited to cartilages; it may also be present in synovial tissue, tendons and bursae. Calcification within the synovial tissues may be so extensive as to mimic synovial chondromatosis (16).

Individuals with CPPD deposition disease often exhibit a *radiologically distinctive arthropathy* (13,14) that resembles osteoarthritis in its reduced cartilage space and the subchondral sclerosis with varying degrees of osteophyte formation. Significantly, the distribution of affected joints differs from ordinary degenerative joint disease in that there is a predilection for the MCP joints, particularly the second

and third, and the interphalangeal joints are often conspicuously spared (Fig 85–8).

Other joints frequently affected in a similar manner in this condition are the elbow, carpal, radiocarpal, and tibiotalar joints. Selective involvement of the retropatellar joint has been suggested to favor this diagnosis.

Another feature of this arthropathy is the widespread occurrence of discrete rarefactions in the subchondral regions which resemble "osteoarthritic cysts" (Fig 85–8). However, these often occur in locations atypical for osteoarthritis. Such cysts may become compressed, resulting in bone fragmentation. When large cysts in weight-bearing joints undergo fragmentation, the resultant deformity may be severe and mimic a neuropathic joint in appearance. It should be emphasized that CPPD deposition may occur in patients with true neuropathic joints or the common variety of osteoarthritis.

Hemochromatosis is frequently associated with a similar distribution of arthropathy (17) and with CPPD deposition disease (18).

Degenerative joint disease. Osteoarthritis (degenerative joint disease) may be primary, or secondary to preexisting disease or trauma which predisposes the articular cartilage to subsequent degeneration.

In primary osteoarthritis there is a predilection for the weight-bearing joints, particularly the knee and hip, as well as

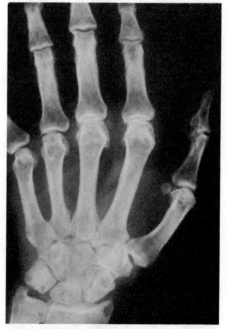

Fig 85–8. Calcium pyrophosphate deposition disease. There are "osteoarthritis-like" changes in the metacarpophalangeal joints associated with small subchondral cyst-like rarefactions and intraarticular soft-tissue calcification. Note the rarefactions in the carpal bones and radial styloid and triangular cartilage calcifications. The opposite side was similarly affected.

the first MTP joint (Fig 85–9), interphalangeal joints of the hands, and the trapezionavicular and the trapeziometacarpal joints (Fig 85–10). Diffuse involvement of the carpal joints, a characteristic feature of RA, does not occur.

Furthermore, whereas the radiocarpal and distal radioulnar joints are commonly involved in RA, they are not affected in primary osteoarthritis.

Other joints usually spared in primary osteoarthritis include the tibiotalar and elbow joints; when these are involved, one should suspect the condition is secondary.

Degenerative joint disease is usually *slowly progressive* with radiographic changes developing gradually over years. If major changes develop within weeks or even months, the diagnosis should be questioned, although an exception to this generalization is *erosive osteoarthritis* (19) in which the finger joints may be altered in a period of months.

The degeneration of articular cartilage is characteristically *segmental*, and therefore, unlike chronic inflammatory diseases, the narrowing of the interosseous space as seen radiologically is also segmental. In the hip the superolateral segment of the articular cartilage is usually affected. In the knee the cartilage of the medial and retropatellar compartments is typically affected although the disease may be limited to one or the other compartment.

It is unusual for the cartilages in both the medial and lateral compartments of the same joint to be affected simultaneously

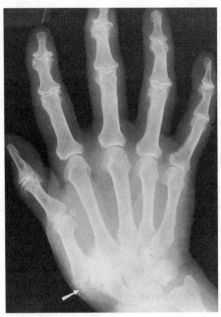

Fig 85–10. Osteoarthritis. Interphalangeal joints are primarily affected, but there is also severe involvement of the trapezio-metacarpal and trapezio-navicular joints. There is osteophyte formation, subchondral sclerosis, and nonuniform narrowing of many of the interphalangeal interosseous spaces.

(20). Occasionally, in small joints, such as in the hand, wrist, and apophyseal joints of the spine, the interosseous space may appear to be uniformly narrowed, particularly when the disease is advanced. As the cartilage degenerates, excessive mechanical stress causes a characteristic sclerosis of the subchondral cortex. Cartilage hyperplasia occurs at the margins of the joints and osteophytes develop at these sites primarily as a result of endochondral bone formation. Thus, the presence of osteophytes and subchondral sclerosis indicates degenerative change in the adjacent articular cartilage.

In advanced disease there may be metaplastic, cartilaginous, and osseous bodies within the joint, particularly the knee, simulating idiopathic synovial chondromatosis.

Cyst-like rarefactions in the subchondral bone are common in osteoarthritis (21), particularly in the hip (Fig 85–11). They are characteristically bordered by thickened trabeculae, seen radiologically as sclerotic margins often sharply demarcated. These characteristically develop adjacent to areas where cartilage degeneration is most severe, although occasionally they are seen at the periphery of the joint near the capsular attachment.

Such cyst-like lesions may collapse causing marked joint deformity (Fig 85–12).

Osteoporosis and soft tissue atrophy are not features of osteoarthritis. Subluxation does not occur, but minimal or moderate

malalignment is frequent and usually reflects intraarticular and paraarticular bone production. Thus, hallux valgus and medial or lateral deviation of the fingers are common, but volar subluxation of the fingers, as occurs in RA, is distinctly unusual.

Degenerative disease may affect the apophyseal and neurocentral (uncovertebral) joints which are synovial lined as well as the discovertebral joints which are fibrocartilaginous. Neurocentral joints are confined to the neck. Apophyseal and discovertebral arthropathies may coexist at the same spinal level but are often independent of one another. Degenerative discovertebral arthritis (degenerative spondylosis) is characteristically associated with loss of mobility, especially in the neck. Severe involvement of the lumbar apophyseal joints may cause spondylolisthesis but this is almost never severe.

Involvement of the neurocentral joints is commonly associated with disc degeneration. As in the joints of the extremities, the apophyseal and neurocentral joints show loss of cartilage space, subchondral sclerosis, and marginal osteophyte formation. In discovertebral joint involvement the disc space narrows uniformly or nonuniformly due to degeneration of the anulus fibrosus.

A "vacuum phenomenon" may cause release of gas into the disc substance; this is significant because its presence virtually

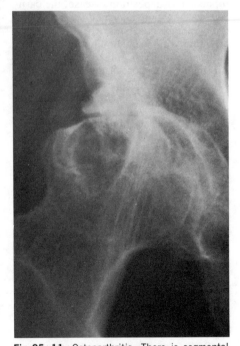

Fig 85–11. Osteoarthritis. There is segmental narrowing of the interosseous space superolaterally with subchondral sclerosis and a cyst-like lesion with thin sclerotic margins in the femoral head. Note osteophyte formation in the femoral head laterally and at the acetabular margins, with typical buttressing of the femoral neck inferiorly. Such buttressing is uncommon in rheumatoid arthritis. Compare with Fig 85–1.

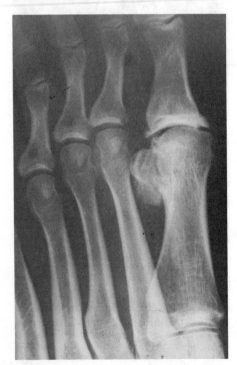

Fig 85–9. Osteoarthritis. First metatarsophalangeal joint is affected with nonuniform narrowing of the interosseous space, subchondral sclerosis, and osteophyte formation.

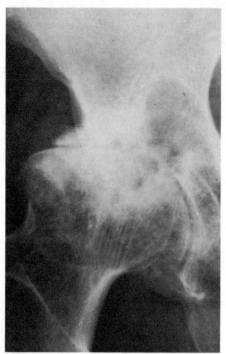

Fig 85–12. Osteoarthritis. Same patient as in Fig 85–11, many years later. Subchondral cyst has collapsed with subsequent flattening of the femoral head. There is further narrowing of the interosseous space, sclerosis, and osteophyte formation.

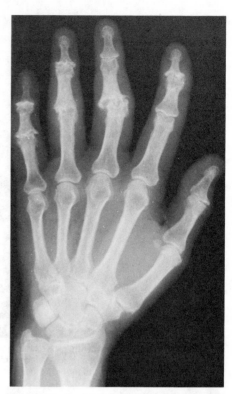

Fig 85–13. Erosive osteoarthritis. There is severe subchondral bone erosion in several interphalangeal joints. The metacarpophalangeal joints are spared. Similar joint changes were present in the opposite hand.

excludes coexisting disc space infection. Osteophytes arise at the discovertebral junction as the result of mechanical stress. Their orientation is limited by the subjacent bulging anulus fibrosus, and hence they tend to be horizontal at their point of origin. This is an important feature in helping to distinguish them from the syndesmophytes of ankylosing spondylitis which tend to be oriented vertically.

Osteoarthritis is common in the sacroiliac joints (22) although it is usually not identified as such radiologically. The changes that may develop are easily differentiated from ankylosing spondylitis. Instead of indistinctness and obliteration of the subchondral cortex typical of spondylitis, there is an accentuation and sclerosis of the subchondral bone. Marginal osteophytes may be identified at the inferior aspect of the joint in profile or they may be visualized en face, particularly superiorly, as focal areas of increased density.

Osteoarthritis is common in the fingers, particularly the distal joints. Frequently, one finds tiny foci of paraarticular ossification within zones of cartilage hyperplasia at the joint margins. A form of interphalangeal osteoarthritis (erosive osteoarthritis) is clinically distinct because of the pronounced articular soft tissue swelling and inflammation and, radiologically, because of the associated severe subchondral bone destruction (Fig 85–13).

The pronounced inflammation and localization to the terminal joints often causes confusion with psoriatic arthritis. Subperiosteal bone apposition may develop in erosive osteoarthritis, but it tends to be minimal to moderate and linear. Fluffy irregular periosteal bone apposition, characteristic of psoriatic arthritis or Reiter's syndrome, does not occur. The condition is easily differentiated from RA in that the MCP joints are not usually affected; there may be uniform narrowing of the interosseous spaces of the MCP joints, but marginal bone erosions do not develop (23). Bony ankylosis of the interphalangeal joints is common in erosive osteoarthritis.

Ankylosing spondylitis. Ankylosing spondylitis primarily affects the vertebral column (24). There is a predilection for sites of ligamentous attachments and fibrocartilaginous joints such as the symphysis pubis and intervertebral and sternomanubrial joints. Extraspinal arthritis occurs in approximately 50% of cases. There is a predilection for the rhizomelic joints (hips and shoulders), but the hands and feet may also be affected.

Destructive arthritis of the feet with radiographically demonstrable bone erosions is relatively uncommon, except for calcaneal erosions; such arthritis is usually a late occurrence.

The earliest changes occur in the sacroiliac joints and consist of blurring of the subchondral bony margins accompanied by an adjacent reactive sclerosis (Fig 85–14). Invariably, both sacroiliac joints are involved although, early in the disease, involvement may be minimally asymmetric. The presence of unilateral sacroiliac arthritis or normal sacroiliac joints is virtually incompatible with the diagnosis.

However, it should be emphasized that the changes in the sacroiliac joints at the onset of the disease may be subtle, and further radiologic examination after an in-

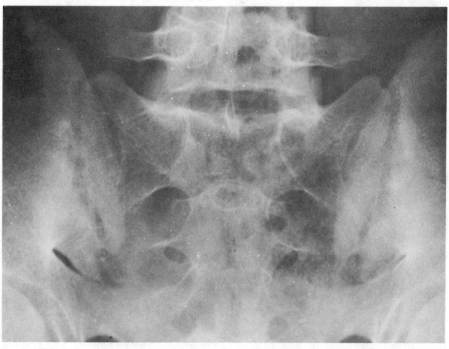

Fig 85–14. Ankylosing spondylitis, sacroiliac joints. Subchondral margins are irregular and indistinct with patchy reactive sclerosis bilaterally.

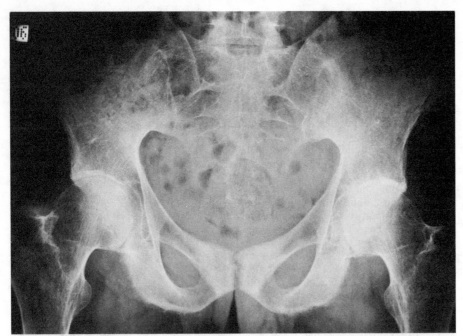

Fig 85–15. Ankylosing spondylitis. The sacroiliac joints are completely ankylosed and the adjacent bone is osteoporotic. There are erosions at the symphysis pubis with reactive sclerosis and fluffy new bone formation at the ischial margins.

terval of several months may be indicated if the disease is strongly suspected on clinical grounds. The interosseous sacroiliac joint spaces become narrowed and obliterated (Fig 85–15).

Reactive sclerosis disappears and generalized rarefaction of the pelvic bones develops as sacroiliac ankylosis ensues.

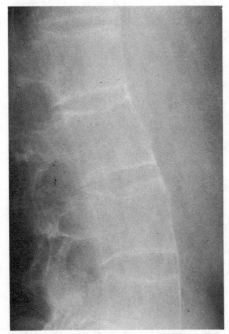

Fig 85–16. Ankylosing spondylitis, lumbar vertebrae, lateral view. Pronounced squaring of the lumbar vertebrae and bridging syndesmophytes. Note narrowing of the intervertebral discs and osteoporosis. Although not shown in this projection, the apophyseal joints were fused.

Unlike those in RA, the bone erosions in this disease, whether vertebral or peripheral, are usually superficial and associated with reactive sclerosis (Fig 85–15), bone proliferation, and ankylosis. Deep erosions with large osteolytic cyst-like lesions, such as occur in rheumatoid arthritis, are distinctly uncommon. These superficial erosions are often overshadowed by bone production which may appear fluffy, particularly at the ischial and femoral trochanteric margins.

Characteristic erosions develop at the anterosuperior and anteroinferior corners of the vertebral bodies, creating an appearance of the corners being planed down. The consequent loss of the usual anterior concavity gives these vertebral bodies a square configuration in the lateral projection (Fig 85–16). This is particularly evident in the lumbar vertebrae which normally have a pronounced concavity anteriorly. Bone apposition within this concavity may also contribute, to some extent, to the squaring.

The reactive sclerosis that develops at the sites of these erosions is the basis for the so-called *shining corners*.

In addition, typical paravertebral ossifications, *syndesmophytes*, develop in the region of the vertebral body erosions and anulus fibrosus and extend vertically, bridging adjacent vertebrae (25) (Figs 85–16 and 85–17). The syndesmophytes, which appear delicate at first, tend to occur at the dorsolumbar and lumbosacral junctions. They may occur at any level, and, as the disease advances, they become generalized and well-defined, giving the appearance known as *bamboo spine*.

The cervical vertebrae may be affected simultaneously with the lower segments, but it is unusual for the cervical region to be involved together with the sacroiliac joints in the presence of a normal dorsolumbar spine.

In addition to bony transformation of the outer laminae of the anulus fibrosus, there is bony ankylosis of the apophyseal joints, costovertebral and costotransverse joints, and ossification of interspinous ligaments and joint capsules. The pelvis, spine, and thorax thus become fixed in a rigid bony union. As bony ankylosis develops, the vertebrae become osteoporotic and the intervertebral disc spaces narrow. Dorsal kyphosis develops and may be severe.

Pathologic fracture of the ankylosed spine is a serious complication of the advanced stages of the disease. These fractures characteristically occur near or through previously ankylosed joints. Such fractures in the lower dorsal or lumbar segments, if unrecognized, may lead to a pseudoarthrosis of the corresponding discovertebral joint which should not be confused with infectious arthritis (26). Atlantoaxial subluxation may be observed but it is much less common than in rheumatoid arthritis (6).

Psoriatic arthritis. Although the distribution of arthritis in psoriasis may be

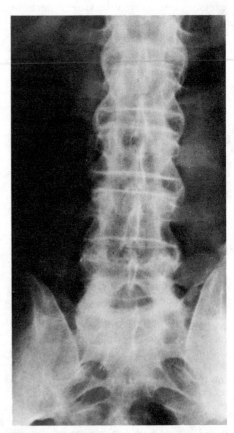

Fig 85–17. Ankylosing spondylitis (frontal view) illustrating well-developed syndesmophytes involving the discovertebral joints of the lumbar spine, giving a "bamboo spine" appearance.

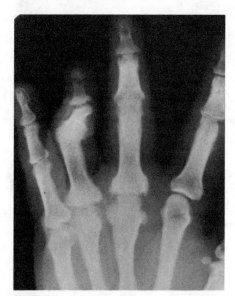

Fig 85–18. Psoriatic arthritis. The joints affected are primarily those of the middle and ring fingers, including terminal joints. Note irregular bone apposition at sites of involvement and absence of osteoporosis.

similar to that of rheumatoid arthritis (27), *two frequently observed patterns* in the hands are significantly different. The first is a predilection for the terminal interphalangeal joints, and the second is a predominant involvement of the joints of a single ray, often with several joints of one hand affected but none in the other (28) (Fig 85–18).

In addition there is a predilection for the interphalangeal joint of the great toe (Fig 85–19); the feet may be more severely involved than the hands. There may be resorption of the terminal tufts of the fingers and of the great toe (Fig 85–19) in association with terminal joint involvement and the terminal phalanx of the great toe may become sclerotic.

Osteoporosis is often absent despite extensive joint destruction. In the early stages, marginal bone erosions at the "bare areas" can be discerned, similar to the sites of erosion in rheumatoid arthritis. However, the pattern of bone erosion may be obscured by coexisting subperiosteal bone apposition, and late in the disease, when joint destruction is severe, the pattern of erosion at the bare areas may no longer be evident. Bone erosion often extends along the diaphysis beyond the capsular attachment, causing a pencil-like tapering of the bone.

Bone apposition near involved joints is characteristic; it may be compact and linear, but more often is poorly defined and irregular, particularly in the active phase of inflammation. Although such bone apposition is not invariably present, it is an important feature which often serves to distinguish this condition from rheumatoid arthritis. Calcaneal erosions are common

at both the posterosuperior and posteroplantar aspects with new bone apposition.

Bilateral symmetric sacroiliac arthritis is common in psoriatic arthritis (29), but often there is unilateral or persistently asymmetric involvement of the sacroiliac joints. Spinal involvement may be indistinguishable from ankylosing spondylitis but in many patients there is a distinctive type of spondylitis (28,30).

Asymmetric large vertebral hyperostoses which bridge adjacent vertebral bodies and commonly spare the anterior surfaces of the vertebrae are characteristic (Fig 85–20). They resemble the large syndesmophytes of ankylosing spondylitis, but differ in that they arise from a broad zone, frequently on the lateral or posterolateral aspects of the vertebral bodies. The intervening intervertebral disc is often normal in height or only minimally narrowed. Unlike the syndesmophytes of ankylosing spondylitis, these bone formations are often not generalized throughout the spine. They appear to be a consequence of focal vertebral osteitis and are common in the lumbar and lower dorsal segments of the spine. Although squaring of the vertebral bodies may be observed, this is not usually as generalized as in ankylosing spondylitis.

The tendency toward *segmental involvement* of the spine is conspicuous and major portions often appear to be skipped. Thus, the cervical spine may be involved in addition to focal areas in the lower dorsal and upper lumbar regions with sparing of the intervening segments. Apophyseal and costovertebral arthritis does occur, but generalized involvement of these articulations is often absent. Atlantoaxial subluxation occurs but is uncommon. Paravertebral, coarse ossifica-

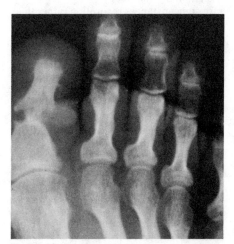

Fig 85–19. Psoriatic arthritis. There is extensive destruction of the interphalangeal joint of the great toe with resorption of the terminal tuft. A similar lesion may be seen in Reiter's syndrome. Note severe destructive changes in the terminal interphalangeal joint of the fifth digit and the lack of osteoporosis. The lesions in the feet in this patient were symmetrical.

tion which seems to be related to the lateral longitudinal ligament rather than to the vertebrae has been described (31).

Reiter's syndrome. Although the arthritis in Reiter's syndrome and psoriatic arthritis may be relatively nonspecific and confused with rheumatoid arthritis or ankylosing spondylitis, the roentgen features in both conditions are often distinct, particularly as the disease progresses (32,33). There is often difficulty in distinguishing *between* psoriatic arthritis and Reiter's disease; this probably represents a true overlap of radiologic manifestations (34).

In Reiter's syndrome there is a predilection for the joints of the lower extremities, particularly the MTP joints (Fig 85–21). The relative sparing of the upper extremities may be conspicuous in the presence of severe destruction of the pedal joints. Occasionally, the spinal involvement is diffuse and similar to ankylosing spondylitis, but in the majority of patients, the spondylitis is similar to that of psoriatic arthritis.

Thus, asymmetric or unilateral sacroiliac arthritis, large asymmetric bony bridges between vertebral bodies, and a tendency toward focal involvement of the spine with skipped segments are characteristic features of Reiter's syndrome. Other similarities to psoriatic arthritis include the predilection for the interphalangeal joint of the great toe and heels and the frequency of periosteal bone apposition near affected joints (Fig 85–21).

Calcaneal erosions characteristically occur at the posterosuperior and posteroinferior aspects, as in psoriatic arthritis, and are frequently associated with reactive bone formation. Early in the disease, one may find articular erosions in the bare areas, but these are often obscured by concomitant new bone formation. Severe bone destruction may occur, particularly in the MTP joints.

Focal periostitis adjacent to involved joints may persist as cortical thickening and irregularity, with relatively little alteration of the adjacent cartilage space. Such cases suggest that the bone and periarticular tissues are as important targets of the inflammation as the cartilage and synovial tissues. Unlike psoriatic arthritis there does not appear to be the predilection for the joints of a single ray or the terminal interphalangeal joints of the hands.

Furthermore, psoriatic patients often show panarthritis of the hands and wrists, but this is rare in Reiter's disease. The hip and sternomanubrial joint are commonly affected in ankylosing spondylitis, but arthritis of these joints is uncommon in Reiter's disease.

Neuropathic joint disease. Neuropathic arthropathy may be monarticular, but polyarticular involvement is common and the pattern of involvement is related to the underlying cause. Thus, upper extremity joints are involved in syringomyelia,

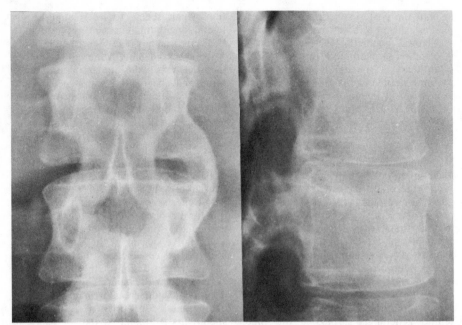

Fig 85–20. Psoriatic spondylitis. Asymmetric, bridging hyperostosis at L1–L2 which arise posterolaterally. Note relative sparing of the anterior vertebral surfaces. The height of the intervening intervertebral disc is minimally reduced. Similar lesions may be seen in Reiter's syndrome.

whereas the lower extremities are more commonly affected in tabes dorsalis, diabetes mellitus, and meningomyelocele. There is a predilection for the tarsal and

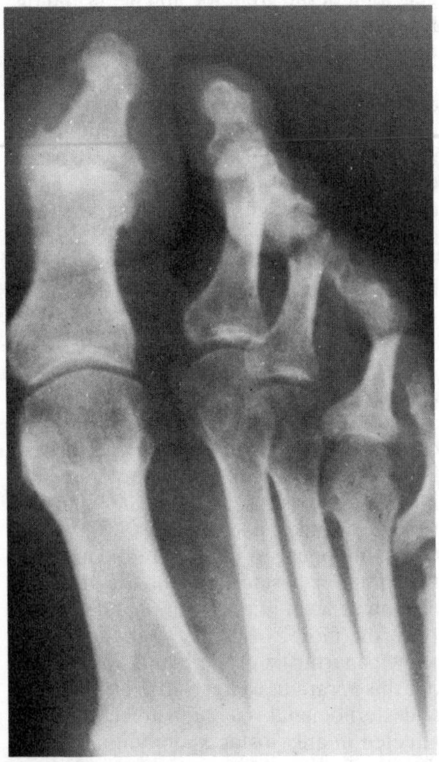

Fig 85–21. Reiter's syndrome. Note involvement of the interphalangeal joint of the great toe, resorption of the terminal tuft and of the fourth and fifth metatarsophalangeal joints, and reactive sclerosis, and subperiosteal bone apposition. The proximal interphalangeal joint of the fifth toe is also affected. Similar lesions may be seen in psoriatic arthritis.

tarsometatarsal joints in diabetic neuropathy.

Soft tissue swelling, often massive, due to persistent or recurrent effusion, is one of the earliest manifestations (35). Osteoporosis is notably absent.

Subluxation is characteristic and although minimal at the onset, gross joint disorganization often ensues (Fig 85–22). Intraarticular fractures are common, and calcification and bone fragments within soft tissues adjacent to the involved joints are typical. The cartilage is destroyed and sclerosis of bone, particularly the subchondral portion, and hypertrophic bone formation are marked.

In some instances resorption rather than hypertrophy of bone is the salient feature, and whether one or the other predominates does not appear to be related to the underlying disease. Subperiosteal bone apposition may be conspicuous and is due to trauma in some cases. However, infection may supervene, particularly with severe joint destruction, and it may be difficult to distinguish features resulting from infection from those due to the underlying neuropathic arthropathy.

The arthropathy is progressive and severe destruction may take place within several weeks (36). Bony ankylosis does not occur. One may observe progressive destruction in a previously normal joint, seemingly triggered by relatively insignificant trauma with or without a fracture.

Infectious arthritis. The radiologic manifestations of infectious arthritis will depend on the causative organism, host resistance, the duration of the inflammation, and the effectiveness of antibiotic therapy. Incomplete treatment may modi-

fy the natural course of the disease and mask typical radiographic features.

Pyogenic arthritis is typified by soft tissue swelling, rapid destruction of cartilage and bone, reactive bone formation due to periosteal involvement, and extensive sequestrum formation. Osteoporosis may not be seen at the outset, but becomes evident within a few days and is always associated with marked regional soft tissue swelling.

Structural alterations may be expected approximately 8–10 days after the onset of symptoms. This timing is an important diagnostic feature; normal roentgenograms several days after the onset of symptoms do not exclude the diagnosis. Rarely is more than one joint affected by pyogenic arthritis unless there is an underlying systemic disease.

The radiologic manifestations of tuberculous arthritis differ significantly from those of pyogenic infection. Any joint may be affected but the knee, hip, and shoulder are commonly involved. Regional osteoporosis is usually present by the time soft tissue and bone lesions are evident. Swelling is less marked than in pyogenic arthritis and may be minimal. Early, the cartilage tends to be preserved, even when there are bone erosions, but it too becomes destroyed late in the disease. Unlike pyogenic arthritis, in which there is early destruction of the subchondral,

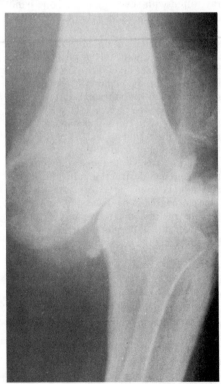

Fig 85–22. Neuropathic joint disease secondary to tabes dorsalis, frontal view of the knee. There is total disorganization of the joint with subchondral sclerosis and fragmentation of the bones. Note the marked soft tissue swelling and subperiosteal bone apposition.

weight-bearing portions of the joint, in tuberculous arthritis, there is a predilection for the marginal or non-weight bearing portions and, in this respect, the disorder resembles rheumatoid arthritis.

Sequestra may develop but are usually small. Unlike pyogenic arthritis, subperiosteal bone apposition is characteristically minimal or, at most, moderate.

Discogenic vertebral sclerosis, presumably secondary to subclinical trauma, may simulate infectious arthritis. Characteristically, the intervertebral disc is reduced in height and the sclerosis occurs anteriorly, contiguous with the vertebral end-plate in 1 or 2 contiguous vertebrae. A zone of rarefaction may be observed within the sclerotic area.

Paraspinal soft tissue swelling is not present. These lesions are common in the lumbar spine particularly at the level of L4–5 and are more frequent in women (37).

1. Martel W: Radiologic considerations in the differential diagnosis of joint disease, Textbook of Rheumatology. WN Kelley, ED Harris Jr, S Ruddy, CB Sledge, eds. Philadelphia, WB Saunders, 1981, pp 580–621
2. Berens DL, Lin R: Roentgen Diagnosis of Rheumatoid Arthritis. Springfield, Charles C Thomas Publisher, 1969
3. Martel W, Hayes JT, Duff IF: The pattern of bone erosion in the hand and wrist in rheumatoid arthritis. Radiology 84:204–214, 1965
4. Martel W. Radiologic manifestations of rheumatoid arthritis with particular reference to the hand, wrist and foot. Med Clin Am 52:655–665, 1968
5. Swezey RL: Dynamic factors in deformity of the rheumatoid arthritic hand. Bull Rheum Dis 22:649–656, 1971
6. Martel W, Page JW: Cervical vertebral erosions and subluxations in rheumatoid arthritis and ankylosing spondylitis. Arthritis Rheum 3:546–556, 1960
7. Martel W: The occipito-atlanto-axial joints in rheumatoid arthritis, Proceedings of an International Symposium. Amsterdam, Excerpta Medical Foundation, 1963, pp 189–209
8. Ansell BM, Kent PA: Radiologic changes in juvenile chronic polyarthritis. Skel Radiol 1:129–144, 1977
9. Martel W, Holt JF, Cassidy JT: Roentgenologic manifestations of juvenile rheumatoid arthritis. Am J Roentgenol 88:400–423, 1962
10. Cassidy JT, Brody GL, Martel W: Monarticular juvenile rheumatoid arthritis. J Pediatr 70:867–875, 1967
11. Martel W: The overhanging margin of bone: a roentgenologic manifestation of gout. Radiology 91:755–756, 1968
12. Martel W, Champion CK, Thompson GR, Carter TL: A radiologically distinctive arthropathy in some patients with the pseudogout syndrome. Am J Roentgenol 109:587–605, 1970
13. Resick D, Niwayama G, Goergen TG, Utsinger PD, Shapiro RF, Haselwood DH, Wiesner KB: Clinical, radiographic and pathologic abnormalities in calcium pyrophosphate dihydrate deposition disease: pseudogout. Radiology 122:1–15, 1977
14. Genant HK: Roentgenographic aspects of calcium pyrophosphate dihydrate crystal deposition disease. Arthritis Rheum 19:307–329, 1976
15. Bocher J, Mankin HJ, Beck RN, Rodnan GP: Prevalence of calcified meniscal cartilage in elderly persons. N Engl J Med 227:1093–1097, 1965
16. Ellamm MH, Krieger MI, Brown N: Pseudogout mimicking synovial chondromatosis. J Bone Joint Surg 57A:863–865, 1975
17. Dymock IW, Hamilton EBD, Laws JW, Laws JW, Williams R: Arthropathy of haemochromatosis: clinical and radiologic analysis of 63 patients with iron overload. Ann Rheum Dis 29:469–476, 1970
18. Twersky J: Joint changes in idiopathic hemochromatosis. Am J Roentgenol 124:139–144, 1975
19. Kidd KL, Peter JB: Erosive osteoarthritis. Radiology 86:640–647, 1966
20. Ahlbäck S: Osteoarthrosis of the knee: a radiographic investigation. Acta Radiol (suppl 277):7–72, 1968
21. Sokoloff L: Osteoarthritis, Bones and Joints. LV Ackerman, HJ Spjut, MR Abell, eds. Baltimore, Williams & Wilkins, 1976, pp 110–129.
22. Resnick D, Niwayama G, Goregen TG: Degenerative disease of the sacroiliac joint. Invest Radiol 10:608–621, 1975
23. Martel W, Snarr JW, Horn JR: The metacarpophalangeal joints in interphalangeal osteoarthritis. Radiology 108:1–7, 1973
24. Berens DL: Roentgen features of ankylosing spondylitis. Clin Orthop 74:21–33, 1971
25. Cruickshank B: Pathology of ankylosing spondylitis. Clin Orthop 74:43–58, 1971
26. Martel W: Spinal pseudoarthrosis: a complication of ankylosing spondylitis. Arthritis Rheum 21:485–490, 1978
27. Peterson CC Jr, Silbiger ML: Reiter's syndrome and psoriatic arthritis: the roentgen spectra and some interesting similarities. Am J Roentgenol 101:860–871, 1967
28. Martel W: Radiologic differential diagnosis of ankylosing spondylitis (Behçet's syndrome). Scand J Rheumatol (suppl 32):141–156, 1980
29. Harview JN, Lester RS, Little AH: Sacroiliitis in severe psoriasis. Am J Roentgenol 127:579–584, 1976
30. Killebrew K, Gold RH, Skolkoff SD: Psoriatic spondylitis. Radiology 108:9–16, 1973
31. Bywaters EGL: Paravertebral ossification in psoriatic arthritis. Ann Rheum Dis 24:313–331, 1965
32. Sholkoff SD, Glickman MG, Steinbach HL: Roentgenology of Reiter's syndrome. Radiology 97:497–503, 1970
33. Martel W, Braunstein EM, Borlaza G, Good AE, Griffin PE Jr: Radiologic features of Reiter's disease. Radiology 132:1–10, 1979
34. Martel W: Radiological manifestations of Reiter's syndrome, Symposium on Reiter's Syndrome. T Bitter, ed. Ann Rheum Dis (suppl 12) 38:23, 1979
35. Katz I, Rabinowitz JG, Dziadiw R: Early changes in Charcot's joints. Am J Roentgenol 86:965–974, 1961
36. Norman A, Robbins H, Milgram JE: The acute neuropathic arthropathy: a rapid, severely disorganizing form of arthritis. Radiology 90:1159–1164, 1968
37. Martel W, Seeger JR, Wicks JD, Washburn RL: Traumatic lesions of the discovertebral junction in the lumbar spine. Am J Roentgenol 127:457–464, 1976

86. Scintigraphy

The 2 isotopes most commonly used for joint imaging are ^{99m}Tc-pertechnetate and ^{99m}Tc-phosphates. The former is mainly bound to serum protein and localizes in inflamed joints because of their increased vascularity and effusions (1). The ^{99m}Tc-labeled phosphates are absorbed by bone directly (2) and include ^{99m}Tc-pyrophosphate and ^{99m}Tc-methylene-diphosphonate.

Technetium pertechnetate scans (^{99m}TcO$_4$). The technique requires care and results should not be overinterpreted (3). In normal joints, the uptake should not exceed the background activity of adjacent tissues. Examples of normal and abnormal joint scans are shown in Fig 86–1. Technetium pertechnetate is not suited to axial joint imaging. Although peripheral joint scans correlate well with clinically apparent synovitis and are more sensitive than x-ray examination, the nonspecificity of scanning is its major drawback. Almost

any joint with pathology shows an abnormal scan. Furthermore, clinicians already seem satisfied with their ability to detect synovitis in peripheral joints by clinical methods.

Nevertheless, in some instances abnormal joint scans provide evidence of clinically obscure joint disease, e.g., steroid-treated early rheumatoid arthritis and polymyalgia rheumatica (3). Normal scans help to confirm a clinical impression of psychogenic rheumatism.

Technetium phosphate scans (^{99m}TcMDP). Technetium-labeled phosphate compounds are primarily used to detect metastatic disease and osteomyelitis. Their use in joint disease is less established. Deeply located joints such as the hips and spinal joints can be evaluated. Although inflamed joints show increased uptake compared with normal ones, the problem is that normal joints show increased uptake as compared with back-

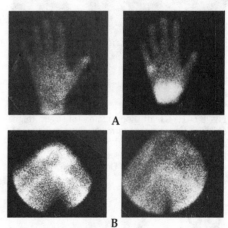

Fig 86–1. Examples of normal controls and abnormal ^{99m}Tc pertechnetate joint scintigrams from rheumatoid arthritis patients. **A,** Left hand of normal person (left) and person with rheumatoid arthritis (right). **B,** Right knee of normal control (left) and person with rheumatoid arthritis (right). (From ref 3).

ground. Therefore, ^{99m}Tc-phosphate scanning is too sensitive to be of value in diagnosing synovitis of peripheral joints.

Favorable reports of detecting early sacroiliitis by enhanced sacroiliac to sacral uptake ratios (4) have been challenged by other reports showing no such discrimination (5). Osteonecrosis of the femoral head may be detected by ^{99m}Tc-phosphate scans before radiologic change. The decreased uptake over the area of avascular bone contrasts with normal or increased uptake of the surrounding bone. Other useful applications of radiolabeled phosphate scans are early detection of osteomyelitis, osteoid osteoma, stress fractures in long bones, and primary bone tumors.

Another nuclide, gallium-67, is used in detection of inflammatory processes because it appears to attach to neutrophilic leukocytes. Again the problem of specificity limits its usefulness since this agent concentrates in several inflammatory processes, including tumors.

To date, the range of circumstances in which scintigraphy has proved useful in rheumatology is narrow, but with improved methods, this may enlarge.

1. McCarty DJ, Polcyn RE, Collins PA, et al: [99m]Technetium scintiophotography in arthritis: technique and interpretation. Arthritis Rheum 13:11–20, 1970

2. Hoffer PB, Genant HK: Radionuclide joint imaging. Semin Nucl Med 6:121–317, 1976

3. Wahner HW, O'Duffy JD: Peripheral joint scanning with technetium pertechnetate: application in clinical practice. Mayo Clin Proc 51:525–531, 1976

4. Lentte BC, Russell AS, Percy JS, et al: The scintigraphic investigation of sacroiliac disease. J Nucl Med 18:529–533, 1977

5. Spencer D, Adams F, Horton PW, Buchanan WW: Scintiscanning in ankylosing spondylitis: a clinical, radiological, and quantitative radioisotoptic study. J Rheumatol 6:426–438, 1979

87. Computed tomography

Computed tomography (CT) has had a profound impact on the diagnosis of space-occupying pathologic processes in medicine. By delineating abnormal masses from normal anatomy, this technique has proved invaluable in judging the extent of tumor invasion of bone or soft tissue (Fig 87–1), in proving recurrence of tumors, and in delineating benign cystic lesions such as meningoceles (1). Although conventional radiography remains more useful in the diagnosis of most diseases of bones and joints, computed tomography is showing promise in the definition of pathology in sites difficult to view radiologically, e.g., the ilium, sacrum, sternum, sternoclavicular joints (2), and spine.

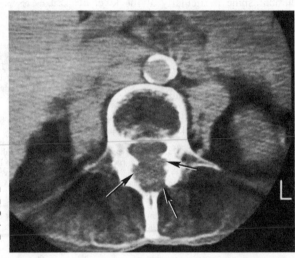

Fig 87–2. CT of lumbar spine in ankylosing spondylitis patient with cauda equina syndrome due to arachnoid cyst shown here invading laminae (**arrows**). (Illustration provided by Dr D O'Duffy)

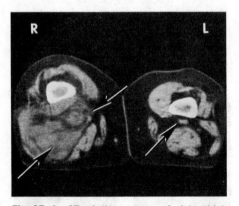

Fig 87–1. CT of liposarcoma of right thigh showing tumor extent (**arrows**), with engulfment of adjacent vessels and nerves. Arrow in left thigh points to neurovascular bundle. (Illustration provided by Dr D O'Duffy)

Preliminary reports of CT in sacroiliitis are conflicting (3,4). Although computed tomography is clearly capable of defining abnormalities in advanced sacroiliitis (1,3,4), conventional x-rays are already of proven value. One study comparing CT with conventional radiographs in early sacroiliitis showed CT as superior (4). Another study of radiologically evident sacroiliitis demonstrated agreement between conventional radiographs and CT with regard to ankylosis, widening, erosions, and sclerosis, but showed no diagnostic advantage for CT (3). However, the newer scanner technology used in the favorable study (4) showed clearer delineation of structures than did that of the study showing equivalence (3).

Examples of CT scans that proved diagnostically useful are shown in Figs 87–1 and 87–2.

1. McLeod RA, Stephens DH, Beabout JW, Sheedy PF, Hattery RR: Computed tomography of the skeletal system. Semin Roent XIII 3:235–247, 1978

2. Destovet JM, Gilula LA, Murphy WA, Sagel SS: Computed tomography of the sternoclavicular joint and sternum. Radiology 138:123–128, 1981

3. Borlaza GS, Seigel R, Kuhns LR, Good AE, Rapp R, Martel W: Computed tomography in the evaluation of sacroiliac arthritis. Radiology 139:437–440, 1981

4. Carrera GF, Foley WD, Kozin F, Ryan L, Lawson TL: CT of sacroiliitis. Am J Radiology 136:41–46, 1981

88. Arthroscopy

Arthroscopy is a diagnostic procedure utilizing a rigid fiberoptic rod-lens telescope of various diameters for direct visualization of intraarticular structures. Thus synovial, meniscal, chondral, and ligamentous lesions can be accurately identified and assessed (1,2). General anesthesia and an operating room are usually used to permit optimal visualization of the joint.

Indications for arthroscopy of the knee, the joint most frequently examined, include:

1. Identification of the site of a surgically correctable lesion; pathologic changes in one compartment in the knee often

result in symptoms referred to the opposite side

2. Identification of significant osteoarthritis complicating meniscal disease and making isolated meniscectomy undesirable

3. Occasional removal of small loose bodies and meniscal tags and partial meniscectomy or patellar shaving

4. Detection of meniscal mimes, lesions that can mimic the features of a torn meniscus, including loose bodies; chondromalacia of the patella or femoral condyles, osteochondral fractures, anterior cruciate ligament lesions, hypermobile or dislocating menisci, partial or complete avulsion of the popliteus tendon, synovial impingement, and synovial plica syndrome.

Plicae represent the remnants of the synovial septae formed during embryologic development of the knee joint. Suprapatellar and mediopatellar plicae are normally present in 20–60% of knees (3). Several factors including trauma induce pathologic changes in plicae and lead to symptoms.

Arthroscopy does not replace the arthrogram in the diagnosis of mechanical internal derangement of the knee; rather, these procedures are complimentary. However, if the arthrogram is equivocal, the need for direct visualization becomes apparent. Other joints besides the knee that can be examined arthroscopically include the shoulder, elbow, hip, and ankle.

Direct visualization of the synovium allows biopsies to be taken from selected areas and may greatly enhance the value of histologic study of this tissue. Photographic documentation of intraarticular structures and pathologic changes is another important benefit of the arthroscopic examination.

Contraindications to arthroscopy include a stiff knee and joint infection. If not cleared by irrigation before the procedure, hemarthrosis may decrease visual clarity. Complications of the procedure are uncommon in skilled hands.

1. Jackson RW, Dandy DJ: Arthroscopy of the Knee. New York, Gruen & Stratton, 1976
2. O'Connor RL: Arthroscopy. Philadelphia, JB Lippincott, 1977
3. Reid GD, Glasgow M, Gordon DA, Wright TA: Pathological plicae of the knee mistaken for arthritis. J Rheumatol 7:573–576, 1980

89. The musculoskeletal examination

A carefully taken, detailed medical history is the most important single element in the evaluation of a patient suspected of having rheumatic disease (1). It is essential for the recognition of systemic disease which may be causing rheumatic symptoms and for the identification of other illnesses that may influence or complicate management. Musculoskeletal symptoms accompany many systemic diseases. Cutaneous manifestations aid in the diagnosis of systemic lupus erythematosus, progressive systemic sclerosis (PSS), dermatomyositis, vasculitis, and psoriatic arthritis. Diseases primarily involving the gastrointestinal tract such as ulcerative colitis, regional enteritis, and Whipple's disease may begin with a disturbance of peripheral joints or spine. Neurologic disorders such as tabes dorsalis and syringomyelia may be responsible for neuropathic arthropathy.

A history of the presence and pattern of joint swelling is important in establishing the presence and type of rheumatic disease. Patients sometimes cannot distinguish between sensations of tightness around a joint and true swelling so that the physician must question the patient closely to establish its presence. The precise localization of the swelling and the time of its appearance and disappearance should be noted. It is helpful to document swelling by questioning an independent observer (e.g., spouse) about its presence and degree. Since certain forms of arthritis, notably gout, ankylosing spondylitis, and systemic lupus erythematosus (SLE) commonly occur in families, complete information is required about arthritic disease in family members.

Since rheumatic symptoms may be a manifestation of some emotional need or disorder, one must assess the psychologic environment of each patient. Detailed information should be obtained concerning the manner in which rheumatic illness has affected the patient's ability to lead a normal life in order to assess the severity of symptoms and to indicate the direction of rehabilitative therapy.

The physician must determine which drugs a patient is taking. Some, such as corticosteroids and immunosuppressive agents, have serious potential side effects and, in the case of corticosteroids, a rapid flare of disease activity may take place if the drug is suddenly discontinued or the dosage reduced. Some medications can produce rheumatic complaints. In particular, a patient with cardiovascular disease who complains of joint pains should be queried carefully about whether he or she is taking hydralazine or procainamide since these may be responsible for the induction of a lupus-like syndrome.

Physical examination. A thorough general physical examination is an essential part of the evaluation since the features of many rheumatic diseases are not limited to the musculoskeletal system. The butterfly rash of systemic lupus erythematosus may be only a dusky reddening over the cheeks and bridge of the nose, easily missed if not specifically sought. Smoothing of the normal wrinkled appearance of the skin may be an early sign of scleroderma. Auscultation of the heart and lungs for the presence of a pleural or pericardial friction rub may indicate involvement of these serous membranes in SLE or rheumatoid arthritis (RA). A careful neurologic examination, including evaluation of mental status, is essential. The psychosis of SLE, the carpal tunnel syndrome of RA (and many other rheumatic disorders), and the trigeminal neuropathy of PSS are important components of these diseases.

The assessment of muscle strength is sometimes difficult in patients with joint diseases since muscle atrophy and weakness occur around painful joints that are not used. Proximal skeletal muscle weakness is indicated by an inability to rise from a sitting position or ascend a steep step without assistance.

The joint examination. A method of systematically recording joint abnormalities is an invaluable aid in determining the extent of joint damage, the overall activity of arthritis, and the response to treatment.

The grading of swelling, tenderness (often done using a scale of 0–4+), and limitation of motion is subjective and will vary among examiners. Grade 1 swelling is not detectable on casual inspection but requires careful palpation to ascertain its presence. When in doubt about the presence of swelling, a grade of 0 to ± should be recorded.

Tenderness is graded according to the amount of steady, even pressure required to elicit a response from the patient as well as the magnitude of the response. Limitation of motion should be carefully measured in terms of the degrees of flexion, extension, or other movement retained or lost.

Gait. Observing how the patient walks is not only helpful diagnostically but also provides a basis for determining treatment such as building up soles of shoes or prescribing canes and crutches.

Specific joints

Shoulder. Swelling of the glenohumoral joint may be difficult to detect because of restriction by overlying tendons and muscles, but an anterior distention can sometimes be seen and felt. The joint capsule and rotator cuff tendons are closely associated. Inflammation of the subacromial bursa usually manifests itself by tenderness just distal to the acromion process. The tendon of the long head of the biceps muscle is easily palpated anteriorly in the

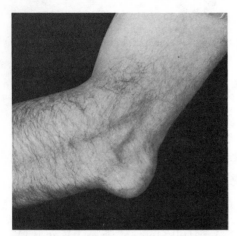

Fig 89—1. Olecranon bursitis in a patient with gout. (From ref 1; reproduced with permission of WB Saunders Company)

bicipital groove between the greater and lesser tubercles. The examiner should observe movement of the scapula and of the humerus. Passive motion with the scapula fixed by the examiner's hand should be compared to active movement since limitation due to pain or muscle weakness is often present. Tears of the rotator cuff are common and can be suspected by inability to raise and hold the arm between 45 and 90 degrees of abduction.

Elbow. Swelling of the elbow should be distinguished from that of the olecranon bursa which overlies the olecranon process and is often affected in rheumatoid arthritis and gout (Fig 89—1). Nodules and tophi often occur in the wall of this bursa. Swelling of the elbow itself is best detected by palpation of the recesses on either side of the olecranon process. Limitation of full extension is an early sign of synovitis. Tenderness in the area of the lateral epicondyle of the humerus is found in tennis elbow.

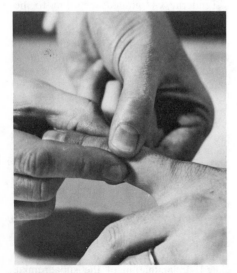

Fig 89—2. A technique for palpation of synovial swelling in a proximal interphalangeal joint. (From ref 1; reproduced with permission of WB Saunders Company)

Wrist. A distinction between swelling of the synovium and the sheath of the extensor tendons may be difficult to perceive and both synovium and sheath are often involved at the same time. Swelling limited to the tendon sheath may be established by failure of applied pressure over the dorsum of the carpus to produce swelling in the area below the head of the ulna where the surface reflection of the synovium is the greatest. Limitation of motion is usually most readily detected in extension.

Hand. There are 15 joints to be examined, and a complete anatomic and functional evaluation of the hand can consume much time. Since the joints are superficially located, swelling is usually detected on inspection. However, careful palpation and ballottement is required to distinguish enlargement due to proliferation of bone (Heberden's and Bouchard's nodes) from that due to synovitis (Fig 89—2). It is useful to record grip strength. A manometer for this purpose, with a modified blood pressure cuff, has been devised.

Hips. So much muscle overlies the hip that swelling is rarely visible. Since patients use the word "hip" to refer to the whole area included by the buttock, upper thigh, and lateral pelvis, one should palpate the region carefully to localize sites of pain and tenderness. The hip joint can be palpated for tenderness just distal to the midpoint of the inguinal ligament. Just below the head of the greater trochanter, the trochanteric bursa can easily be felt.

Before testing range of motion, one should observe the resting position of the thighs and pelvis as the patient lies supine on the examining table. Any discrepancy in leg length should be noted. One should test the range of flexion, extension, abduction, adduction, and rotation, both internal and external. In testing flexion, it is important to immobilize the pelvis. Flexion contracture of the hip is demonstrated by having the patient flex the contralateral thigh while lying supine.

Knee. Careful palpation for the presence of small amounts of fluid is essential. Swelling in the prepatellar bursa or the popliteal bursa must be distinguished from that in the knee joint. Palpation of the areas medial and lateral to the patella can provide information about hypertrophy of the synovium. Large effusions can be detected by ballotting the patella after compressing the suprapatellar bursa so as to upwardly displace the fluid that it contains. Probably the most sensitive means of detecting small amounts of fluid is by the bulge sign, illustrated in Figs 89—3 and 89—4 (2). Localization of tenderness is especially important in tears of the menisci and the collateral ligaments. Limitation of motion usually first affects extension.

Ankle and subtalar joints. The ankle is the articulation of the distal tibia and fibula with the talus whereas the subtalar joint

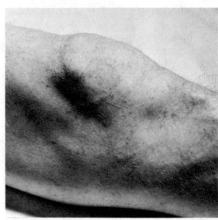

Fig 89—3. Bulge sign for demonstrating a small synovial effusion of the knee. View of the medial aspect of the left knee showing depressed (shaded) area after this side of the joint has been stroked to move the fluid to the other side. (From ref 2; reproduced with permission of the editor)

involves the talus, calcaneus, and part of the navicular. Flexion and extension of the foot take place at the ankle while inversion and eversion involve the subtalar joint.

Swelling of the ankle itself is sometimes difficult to distinguish from edema of the overlying soft tissues, and both may be present simultaneously. Synovial swelling is most marked anteriorly and just below the malleoli. Limitation of motion is usually most apparent on dorsiflexion and inversion of the foot.

Foot. Both swelling and limitation of motion may be difficult to detect in the toes. Inflammation of the first metatarsophalangeal (MTP) joint is characteristic of gouty arthritis and may be associated with such intense heat, redness, and periarticular edema to suggest cellulitis. Hallux valgus (lateral deviation of the main axis of the great toe) may occur alone or as part of a chronic polyarthritis. Tenderness of the

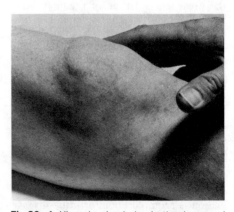

Fig 89—4. View showing bulge in the depressed area seen in Fig 89—3, created by stroking the lateral aspect of knee to move the fluid back into the medial aspect of the knee. (From ref 2; reproduced by permission of the editor)

MTP joints is an important early sign of rheumatoid arthritis and is detected by the application of pressure over the individual MTP joints or by compression of the forefoot.

Spine. The presence of muscle spasm of lateral curvature and of flattening of the lumbar curve is helpful in the diagnosis of spinal disease that can be discerned on inspection. A careful assessment of range of motion of the cervical and lumbar vertebrae as well as measurement of chest expansion should be carried out in patients with back or radicular symptoms.

The Schober test is used to estimate lumbar flexion. With the patient standing erect, a mark is made on the middle of the back at the level of the posterior iliac spines (approximately L5) and at a point 10 cm above. The change (increase) in the distance between these 2 points is measured on maximum anterior flexion of the lumbar vertebrae. Limitation of lumbar flexion is indicated by an increase of less than 3 cm (3).

The diagnosis of most forms of spondylitis is aided more by roentgenographic examination (see Section 85) than by physical examination.

1. Polley HF, Hunder GG: Rheumatologic Interviewing and Physical Examination of the Joints, ed 2. Philadelphia, WB Saunders, 1978
2. Hunder GG, Polley HF: Detecting small effusions of the knee. Postgrad Med 40:689–692, 1966
3. Moll JMH, Wright V: Normal range of spine mobility: an objective clinical study. Ann Rheum Dis 30:381–386, 1971

90. Examination of synovial fluid

Careful evaluation of joint fluid (synovia) is one of the most important steps in the differential diagnosis of arthritis (1–3). Prompt overall examination alone often permits separation into 4 distinct categories of differing pathophysiology, namely:

I. Noninflammatory
II. Inflammatory
III. Infectious, especially bacterial infection, or
IV. Hemorrhagic

Several simple laboratory tests should also be performed to confirm the suspected classification and to further assist in establishing a specific diagnosis (Table 90–1).

Group I synovial fluids are seen most often in osteoarthritis or traumatic arthropathies. In these situations, synovial thickening is usually minimal on physical examination, but effusions may occur, varying from a few milliliters to over 100 ml. The synovia is clear; print may be read through it when it is placed in a glass tube. A yellowish tint is often noted in pathologic conditions (believed due to xanthochromia), whereas normal joint liquor is nearly colorless.

These fluids are sticky to touch due to high viscosity and drip from the syringe (*after* removal of the needle) with stringing out to 3–5 cm. A single drop placed between two fingertips forms a long string when the fingers are separated, and an excellent "mucin clot" forms when a drop of group I synovia is placed in a tube of dilute acetic acid. Dilution by capillary leakage in traumatic states may diminish the viscosity.

The total white blood cell count in group I synovial fluids is almost always less than 2000/mm³ and the proportion of mononuclear elements is usually greater than 50%.

At times, obviously inflammatory disorders may produce a group I fluid. This happens occasionally in acute rheumatic fever and systemic lupus erythematosus and nearly always in arthritis or periarthritis associated with erythema nodosum.

Group II fluids are grossly opaque due to cellular debris; although light can be seen through these specimens, it is seldom possible to read print clearly. The white cell count varies from 5,000–75,000/mm³, with the majority of cells being polymorphonuclear leukocytes (PMNs). Viscosity is reduced, because of the breakdown of mucopolysaccharides by the lysosomal enzymes of PMNs.

The fluid drips like water and the mucin test results in fragmented bits of mucopolysaccharide gel rather than a tight, ropy clot. When the white cell count is performed, the fluid must be diluted with saline rather than acetic acid, since the latter coagulates mucopolysaccharide and makes counting the cells impossible.

In crystal-induced disease the responsible crystals (monosodium urate monohy-

Table 90–1. Examination of the synovial fluid

	Normal	Group I Noninflammatory	Group II Inflammatory	Group III Septic
Gross appearance	Transparent, clear	Transparent, yellow	Opaque or translucent, yellow	Opaque, yellow to green
Viscosity	High	High	Low	Variable
White cells/mm³	<200	<200	5,000–75,000	>50,000, often >100,000
Polymorphonuclear leukocytes	<25%	<25%	>50%	>75%
Culture	Negative	Negative	Negative	Often positive
Glucose (mg/dl)	Nearly equal to blood	Nearly equal to blood	>25, lower than blood	>50, lower than blood
Associated conditions		Degenerative joint disease Trauma* Neuropathic arthropathy* Hypertrophic osteoarthropathy† Pigmented villonodular synovitis* SLE† Acute rheumatic fever† Erythema nodosum	Rheumatoid arthritis Connective tissue diseases (SLE, PSS, DM/PM) Ankylosing spondylitis Other seronegative spondylarthropathies (psoriatic arthritis, Reiter's syndrome, arthritis of chronic inflammatory bowel disease) Crystal-induced synovitis (gout or pseudogout) Acute rheumatic fever	Bacterial infections Compromised immunity (disease or medication related) Other joint disease

* May be hemorrhagic.
† Group I or II.
SLE = Systemic lupus erythematosus; PSS = progressive systemic sclerosis; DM/PM = dermatomyositis/polymyositis.

drate in gout and calcium pyrophosphate dihydrate in pseudogout) can be seen intra- and extracellularly on microscopic examination of a thin (1-drop) wet preparation of joint fluid using low light and high magnification. Special techniques using polarizing lenses (crystals are able to rotate light) and a first order red compensator assist in identification and permit definitive characterization of these crystals. Oxalate tubes should not be used to collect anticoagulated specimens when crystal-induced arthropathy is suspected since artifactual crystals of calcium oxalate may be formed. Corticosteroid and cholesterol crystals may also be a source of confusion, but can be recognized by their distinct appearance.

Group II noncrystal-induced inflammatory fluids most commonly occur in one of 2 broad disease categories: 1) rheumatoid arthritis or one of the other connective tissue diseases, and 2) ankylosing spondylitis or one of its variants (the seronegative spondylarthropathies). Unfortunately, synovial fluid examination alone seldom serves to distinguish these conditions. In rheumatoid arthritis (RA) and systemic lupus erythematosus complement levels are reduced in the synovia compared with simultaneous serum values (often <30%), while in Reiter's syndrome, the complement level in synovial fluid tends to be normal or elevated. Total immunoglobulin levels in joint fluid may also be elevated in RA.

Cytoplasmic inclusions are frequently present in the polymorphonuclear cells in fluids from patients with rheumatoid arthritis. These inclusions have been shown to contain IgG and IgM (rheumatoid factor), but unfortunately are not specific for RA.

Group III (septic) synovial effusions have a frankly purulent gross appearance, and no light can penetrate these thick fluids. The white cell count is dramatically elevated, with over 50,000/mm^3 (almost all PMNs) being the rule. One exception is tuberculous arthritis, in which the total count may be lower and the proportion of mononuclear cells, especially lymphocytes, higher (30–50%). Partially treated infections and early infections with less virulent agents such as gonococci can also produce lower leukocyte counts.

The glucose level in these fluids is sharply reduced and is often found to be 10 mg/dl or less. Both bacteria and polymorphonuclear leukocytes are responsible for excessive glucose utilization. There is an inverse linear relationship between total white cell count and glucose concentration; thus a slight reduction in glucose concentration may be found in group II effusions.

A general guideline is that a synovial fluid glucose concentration less than half that of the contemporaneous blood glucose level is highly suggestive of bacterial infection. The validity of this relationship depends on prompt processing of the specimen since leukocyte metabolism of carbohydrate in vitro may lead to a spurious low glucose value.

Gram stains are occasionally positive for the infecting microorganism, and culture frequently leads to a precise diagnosis. Unfortunately, in a fairly high proportion of infected synovial fluids, the offending agent is impossible to identify in culture because the few organisms are fastidious in their culture requirements; this is especially true in gonococcal infection.

Group IV or hemorrhagic synovial fluid accumulations may occur due to either systemic conditions or localized articular problems. Hemophilia, other congenital or acquired hemorrhagic diathesis, or overanticoagulation are systemic causes of hemarthrosis, while trauma, villonodular synovitis, and neuropathic arthropathy are more localized processes responsible for bloody synovial fluid.

It should be emphasized that there is overlap in the synovial fluid classification system presented here. Therefore, it is important that diagnostic decisions be based on all available data, including setting, history and physical examination, and other pertinent laboratory and/or roentgenographic data. Nevertheless, certain findings in synovia, such as the positive identification of microorganisms or crystals, are essential to accurate diagnosis and the development of an appropriate therapeutic plan.

1. Ropes MW, Bauer W: Synovial Fluid Changes in Joint Disease. Cambridge, Harvard University Press, 1953
2. McCarty DJ Jr: Synovial fluid, Arthritis and Allied Conditions. Ed 9. DJ McCarty, Jr., ed. Philadelphia, Lea & Febiger, 1979, pp 51–69
3. Schumacher HR: Synovial fluid analysis, Textbook of Rheumatology. WN Kelley, ED Harris, S Ruddy, C Sledge, eds. Philadelphia, WB Saunders, 1981, pp 568–579

91. Clinical pharmacology of the antirheumatic drugs

Drugs are given to patients with rheumatic diseases, first to relieve their symptoms and second, when possible, to arrest the disease progression. To achieve the best results, the correct drug must be given in the exact dose to the right patient at the appropriate point in the disease course at the optimal time of day.

A distinction must be made between nonspecific or symptomatic drugs and those with a more fundamental action dependent on the nature of the underlying disease process. Analgesics relieve pain, regardless of its cause and antiinflammatory drugs have effect in any inflammatory disorder. Both work quickly. Analgesics are effective within minutes of administration and their action lasts for 4–8 hours. Antiinflammatory drugs are effective within a few days of the start of treatment.

The action of a more specific drug is dependent on the nature of the underlying disease process: penicillamine is not effective in gout, and allopurinol is useless in rheumatoid arthritis. Some drugs take months to achieve their benefits, which may include improvement in nonarticular features and a more favorable outcome of the disease.

Simple analgesics

Analgesic drugs are of limited value in arthritis, and drugs with additional antiinflammatory activity are more effective than potent narcotics. Nevertheless, simple analgesics are used for patients with mild or intermittent pain in whom regular treatment is not required and as a supplement to regular therapy with other drugs. Aspirin (600 mg) may be used in this way and alternatives include acetaminophen (1 gm) and the combinations of dextropropoxyphene with acetaminophen. In low doses, these compounds are well tolerated.

Aspirin and other salicylates

Aspirin represents the beginning of the antiinflammatory era and has continued to be the mainstay of antiinflammatory therapy for many years (1). A drawback is the dose—at least 3.6 gm daily—required to achieve good results in inflammatory conditions such as rheumatoid arthritis. This amount of medication is inconvenient, requiring the patient to swallow large numbers of pills and can be associated with a high frequency of side effects.

Some patients with rheumatoid arthritis cannot tolerate plain aspirin in full dosage. Withdrawals occur mainly because of gastric intolerance (nausea, epigastric pain, indigestion) or tinnitus and deafness. Aspirin has a number of other important side effects, including occult gastric bleeding which may lead to anemia, occasional hematemesis or melena, aggravation of allergic rhinitis or asthma, and hypersensitivity reactions. Aspirin is dangerous for patients taking oral anticoagulants, may enhance the action of oral antidiabetic drugs, and inhibits the uricosuric action of probenecid.

Numerous attempts have been made to overcome the problems of aspirin therapy. The gastric tolerance can be improved and the frequency of microbleeding decreased by taking the drug with food or milk or by using buffered, microencapsulated, or enteric coated preparations. Nonacetylated salicylate preparations have similar advantages, but may be less potent antiinflammatory agents. Choline salicylate is a solution some patients prefer and is not associated with gastric microbleeding. A similar preparation in solid form, a combination of choline and magnesium salicylate, has been shown to require only twice a day administration. Also available is a salicylic acid ester absorbed in the small intestine, which then releases salicylate.

Although these sophisticated formulations are kind to the stomach, they do not avoid other problems such as tinnitus and deafness. Plain aspirin is cheap, but some aspirin-containing preparations are almost as costly as newer drugs of other types.

Nonsteroidal antiinflammatory drugs (2–6)

Classification. A chemical classification of this rapidly growing class of drugs is shown in Table 91–1. It is of little value to the clinician since drugs of similar chemical type may have quite different properties, whereas drugs of a different chemical type may behave in the same way.

Sulindac is a chemical relative of indomethacin but resembles propionic acid derivatives, in having a slightly less potent antiinflammatory effect, but causing fewer side effects than indomethacin. Within the group of propionic acid derivatives are drugs with widely different properties, short and long plasma half-lives, prominent analgesic and prominent antiinflammatory potency, excellent tolerance, and adverse effects affecting particularly the stomach or the skin. All indene derivatives do not cause headaches and all pyrazole derivatives do not cause blood dyscrasias. Thus, it is difficult to devise a classification on clinical grounds. There is some justification for separating the older drugs, aspirin, phenylbutazone, and indomethacin from the newer, often better tolerated compounds.

There are also particular uses for antiinflammatory drugs. Examples of these are shown in Table 91–2. The most obvious way of using these drugs is to give regular therapy for a chronic disease like rheumatoid or osteoarthritis. The aim is usually an antiinflammatory effect.

But the nonsteroidal antiinflammatory drugs are also analgesics and can be given on demand for pain that is intermittent or variable. Some compounds are particular-ly useful for night pain and morning stiffness which are frequent problems in inflammatory arthropathies. A night dose can be added to regular daytime therapy. In self-limited diseases like gout, a rapid antiinflammatory action is required. A large initial dose of an antiinflammatory drug is usually given, then reduced as the pain improves.

Dosage schedule may also influence choice. Once-a-day dosage is especially convenient for long-term antiinflammatory therapy in chronic diseases. More frequent dosing is likely to be preferred by patients with more severe pain and less active inflammation.

The use of some of these drugs has been established in children. Others, like phen-

Table 91–1. A partial list of nonsteroidal antiinflammatory drugs

Salicylates
*Aspirin
*Numerous other salicylates
*Diflunisal (Dolobid)

Indoles
*Indomethacin (Indocin, Indocid)
*Sulindac (Clinoril)
*Tolmetin (Tolectin)
*Zomepirac (Zomax)

Pyrazoles
*Phenylbutazone (Butazolidin)
*Oxyphenbutazone (Tandearil)
Azapropazone (Rheumox)
Feprazone (Methrazone)

Fenamates
*Mefenamic acid (Ponstel)
*Meclofenamate sodium (Meclomen)
Flufenamic acid (Meralen)
Tolfenamic acid (Clotam)
Clofenamic acid

Proprionic acid derivatives
*Ibuprofen (Motrin, Bufren)
*Naproxen (Naprosyn)
*Fenoprofen calcium (Nalfon, Fenpron)
Flurbiprofen (Froben, Ansaid)
Ketoprofen (Alrheuma, Orudis)
Fenbufen (Cinopal, Lederfen)
Carprofen (Ridamyl)
Pirprofen (Rengasil)

Phenylacetic acid derivatives
Fenclofenac (Flenac)
Diclofenac (Voltaren, Voltarol)

Oxicams
*Piroxicam (Feldene)
Isoxicam (Maxicam)

* Approved for use in the United States as of 1982.

Table 91–2. A selection of nonsteroidal antiinflammatory drugs with appropriate dosage

Drug	Dosage
Aspirin	600–1,500 mg 4 times daily or 600 mg as required for pain
Azapropazone	600 mg twice a day
Benorylate	10 ml (4 gm) twice a day or suspension of 1.5 gm 3 times a day using tablets
Choline magnesium trisalicylate	1 gm twice a day for osteoarthritis; 1.5 gm twice a day for rheumatoid arthritis
Diflunisal	500 mg immediately then 250 or 50 mg twice a day
Fenbufen	300 mg in morning, 600 mg at night (night dose only may be enough)
Fenclofenac	300 mg twice a day
Fenoprofen	600 mg 3 times a day or 300 mg as required for pain
Feprazone	200 mg twice a day
Flurbiprofen	50 mg in morning, 100 mg at night
Flufenamic acid	200 mg 3 times a day
Ibuprofen	400 mg 3 times a day or up to 600 mg 4 times a day as required for pain
Indomethacin	25–50 mg 3 times a day, 75–100 mg at night for night pain/morning stiffness
Indomethacin slow release	75 mg at night or twice a day
Indoprofen	200 mg 3 times a day or 200 mg as required for pain
Ketoprofen	100 mg twice a day
Meclofenamate sodium	50–100 mg 3 or 4 times a day
Mefenamic acid	500 mg 3 times a day or 500 mg as required for pain
Naproxen	500 mg twice a day
Phenylbutazone	100 mg 3 times a day. Not more than 7 days
Piroxicam	20 mg daily morning or night
Sulindac	200 mg twice a day
Tolmetin sodium	400 mg 3 times a day
Zomepirac	100 mg 3 times a day or 100 mg as required for pain

Note: Lower doses are used for osteoarthritis and milder conditions. Doses must often be increased to the maximum allowed for active rheumatoid arthritis.

ylbutazone, must be avoided. Some are particularly suitable for patients with a history of indigestion, and others are especially likely to cause trouble. Some can usually be given with anticoagulants and others cannot.

Pharmacology and mode of action. All the nonsteroidal antiinflammatory drugs are inhibitors of the cyclooxygenase pathway of arachidonic acid breakdown. Their potency in this respect varies and does not correlate with analgesic or antiinflammatory efficacy. They also act to a variable extent on cellular aspects of inflammation. It is therefore likely that their clinical actions depend on effects at several stages in the complex process of inflammation, but these are not yet clearly defined.

Pharmacokinetics. Plasma levels of most antiinflammatory drugs are not helpful in determining either efficacy or toxicity and are therefore of no practical value.

The exception is aspirin. There is some correlation between plasma salicylate levels and antiinflammatory efficacy. Since the aspirin dosage required to achieve optimal efficacy varies widely, it may be useful to monitor salicylate levels, aiming for a value between 20 and 30 mg/100 ml. Plasma levels are also useful in children who may have very high levels without the usual warning of tinnitus and deafness. Plasma half-life is of some importance in determining the dosage regimen of a drug (Table 91–3).

Compounds with long plasma half-lives like piroxicam can be given once daily and achieve relief of symptoms over 24 hours for many patients. Piroxicam can also be given either in the morning or at night with equal efficacy, whereas compounds with short plasma half-lives must be given at night to achieve optimal relief of morning stiffness.

Compounds with short plasma half-lives do not require the very frequent dosing that their plasma level profiles might suggest. In many cases, adequate antiinflammatory efficacy can be achieved with twice daily dosing, and more frequent administration is desirable only for analgesia. All the nonsteroidal antiflammatory

Table 91–3. Plasma half-lives of nonsteroidal antiinflammatory drugs

Compound	Plasma half-life (hrs)
Indomethacin	2–3
Sulindac	18 (sulfide)
Tolmetin	1–3
Mefenamic acid	3–4
Flufenamic acid	9
Ibuprofen	2
Naproxen	12–15
Fenoprofen calcium	3
Flurbiprofen	4
Ketoprofen	1–35
Piroxicam	45
Diflunisal	8–12

drugs are well absorbed from the stomach and all are highly protein bound.

Factors affecting choice. Choice is determined by aspects of the patients as well as the aspects of the drug. These are discussed in the following sections.

Efficacy. There are no important differences in the efficacy of the currently available compounds. The major factor that determines the success or failure of treatment is individual response variation: one patient responds well to one drug and one to another. About 20% of patients fail to benefit from any one nonsteroidal antiinflammatory drug. Of the remaining patients some will improve slightly, some moderately, and some very well, the degree of response being normally distributed. Because of this phenomenon, it is often necessary to try a number of different drugs before finding the one that produces optimal efficacy for a particular patient.

Nonsteroidal antiinflammatory drugs relieve pain and stiffness, reduce swelling, and improve function. They have no proven effect on the disease outcome.

Tolerance. The occurrence of side effects, like efficacy, is determined mainly by individual variation. Some people have them, others don't. Apart from indigestion and other minor gastric disturbances, side effects are unusual with these drugs. But because large numbers of patients take antiinflammatory drugs, even rare reactions are important. Adverse effects common to all these drugs include gastric irritation, rashes, aggravation of asthma and allergic rhinitis, and renal effects in compromised patients. Other reactions are peculiar to certain compounds.

Gastric problems. The most common gastric problems are epigastric pain, nausea, and indigestion. The incidence varies widely, highest with plain aspirin and lowest with the newer compounds like propionic acid derivatives.

Peptic ulceration is rare with nonsteroidal antiinflammatory drugs. Support for such drugs in the etiology of peptic ulcers comes from studies showing differences in the site of ulcers in patients taking or not taking this medication. Patients taking antiinflammatory drugs are more likely to have ulcers around the pylorus and less likely to have duodenal ulcers. The most important therapeutic point is that such ulcers may heal simply on withdrawal of medication.

Gastric bleeding may be overt or occult. Hematemesis and melena are probably rare events and usually due to gastric erosion which can be demonstrated on gastroscopy. Occult bleeding is an occasional problem and large amounts of blood loss may contribute to the anemia of rheumatoid arthritis.

Asthma–allergic rhinitis. Aspirin aggravates asthma or allergic rhinitis in about 10% of sufferers. Other nonsteroidal antiinflammatory agents may have the same effect.

Rashes. An allergic type of generalized maculopapular rash occurs occasionally with any antiinflammatory drug and more with some than others. It resolves rapidly with withdrawal of medication. Angioneurotic edema is rare, but if it occurs with one drug, it usually occurs with all. Stevens-Johnson syndrome is a very rare side effect of nonsteroidal antiinflammatory drugs.

Renal effects. Prostaglandins become important in maintaining renal blood flow in edematous patients, for example, in cirrhosis, cardiac failure, or nephrotic syndrome. In such patients the use of a nonsteroidal antiinflammatory drug may aggravate edema, antagonize diuretics, raise serum creatinine, and cause reversible acute renal failure. Interstitial nephritis can occur and explains some bouts of renal failure.

Hepatic effects. Drug-induced hepatitis, sometimes cholestatic, is described as a rare side effect of some nonsteroidal antiinflammatory drugs. Raised transaminase levels may occur with aspirin therapy, particularly in juvenile arthritis and systemic lupus erythematosus. Usually minor, often transient and unimportant abnormalities of liver function test results occasionally occur with other compounds.

Tinnitus and deafness. Tinnitus and deafness occur with salicylates except diflunisal. These are a dose-related phenomenon but occur at widely differing doses in different patients.

Tinnitus and deafness are an indication to reduce the dose. Headaches and confusion, also dose-related, occur with indomethacin. They are best avoided by giving the drug at night. Central nervous system symptoms may also occur with the other nonsteroidals.

Other side effects. Agranulocytosis and aplastic anemia are very rare complications of treatment with phenylbutazone and oxyphenbutazone, with an estimated frequency of 1 in 66,000 prescriptions, but with a fatality rate up to 50%. These complications are unlikely to occur within the first week of treatment, and it is therefore recommended that phenylbutazone therapy be restricted to this duration. Aplastic anemia is more common after prolonged treatment in elderly patients, while agranulocytosis occurs most often within the first month of treatment in younger patients.

Blood dyscrasias have been reported rarely with other antiinflammatory drugs and their relationship to treatment therefore remains doubtful.

Diarrhea is a complication of treatment with mefenamic acid and less often with other fenamates. Mefenamic acid also rarely causes hemolytic anemia.

Safety. Death is not usually associated with nonsteroidal antiinflammatory drug therapy but may occur from hematemesis and melena or from aplastic anemia with phenylbutazone. The latter is rare but should remind the prescriber of the potential hazard of the prescription and of the need to balance risk with benefit. Nonsteroidal antiinflammatory drugs are not completely safe and should not be used for trivial aches and pains, especially in the elderly.

Convenience. Once-a-day medication is convenient and improves compliance especially in elderly patients who may require other drugs. Patients with intermittent or variable symptoms and those in whom the major requirement is analgesia, rather than an antiinflammatory effect, may do better with more frequent dosing and a more flexible schedule.

Cost. Aspirin is cheap. The newer nonsteroidal antiinflammatory drugs are much more expensive. Costs vary with the source and nature of the treatment, but as a rough guide, one day's treatment with a generic brand of aspirin (3.6 gm) costs 15¢ while a single 20 mg dose of piroxicam costs just over a dollar. The cost of alternative compounds is very similar. As aspirin formulations become more sophisticated, they also become more expensive.

Indications. Nonsteroidal antiinflammatory drugs are used for the relief of symptoms in a wide range of diseases including rheumatoid and osteoarthritis, ankylosing spondylitis, gout, other inflammatory arthropathies such as psoriatic arthropathy and reactive arthritis, and soft tissue rheumatism including traumatic lesions and sports injuries.

All the available compounds are effective in rheumatoid and osteoarthritis and suitable for their treatment, except phenylbutazone which should be avoided altogether. High-dose aspirin is a reasonable alternative in rheumatoid arthritis, less suitable for osteoarthritis because of side effects, and inconvenient and less effective than other drugs in ankylosing spondylitis and gout. In these diseases indomethacin remains a good first choice with newer drugs like naproxen or piroxicam available as alternatives.

The propionic acid derivatives seem to be particularly useful in sports injuries, and their favorable therapeutic ratio supports their use in such conditions. Drugs of this type are not usually helpful in frozen shoulders or tennis elbows. Safety is a major consideration in juvenile arthritis, though aspirin is particularly valuable for its systemic antipyretic action.

Special problem patients. The most common problem patient is one with a delicate stomach, with or without structural lesions such as peptic ulcer or hiatus hernia. The newer drugs like naproxen or ibuprofen can often be used in such patients without danger or intolerance. Sometimes drugs can be tolerated if given in a different formulation, such as a coating on

aspirin, by suppository at night, or with meals, antacids, or cimetidine.

Many nonsteroidal antiinflammatory drugs are excreted by the kidney, so that reduction in dosage may be appropriate for patients in renal failure. Borderline renal function is an indication for great caution with these drugs because a minor degree of impairment of renal function may be critical.

Elderly patients are particularly at risk from serious toxicity such as hematemesis and from the blood dyscrasias of phenylbutazone. Fluid retention and interactions with other drugs are also more likely to cause trouble.

Drug interactions and combinations. Aspirin and phenylbutazone should usually not be given with anticoagulants or sulfonylurea antidiabetic drugs. Most of the alternatives have been shown to be safe with these drugs, but occasional patients receiving anticoagulants may show a rise in prothrombin time when antiinflammatory drugs are started. The prothrombin time should therefore be measured daily for the first 5 days of such combination therapy.

Nonsteroidal antiinflammatory drugs can be given safely with simple analgesics and with gold and penicillamine-like drugs. The combination of one antiinflammatory drug with another is usually pointless. The exception is the use of one drug for regular daytime treatment and another at night to relieve night pain and morning stiffness.

Selection, choice, and dosage. A selection of drugs with appropriate dosages is given in Table 91–2. The dosage depends in part on the aim of treatment. With little difference in efficacy between the drugs, safety and tolerance become the major factors in choice, with convenience the next. If cost is a major consideration, aspirin will remain the front runner; if not, some of the modern well-tolerated drugs with convenient dosage schedules such as piroxicam or naproxen will be favored.

Corticosteroids

Corticosteroids are naturally occurring hormones or synthetic analogs with potent antiinflammatory activity. They will therefore relieve pain in inflammatory arthropathies. Unfortunately, other metabolic effects of corticosteroids, including weight gain, diabetes mellitus, osteoporosis, thin skin, and other features of Cushing's syndrome, will occur with excessive doses and especially with prolonged therapy (7). Therefore, corticosteroids can seldom be used for symptomatic relief, but they are used to control systemic manifestations of disease such as vasculitis and for local injection into joints or soft tissues (see Section 93).

Choice. A list of compounds with equivalent doses is given in Table 91–4. For

Table 91–4. Equivalent doses of corticosteroids representing approximately the daily natural production rate

Corticosteroid	Dosage
Cortisone	25 mg
Hydrocortisone	20 mg
Prednisone or prednisolone	5 mg
Methylprednisolone	4 mg
Dexamethasone	0.75 mg
Betamethasone	1 mg
Paramethasone	2 mg
Triamcinolone	4 mg

systemic administration there is no reason to use anything but prednisone or prednisolone. Prednisolone, for example, is available as tablets, enteric coated for the delicate stomach, and for intravenous or intramuscular injection. For intraarticular injection, a highly insoluble compound such as triamcinolone hexacetonide is desirable. The local action of such a compound is prolonged in comparison with the more soluble hydrocortisone which rapidly disappears from the joint into the systemic circulation.

Prednisolone is well absorbed from the stomach with a plasma half-life of 3–4 hours. The half-life of its biological effects is much longer, 18–36 hours, so that it is unnecessary to give the drug more than once or twice a day. It is metabolized in the liver.

Indications and dosage. Corticosteroids are seldom used in rheumatoid arthritis because the dose required to control the symptoms and the prolonged course of the disease will almost inevitably lead to the problems of Cushing's syndrome. A safe dose, 7.5 mg of prednisolone daily, usually shows disappointing results. It can be used at night to relieve morning stiffness but is no more effective than indomethacin. The exception is in elderly patients with explosive disease. They often respond dramatically to 7.5 mg or 10 mg daily of prednisolone and poorly to alternatives.

Corticosteroid therapy is mandatory and urgent in temporal arteritis, both to control symptoms and to prevent complications like blindness. It is also usually needed for control of symptoms in polymyalgia rheumatica. A daily dose of 15 mg of prednisolone is usual in polymyalgia and 40 mg in temporal arteritis. After a few months, a dosage reduction program is begun with small increments over 2 to 4 years.

Corticosteroids may be required in connective tissue disorders such as polymyositis, systemic lupus erythematosus, and polyarteritis nodosa, the dose depending on the severity of symptoms.

Alternate day dosage of prednisolone causes less pituitary suppression than daily therapy and is therefore desirable in children to preserve growth. Adrenocorticotropic hormone (ACTH) has the same advantage but all the other disadvantages of corticosteroids. It must be given by injection, and dosage is more difficult to regulate. It is sometimes used in a difficult case of acute gout, to speed the remission produced by hospitalization in rheumatoid arthritis, and in resistent frozen shoulder or shoulder–hand syndrome. Dosage is 40–80 units twice weekly by intramuscular injection.

"Specific" drugs for rheumatoid arthritis

The slow acting or remission-inducing compounds (4,5,8,9) produce a gradual suppression of the symptoms and signs of rheumatoid arthritis (RA) (see Section 12), which reaches a plateau after 4–6 months of treatment. They are also useful for the extraarticular features of RA and make possible a reduction in the requirements for symptomatic remedies, including corticosteroids. To a variable extent, these compounds are capable of retarding disease progression, as judged by radiographic changes (erosions). Their mode of action is unknown.

Immunosuppressive drugs have this type of action (5,9–16) and are considered in Section 92. Persistence of uncontrolled active disease, despite adequate antiinflammatory therapy, is the principal indication for the use of drugs of this type. Because of their potential toxicity, they should be given only to patients with more severe or progressive disease. If possible, they should be used before irreversible changes have occurred in joints.

Since all drugs of this type work slowly, it is necessary to continue analgesic and antiinflammatory therapy until the patient responds. Concomitant use of drugs such as phenylbutazone, which can cause marrow suppression, should be avoided. Dosage can be gradually reduced as the patient improves.

Gold-containing compounds. Two gold-containing compounds are now available for use in rheumatoid arthritis—aurothioglucose and aurothiomalate (4,5,8,9,17). Both must be given by intramuscular injection. Aurothioglucose is as effective as aurothiomalate and has a lower frequency of adverse reactions. A gold compound suitable for oral use is under active investigation (18).

An initial test dose containing 10 mg of gold should be given, although reactions are uncommon. Thereafter, the patient receives 50 mg weekly until a beneficial response is obtained, usually 3–4 months. The intervals between the injections are then increased to 2 weeks and later to 3 or 4 weeks. Because the relapse that follows lowering of the dose may be delayed for several months, dosage should not be reduced more often than once in 3 months.

If there is a return of symptoms, the dose can be increased with weekly injections until control is regained. It is important to avoid a full return of the disease since second courses of gold are not usually effective. Many therapists obtain a complete blood count and urinalysis before each dose. Others obtain these tests biweekly.

The most common adverse reaction to chrysotherapy is a rash, occurring in about 30% of patients, most often in the first 6 months, and requiring temporary cessation of treatment. Rashes are occasionally severe and rarely exfoliative. Proteinuria occurs later and may require withdrawal of treatment. Agranulocytosis, aplastic anemia, or thrombocytopenia are rare but potentially fatal reactions that preclude any further administration of gold-containing compounds. Other rare reactions that are nevertheless important to keep in mind are colitis, fibrosing alveolitis, and cholestatic jaundice.

Auranofin is a gold salt that can be given orally (18). It differs from the injectable gold salts in several other respects. It is active in adjuvant arthritis but in no other models of inflammation. Effective plasma levels in humans are lower than those achieved with injected gold salts. Trials to date suggest that auranofin is slightly less effective than injected gold salts in rheumatoid arthritis but certainly causes fewer side effects and is much safer. The optimal dose is 3 mg twice daily. The most common side effect is diarrhea, which is usually mild and transient. Occasional rashes occur but no aplastic anemia has been reported so far. It is not yet approved for use in the United States at the time of this writing.

Penicillamine. This agent has clinical effects similar to those of the gold-containing compounds (4,5,9,19,20). Both have been found to be effective in retarding disease progression as judged by radiographic study.

Penicillamine should be given in an initial dose of 250 mg a day and then increased in amount after 1–2 months to 500 mg a day. No further increase should be made until the patient's response can be assessed. Occasional patients require doses up to 1 gm a day. Urinalysis and full blood count including platelets should be performed at least monthly.

Penicillamine has many side effects, and it is essential that these be managed correctly if the patient is to be treated safely and the drug continued. The earliest problem is often nausea or vomiting; this may often be avoided by keeping the dose at a low level and gradually increasing it as tolerance improves. Acute febrile reactions rarely occur after the first few doses, and patients with these effects may need to start with very small quantities of the drug. Loss of taste occurs after about 6 weeks and improves after a further 6

weeks, regardless of whether treatment is continued.

Early rashes appear within the first few months and resemble those that occur with ampicillin. The drug should be stopped and restarted at a low dose when the rash has cleared. Late rashes occur after 6 months or more of treatment and are quite different. The lesions are raised with a scaly surface and usually resistant to all forms of local treatment. If the rash is troublesome, the drug must be stopped.

Proteinuria occurs from the fourth month onward and is associated with deposition of immune complexes in the glomerulus. This is not usually accompanied by any impairment of renal function, however, and the proteinuria tends to decrease gradually over 12–18 months whether or not the drug is stopped. If the proteinuria is modest (less than 2 gm per 24 hours) and if renal function remains normal, the drug may be continued.

Mouth ulcers are another occasional problem. Thrombocytopenia may occur at any time and develops suddenly but is usually benign. The drug should be stopped if the count falls below 100,000 platelets/mm^3; rapid recovery after discontinuation is the rule. Treatment can be restarted at a low dose and maintained at a level below that which led to thrombocytopenia. Rarely, there is a gradual marrow suppression with thrombocytopenia, neutropenia, and anemia. This is much more serious than thrombocytopenia alone and has led to a few fatalities. Treatment must be stopped in this situation.

Rarer but increasingly reported side effects that demand withdrawal of treatment include myasthenia gravis, Goodpasture's syndrome, pemphigus, polymyositis, and drug-related lupus, which can occur after about 2 years of treatment. The lupus-like syndrome usually presents as a recurrence of joint symptoms with a high titer of serum antinuclear antibody.

Hydroxychloroquine. This drug has been said to have an action similar to gold in rheumatoid arthritis though it has not been shown to alter the radiologic progression of the disease (4,5,9). Hydroxychloroquine is used in doses of 200–400 mg daily. The biggest problem is retinopathy but this is dose-related and can be avoided by restricting the dosage. Nevertheless eyes must be examined at least every 6 months. Once symptoms of impaired vision have occurred, the defect is irreversible and may even progress. Apart from this problem, the drug is well tolerated.

Chloroquine is reputed to aggravate psoriasis but some patients with psoriatic arthritis may benefit from its use.

1. Dromgoole SH, Furst DE, Paulus HE: Rational approaches to the use of salicylates in the treatment of rheumatoid arthritis. Semin Arthritis Rheum 11:257–283, 1981
2. Huskisson EC, ed: Anti-rheumatic drugs. Clin Rheum Dis 5:351–736, 1979

3. Simon LS, Mills JA: Nonsteroidal antiinflammatory drugs. N Engl J Med 30:1179–1185, 1237–1243, 1980

4. Craig GL, Buchanan WW: Antirheumatic drugs: clinical pharmacology and therapeutic use. Drugs 20:453–484, 1980

5. Hunder GG, Bunch TW: Treatment of rheumatoid arthritis. Bull Rheum Dis 32:1–7, 1982

6. Brezin JH, Katz SM, Schwartz AB, et al: Reversible renal failure and nephrotic syndrome associated with non-steroidal anti-inflammatory drugs. N Engl J Med 301:1271–1273, 1979

7. Garber EK, Fan PT, Bluestone R: Realistic guidelines of corticosteroid therapy in rheumatic disease. Semin Arth Rheum 11:231–256, 1981

8. The Cooperating Clinics Committee of the American Rheumatism Association: A controlled trial of gold salt therapy in rheumatoid arthritis. Arthritis Rheum 16:353–358, 1973

9. Bunch TW, O'Duffy JD: Disease-modifying drugs for progressive rheumatoid arthritis. Mayo Clinic Proc 55:161–179, 1980

10. Cooperating Clinics Committee of the American Rheumatism Association: A controlled trial of cyclophosphamide in rheumatoid arthritis. N Engl J Med 283:883–889, 1970

11. Townes AS, Sowa JM, Shulman LE: Controlled trial of cyclophosphamide in rheumatoid arthritis. Arthritis Rheum 19:563–573, 1976

12. Gerber LN, Steinberg AD: Clinical use of immunosuppressive drugs. Drugs 11:14–35, 1976

13. Dwosh IL, Stein HB, Urowitz MB, Smythe HA, Hunter T, Ogryzlo MA: Azathioprine in early rheumatoid arthritis: comparison with gold and chloroquine. Arthritis Rheum 20:685–692, 1977

14. Williams JH, Reading JC, Ward JR, O'Brien WM: Comparison of high and low dose cyclophosphamide therapy in rheumatoid arthritis. Arthritis Rheum 23:521–527, 1980

15. Woodland J, DeSaintonge DMC, Evans SJN, Sharman VL, Currey HLF: Azathioprine in rheumatoid arthritis: double-blind study of full versus half doses versus placebo. Ann Rheum Dis 40:355–359, 1981

16. DeSilva M, Hazleman BL: Long-term azathioprine in rheumatoid arthritis: a double-blind study. Ann Rheum Dis 40:560–563, 1981

17. Gottlieb NL: Chrysotherapy. Bull Rheum Dis 27:912–917, 1977

18. Berglöf F-E, Berglöf K, Walz DT: Auranofin: an oral chrysotherapeutic agent for the treatment of rheumatoid arthritis. J Rheumatol 5:68–74, 1978

19. Multicentre Trial Group: Controlled trial of D-penicillamine in severe rheumatoid arthritis. Lancet 1:275–280, 1973

20. Jaffe IA: D-penicillamine. Bull Rheum Dis 28:948–952, 1978

92. Principles in the use of immunosuppressive agents

Aberrant immune responses are generally considered to constitute important pathogenic factors in many of the connective tissue disorders. This belief has led to the increasing use of immunosuppressive drugs, agents designed to nonspecifically inhibit immune reactions. These drugs, referred to collectively as immunoregulatory agents, were originally introduced as antineoplastic compounds. Shortly thereafter, they were found to possess significant immune inhibitory activities. Although there are many drugs that have immunosuppressive properties, drugs of only 3 major categories—alkylating agents, purine analogs, and folic acid antagonists—are commonly used in the treatment of rheumatic disorders. This section will concentrate on the activities of agents of these classes. Others are considered in comprehensive reviews of drug-induced immunosuppression (1–9).

Immunoregulatory drugs exert both their antineoplastic and immunosuppressive activities by virtue of their capacity to inhibit cellular metabolic pathways or to kill proliferating cells. Some of their immune inhibitory properties are believed to result from a reduction in pools of immunologically competent lymphocytes (10). In experimental studies, the conditions required for immunosuppression have been delineated (1); in contrast, the factors necessary to achieve maximal effectiveness in clinical situations have not. In fact, the actual mechanisms through which these drugs act in many immunological disorders have not been fully defined. Furthermore, there are comparatively few controlled clinical trials ascertaining beneficial effects, and those available often present conflicting data (3,6,7).

Nevertheless, there is general agreement that, in selected patients, immunosuppressives are of significant therapeutic value. Those rheumatic disorders in which there are sufficient preliminary data available to ascertain effectiveness are rheumatoid arthritis, systemic lupus erythematosus, polyarteritis and other vasculitidies, Wegener's granulomatosis, polymyositis, psoriatic arthritis, chronic active hepatitis, inflammatory bowel diseases, autoimmune hemolytic anemia, and immune thrombocytopenia.

Clinical effects. Although each immunosuppressive possesses unique pharmacologic properties, all share activities which are of clinical importance. These common characteristics include:

1. The cytolytic and metabolic inhibitory activities of these drugs are not limited to immunologically competent lymphocytes or their progeny. These agents can be considered as nonselective "cell poisons" which are potentially able to affect the function of any cell and to impair the generation of several types of normal cells. These inhibitory properties are particularly evident in those cellular systems that depend on a rapid rate of renewal for homeostasis. These include bone marrow, gastrointestinal epithelium, and germinal centers of the gonads. As described below, much of the major toxicity associated with the immunosuppressive therapy results from the decreased rate of new cell formation in these tissues.

2. Cytotoxic drugs do not selectively inhibit a single immune response; rather, they serve to impair responses to a wide spectrum of antigens. Although the extent of immune inhibition is not uniform, the overall effect is to compromise the immune defense system. This results in an iatrogenic immune deficiency syndrome with all its attending consequences.

3. The clinical effectiveness of immunosuppressive therapy is very inconsistent and unpredictable. Several factors contribute to the difficulty in ascertaining therapeutic activity. In most disorders, the pathologic immune reactions have not been identified; thus, it is not possible to measure specific immunosuppression. Furthermore, there is no agreement as to suitable laboratory measures of overall immune inhibitory activity. Thus, the effectiveness of immunosuppressive therapy is based primarily on changes in clinical status. The changes in disease activity usually occur at a slow rate and generally require several months of treatment to assess clinical response. Controlled studies are essential in the evaluation of immunosuppressive drugs to differentiate changes in clinical disease status occurring as a result of the natural history of the disease from changes induced by immunosuppression.

General considerations of immunosuppression. The effects of immunoregulatory drugs on immunologically competent lymphocytes depend on 2 interrelated variables: the cell cycle specificity of the agent and the proliferative status of the target cells.

Cycle specificity. The cycle specificity is defined as the ability of an agent to exert cytotoxic activities according to the phase of the mitotic cycle (Table 92–1). Certain drugs act selectively in that they have no adverse effects on proliferating cells that are not in the vulnerable phase of their mitotic cycle. Cellular depletion is primarily restricted to tissues in which a high proportion of cells are actively replicating. By contrast, areas in which there is a slow rate of cell turnover, such as peripheral lymphoid, organs are not acutely depopulated. Agents showing these selective cytotoxic activities are designated as **phase-specific**; examples include methotrexate, which acts principally in the S phase of the cell cycle involving DNA synthesis, and vincristine which affects the M, or mitosis, phase.

Other drugs exert cytotoxic effects during several phases of the mitotic cycle. With respect to their immunosuppressive activitites, these compounds can deplete

Table 92–1. Classification of immunosuppressive agents

Phase-specific agents: drugs capable of exerting cytotoxic activity during a discrete phase of the mitotic cycle (e.g., methotrexate, vincristine)
Cycle-specific agents: drugs that are toxic to both intermitotic and actively cycling cells; maximum cytotoxicity is directed against proliferating cells (e.g., cyclophosphamide, chlorambucil)
Cycle nonspecific agents: agents that exert uniform cytotoxic activity for all cells regardless of their proliferative activities; these are equally effective against intermitotic and cycling cells (e.g., x-irradiation)

intermitotic cells, including immunologically competent lymphocytes. Based on their comparative toxicities for intermitotic and cycling cells, 2 groups of agents are distinguished, **cycle specific** and **cycle nonspecific**. The cycle specific group has greater cytotoxic activities against proliferating cells, whereas the cycle nonspecific group possesses uniform toxicities for all cells, regardless of their replicative status. Cyclophosphamide is the principal cycle specific compound used for clinical immunosuppression; x-irradiation represents an example of a cycle nonspecific mode of treatment.

Proliferative status. The proliferative status of immunologically competent cells represents the second factor that influences both lymphocytotoxicity and immunosuppression. The proliferative activities of lymphoid cells are primarily defined by their temporal relation to antigenic exposure (11,12). In the absence of an appropriate immunogen, responsive lymphocytes populate peripheral tissues in an intermitotic state. Shortly after stimulation, these responsive cells undergo rapid proliferative expansion that is followed by differentiation into mature immunologic effectors. In the T cell system, these are small intermitotic lymphocytes. Effectors in the B cell system are end-stage plasma cells lacking the capacity for further replication. Arbitrarily, the period between initial antigenic exposure and the development of differentiated effectors is designated as the *induction phase*; once effectors are formed, the reaction is considered to have entered an *effector phase*.

The kinetic characteristics of lymphocytes constitute the dominant factor determining the immunosuppressive activities of different cytotoxic drugs (13,14). In animal experiments, phase-specific agents are highly effective if their period of administration coincides with the induction phase of the response. However, they have no inhibitory activity if therapy is restricted to the interval prior to antigenic challenge. Furthermore, these drugs are, at best, minimally active during the established phase. Although cycle-specific drugs display maximum immunosuppressive activity during the induction phase, they are also active both before the antigen is present and once a reaction has entered an established phase.

Immunosuppressive drugs can have differential effects on the immune system leading to selective inhibition of humoral or cell-mediated responses. Cyclophosphamide is more potent in its ability to inhibit humoral immunity (15,16), whereas azathioprine has been considered to be more effective against cellular reactions (17). Furthermore, drug therapy can at times paradoxically enhance certain immune responses. Six-mercaptopurine (6-MP) given before antigen challenge can heighten antibody responses (18), whereas cyclophosphamide has been shown to augment certain cell-mediated reactions (19–21). The principal activities of these 2 immunosuppressives are summarized in Table 92–2.

Azathioprine. Azathioprine, a purine analog, is a nitroimidazole derivative of the antileukemic agent, 6-mercaptopurine (17). In vivo, azathioprine is converted into 6-MP by splitting off the imidizole group. This conversion significantly augments the immunosuppressive activity while reducing toxicity. The 6-MP is subsequently oxidized to thiouric acid by xanthine oxidase enzymes. Inhibition of xanthine oxidases with drugs such as allopurinol significantly decreases drug metabolism and enhances toxicity.

Azathioprine, or 6-MP, is incorporated into RNA as the ribonucleotide thioinosinic acid. This results in an interference with the interconversion of purine nucleotides and, by feedback inhibition, reduces purine biosynthesis. The 6-MP-ribonucleotide may also inhibit DNA synthesis.

As immunosuppressants, both 6-MP and azathioprine are highly effective if administered during the induction phase (14,22,23). This observation correlates with the clinical effectiveness in suppressing renal transplant rejection reactions. By contrast, if the immune effectors are in a nonproliferative phase of their cell cycle, these drugs are relatively ineffective as immunosuppressants (13,22,23). In clinical trials, it appears that this drug has significant therapeutic activity in several immunologically related disorders including rheumatoid arthritis (24–26), polymyositis (27), and psoriatic arthritis (28,29). Azathioprine is administered orally in doses of 1.5–2.5 mg/kg/day.

Cyclophosphamide. Cyclophosphamide, a cycle-specific alkylating agent, acts primarily by crosslinking complimentary DNA strands (9). Depending on the extent of cellular injury, affected cells can be killed immediately, sustain injuries that are subsequently lethal when the cell enters mitosis, or if repair can be effected, leave the cell intact. In contrast to azathioprine, cyclophosphamide is capable of depleting pools of intermitotic lymphocytes. This is reflected by a reduction in the blood lymphocyte concentration; the magnitude of this effect is dose-dependent.

In addition, cyclophosphamide inhibits the proliferative capacity of residual lymphocytes in vitro (13,30). However, it does not impair those activities that are independent of cellular replication. Thus, lymphocytes surviving cyclophosphamide therapy are capable of reacting normally in assays which assess cytotoxicity (31) and the release of lymphokines (30).

In animal studies, cyclophosphamide appears to be the single most effective cytotoxic immunosuppressant (1). It exerts inhibitory activities at all stages of the immune response. Experimentally, the maximum immunosuppressive activity occurs if drug therapy coincides with the induction period.

In general, humoral immune responses are suppressed to a greater extent than cell-mediated reactions (15,16,19,32). This finding correlates with observations indicating that this agent exerts a more sustained toxic effect on B lymphocytes compared with that on T cells (33–36). Recent studies have also emphasized that cyclophosphamide is capable of eliminating certain suppressor cells (19–21, 37,38). This cellular effect has been implicated as a factor leading to augmentation of certain cell-mediated responses.

Pharmacologically, cyclophosphamide is inactive until it is metabolized by the liver (39). The active moiety has not been identified; however, it is present in the

Table 92–2. Comparison of effects of cyclophosphamide and azathioprine

Effects	Cyclophosphamide	Azathioprine
Decreased primary immune responses	+++	+++
Decreased secondary immune responses	++	+
Decreased immune complexes in NZB/W mice	++	0
Antiinflammatory effects	+	++
Decreased delayed hypersensitivity	± to ++	++
Lymphopenia	+++	±
Inhibition of mitogenic responses	+++	0
Selectivity for B lymphocytes	++	0

circulation for only a brief interval. Cyclophosphamide has been effectively used in rheumatoid arthritis, Wegener's granulomatosis, and other connective tissue diseases (3,6,40). However, there is still debate regarding its ability to alter the course of lupus nephritis (41,42). Results of studies of cyclophosphamide combined with azathioprine or given as intermittent, intravenous therapy are inconclusive (43).

The drug can be administered either orally or parenterally. The usual oral dose is 1.5–2.5 mg/kg/day. It can be given in the form of bolus therapy; a typical dose schedule is 10–15 mg/kg administered intravenously at 3–4 week intervals.

Chlorambucil. Chlorambucil is an alkylating agent which has properties similar to cyclophosphamide. Few clinical studies evaluating this drug in the treatment of rheumatic diseases are available. The usual oral dose is 0.05 to 0.20 mg/kg/day.

Methotrexate. Methotrexate is a folic acid analog which binds the enzyme folic acid reductase with a far greater affinity than the natural substrate dihydrofolic acid. The binding prevents 1 carbon transfer required for thymidine, and thus DNA, synthesis. Therefore, methotrexate has its greatest effect on proliferating cells with little alteration of resting cells. In animal models, it has proved to be a highly effective immunosuppressant, capable of impairing both humoral and cell-mediated responses.

Uncontrolled clinical studies suggest the drug is of benefit in rheumatoid arthritis (44,45), psoriasis, psoriatic arthritis (29,46), and polymyositis (47). The usual oral dose is 5–30 mg weekly, frequently given as 3 divided doses separated by 12 hours. The drug can also be given intravenously in doses of 15–50 mg weekly. The metabolic block induced by methotrexate can be overcome by the administration of folinic acid.

Toxicity. Immunosuppressants are capable of causing several severe or even potentially fatal toxic reactions (Table 92–3) (48). The most prominent acute side effects involve those tissues with a rapid rate of cell renewal, i.e., those in the hematopoietic, gastrointestinal, and reproductive systems.

The ability of these drugs to interfere with the generation of hematopoietic precursors probably represents their most serious acute toxicity. Therapy can lead to neutropenia and/or thrombocytopenia, either of which may be of sufficient severity to result in severe and potentially fatal infection or bleeding. Because of the interval required for maturation of hematopoietic precursors, neutropenia and thrombocytopenia are not immediately evident after drug administration. Typically, the nadir in blood neutrophil counts occurs 10–14 days after a single injection of a cytotoxic drug. Platelet depression is most prominent after 7–10 days. With daily

Table 92–3. Toxicity of immunosuppressive drugs

Bone marrow depression (neutropenia, thrombocytopenia, anemia)
Gastrointestinal disturbances
Infections resulting from generalized depression of immune reactivity
Increased risk of teratogenesis
Increased risk of malignancies
Selective toxicities:
  azathioprine—hepatic dysfunction
  cyclophosphamide—alopecia, hemorrhagic cystitis, gonadal dysfunction
  methotrexate—stomatitis, megaloblastic anemia, hepatitis/cirrhosis

therapy, the effects tend to be cumulative. Careful attention to blood counts, with prompt adjustment in dosage can serve to minimize the risks of these toxicities.

Gastrointestinal manifestations are common and often represent a source of considerable discomfort to the patient. Major symptoms include abdominal pain, nausea, vomiting, and diarrhea. These drugs also possess teratogenic properties and, unless essential, they should not be used during pregnancy.

Immunosuppressive therapy has been associated with serious long-term side effects. Because these drugs compromise the immune defense system, patients who are treated with them tend to be vulnerable to opportunistic infections, such as *Pneumocystis carinii*, cytomegalic inclusion virus, and disseminated fungal diseases. Another potential consequence of impairment of the immune system is an increased risk of neoplasia (49). In particular, patients receiving immunosuppressants after renal transplantation show a frequency of lymphoma which has been estimated to be about 100 times that of an age-matched population. Furthermore, certain drugs, particularly the alkylating agents, may be leukemogenic.

In addition to the general toxicities that apply to all agents, each drug possesses certain unique side effects. Cyclophosphamide can produce alopecia, gonadal fibrosis, infertility, and hemorrhagic cystitis. The latter, due to an unidentified toxic metabolite, may produce massive hematuria; chronic drug use leads to an increased risk of bladder fibrosis and transitional cell carcinoma. Azathioprine has been rarely noted to cause a toxic hepatitis. Methotrexate may cause stomatitis, a megaloblastic anemia, and in some cases, hepatitis which may progress to cirrhosis.

Toxicity associated with therapy is of major clinical importance. Any decision regarding the institution of immunosuppressive therapy must entail careful considerations of the risk/benefit ratios. Because of the serious side effects, it is advisable to restrict immunosuppressive therapy to those patients with severe or potentially life-threatening diseases.

Corticosteroids. In addition to their antiinflammatory properties, corticosteroids also possess significant immune-modulating activities (50). Unfortunately, there has been considerable misunderstanding regarding the effects of these drugs on immune reactivity. This results primarily from the failure to identify species differences in susceptibility of lymphocytes to corticosteroid-induced lysis. In mice and rats, 2 animal species frequently used for immunologic studies, corticosteroids cause extensive lympholysis. In contrast, normal human lymphocytes are comparatively resistant to direct destruction by steroids. Because of these differences, animal studies may not yield data directly applicable to the clinical usage of these agents. The effects of corticosteroids on lymphocytes and immunity are summarized in Table 92–4.

Clinical studies indicate that the major effect of corticosteroids is to cause a transient redistribution of lymphocytes (51,52). Following a single injection, the blood lymphocyte count decreases, a result of a sequestration of these cells in tissue reservoirs. There is evidence suggesting that the major site of lymphocyte entrapment is the bone marrow. The nadir in the blood lymphocyte count is observed after 4–6 hours. Both T and B cells are affected; the T cells are more greatly reduced than B cells. Within 14 hours, the number of blood lymphocytes returns to normal. This redistribution effect recurs with each dose of corticosteroid. Although normal lymphocytes are comparatively resistant to lysis, certain neoplastic lymphoid cells, such as those in acute lymphoblastic leukemia, are highly sensitive.

Although their immunosuppressive activities have not been completely defined, corticosteroids are capable of suppressing both humoral and cell-mediated immune reactions. Continued administration of these agents decreases the serum concentrations of immunoglobulins (53); this effect appears to result primarily from de-

Table 92–4. Effects of corticosteroids on the immune reaction

Lymphocytes
  human lymphocytes resistant to corticosteroid-induced lysis
  transient lymphopenia due to sequestration of cells
  T cells reduced more than B cells
Humoral immune responses
  serum immunoglobulins modestly reduced
  antibody titers not acutely altered
  modification of reactions due to:
    impaired release of lyosomal enzymes and/or chemical mediators
    inhibition of phagocytosis
Cellular immunity
  impaired delayed responses; develops slowly
  mechanisms for immunosuppression not defined

creased immunoglobulin synthesis (53,54). However, antibody titers to specific antigens are not immediately altered (55).

In many autoimmune diseases, corticosteroids appear to act either by interfering with phagocytic activities and thereby limiting the cellular uptake of antigen–antibody complexes (56,57) or by impairing the release of lysosomal enzymes and other intracellular mediators which are responsible for tissue injury (58). The former mechanism may account for the beneficial effects of corticosteroids in disorders such as autoimmune hemolytic anemia. The latter effect serves to limit tissue injuries resulting from the deposition of toxic immune complexes.

Cell-mediated responses are also impaired by corticosteroids. It is well known that these compounds can cause cutaneous anergy. However, suppression of cutaneous delayed hypersensitivity tends to develop slowly. In general, skin test reactivity is lost after 10–14 days of therapy (50). The impaired cellular responses observed with corticosteroid therapy may be of prime importance in the predisposition of patients to tuberculosis and other infections due to intracellular pathogens. At present, the mechanisms responsible for impaired cell responses have not been fully defined; they probably result from a blockade at the level of lymphocyte–macrophage interaction.

1. Makinadon T, Santos GW, Quinn RP: Immunosuppressive drugs. Pharmacol Rev 22:189–247, 1970
2. Steinberg AD, Plotz PH, Wolff SM, Wong VG, Agus SG, Decker JL: Cytotoxic drugs in treatment of nonmalignant diseases. Ann Intern Med 76:619–642, 1972
3. Skinner MD, Schwartz RS: Immunosuppressive therapy. New Engl J Med 287:221–227, 281–296, 1972
4. Decker JL, Bertino JR, Hurd ER, Steinberg AD: Cytotoxic drugs in rheumatic diseases. Arthritis Rheum 16:79–96, 1973
5. Kaplan SR, Calabresi P: Immunosuppressive agents. New Engl J Med 289:952–955, 1234–1236, 1973
6. Gerber NL, Steinberg AD: Clinical use of immunosuppressive drugs. Drugs 11:14–35, 90–112, 1976
7. Bach JF: The Mode of Action of Immunosuppressive Agents. Amsterdam, Elsevier-North Holland, 1975
8. Chabner BA, Myers CE, Coleman CN, Johns DG: The clinical pharmacology of antineoplastic agents. New Engl J Med 292:1107–1113, 1159–1168, 1975
9. Webb DR, Winkelstein A: Immunosuppression and immunopotentiation, Basic and Clinical Immunology. Ed 2. HH Fudenberg, DP Stiles, JL Caldwell, JV Wells, eds. Los Altos, CA, Lange Medical Publications, 1978, pp 308–321
10. Winkelstein A, Kift BL, Sternkopf EJ: The effect of cytotoxic immunosuppressants on in vivo and in vitro parameters of T cell function, Proceedings of Conference on Immunopharmacology. NE Rosenthale, HC Mansmann Jr, eds. New York, Spectrum Publications, 1975, pp 213–229
11. Craddock CG, Longmire R, McMillan R: Lymphocytes and the immune response. New Engl J Med 285:324–331, 378–384, 1971
12. Winkelstein A, Rabin BS: Lymphocyte biology. Bull Rheum Dis 25:816–821, 822–827, 1974
13. Winkelstein A: Effect of cytotoxic immunosuppressants on tuberculin sensitive lymphocytes in guinea pigs. J Clin Invest 56:1587–1596, 1975
14. Lin HS: Schedule-dependent effects of phase-specific cytotoxic agents on production of hemolytic plaque-forming cells. J Natl Cancer Inst 56:95–99, 1976
15. Leppner GH, Calabresi P: Selective suppression of humoral immunity by antineoplastic drugs. Annu Rev Pharmacol Toxicicol 16:367–379, 1976
16. Otterness IG, Chang YH: Cooperative study of cyclophosphamide, 6-mercaptopurine, azathioprine and methotrexate. Clin Exp Immunol 26:346–354, 1976
17. Elion GB: Immunosuppressive agents. Transplant Proc 9:975–979, 1977
18. Chanmougan D, Schwartz RS: Enhancement of antibody synthesis by 6-mercaptopurine. J Exp Med 124:363–378, 1966
19. Turk JL, Parker D, Poulter LW: Functional aspects of the selective depletion of lymphoid tissues by cyclophosphamide. Immunology 23:493–501,1972
20. LaGrange PH, Mackaness GB, Miller TE: Potentiation of T cell mediated immunity by selective suppression of antibody formation with cycloprosphamide. J Exp Med 139:1529–1539, 1974
21. Askenase PW, Hayden BJ, Gerson RK: Augmentation of delayed-type hypersensitivity by doses of cyclophosphamide which do not affect antibody responses. J Exp Med 141:697–702, 1975
22. Winkelstein A, Craddock CG, Lawrence JS: Cell replication in the primary hemolysin response: the effect of six mercaptopurine. J Reticulendothel Soc 9:307–322, 1971
23. Phillips SM, Zweiman B: Mechanisms in the suppression of delayed hypersensitivity in the guinea pig by 6-mercaptopurine. J Exp Med 137:1494–1510, 1973
24. Hunter T, Urowitz MB, Gordon DA, Symthe HA, Ogryzlo MA: Azathioprine in rheumatoid arthritis: a long-term followup study. Arthritis Rheum 18:15–25, 1975
25. DeSilva M, Hazelman BL: Long-term azathioprine in rheumatoid arthritis: a double-blind study. Ann Rheum Dis 40:560–563, 1981
26. Woodland J, Chaput de Saintonge DM, Evans SJW, Sharman VL, Currey HLF: Azathioprine in rheumatoid arthritis: a double-blind study of full versus half doses versus placebo. Ann Rheum Dis 40:355–359, 1981
27. Bunch TW: Prednisone and azathioprine for polymyositis: long-term followup. Arthritis Rheum 24:45–48,1981
28. Baum J, Hurd E, Lewis D, Ferguson JL, Ziff M: Treatment of psoriatic arthritis with 6-mercaptopurine. Arthritis Rheum 16:139–147, 1973
29. McDonald CJ: The uses of systemic chemotherapeutic agents in psoriasis. Pharmacol Ther 14:1–24, 1981
30. Winkelstein A: Differential effects of immunosuppressants on lymphocyte function. J Clin Invest 52:2293–2299, 1973
31. Winkelstein A, Brizzi J, Kift BL: The effect of cyclophosphamide on mitogen-induced and antibody-dependent cytotoxicity in guinea pigs. J Immunopharmacol 1:139–156, 1979
32. Salvin SB, Smith RF: The specificity of allergic reactions. IV. Immunologic unresponsiveness, delayed hypersensitivity and circulating antibody to proteins and hapten-protein conjugates in adult guinea pig. J Exp Med 119:851–868, 1964
33. Poulter LW, Turk JL: Proportional increase in theta carrying lymphocytes in peripheral lymphoid tissues following treatment with cyclophosphamide. Nature 238:17–18, 1972
34. Stockman GD, Heim LR, South MA, Trenton JJ: Differential effect of cyclophosphamide on the B and T compartments of adult mice. J Immunol 110:277–282, 1973
35. Fauci AS, Dale DC, Wolff SM: Cyclophosphamide and lymphocyte subpopulations in Wegener's granulomatosis. Arthritis Rheum 17:355–361, 1974
36. Hurowitz DA: Selective depletion of Ig-bearing lymphocytes by cyclophosphamide in rheumatoid arthritis and systemic lupus erythematosus: guidelines for dosage. Arthritis Rheum 17:363–374, 1974
37. Gershon RK: T cell control antibody production. Contemp Topics Immunobiol 3:1–40, 1974
38. Zembala M, Asherson GL: The effect of cyclophosphamide and irradiation on cells which suppress contact sensitivity in the mouse. Clin Exp Immunol 23:554–561, 1976
39. Gershwin ME, Goetzl EJ, Steinberg AD: Cyclophosphamide: use in practice. Ann Intern Med 80:531–540, 1974
40. Cooperating Clinics Committee of the American Rheumatism Association: A controlled trial of cyclophosphamide in rheumatoid arthritis. New Engl J Med 283:883–889, 1970
41. Klippel JH: Studies in the treatment of lupus nephritis. Ann Intern Med 91:599–602, 1979
42. Donadio JV Jr, Holley KE, Ferguson RH, Illstrup DM: Treatment of lupus nephritis with prednisone and cyclophosphamide. New Engl J Med 299:1151–1155, 1978
43. Dinant HJ, Decker JL, Klippel JH, Balow JE, Plotz PH, Steinberg AD: Alternative modes of cyclophosphamide and azathioprine therapy in lupus nephritis. Ann Intern Med 96:728–736, 1982
44. Wilkins RF, Watson MA, Paxson CS: Low dose pulse methotrexate therapy in rheumatoid arthritis. J Rheumatol 7:501–505, 1980
45. Michaels RM, Nashel DJ, Leonard A, Sliwinski AJ, Derbes SJ: Weekly intravenous methotrexate in the treatment of rheumatoid arthritis. Arthritis Rheum 25:339–341, 1982
46. Roenigk HH Jr, Aurbach R, Maibach HI, Weinstein GD: Methotrexate guidelines revised. J Am Acad Dermatol 6:145–155, 1982
47. Metzger AL, Bohan A, Goldberg LS, Bluestone R, Pearson CM: Polymyositis and dermatomyositis: combined methotrexate and corticosteroid therapy. Ann Intern Med 81:182–189, 1974
48. Schein PS, Winokur SH: Immunosuppressive and cytotoxic chemotherapy: long-term complications. Ann Intern Med 82:84–95, 1975
49. Penn I, Starzl TE: Immunosuppression and cancer. Transplant Proc 5:943–947, 1973
50. Claman HN: Corticosteroids and lymphoid cells. New Engl J Med 287:388–397, 1972
51. Fauci AS, Dale DC: The effect of in vivo hydrocortisone on subpopulations of human lymphocytes. J Clin Invest 53:240–246, 1974
52. Yu DTY, Clements PJ, Paulus HE, Peter JB, Levy J, Barnett EV: Human lymphocyte subpopulations: effect of corticosteroids. J Clin Invest 53:565–571, 1974
53. Butler WT: Corticosteroids and immunoglobulin synthesis. Transplant Proc 7:49–53, 1975
54. McMillan R, Longmire R, Yelenosky R: The effect of corticosteroids on human IgG synthesis. J Immunol 116:1592–1595, 1976
55. Tuchinda M, Newcomb RW, DeVald BL: Effect of prednisone treatment on the human immune response to keyhole limpet hemocyanin. Int Arch Allergy 42:533–544, 1972
56. Rinehart JJ, Balcerzak SP, Sagone AL, LoBuglio AF: Effects of corticosteroids on human monocyte function. J Clin Invest 54:1337–1343, 1974
57. Schreiber AD, Parsons J, McDermott P, Cooper RA: Effect of corticosteroids on the human monocyte IgG and complement receptors. J Clin Invest 56:1189–1197, 1975
58. Fauci AS, Dale DC, Balow JE: Glucocorticosteroid therapy: mechanisms of action and clinical considerations. Ann Intern Med 84:304–315, 1976

93. Intraarticular injection

Intraarticular injection has played an important role in the management of arthritis since hydrocortisone was introduced for this purpose in 1951 (1–3). Other drugs and preparations, including phenylbutazone, sodium salicylate, urokinase, and benzyl salicylate in oil, have also exerted antiphlogistic effects when injected directly into inflamed joints. However, these compounds offer no therapeutic advantage and are irritating compared with steroids (4). Other agents, such as osmic acid (5) and radioisotopes (6), have been injected intraarticularly to necrose inflamed synovium, but are not generally used in the United States. The antibiotic, rifamycin, has also been used and may be effective in inhibiting protein synthesis (7).

Rationale and advantages. The major objective of intrasynovial therapy is to enter a joint space, tendon sheath, or bursa, remove any excess fluid, and instill the corticosteroid suspension that will provide the most effective relief of pain and promote resolution of inflammation for the longest time. Reaccumulation of effusion may be inhibited in part by a local effect on vascular permeability (8). Systemic "spillover" after absorption of the locally injected corticosteroid may occur, varying with the amount and solubility of the preparation administered.

Advantages of local injection consist of the minimization of the hazards inherent in systemic administration of corticosteroids and the direct application of potent medication to a confined site of disease. Arthrocentesis also permits the aspiration of synovial fluid as a useful diagnostic aid.

Indications. It is important to remember that intrasynovial therapy is an adjunctive measure and except for certain regional problems such as traumatic synovitis or olecranon bursitis, it constitutes only one

part of a comprehensive treatment program.

The indications for intrasynovial treatment are summarized in Table 93–1. Although intrasynovial therapy is essentially palliative, it frequently provides striking and sometimes durable relief of pain and disability. This form of therapy is especially useful in patients with rheumatoid arthritis in whom troublesome involvement is limited to only one or a few peripheral joints.

Contraindications and complications. Infection in the vicinity of the site to be injected or a generalized infection is a contraindication to the local instillation of a corticosteroid. However, in some patients with infections, intraarticular therapy may be carried out along with appropriate antibiotic therapy if the indication is deemed urgent. The risk of provoking serious bleeding in patients receiving anticoagulants must be considered.

Badly damaged joints of the lower extremities, such as an unstable knee, should not be injected with corticosteroids unless there is a relatively large inflammatory effusion and the patient will cooperate by adhering to a nonweight-bearing schedule for several weeks after the injection.

Despite some systemic effects, the morphologic changes of hypercortisonism or other undesirable metabolic effects of corticosteroids rarely occur as a consequence of intrasynovial injections. The frequency of an infection of the joint as an aftermath of local injection is extremely small. Local adverse reactions are minor. The so-called post-injection flare begins shortly after injection. This usually subsides within a few hours, but may rarely persist as long as 48–72 hours. Some of these reactions represent synovitis due to corticosteroid

ester crystals. Some mild synovial fluid leukocytic reaction appears to occur after most injections but has no effect on subsequent response (7). Another infrequent complication is localized atrophy of the skin or subcutaneum.

It has been suggested that the relief after the introduction of corticosteroid leads to "overuse" of the involved joint, causing additional cartilage and bone deterioration, giving rise to a so-called Charcot-like steroid arthropathy. Study of the joints of rabbits indicates that frequently repeated injections of soluble corticosteroids may interfere with protein synthesis in articular cartilage. The joints of monkeys injected intrasynovially with corticosteroids appear to respond differently, however (9). The harmful effect on cartilage observed in rabbits was not demonstrated. In addition, a recent investigation of patients who received frequently repeated corticosteroid injections into the knees did not support the contention that corticosteroids inevitably lead to acclerated joint destruction (10).

Table 93–1. Indications for intrasynovial corticosteroid therapy

1. For relief of synovitis in tendon sheaths, bursae, or joints in inflammatory, non-infectious arthropathies, or tenosynovial disorders
2. To suppress and control inflammation when one or only a few peripheral joints are inflamed, provided infection has been excluded as the cause
3. In a few particularly troublesome inflamed joints in a patient with otherwise well controlled polyarthritis
4. To facilitate a rehabilitative and physical therapy program
5. To support the patient with rheumatoid arthritis and other active joint inflammation pending the effects of other systemic, disease-remitting therapy, such as chrysotherapy
6. When systemic therapy is contraindicated

Table 93–2. Injectable corticosteroids

Repository preparation	Quantity per ml
Hydrocortisone tertiary butyl acetate	50 mg
Prednisolone tertiary butyl acetate	20 mg
Dexamethasone acetate	8 mg
Betamethasone acetate and disodium phosphate	3, 6 mg
Methylprednisolone acetate	20, 40, 80 mg
Triamcinolone acetonide	40 mg
Triamcinolone diacetate	40 mg
Triamcinolone hexacetonide	20 mg

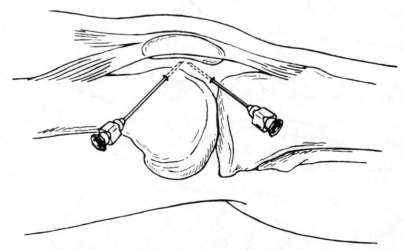

Fig 93–1. Arthrocentesis of knee (medial approach). (Illustration provided by Dr D Neustadt)

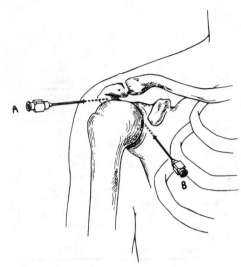

Fig 93–2. A, Injection of subacromial bursa or supraspinatus tendon; **B**, anterior approach for injection of glenohumeral joint. (Illustration provided by Dr D Neustadt)

Choice of drug. Hydrocortisone and a variety of available repository preparations are listed in Table 93–2.

All corticosteroids, with the exception of cortisone and prednisone, exert a prompt and significant antiphlogistic effect when injected into an inflamed joint. The most soluble corticosteroid suspension is absorbed rapidly and has a short duration of effect. The duration of action of the less readily soluble tertiary-butylacetate (TBA) ester is more prolonged. Although an occasional patient may obtain greater benefit from one derivative than another, no single corticosteroid has been shown to have a convincing margin of superiority with the possible exception of triamcinolone hexacetonide (2).

Dosage and administration. The dose of any microcrystalline suspension used for intrasynovial injection must be arbitrarily selected. The following is a useful guide: for small joints of the hand and feet, 2.5–15 mg of prednisolone suspension or equivalent; for medium size joints such as the wrists and elbows, 10–20 mg; for the knee, ankle, and the shoulder, 20–50 mg; and for the hip 25–50 mg. Occasionally it is necessary to give larger amounts to obtain optimal results.

The longer the intervals between intraarticular injections, the better. A 4 week minimum is suggested in general and an interval of 8–12 weeks for weight-bearing joints. After knee injections, the patient can be advised to remain at bed rest for a few days with the exception of bathroom visits and meals. Crutches may then be prescribed to be used with 3-point gait to protect the injected joint for 2–4 weeks. This routine facilitates a sustained improvement and avoids the hazard of overworking the injected joint.

Techniques and general considerations. Arthrocentesis is easily and relatively painlessly performed in a joint distended with fluid or one in which synovial proliferation is present. The preferred site of entry for most joints is the extensor surface, avoiding the large nerves and major vessels, which are usually present on the flexor surface. A local anesthetic is sometimes desirable, especially when entering a relatively "dry" joint, in which only a small amount of fluid is present. Aspiration of as much synovial fluid as possible before instillation of the corticosteroid suspension reduces the dilution factor. Gentle manipulation, carrying the joint through its excursions of motion, facilitates diffusion of the injected medication.

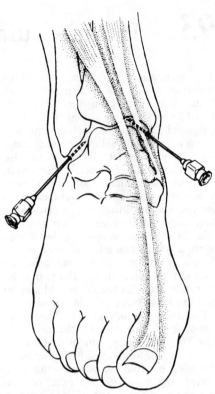

Fig 93–4. Arthrocentesis of ankle joint (medial and lateral approaches). (Illustration provided by Dr D Neustadt)

Specific joints. The joints frequently requiring injection are the knee, shoulder, elbow, wrist, ankle, and small joints of hands and feet. Less commmonly injected joints include the hip and temporomandibular joint.

The knee. The knee joint contains the largest synovial space in the body and is the most commonly aspirated and injected joint. Aspiration of the knee is usually carried out with the leg extended as much as possible. The joint is usually entered medially or laterally beneath the undersurface of the patella (Fig 93–1). The less frequently employed infrapatellar route is useful when the knee cannot be fully extended and only minimal fluid is present.

The shoulder. The anterior approach to the glenohumeral joint is the simplest entry. The needle is directed mediodorsally in the groove between the medial aspect of the humeral head at a point just inferior to the tip of the coracoid process (Fig 93–2).

The posterior approach is sometimes preferred because it is out of the patient's line of vision. Internal rotation of the shoulder with adduction of the patient's arm across the chest wall and with the hand resting on the opposite shoulder eases the task of insertion which is made just below (1–2 cm) the posterolateral angle of the posterior aspect of the acromion.

Supraspinatus tendon and subacromial bursa. The lateral approach is used, sliding the needle below the lateral aspect of the acromion just superior to the greater

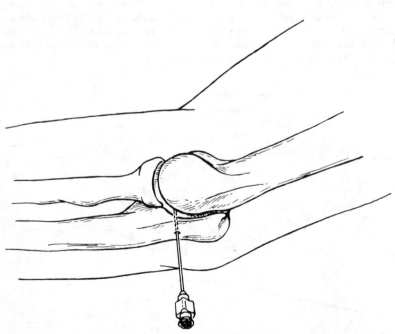

Fig 93–3. Arthrocentesis of elbow. (Illustration provided by Dr D Neustadt)

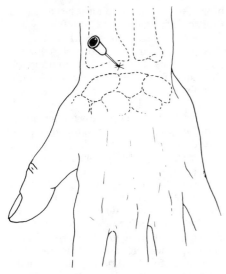

Fig 93–5. Arthrocentesis of the wrist (radial approach). (Illustration provided by Dr D Neustadt)

tuberosity and head of the humerus (Fig 93–2).

The elbow. This joint can usually be readily entered via the posterolateral approach. With the joint incompletely extended and held in a relaxed position, the bulge of the synovial effusion is noted posterolaterally, just outside the olecranon process and inferior to the lateral humeral epicondyle. The needle is introduced just lateral to the olecranon process and just below the lateral epicondyle. The needle is directed medially, proximal to the radial head. The radial head can be easily identified by pronating and supinating the forearm (Fig 93–3).

The ankle (tibiotalar joint). The ankle joint may be difficult to enter. The usual point of entry is just medial to the extensor hallucis longus tendon (Fig 93–4). A lateral approach can be used by directing the needle just inside the fibula.

The wrist joint. Radial or lateral entry is made on the dorsum of the wrist with the hand slightly flexed, most commonly at a point on the dorsum just lateral to the extensor tendon of the thumb (Fig 93–5). The ulnar or medial entry of the joint space may be made by inserting the needle into the space just below the lateral ulnar margin in the palpable gap between this border and the carpus. The dorsal approach avoids the radial artery and the ulnar and median nerves.

Joints of the hands and feet. The carpometacarpal joint of the thumb is commonly affected in osteoarthritis. With the thumb adducted and held in flexion within the palm, injection is carried out from the dorsal side, inserting the needle at the point of maximum tenderness. The metacarpophalangeal and interphalangeal joints are entered on the dorsal surface, the needle being inserted beneath the extensor tendon from either the lateral or medial side.

Other conditions that may respond to intrasynovial therapy include carpal tunnel syndrome, trigger fingers, deQuervain's and other forms of tenosynovitis, trochanteric and gluteal bursitis, bicipital and achilles tendinitis, plantar fasciitis, epicondylitis, and ganglia. Techniques and special procedures for successful injection of these problems are available (2).

1. Hollander JL: Arthrocentesis and intrasynovial therapy, Arthritis and Allied Conditions, ed 9. DJ McCarty, Jr, ed. Philadelphia, Lea & Febiger, 1979, pp 402–414.
2. Steinbrocker O, Neustadt DH: Aspiration and Injection Therapy in Arthritis and Musculoskeletal Disorders. Hagerstown, Maryland, Harper & Row, 1972
3. Editorial: Intra-articular steroids. Br Med J 1:600–601, 1978
4. Neustadt DH, Steinbrocker O: Observations on the effects of intra-articular phenylbutazone. J Lab Clin Med 47:284–288, 1956
5. Sheppard H, Ward DJ: Intraarticular osmic acid in rheumatoid arthritis: 5 years experience. Rheum Rehab 19:25–29, 1980
6. Lee P: The efficacy and safety of radiosynovectomy. J Rheumatol 9:165–167, 1982
7. Caruso I, Montrone F, Fumagelli M, et al: Rheumatoid knee synovitis successfully treated with intraarticular rifamycin SV. Ann Rheum Dis 41:232–236, 1982
8. Eymontt MJ, Gordon GV, Schumacher HR, Hansell JR: The effects on synovial premeability and synovial fluid leukocyte counts in symptomatic osteoarthritis after intraarticular corticosteroid administration. J Rheumatol 9:198–203, 1982
9. Gibson T, Burry HC, Poswillo D: Effect of intraarticular corticosteroid injections on primate cartilage. Ann Rheum Dis 36:74–79, 1976
10. Balch HW, Gibson JMC, El-Ghobarey AF: Repeated corticosteroid injections into knee joints. Rheum Rehab 16:137–140, 1977

94. Surgical management of arthritis

Although the general consequences of joint damage due to arthritis are similar, significant differences exist between that caused by osteoarthritis and rheumatoid arthritis. Indeed, there are unique surgical aspects to many of the joint diseases. In some instances, these unique features place the patient at special risk from surgery; in others, they jeopardize the eventual result. These features serve to emphasize 2 philosophical points: 1) the surgeon who operates on patients with arthritis, especially on those with rheumatoid arthritis, should be familiar with the special technical aspects necessitated by the unusual requirements of the patient with multiple joint involvement, and 2) the surgeon should be part of a team composed of rheumatologist, nurses, therapists, social workers, as well as the patient.

The fact must be emphasized that the surgical patient with rheumatoid arthritis is frequently weak and discouraged and must face the prospect of a series of operations before achieving reasonable functional independence. Often the patient has excessive expectations with regard to the outcome of surgery (1). By participating in the planning and timing of the surgical events, the patient can better comprehend the duration of treatment, the necessity of prolonged physical therapy, and the eventual realistic goal of the procedure.

Since relief of pain is the most consistent effect of reconstructive surgery, pain is the primary indication for most operative interventions. Restoration of motion and function, distinct from relief of pain, is less predictable and requires careful assessment of each patient's disability before improvement can be anticipated.

Some surgical procedures in rheumatoid arthritis are prophylactic as well as therapeutic (e.g., synovectomy, fusion of the first and second cervical vertebrae, fusion of the base of the thumb). The patients should understand the preventive aspects so that there will be no disappointment when the therapeutic result does not seem to justify the pain and inconvenience of surgery (1).

The surgical patient with rheumatoid arthritis has an average length of hospitalization of about 18 days and may require 2 to 6 or more major procedures. Without putting a dollar value on the "quality of life," can such extensive procedures be justified by society? One recent study of 16 patients undergoing bilateral hip and knee replacement showed that none of those patients returned to work after this expensive series of operations involving an average of 3 months of hospitalization (2).

Though precise data are not yet available, preliminary studies strongly suggest that society does benefit in terms of decreased need for home help, home modifications, hospitalization or confinement to an institution because of loss of independent functional capacity, and release of the spouse from his or her helping role, allowing the spouse's return to the work force. For many individual patients, however, the goal must be relief of pain, restoration of some functional independence, and a qualitative improvement in their existence without the expectation of pure economic justification (3).

Certainly the major single advance in the care of patients with arthritis has been the development of total joint replacement (4). The concepts initially involved in replacement of the arthritic hip have now been expanded to cover most of the other appendicular joints. In patients with osteoarthritis, there are numerous alternatives to joint replacement, many of which are preferable, especially in younger patients. In patients with rheumatoid arthritis, procedures such as arthrodesis, synovectomy, repair of ruptured tendons, and other nonprosthetic procedures still play an important role. For predictable relief of pain and restoration of function, however, joint replacement surgery has revolutionized the outlook for patients with multiple joint involvement. The special problems presented by patients with rheumatoid arthritis deserve emphasis and serve to illustrate many principles applicable to patients with osteoarthritis.

Preoperative evaluation

Medical considerations. The first consideration is whether a painful joint in a patient with arthritis requires surgery. If synovitis is the cause of the patient's pain and disability, medical management with drugs and physical modalities is appropriate. If it can be determined that structural damage to the joint is the problem, then it is unrealistic to expect that medication will be sufficient.

A trial of antiinflammatory medication and physical therapy is appropriate, particularly for the weight-bearing joints where the use of crutches may allow acute disabling symptoms to subside to an acceptable level, even in the presence of structural damage. If these measures fail and structural damage can be demonstrated on physical examination or by radiographic examination, arthrodesis or arthroplasty can be considered. It is better to perform surgery on each joint as it becomes destroyed than to wait until the patient has a multitude of badly damaged joints requiring prolonged hospitalization, multiple anesthetics, and a series of debilitating surgical procedures.

General operative risk should be assessed, especially consideration of the systemic manifestations of the rheumatic diseases. The patient should be in optimal medical condition and, when being treated with corticosteroids, should be taking the lowest possible maintenance dose. Sources of infection should be identified and eradicated to prevent postoperative hematogenous seeding of the operative site. Carious teeth should be cared for, and if necessary, extracted before surgery on the joints.

Urinary tract infections should be identified and treated. Many women have asymptomatic bacteriuria, and urine culture before surgery is an absolute requirement. In men, prostatic hypertrophy, if severe, should be treated before surgery to avoid postoperative catheterization with its attendant risk of infection and bacterial seeding. It is useful to determine if the patient is able to void in the supine position. Frequently, preoperative practice at supine voiding will facilitate this function in the postoperative period.

Patient cooperation. Most difficult to evaluate is the patient's motivation and ability to participate meaningfully in the postoperative program. Patients should be evaluated by physical and occupational therapists, both to assess their ability to participate in the program and to determine what special requirements they may present during the postoperative period. Instruction in crutch ambulation before surgery shortens the need for training in the postoperative instruction period.

If multiple procedures are envisioned, it is often useful to perform a simple procedure first in order to assess the ability of the patient to follow the postoperative program. If both hips and knees require surgery, the hip can be used for this assessment. The relief of pain and improvement in function following hip arthroplasty are essentially independent of the patient's cooperation. The postoperative period is characterized by minimal pain. If the patient is unable to cooperate with a therapy program following hip replacement, it is unlikely that he or she will be able to participate in the postoperative program following a more painful arthroplasty that requires maximal patient cooperation.

The arthritis patient. Patients with **rheumatoid arthritis** or other systemic rheumatic diseases pose certain special problems that can influence the results and risks of surgery. The patient with rheumatoid arthritis frequently has multiple joints involved, each interfering with the function of the others. The rheumatoid patient undergoing surgery is on the average 10 years younger than the patient with osteoarthritis undergoing similar procedures and therefore has longer to live with a prosthetic joint (5). This means that there will be more time for complications to appear, such as delayed infection, late loosening, and wear of the component parts.

Much has been written of the increased susceptibility to infection in patients with rheumatoid arthritis (6,7), and it has been demonstrated that the patient undergoing total hip replacement does have a significantly increased risk of late hematogenous seeding of the prosthetic joint (8).

Approximately 10% of patients coming to surgery are on corticosteroid therapy, which some studies show increases the risk of infection (9). Steroids can also produce friable, easily torn skin. Because of this, the nursing staff must be cautioned to handle patients very carefully while they are sedated or anesthetized.

Aspirin, used by almost all patients, may produce difficulties with intraoperative and postoperative bleeding. Aspirin therapy may be discontinued a week before surgery and replaced with pure analgesics if there have been coagulation problems. In patients taking immunosuppressive drugs, the effect of these agents on postoperative infection must be considered (10,11).

In spite of controversy about the effect of penicillamine on wound healing (12–14), most experienced surgeons are of the opinion that healing of patients receiving this compound is definitely delayed. Thus, penicillamine therapy may delay the postoperative rehabilitation program until wound healing is satisfactory.

Both clinical and laboratory evidence suggests that the rheumatoid process is perpetuated in a given joint by retention of articular cartilage (15,16). Whether this is because of sequestered antigen–antibody complexes, the continued release of cartilage breakdown products that produce synovial inflammation, or undiscovered factors in unknown. It has been frequently observed, however, that patients in whom the patellar cartilage is retained after total knee replacement will have involvement of the prosthetic joint in systemic exacerbations of the disease. However, patients in whom all cartilage has been removed will not experience involvement of the prosthetic knee in such flare-ups.

The patient with **juvenile arthritis** presents certain unique features that directly influence the expected results of surgical intervention. As in patients with ankylosing spondylitis, there appears to be a much greater involvement of the soft tissues surrounding the joint in many of these individuals with the result that the ultimate range of motion achieved after joint arthroplasty is less than would be predicated from the range achieved at surgery (17).

Following arthroplasty, there is a progressive loss of motion in these patients, and the effect of this loss on ultimate functional capacity must be anticipated (18). The young age at which some patients with juvenile arthritis undergo arthroplasty exposes their prosthetic joints to both greater functional demands and a longer period of exposure to late complications, such as infection and loosening (19). In addition, some of these patients have severe micrognathia, which may make intubation difficult and/or produce postoperative respiratory problems (20).

The patient with **ankylosing spondylitis** has diminished chest excursion and is therefore at greater risk for postoperative pulmonary problems. Because of rigidity of the cervical spine, intubation is extremely difficult. Sometimes preoperative tracheostomy is required before an anesthetic agent can be delivered. Ossification in the anulus fibrosus and spinal ligaments can create great difficulty in carrying out spinal anesthesia; careful assessment by the anesthesiologist is useful in choosing the appropriate type and route of anesthetic and in anticipating difficulties.

Following total hip replacement, the patient with ankylosing spondylitis frequently fails to regain the same range of motion achieved by patients with rheumatoid arthritis or osteoarthritis (21). This is due not only to the increased involvement of the periarticular soft tissues seen in this disease, but also to an increased frequency of heterotopic ossification in the muscles and capsules surrounding the hip joint (22). Although the range of motion achieved may be only 65 degrees of hip flexion, this is often a significant improvement in the patient's function and independence (23). If advised of this preoperatively, the patient can make a more informed decision regarding the desirability of surgery and is less likely to experience disappointment in the postoperative period.

Patients with **psoriatic arthritis** sometimes have skin involvement in the area of the proposed surgical incision. Several papers report the frequent contamination of psoriatic skin by microorganisms and suggest an increased risk of infection following incision through such skin (24–26). It would appear to be desirable to clear up the skin in the operative site by appropriate local therapy before surgery.

The arthropathies related to **chronic inflammatory intestinal disease** pose a special threat of postoperative infection because of both late hematogenous seeding from a focus of infection in the bowel and the occasional source of contamination from the colostomy in proximity to the incision for hip replacement.

Systemic lupus erythematosus presents a very difficult problem for both the patient and the physician. The patients are often young and under treatment with large doses of corticosteroids and may have a near-normal life expectancy when they develop osteonecrosis (27). To implant a prosthetic joint in a young patient invites the long-term failures related to wear and loosening; to do so in a patient on long-term treatment with corticosteroids adds the further risk of infection. Renal involvement in these patients may limit their life expectancy.

In these young patients, prosthetic replacement may well be justified to relieve pain and improve the quality of life for the remaining years. On the other hand, in the patient with a normal life expectancy, there will almost certainly be late problems following joint replacement in the third and fourth decades. The development of avascular necrosis of a femoral condyle in these patients results in pain,

deformity, and functional loss. It may be better to accept the lesser benefit from a high tibial osteotomy than to carry out joint replacement surgery with the high probability of eventual complication.

Individual joints. In addition to the systemic problems presented by patients with rheumatoid arthritis, the involvement of multiple joints often creates special difficulties. Since the patient will require crutches after lower extremity surgery, it is essential to evaluate the patient's ability to use crutches before the operation. If there is extensive involvement of the shoulder, elbow, or wrist, axillary crutches may not be appropriate. Forearm crutches will sometimes be a suitable alternative, particularly if involvement of the wrist or elbow makes the use of axillary crutches painful.

Occasionally, it will be necessary to perform arthrodesis of the **wrist** before surgery on the lower extremities so that the patient will be able to use forearm crutches in the postoperative period.

In addition, patients who do not have 100 degrees of **knee** flexion find it difficult to arise from a seated position without applying major force to the upper extremity. If the upper extremities are unable to cope with these forces, special attention must be directed to obtaining maximal hip and knee flexion after surgery to minimize the need for upper extremity assistance (2).

The **elbow and shoulder** require arthroplasty less often than the weight-bearing joints of the lower extremity. Indeed, relieving the patient of the need to use crutches by performing arthroplasties of the hips and knees often diminishes shoulder pain to a tolerable level. The shoulder achieves great compensatory motion by virtue of the mobile scapula. Unremitting pain, however, may suggest the need for shoulder arthroplasty. In some patients, pain or lack of motion with the attendant difficulty in placing the hand in a functional position requires surgical treatment of the elbow; synovectomy (with or without radial head excision) may be adequate (28). If pain is relieved after synovectomy or if motion is insufficient, elbow replacement is appropriate.

Both **hips** of patients with rheumatoid arthritis are usually affected, even though only one may require arthroplasty. Involvement of the contralateral hip will handicap the patient's postoperative recovery and may diminish the ultimate range of motion achieved in the operated hip. If it is obvious that both hips will require arthroplasty, it is preferable to carry out both procedures during the same hospitalization to facilitate functional recovery. Except under unusual circumstances such as extremely difficult and hazardous intubation, it is rarely justifiable to carry out bilateral total hip replacements during the same anesthetic (29).

Patients undergoing hip or knee arthroplasty are sometimes disappointed to find that painful **foot** deformities prevent comfortable ambulation after their extensive surgical procedures. In addition, the plantar surface of the feet and dorsum of the toes are subject to skin breakdown because of rheumatoid deformities. These may become sources of bacterial contamination following arthroplasty of more proximal joints. These areas of skin breakdown should be healed before surgery on proximal joints in order to prevent spread of infection. This can often be achieved by shoe modifications and protective footwear but may require surgical correction.

The **temporomandibular joint** is frequently involved in juvenile arthritis as well as in adult rheumatoid arthritis. In the child, temporomandibular joint dysfunction combined with micrognathia may cause difficulties with intubation and respiration following extubation (20). Careful preoperative analysis by the anesthesiologist will prevent some of these difficulties, and fiberoptic intubation will minimize trauma and postoperative laryngeal edema.

The **cervical spine** is involved significantly in 30–40% of patients with rheumatoid arthritis (30–32). Although this is usually not apparent to the patient, it should be considered in the preoperative evaluation to avoid the potentially disastrous consequences of excessive manipulation of the neck during intubation. In the patient with marked C1–2 instability, the medullary respiratory center and long spinal tracts may sustain damage when the neck is manipulated during intubation. While spinal anesthesia is being administered, the patient is often asked to "curl up" to facilitate insertion of the spinal needle. Flexion of the cervical spine in the presence of C1–2 instability should be avoided during this maneuver.

Operative versus nonoperative treatment. In some instances of advanced age, increased risk factors, lack of patient motivation, or relatively minor pain, it may be suggested that the patient should accept limited function rather than undergo a complex and potentially dangerous surgical procedure. The wrist is a good example of this dilemma. Three options are available: splinting, arthrodesis, or arthroplasty. Arthrodesis provides a stable, painless wrist but jeopardizes function to some extent, particularly in the performance of personal hygienic chores (33). For this reason, patients with bilateral involvement are often advised to have a wrist arthroplasty, using some form of prosthetic implant (34). Such prostheses carry the obvious risk of breakage, loosening, and infection. For some patients, prostheses or fusion are indicated, but others would be better served by the use of a wrist splint, worn at night and during work but removed when flexibility is required (35).

Similarly, painful foot and ankle deformities are often best managed by special shoes and inserts that minimize pressure points or an orthosis to splint the ankle and correct heel valgus.

Although more than 90% of patients undergoing joint replacement experience pain relief and improved function, all such procedures must still be considered evolutionary. Changes in design, surgical technique, and materials continue, with improvements coming rapidly in some joints and more slowly in others such as the hip. For this reason, such surgery should be delayed as long as possible in patients who continue to function at a satisfactory level with tolerable discomfort. The old and reliable procedures such as fusion and osteotomy should be used when appropriate, especially in younger patients. When joint replacement is required, the special needs and problems of the arthritis patient must be considered. There is a close relationship between the technical expertise with which an arthroplasty is performed and its immediate and ultimate functional result.

Functional analysis of large number of patients who have undergone arthroplasty will determine the appropriate indications for surgery and choice of prosthetic designs, but medical judgment in selecting patients for surgery as well as the precise surgical technique in carrying out the operation will remain the dominant requirements for success in the surgical management of arthritis.

1. Burton KE, Wright V, Richards J: Patient's expectations in relation to outcome of total hip replacement surgery. Ann Rheum Dis 38:471–474, 1979
2. Jergesen HE, Poss R, Sledge CB: Bilateral total hip and knee replacement in adults with rheumatoid arthritis: an evaluation of function. Clin Orthop 137:120–128, 1978
3. Johnson KA: Arthroplasty of both hips and both knees in rheumatoid arthritis. J Bone Joint Surg 57A:901–904, 1975
4. Charnley J: Low Friction Arthroplasty of the Hip: Theory and Practice. Berlin, Springer-Verlag, 1979
5. Poss R, Ewald FC, Thomas WH, Sledge CB: Complications of total hip replacement arthroplasty in patients with rheumatoid arthritis. J Bone Joint Surg 58A:1180, 1976
6. Gristina AG, Rovere GD, Shoji H: Spontaneous septic arthritis complicating rheumatoid arthritis. J Bone Joint Surg 56A:1180–1184, 1974
7. Kellgren JH, Ball J, Fairbrother RW, Barnes KL: Suppurative arthritis complication rheumatoid arthritis. Br Med J 1:1193–1200, 1958
8. Poss R: Personal communication
9. Garner RW, Mowat AG, Hazelman BL: Wound healing after operations on patients with rheumatoid arthritis. J Bone Joint Surg 55B:134–144, 1973
10. Foker JE, Schwartz R, Smith DC, Matas A: Surgical problems in immunodeficient and immunosuppressed children. Surg Clin N Am 59:213–221, 1979
11. O'Loughlin JM: Infections in the immunosuppressed patient. Med Clin N Am 59:495–501, 1975
12. Burry HC: Penicillamine and wound healing—a potential hazard? Postgrad Med J (Aug supplement) 75–76, 1974
13. Deshmukh K, Nimni ME: A defect in the intramolecular and intermolecular crosslinking of collagen caused by penicillamine. J Biol Chem 244:1787–1795, 1969
14. Schorn D, Mowat AG: Penicillamine in rheumatoid arthritis: wound healing, skin thickness, and osteoporosis. Rheumatol Rehabil 16:223–230, 1977
15. Cooke TD, Richer S, Hurd E: Localization of antigen–antibody complexes in intra-articular collagenous tissues. Ann New York Acad Sci 256:10–24, 1975
16. Ohno O, Cooke TD: Electron microscopic morphology of immunoglobulins aggregates and their interactions in rheumatoid articular collagenous tissues. Arthritis Rheum 21:516–527, 1978
17. Bisla RS, Inglis AE, Ranawat CS: Joint replacement surgery in patients under thirty. J Bone Joint Surg 58A:1098–1104, 1976
18. Singsen BH, Isaacson AS, Burnstein BH, Patzakis MJ, Kornreich HK, King KK, Hanson V: Total hip replacement in children with arthritis. Arthritis Rheum 21:401–406, 1978
19. Sledge CB: Joint replacement surgery in juvenile rheumatoid arthritis. Arthritis Rheum 20:567–572, 1977
20. Conway W, Bauer G, Barns M: Hypersomnolence and intermittent upper airway obstruction: occurrence caused by micrognathia. JAMA 237:2740–2744, 1977
21. Bryan JS, Scott WT, Bickel WH: Surgery of Rheumatoid Arthritis. RL Cruess, NW Mitchell, eds., Philadelphia, JB Lippincott, 1971, pp 63–68
22. Ritter MA, Vaughan RB: Ectopic ossification after total hip arthroplasty: predisposing factors, frequency and effect on results. J Bone Joint Surg 59A:345–351, 1977
23. Williams E, Taylor AR, Arden GP: Arthroplasty of the hip in ankylosing spondylitis. J Bone Joint Surg 59B:393–397, 1977
24. Aly R, Maibach HI, Mandel A: Bacterial flora in psoriasis. Br J Dermatol 95:603–606, 1976
25. Lambert JR, Wright V: Surgery in patients with psoriasis and arthritis. Rheumatol Rehabil 18:35, 1979
26. Marples RR, Heaton CL, Kligman AM: Staphylococcus aureus in psoriasis. Arch Dermatol 107:568–570, 1973
27. Griffiths ID, Maini RN, Scott JT: Clinical and radiological features of osteonecrosis in systemic lupus erythematosus. Ann Rheum Dis 38:413–422, 1979
28. Copeland SA, Taylor JG: Synovectomy of the elbow in rheumatoid arthritis. J Bone Joint Surg 61B:69–73, 1979
29. Head WC, Paradies LH: Ipsi-lateral hip and knee replacements as a single surgical procedure. J Bone Joint Surg 59A:352–354, 1977
30. Nakano KK: Neurologic complications of rheumatoid arthritis. Orthop Clin N Am 6:861–880, 1975
31. Rana NA, Hancock DO, Taylor AR, Hill AGS: Upward translocation of the dens in rheumatoid arthritis. J Bone Joint Surg 55B:471–477, 1973
32. Rana NA, Hancock DP, Taylor AR, Hill AGS: Atlantoaxial subluxation in rheumatoid arthritis. J Bone Joint Surg 55B:458–470, 1973
33. Millender LH, Nalebuff EA: Arthrodesis of the rheumatoid wrist: an evaluation of 60 patients and a description of a different surgical technique. J Bone Joint Surg 55A:1026–1034, 1973
34. Volz RG: Total wrist arthroplasty: a new approach to wrist disability. Clin Orthop 128:180–189, 1977
35. Convery FR, Minteer MA: The use of orthoses in the management of rheumatoid arthritis. Clin Orthop 102:118–125, 1974

95. Rehabilitative and restorative therapy of patients with rheumatic diseases

An **impairment** is the specific joint disorder that afflicts a patient. A **handicap** is the extent to which the joint impairment *impedes* function. **Disability** is the extent to which a handicap *prevents* function. An office worker with osteoarthritis in one knee (the impairment), may have to park close to his place of work and walk slowly with a cane (handicap), but because he is working full time, he has *no disability* (1).

Objectives. Comprehensive therapeutic programs for arthritis patients should attempt to restore patients to their highest level of social and vocational function. Successful rehabilitation can often be achieved and may ideally consist of restoration to full employment and social participation, or (less dramatic but equally important) enhanced independence in self-care for the severely involved arthritic, or both (2).

Rehabilitative therapies combine medical management and, when appropriate, judicious surgical intervention with as wide a range of supporting services as may be required to restore a patient to optimal function. Practical considerations and economic realities will define the perimeters and "fence in" that range.

The health care team is usually made up of primary physicians, rheumatologists, physiatrists, occupational therapists, physical therapists, and nurses. It frequently includes psychiatrists, psychologists, dieticians, patient educators, and social workers. It always involves the patient and should extend to his family as well (1).

The rehabilitative setting may include the doctor's office, ambulatory care center, acute care hospital, rehabilitative facilities, pain center, and the patient's home, place of work and recreational settings (1,3,4).

Evaluation of function. All therapy must ultimately be measured in terms of its effectiveness. Costs and risks are weighed against results. A variety of criteria have been used to assess function, but none have been universally accepted (4). A subjective functional assessment for rheumatoid arthritis has recently been validated and may prove to be the most practical means of globally assessing function (5). At present the ARA Database uses criteria that measure walking time and attempts to quantify aspects of upper and lower extremity function, compliance, and self-care (1,6,7).

The relief of pain and maintenance of joint function with minimization of exposure to drug side effects and/or surgical complications is an implicit charge of conservative treatments and rehabilitative therapies.

The judicious use of rest, exercise, and "modalities" may greatly facilitate recovery from joint disorders. Their injudicious prescription or application results in a hodgepodge of ritualized procedures that may at the least provide false hopes and frustrations to the patient, and at worst compound the problem and delay institution of appropriate treatment.

Rationale for rest and exercise. Joint inflammation is often aggravated by joint use. In rheumatoid arthritis and other destructive arthropathies, aggravated joint inflammation results not only in greater pain and disability but also causes progressive joint and tendon damage (8). Joint rest by means of immobilization can reduce joint inflammation. Immobilization (splinting) must be prescribed for short periods (3–4 weeks) and in relatively acute disorders to avoid the functional problems associated with loss of motion or the complications of joint ankylosis and disuse muscle atrophy (9,10). Temporary joint rest achieved by the use of removable braces, corsets, or static "working" splints, or by rest periods (with specified postures, e.g., prone position to prevent hip flexion contracture) can relieve pain and inflammation and improve function (1,11,12). Atrophy and loss of motion from disuse must be compensated for by specific exercises designed to avoid exacerbation of the original joint problem (1).

Rest is an extremely useful adjunct for chronic generalized active inflammatory joint disease or severely painful degenerative joint disorders. This does not mean absolute bedrest, rather it means the provision of sufficient time in chairs, couches, or bed, and deliberate pacing (work alternating with rest or change of activities) to allay fatigue and minimize joint strain. Patients with moderately severe joint disease should have 8–10 hours of rest at night and 1–2 hour rest periods during the day. Posture and position, whether lying, sitting, or standing, require specific recommendations to encourage desired joint alignment. Attention to table and chair height, back and seat support in chairs and cars, bed height, and firmness of mattress (or added support by properly selected bed boards) can be major factors in restoring patients to function.

Exercise therapy. Pain and disuse lead to muscle atrophy and loss of joint mobility. Joint cartilage nutrition and bone mineralization are dependent on joint movement and muscle action. Weak muscles result in poorly coordinated stressful movements, increased pain, loss of function, and potential worsening of joint disorders.

Stretching exercises maintain or increase joint mobility. They may also be used to relieve pain secondary to muscle cramps or chronically tensed muscles, e.g., the use of pelvic tilts by patients with low back pain after prolonged sitting in an improperly designed chair or car seat (1).

Maintaining joint motion. During the acute phases of disorders capable of producing irreversible joint damage, gentle assisted range of motion exercises carried out once or twice a day just to the point of pain will help minimize contractures. Acutely inflamed joints should be positioned and/or splinted when not being exercised to assure maximum function in case some degree of unavoidable contracture cannot be subsequently overcome (1).

In subacute or chronic joint disease with irreversible deformity, active or active-and-assisted stretching exercises are prescribed to minimize further loss of joint mobility. This regimen should consist of 3–5 warmup stretches followed by 1–2 maximally tolerated stretches once or twice daily (1).

One cannot usually rely on the patient's daily activities as a substitute for prescribed exercises. Patients quickly learn to avoid painful or fatiguing motions during activity and consequently avoid precisely those movements required in therapeutic exercises to improve mobility and strength.

When increased mobility is the goal in subacute or chronic inflammatory joint disorders or in mild to moderately severe degenerative joint disease, stretching exercises must be tailored to the patient's tolerance. In general, some mild diffuse aching is to be expected during or after an exercise session. Reassessment of the exercise program is demanded if the patient experiences acute focal pain, pain that persists longer than 2 hours, or pain on the day after exercise that is greater than can be accounted for by an unaccustomed increase in joint usage.

For potentially reversible subacute joint involvements, stretching exercises should initially be performed 2–3 times a day. Each session should consist of 5 warmup exercises followed by 2–5 "good" stretches. As pain tolerance and chronicity permit, these sessions may be increased in frequency, with 5–10 warmups and 3–5 maximal stretches per affected joint area (1). The application of local heat (warm tub, shower, hot packs) and/or a warming of the muscles by mild activity helps to relieve protective painful muscle spasm and enhance the ability to stretch.

Patients with morning stiffness should be instructed to exercise in the forenoon, with full analgesic medication, and before late afternoon fatigue or stiffness occurs if they are to get maximum benefits from exercise therapy.

Although true polymyositis is sometimes encountered and steroid myopathy is not rare, most muscle weakness commonly associated with joint disease is a consequence of the relative disuse caused by painful inhibition of joint motion. The goals of strengthening exercises are to increase the strength and endurance of specific muscle groups to facilitate function (1).

Activity. Forceful muscle contractions are necessary to increase strength (2). Since motion of arthritic joints is usually painful, the strategy for muscle strengthening requires careful planning if sufficient force to increase strength is to be generated. Muscle fibers of type I (aerobic, oxidative, long endurance, repetitive, jogging contractions) and type II (anaerobic, glycolytic, short duration, low endurance, forceful, weight lifting contractions) are fairly randomly distributed throughout the muscles (13).

Type I fibers (red, myoglobin-rich) consist of at least 2 subsets, one with smaller, slower responding motor units and the other with motor units intermediate between the former and type II fibers (13). Type II fibers can be stimulated to increase static strength and static holding endurance by brief (6 second) isometric contractions at two-thirds muscle strength performed once daily. In the presence of arthritis, contractions can approach the requisite force by designing the exercises so that the joint is placed in its midrange and in a position of comfort to minimize painful inhibition of muscle contractions (13,14).

Successful isometric strengthening of appropriate muscle groups facilitates activities of daily living by providing the static strength and endurance for such activities as arising from a chair to take a few steps or for pouring and drinking a cup of tea (1). When inflammation subsides, the strength and coordination thus achieved will facilitate the repetitive movements requisite to gain the dynamic (aerobic) endurance for work and recreational activities (1,13). For many patients, and particularly for those with multiple joint involvement or severe disease, the buoyancy of water makes swimming the best all around exercise, provided attention is given to the proper selection of strokes and to avoidance of chilling or excessive fatigue.

Activities of daily living. Although prescribed medications, rest, splinting, and exercise are essential for ultimate optimal disease control and restoration of function, the patient with arthritis often has immediate functional needs to meet. Joint protection, energy conservation, and the use of proper body mechanics are the major components of a properly designed arthritis regimen (15). The patient must be taught how to perform essential grooming and hygienic activities so that the joints are not overstressed and so that he or she can, if possible, perform these and other essential tasks without assistance.

A raised toilet seat or long-handled shoehorn are two examples of simple devices that permit independence for patients with back pain or hip and knee disease. Other items patients will find useful in daily activities can be found in the *Self-Help Manual for Patients with Arthritis* available from the Arthritis Foundation. For some patients, rearrangement of household and work areas, modification of automobiles, and elimination of architectural barriers may be needed to permit full participation in daily activities (1,4,15,16).

Physical therapy. Physical agents such as infrared, ultraviolet, and short wave irradiations are used primarily for pain relief or as an adjunct to exercise. Relief of protective, pain-induced tonic muscle contractions by heat, cold, and/or massage (manual or mechanical) is often helpful to assure that exercise therapy can accomplish its goals of stretching and strengthening. Infrared irradiation is administered in various ways including hot packs, paraffin, mud baths, showers, tub baths, and heat lamps.

Studies of the efficacy of these modalities are meager and criteria for selection among them are empirical (1,17,18). In general, cold applications are useful in the case of acute trauma and inflammation; moist heat and/or miscellaneous modalities including paraffin, steam, and baths in various media are used in subacute to chronic disorders. For focal and chronic myalgias and neuralgic or arthritic disorders, deep heating by short wave diathermy (and particularly for focal lesions by ultrasound irradiation) is widely used, but convincing studies of efficacy are not available (1,17,18).

The value of traction in pain relief in acute arthritis of the hip is well accepted. Traction for relief of pain associated with cervical or lumbar disc disease (with or without radiculopathy) is less clearly established as useful. Both cervical and lumbar traction can be administered by a variety of techniques, many involving forces insufficient to achieve vertebral separation (1,19,20). Both cervical and lumbar traction may provide relief by enforcing rest and/or stretching tonically contracting paraspinal muscles. Simplified techniques for home cervical traction are readily taught (1). Horizontal pelvic traction for lumbar disc disease usually requires forces equal to 50% of the body weight and a friction free sliding component in the traction table to achieve even minimal vertebral separation (19).

The recent introduction of acupuncture has stimulated considerable research in pain control mechanisms. Acupuncture has not been shown to affect the course of arthritic disorders and no specificity to the location of needles has been demonstrated. Nonetheless, an apparent enhanced placebo counterirritant reaction mediated in part by enkaphalin and endorphin polypeptide neurotransmitters may be evoked by acupuncture, dry needling, and a variety of transcutaneous nerve stimulation devices as well as by old-fashioned massage, salves, balms and plasters (1,21). In this category, one can also place various biofeedback and relaxation techniques advocated for relief of psychic tension and muscle relaxation to reduce pain.

There is little question that some or all of these procedures may be helpful to some individuals suffering from joint pain, but the cost and amount of effort to achieve these nonspecific effects must be carefully weighed against the role of what, for the moment, appear to be more specific rational and quantifiable alternative forms of therapy.

Psychosocial factors. The holistic approach to joint disease treatments incorporates the best elements of comprehensive medical, surgical, and psychosocial management. The term *holistic* is often debased to describe any one of a variety of nonmedical "natural" dietary or mystical health cults or fads that may be in vogue. The pain management centers designed to treat conditions associated with refractory pain (of which arthritis and back pain constitute a major portion) rely heavily on a multifaceted approach including psychologic and social manipulation, relaxation therapies (biofeedback meditation), and operant conditioning to modify pain dependent behavior (22).

The ultimate form and place of pain management centers remain to be determined, but at present they are proliferating and appear to be fulfilling a need in the management of some patients with refractory pain.

Whatever the eventual status of these centers may be, the need for careful patient and family education regarding the nature and treatment of arthritis is clear. Such education should be carefully planned and, where necessary, coordinated with psychologic and social supportive therapy (1,4,23,24).

Successful arthritis rehabilitation requires a detailed understanding of the nature of rheumatic disorders by all members of the health care team, an informed patient and family, and a highly individualized and carefully planned and modulated treatment regimen (24).

1. Swezey RL: Arthritis. Rational Therapy and Rehabilitation. Philadelphia, WB Saunders, 1978
2. Robinson HS: Prognosis: return to work—arthritis, Total Management of the Arthritic Patient. GE Ehrlich, ed, Philadelphia, JB Lippincott, 1973, pp 183–192
3. Boyle RW: The Therapeutic Gymnasium, Therapeutic Exercises. S Licht, ed. Baltimore, Waverly Press, Inc, 1961, p 257.
4. Swezey RL: Arthritis rehabilitation: staff, facilities, and evaluation, Rehabilitation Management of Rheumatic Conditions, ed 2. GE Ehrlich, ed, Baltimore, Williams & Wilkins, 1980, pp 1–28
5. Meenan RF, Gertman PM, Mason JH: Measuring health status in arthritis: the arthritis impact scales. Arthritis Rheum 23:146–152, 1980
6. Hess EV: A uniform database for rheumatic disease. Arthritis Rheum 10:645–648, 1976
7. Robinson HS, Bashall DA: Functional assessment, Total Management of the Arthritic Patient. GE Ehrlich. ed. Philadelphia, JB Lippincott, 1973, pp 241–252
8. Swezey RL: Dynamic factors in deformity of the rheumatoid hand. Bull Rheum Dis 22:649–656, 1971
9. Partridge REH, Duthie JJR: Controlled trial of the effect of complete immobilization of the joints in rheumatoid arthritis. Ann Rheum Dis 22:91–99, 1965
10. Gault SJ, Spyker MJ: Beneficial effect of immobilization of joints in rheumatoid and related arthritidies: a splint study using sequential analysis. Arthritis Rheum 12:34–44, 1969
11. Malick MH: Manual on Static Hand Splinting, Vol 1, Pittsburgh, Harmarville Rehabilitation Center, 1972
12. Bennett RL: Rheumatoid wrist and hand slip-on splints. Arthritis and Physical Medicine, S Licht, Ed. Baltimore, Waverly Press, 1969, pp 482–491
13. Edington DW, Edgerton VR: The Biology of Physical Activity. Boston, Houghton Mifflin, 1976
14. Müller EA: Influence of training and inactivity on muscle strength. Arch Phys Med 41:449–462, 1970
15. Cordery J: The Conservation of Physical Resources as Applied to the Activities of Patients with Arthritis and the Connective Tissue Diseases. Study Course III, Third International Congress, World Federation of Occupational Therapists, Dubuque, Iowa, William C. Brown, 1962, p. 22
16. Lowman EW, Klinger JL: Aids to Independent Living. Self-Help for the Handicapped. New York, McGraw-Hill, Inc, 1961
17. Lehman JF, Warren CG, Scham SM: Therapeutic heat and cold. Clin Orthop 99:207–245, 1945
18. Lehmann JR, DeLateur BJ: Heat and cold in the treatment of arthritis, Arthritis and Physical Medicine. S Licht, ed. Baltimore, Waverly Press, 1969, p 315
19. Judovich BD, Nobel GR: Traction therapy, a study of resistance forces. Am J Surg 93:108–114, 1957
20. Colachis SC Jr, Strohn BR: A study of traction forces and angle of pull on vertebral interspaces in the cervical spine. Arch Phys Med Rehab 46:815–819, 820–830, 1965
21. Reuler JR, Girard DE, Nardone DA: The chronic pain syndrome: misconceptions and management. Ann Intern Med 93:588–596, 1980
22. Fordyce WE, Fowler RS, Lehmann JF, DeLateur BJ, Sand PL, Trieschmann RB: Operant conditioning in the treatment of chronic pain. Arch Phys Med Rehab 54:399–408, 1973
23. Swanson DW, Swenson WM, Maruta T, McPhee MC: Program for managing chronic pain. Mayo Clin Proc 51:401–408, 1976
24. Davis MS: Variations in patients compliance with doctor's advice: an empirical analysis of patters of communication. Am J Pub Health 58:274–288, 1968

96. Psychosocial aspects of rheumatic disease— a patient speaks

Henrietta Aladjem

When I was first diagnosed as having systemic lupus erythematosus (SLE or lupus), it was a frightening experience. I had never heard the word lupus before or known of anyone who had anything similar to what I had. I was told that I was suffering from a rare, mysterious disease that affects predominantly blue-eyed blonds with a pinking complexion like mine.

At that time in the history of medicine (1953), lupus was considered uniformly fatal. When I didn't die, the physicians questioned the diagnosis.

On my own, all I could find out about the disease was that lupus comes from the Latin and it means *wolf*, and erythema from the Greek, means literally to be red. The first thing that came to mind, was— What do the wolf and lupus have in common? The question kept hammering away in my mind. The very sound of the disease was lethal because of identification with the predator.

Unfortunately, even today, patients read or hear that lupus is invariably a fatal illness; this leads to great anxiety. Similarly a patient may be told that she or he has arthritis which leads to ungrounded fears of disabling deformities. And physicians observe that, when one adds to these natural fears and anxieties to a frank organic psychosis, one gets a hyperirritable, confused person who is afraid of living and afraid of dying.

Help with such fears requires much of the physician's time and a real understanding of the patient's stresses.

Lupus is no longer a rare disease, and it is far from being fatal. Physicians stress that the past few decades have been an exciting time for research regarding better understanding of the pathogenesis and pathophysiology of lupus. The medical community feels that today the major problems facing patients and physicians are those of chronic disease with both complications of the disease and therapy.

But do the physicians know what this disease does to a human life? Without knowing this, can they properly treat the patient?

To me, lupus remains a disease with a name that's difficult to pronounce and more difficult to live with. It is a disease with an unpredictable prognosis and symptoms that are difficult to explain. It is intermittent, recurrent, and it nibbles away at the will to live and the ability to cope. It can threaten life and it can prevent the patient from functioning like a normal human being.

I have spent many hours at medical libraries searching for literature on the psychosocial and emotional problems of the lupus patient. I found that such problems were rarely mentioned in the psychiatric literature and when they are, focus is directed toward SLE with central nervous system involvement. I could not find anything to reflect the fears and apprehensions of the individual—of human suffering—the very core of the disease. In lupus the body and the soul are enmeshed in a sense of pain and desperation that makes it difficult for the physicians to distinguish whether they are dealing with a neurotic who has developed lupus or a lupus patient who has developed a neurosis because of the disease. Some physicians say it is difficult to tell for sure in some patients. This makes one wonder if many young women who are so-called neurotics do not have a touch of lupus.

Physicians often ask me, "When did your lupus begin?" There are so many beginnings, so many experiences, I never know how to explain the symptoms so they wouldn't judge me a fool. Looking into the distant past I wonder whether the disease was inherited. In adolescence, my parents attributed some of my afflictions to a delicate constitution; constant strep throats, susceptibility to colds, recurring pneumonia, and the overreaction to mosquito bites. In my case, sunlight affected my skin. My skin needed protection from heat, cold, wind, ultraviolet light—anything that touched it. The rash that I got from the sun or the blue blotches from the cold induced parallel changes in my system. The skin reaction was more spectacular, while the reaction of the internal organs was more dangerous.

The drugs I took, instead of helping, caused more problems that were rarely interpreted correctly. The reaction should have been perceived as a warning signal from nature, not just for one drug, but for all.

The patient with lupus is concerned not only with the immediate side effects of the drugs, but also with side effects that may appear years after a specific drug was taken. Medications with well-established toxicities are frequently used in the management of this disease. This has evolved because of the frequency of a life-threatening situation or because the restrictions placed on the seriously ill patient become unacceptable to her and her family. The lupus patient remains a consumer of the most experimental nature.

Very often the drugs prescribed by the physician depend on which research center you go to and who is the attending physician.

The lupus patient is a bewildered human being who is besieged by physical, emotional, and economic problems. The patient becomes ruled by fears—fears that others will find out that one is struck by a mysterious illness, fear of being cut off from the human flow of life, fears of not being able to do the things one was trained to do. One gets worse and then gets better without obvious cause. And there are times when the patient is the only person who is sure that she is really sick but doesn't know what is wrong. You try to tell the doctor about the transient nodules under your elbows, the migratory pains and aches, the inflammation that comes and goes unpredictably, particularly swelling and reddening of the soles of your feet that are present one day and by the next day may have disappeared. You watch the doctor's expression change from an attentive one to one of obvious annoyance, and there are moments when you begin to wonder whether what you are trying to tell him is even true.

The symptoms of the patient are often insidious and they can confuse even the most knowledgeable physician.

Most lupus patients, if not all of them, experience an intense fatigue. The lupus fatigue is unique—it absorbs the whole person. It doesn't act like an organic, psychologic, or physiologic fatigue. It doesn't respond to drugs, rest and relaxation, or psychiatric help. You cannot call it malaise or even lethargy. You feel depleted of energy and spiritually exhausted, to the point where even brushing your teeth becomes a difficult chore. At times the sense of futility is so great that one becomes tempted to "give up" or give in to permanent sleep. What keeps one going is the need to help one's children, attend to a job, or the moral responsibility one feels for life itself.

The lupus patients I know don't believe the physicians can even begin to imagine the physical and psychologic desperation created by the lupus fatigue.

The need for linking the lupus fatigue to our profound depression is becoming more and more urgent as observations reveal its damaging effect in many, and to a certain degree, perhaps in all. Many lupus patients describe this fatigue as their first symptoms of lupus. They claim that they experience this symptom even when their physicians tell them that they are in remission.

Lupus is not just another chronic disease.

What makes it so difficult is that the symptoms come and go unpredictably, and the patient doesn't show any signs of deterioration. The people around you see you well one moment and distressed the next and they can become distrustful and feel that you may be a hypochondriac or even worse—a person who will always find excuses for poor performance.

When emphasis on neurosis is accentuated by the physician, it becomes destructive to the whole family because this implies that the person has control over her illness which she absolutely does not.

And the patient makes the mistake of thinking that she caused all the difficulties when it is really the illness.

In the early 1970s the American Rheumatism Association established preliminary criteria for SLE based on the presence of 4 or more of 14 manifestations. The Criteria will be expanded as new information comes in. *Lupus fatigue should be placed high on the list.*

As for me, I was fortunate. I had good doctors; they cared and they wanted to help me. They stuck by me and gave me courage. We interacted as people. The physician became the *person* who could help me, and I the *person* who needed to be helped. Even though I was told from the beginning that they didn't know of any cure, I was encouraged to believe that the will to live and the desire to cope were regenerating forces playing an important role in fighting lupus. In my case, what medical science could not do, the doctors achieved with their humanity.

For the past 15 years, I have been in complete remission. I have a checkup once a year, and I am on no medication. When patients ask me what am I doing to stay well, I tell them that I am a living example of Osler's aphorism: If you want to live a long life, get a chronic disease and learn how to take care of it. The secret is to reach and alter the whole way of life, by probing for and correcting all the various noxious influences—diet, medication, general hygiene, proper medical attention and rest, and we must learn to avoid stress to any extent possible.

And finally, when patients ask me if I still take the nicotinamide, I tell them yes I do—for sentimental reasons. But I am realistic, I know that the predisposition to lupus will always be present, as well as the lack of resistance to infections, severe reactions to drugs, and the sun will always be my enemy.

And I would like to add a sentence in the words of Dr. Rene Dubos: "The hope in the future likes in the physician's willingness to listen to the patient, and the patient's courage to reject medical science without humanity."

Appendixes

1. Criteria for the diagnosis and classification of the rheumatic diseases

The criteria presented in the following sections have been developed with several different purposes in mind. For a given disorder, one may have criteria for: 1) classification of groups of patients (e.g., from population surveys, selection of patients for therapeutic trials, or analysis of results of interinstitutional patient comparisons), 2) diagnosis of individual patients, 3) estimations of disease frequency and/or severity (epidemiologic surveys) including remission, and 4) assistance in determination of prognosis.

The criteria are variously described as "diagnostic criteria," "criteria for guidance in the diagnosis," and "preliminary criteria for the classification." The original intention was to propose criteria as guidelines for *classification* of disease syndromes for the purpose of assuring correctness of diagnosis in patients taking part in clinical investigation rather than for individual patient diagnosis. However, the proposed criteria have in fact been used as guidelines for patient diagnosis as well as for research classification. One must be cautious in such application since the various criteria are derived from the use of analytic techniques that allow the minimum number of variables to achieve the best group discrimination, rather than to attempt to arrive at a diagnosis in each patient, regardless of the amount of information needed.

The proposed criteria are empiric and not intended to include or exclude a particular diagnosis in any individual patient. They are valuable in offering a standard to permit comparison of groups of patients from different centers which take part in various clinical investigations including therapeutic trials.

The ideal criterion is absolutely sensitive, i.e., all patients with the disorder show this physical finding or the positive laboratory test, and absolutely specific, i.e., the positive finding or test is never present in any other disease. Unfortunately, few such criteria or sets of criteria exist. Usually the greater the sensitivity of a finding, the lower is its specificity, and vice-versa. When criteria are established empirically, as in the modified Jones criteria for rheumatic fever or the American Rheumatism Association criteria for rheumatoid arthritis, attempts are made to select reasonable combinations of sensitivity and specificity.

Existing criteria derive from an incomplete concept of disease and imperfect diagnostic technology which will require many years for full refinement and accuracy. Thus, criteria are expected to change as improved knowledge and techniques become available in the different disease areas and as concepts of pathophysiology change. This is a vital and dynamic area of research in which rheumatology leads other disciplines in medicine.

2. Criteria for the classification of rheumatoid arthritis

Diagnostic Criteria for Rheumatoid Arthritis

A. Classic rheumatoid arthritis

This diagnosis requires 7 of the following criteria. In criteria 1 through 5 the joint signs or symptoms must be continuous for at least 6 weeks. Any one of the features listed under Exclusions will exclude a patient from this and all other categories.

1. Morning stiffness
2. Pain on motion or tenderness in at least 1 joint (observed by a physician)
3. Swelling (soft tissue thickening or fluid, not bony overgrowth alone) in at least 1 joint (observed by a physician)
4. Swelling (observed by a physician) of at least 1 other joint (any interval free of joint symptoms between the 2 joint involvements may not be more than 3 months)
5. Symmetric joint swelling (observed by a physician) with simultaneous involvement of the same joint on both sides of the body (bilateral involvement of proximal interphalangeal, metacarpophalangeal, or metatarsophalangeal joints is acceptable without absolute symmetry). Terminal phalangeal joint involvement will not satisfy this criterion
6. Subcutaneous nodules (observed by a physician) over bony prominences, on extensor surfaces, or in juxtaarticular regions
7. Roentgenographic changes typical of rheumatoid arthritis (which must include at least bony decalcification localized to or most marked adjacent to the involved joints and not just degenerative changes). Degenerative changes do not exclude patients from any group classified as having rheumatoid arthritis.
8. Positive agglutination test—demonstration of the "rheumatoid factor" by any method which, in 2 laboratories, has been positive in not over 5% of normal controls, or positive streptococcal agglutination test. [The latter is now obsolete.]
9. Poor mucin precipitate from synovial fluid (with shreds and cloudy solution). (An inflammatory synovial effusion with 2,000 or more white cells/mm³, without crystals can be substituted for this criterion.)
10. Characteristic histologic changes in synovium with 3 or more of the following: marked villous hypertrophy; proliferation of superficial synovial cells often with palisading; marked infiltration of chronic inflammatory cells (lymphocytes or plasma cells predominating) with tendency to form "lymphoid nodules"; deposition of compact fibrin either on surface or interstitially; foci of necrosis.
11. Characteristic histologic changes in nodules showing granulomatous foci with central zones of cell necrosis, surrounded by a palisade of proliferated mononuclear and peripheral fibrosis and chronic inflammatory cell infiltration

B. Definite Rheumatoid Arthritis

This diagnosis requires 5 of the above criteria. In criteria 1 through 5 the joint signs or symptoms must be continuous for at least 6 weeks.

C. Probable Rheumatoid Arthritis

This diagnosis requires 3 of the above criteria. In at least one of criteria 1 through 5 the joint signs or symptoms must be continous for at least 6 weeks.

D. Possible Rheumatoid Arthritis

This diagnosis requires 2 of the following criteria and total duration of joint symptoms must be at least 3 months.

1. Morning stiffness
2. Tenderness or pain on motion (observed by a physician) with history of recurrence or persistence for 3 weeks
3. History or observation of joint swelling.
4. Subcutaneous nodules (observed by a physician)
5. Elevated sedimentation rate or C-reactive protein
6. Iritis [of dubious value as a criterion except in juvenile arthritis]

E. Exclusions

1. The typical rash of systemic lupus erythematosus (with butterfly distribution, follicle plugging, and areas of atrophy)
2. High concentration of lupus erythematosus cells (4 or more in 2 smears prepared from heparinized blood incubated not over 2 hours) [or other clearcut evidence of systemic lupus erythematosus.]
3. Histologic evidence of periarteritis nodosa with segmental necrosis of arteries associated with nodular leukocytic infiltration ex-

tending perivascularly and tending to include many eosinophils

    4. Weakness of neck, trunk, and pharyngeal muscles or persistent muscle swelling or dermatomyositis

    5. Definite scleroderma (not limited to the fingers). [This is an arguable point.]

    6. A clinical picture characteristic of rheumatic fever with migratory joint involvement and evidence of endocarditis, especially if accompanied by subcutaneous nodules or erythema marginatum or chorea. (An elevated antistreptolysin titer will not rule out the diagnosis of rheumatoid arthritis.)

    7. A clinical picture characteristic of gouty arthritis with acute attacks of swelling, redness, and pain in 1 or more joints, especially if relieved by colchicine or accompanied by urate crystals

    8. Tophi

    9. A clinical picture characteristic of acute infectious arthritis of bacterial or viral origin with: an acute focus of infection or in close association with a disease of known infectious origin; chills; fever; and an acute joint involvement, usually migratory initially (especially if there are organisms in the joint fluid or response to antibiotic therapy)

    10. Tubercule bacilli in the joints or histologic evidence of joint tuberculosis

    11. A clinical picture characteristic of Reiter's syndrome with urethritis and conjunctivitis associated with acute joint involvement, usually migratory initially

    12. A clinical picture characteristic of the shoulder–hand syndrome with unilateral involvement of shoulder and hand, with diffuse swelling of the hand followed by atrophy and contractures

    13. A clinical picture characteristic of hypertrophic osteoarthropathy with clubbing of fingers and/or hypertrophic periostitis along the shafts of the long bones especially if an intrapulmonary lesion (or other appropriate underlying disorder) is present

    14. A clinical picture characteristic of neuroarthropathy with condensation and destruction of bones of involved joints and with associated neurologic findings

    15. Homogentisic acid in the urine, detectable grossly with alkalinization

    16. Histologic evidence of sarcoid or positive Kveim test

    17. Multiple myeloma as evidenced by marked increase in plasma cells in the bone marrow, or Bence-Jones protein in the urine

    18. Characteristic skin lesions of erythema nodosum

    19. Leukemia or lymphoma with characteristic cells in peripheral blood, bone marrow, or tissues

    20. Agammaglobulinemia

It should be noted that these criteria were developed before the new classification of rheumatic diseases adopted by the American Rheumatism Association in 1963, in which ankylosing spondylitis, psoriatic arthritis, and arthritis associated with ulcerative colitis and regional enteritis are listed as distinct from rheumatoid arthritis.

1. Ropes MW, Bennett GA, Caleb S, Jacox R, Jessar RA: 1958 Revision of diagnostic criteria for rheumatoid arthritis. Bull Rheum Dis 9:175–176, 1958

2. Blumberg B, Bunim JJ, Calkins E, Pirani CL, Zvaifler NJ: ARA nomenclature and classification of arthritis and rheumatism (tentative). Arthritis Rheum 7:93–97, 1964

Proposed Criteria for Clinical Remission in Rheumatoid Arthritis*

Five or more of the following requirements must be fulfilled for at least 2 consecutive months:

1. Duration of morning stiffness not exceeding 15 minutes
2. No fatigue
3. No joint pain (by history)
4. No joint tenderness or pain on motion
5. No soft tissue swelling in joints or tendon sheaths
6. Erythrocyte sedimentation rate (Westergren method) less than 30 mm/hour for a female or 20 mm/hour for a male

---

* These criteria are intended to describe either spontaneous remission or a state of drug-induced disease suppression, which simulates spontaneous remission. To be considered for this designation a patient must have met the ARA criteria for definite or classic rheumatoid arthritis at some time in the past.

No alternative explanation may be invoked to account for the failure to meet a particular requirement. For instance, in the presence of knee pain, which might be related to degenerative arthritis, a point for "no joint pain" may not be awarded.

Exclusions: Clinical manifestations of active vasculitis, pericarditis, pleuritis or myositis, and unexplained recent weight loss or fever attributable to rheumatoid arthritis will prohibit a designation of complete clinical remission.

These criteria are based on data provided by 35 rheumatologists on 175 rheumatoid arthritis (RA) patients considered to be in complete remission and 169 patients considered to be in partial remission or to have active disease. In this study sample,

5 or more criteria points yielded a 72% sensitivity for clinical remission and 100% specificity in discriminating RA patients with active disease.

The purpose of these criteria is to encourage uniformity in definition and use of the term *remission*. The criteria may be applied to individual patients or as an endpoint in therapeutic trials. They do not attempt to define a total absence of all articular and extraarticular inflammation and immunologic activity related to RA. Indeed, this could be documented only by extraordinary measures. The criteria deal with complete "clinical" remission, indicating a level of minimal disease activity that can be defined using readily available information and convenient measurements.

The concept of remission also includes a time dimension. A period of 2 months was chosen because 90% of the patients studied had been in remission for at least this long.

The majority of patients entering the study had received "remission-inducing" drugs. Although the inclusion of patients in spontaneous remission was actively solicited, few were identified. This may indicate that natural remissions are rare, or that such patients are lost to followup by rheumatologists. No differences in clinical characteristics and course were identified when spontaneous and drug-induced remissions were compared. Therefore, a qualification has been included, noting that the proposed criteria are also intended to describe a state of drug-induced disease suppression that simulates remission.

Substantial variation was found in the concept of remission among rheumatologists. Some define the term in a rigid, absolutist manner. Others use it in a relative fashion to describe patients who have improved considerably, have essentially no symptoms, and have achieved as low a level of objective findings as could be expected in view of the prior course. The proposed criteria attempt to reach a consensus. They have not yet been tested in prospective studies or in other population groups and, therefore, are considered preliminary.

1. Pinals RS, et al: Preliminary criteria for clinical remission in rheumatoid arthritis. Arthritis Rheum 24:1308–1315, 1981

3. Criteria for determination of progression of rheumatoid arthritis and of functional capacity of patients with the disease

Classification of Progression of Rheumatoid Arthritis (1)

Stage I, Early
*1. No destructive changes on roentgenographic examination
2. Roentgenologic evidence of osteoporosis may be present.

Stage II, Moderate
*1. Roentgenologic evidence of osteoporosis, with or without slight subchondral bone destruction; slight cartilage destruction may be present.
*2. No joint deformities, although limitation of joint mobility may be present.
3. Adjacent muscle atrophy
4. Extraarticular soft tissue lesions, such as nodules and tenosynovitis may be present.

Stage III, Severe
*1. Roentgenologic evidence of cartilage and bone destruction, in addition to osteoporosis
*2. Joint deformity, such as subluxation, ulnar deviation, or hyperextension, without fibrous or bony ankylosis.
3. Extensive muscle atrophy
4. Extraarticular soft tissue lesions, such as nodules and tenosynovitis may be present.

Stage IV, Terminal
*1. Fibrous or bony ankylosis
2. Criteria of stage III

*The criteria prefaced by an asterisk are those that must be present to permit classification of a patient in any particular stage or grade.

Classification of Functional Capacity in Rheumatoid Arthritis (1)

Class I: Complete functional capacity with ability to carry on all usual duties without handicaps
Class II: Functional capacity adequate to conduct normal activities despite handicap of discomfort or limited mobility of 1 or more joints
Class III: Functional capacity adequate to perform only few or none of the duties of usual occupation or of self care
Class IV: Largely or wholly incapacitated with patient bedridden or confined to wheelchair, permitting little or no self care

1. Steinbrocker O, Traeger CH, Batterman RC: Therapeutic criteria in rheumatoid arthritis. JAMA 140:659–662, 1949

4. Criteria for the diagnosis of juvenile rheumatoid arthritis

I. General

The JRA Criteria Subcommittee in 1982 again reviewed the 1977 Criteria (1) and recommended that *juvenile rheumatoid arthritis* be the name for the principal form of chronic arthritic disease in children and that this general class should be classified into 3 onset subtypes: systemic, polyarticular, and pauciarticular. The onset subtypes may be further subclassified into subsets as indicated below. The following classification enumerates the requirements for the diagnosis of JRA and the 3 clinical onset subtypes and lists subsets of each subtype that may be useful in further classification.

II. General criteria for the diagnosis of juvenile rheumatoid arthritis:

A. Persistent arthritis of at least 6 weeks duration in 1 or more joints
B. Exclusion of other causes of arthritis. (See list of exclusions).

III. JRA onset subtypes

The onset subtype is determined by manifestations during the first 6 months of disease and remains the principal classification, although manifestations more closely resembling another subtype may appear later.

A. Systemic onset JRA: This subtype is defined as JRA with persistent intermittent fever (daily intermittent temperatures to 103°F or more) with or without rheumatoid rash or other organ involvement. Typical fever and rash will be considered probable systemic onset JRA if not associated with arthritis. Before a definite diagnosis can be made, arthritis, as defined, must be present.

B. Pauciarticular onset JRA: This subtype is defined as JRA with arthritis in 4 or fewer joints during the first 6 months of disease. Patients with systemic onset JRA are excluded from this onset subtype.

C. Polyarticular JRA: This subtype is defined as JRA with arthritis in 5 or more joints during the first 6 months of disease. Patients with systemic JRA onset are excluded from this subtype.

D. The onset subtypes may include the following subsets:

1. Systemic onset (SO)
   a. Polyarthritis
   b. Oligoarthritis
2. Oligoarthritis (OO) (Pauciarticular onset)
   a. Antinuclear antibody (ANA) positive-chronic uveitis
   b. RF positive
   c. Seronegative B27 positive
   d. Not otherwise classified
3. Polyarthritis (PO)
   a. Rheumatoid factor (RF) positivity
   b. Not otherwise classified

IV. Exclusions
A. Other rheumatic diseases
   1. Rheumatic fever
   2. Systemic lupus erythematosus
   3. Ankylosing spondylitis
   4. Polymyositis and dermatomyositis
   5. Vasculitic syndromes
   6. Scleroderma
   7. Psoriatic arthritis
   8. Reiter's syndrome
   9. Sjögren's syndrome
   10. Mixed connective tissue disease
   11. Behçet's syndrome
B. Infectious arthritis
C. Inflammatory bowel disease
D. Neoplastic diseases including leukemia
E. Nonrheumatic conditions of bones and joints
F. Hematologic diseases
G. Psychogenic arthralgia
H. Miscellaneous
   1. Sarcoidosis
   2. Hypertrophic osteoarthropathy
   3. Villonodular synovitis
   4. Chronic active hepatitis
   5. Familial Mediterranean fever

V. Other proposed terminology

Juvenile chronic arthritis (JCA) and juvenile arthritis (JA) are new diagnostic terms currently in use in some places for the arthritides of childhood. The diagnoses of JCA and JA are not equivalent to each other, nor to the older diagnosis of juvenile rheumatoid arthritis or Still's disease. Hence reports of studies of JCA or JA cannot be directly compared with one another nor to reports of JRA or Still's Disease. JCA is described in more detail in a report of the European Conference on the Rheumatic Disease of Children (2) and juvenile arthritis in the report of the Ross Conference (3).

1. JRA Criteria Subcommittee of the Diagnostic and Therapeutic Criteria Committee of the American Rheumatism Association: Current proposed revisions of the JRA criteria. Arthritis Rheum 20(suppl)195–199, 1977
2. Ansell BW: Chronic arthritis in childhood. Ann Rheum Dis 37:107–120, 1978
3. Fink CW: Keynote address: Arthritis in childhood, Report of the 80th Ross Conference in Pediatric Research. Columbus, Ross Laboratories, 1979, pp 1–2

5. Jones criteria for guidance in the diagnosis of rheumatic fever

Jones criteria (revised) for guidance in the diagnosis of rheumatic fever (1)

Major manifestations	Minor manifestations
Carditis	Clinical
Polyarthritis	Fever
Chorea	Arthralgia
Erythema marginatum	Previous rheumatic fever
Subcutaneous nodules	or rheumatic heart disease

Plus

Supporting evidence of preceding streptococcal infection:
increased ASO or other streptococcal antibodies
positive throat culture for group A streptococcus
recent scarlet fever

*The presence of 2 major criteria, or of 1 major and 2 minor criteria, indicates a high probability of the presence of rheumatic fever if supported by evidence of a preceding streptococcal infection. The absence of the latter should make the diagnosis suspect, except in situations in which rheumatic fever is first discovered after a long latent period after the antecedent infection (e.g., Sydenham's chorea or low-grade carditis).

1. Stollerman GH, Markowitz M, Taranta A, Wanamaker LW, Whittemore R: Jones criteria (revised) for guidance in the diagnosis of rheumatic fever. Circulation 32:664–668, 1965

6. Revised criteria for the classification of systemic lupus erythematosus

1982 Revised Criteria for Classification of Systemic Lupus Erythematosus*

Criterion		Definition
1. Malar rash		Fixed erythema, flat or raised, over the malar eminences, tending to spare the nasolabial folds
2. Discoid rash		Erythematous raised patches with adherent keratotic scaling and follicular plugging; atrophic scarring may occur in older lesions
3. Photosensitivity		Skin rash as a result of unusual reaction to sunlight, by patient history or physician observation
4. Oral ulcers		Oral or nasopharyngeal ulceration, usually painless, observed by a physician
5. Arthritis		Nonerosive arthritis involving 2 or more peripheral joints, characterized by tenderness, swelling, or effusion
6. Serositis	a)	Pleuritis—convincing history of pleuritic pain or rub heard by a physician or evidence of pleural effusion *OR*
	b)	Pericarditis—documented by ECG or rub or evidence of pericardial effusion
7. Renal disorder	a)	Persistent proteinuria greater than 0.5 grams per day or greater than 3+ if quantitation not performed *OR*
	b)	Cellular casts—may be red cell, hemoglobin, granular, tubular, or mixed
8. Neurologic disorder	a)	Seizures—in the absence of offending drugs or known metabolic derangements; e.g., uremia, ketoacidosis, or electrolyte imbalance *OR*
	b)	Psychosis—in the absence of offending drugs or known metabolic derangements, e.g., uremia, ketoacidosis, or electrolyte imbalance
9. Hematologic disorder	a)	Hemolytic anemia—with reticulocytosis *OR*
	b)	Leukopenia—less than $4,000/mm^3$ total on 2 or more occasions *OR*
	c)	Lymphopenia—less than $1,500/mm^3$ on 2 or more occasions *OR*
	d)	Thrombocytopenia—less than $100,000/mm^3$ in the absence of offending drugs
10. Immunologic disorder	a)	Positive LE cell preparation *OR*
	b)	Anti-DNA: antibody to native DNA in abnormal titer *OR*
	c)	Anti-Sm: presence of antibody to Sm nuclear antigen *OR*
	d)	False positive serologic test for syphilis known to be positive for at least 6 months and confirmed by *Treponema pallidum* immobilization or fluorescent treponemal antibody absorption test
11. Antinuclear antibody		An abnormal titer of antinuclear antibody by immunofluorescence or an equivalent assay at any point in time and in the absence of drugs known to be associated with "drug-induced lupus" syndrome

* The proposed classification is based on 11 criteria. For the purpose of identifying patients in clinical studies, a person shall be said to have systemic lupus erythematosus if any 4 or more of the 11 criteria are present, serially or simultaneously, during any interval of observation.

1. Tan EM, Cohen AS, Fries JF, Masi AT, McShane DJ, Rothfield NF, Schaller JG, Talal N, Winchester RJ: The 1982 revised criteria for the classification of systemic lupus erythematosus (SLE). Arthritis Rheum 25:1271-1277, 1982

7. Criteria for the classification of acute gouty arthritis

Classification criteria for acute gouty arthritis (gout)

A. The presence of characterisitc urate crystals in the joint fluid, or

B. A tophus proved to contain urate crystals by chemical means or polarized light microscopy, or

C. The presence of 6 of the following 12 clinical, laboratory, and x-ray phenomena listed below:

   1. More than one attack of acute arthritis

   2. Maximal inflammation developed within 1 day

   3. Attack of monarticular arthritis

   4. Joint redness observed

   5. First metatarsophalangeal joint painful or swollen

   6. Unilateral attack involving first metatarsophalangeal joint

   7. Unilateral attack involving tarsal joint

   8. Suspected tophus

   9. Hyperuricemia

   10. Asymmetric swelling within a joint (roentgenogram)

   11. Subcortical cysts without erosions (roentgenogram)

   12. Negative culture of joint fluid for microorganisms during attack of joint inflammation

---

1. Wallace SL, Robinson H, Masi AT, Decker JL, McCarty DJ, Yü T-F: Preliminary criteria for the classification of the acute arthritis of primary gout. Arthritis Rheum 20:895–900, 1977

8. Preliminary criteria for classification of progressive systemic sclerosis (scleroderma)

For the purposes of classifying patients in clinical trials, population surveys, and other studies, a person shall be said to have progressive systemic sclerosis (scleroderma), if the one major or 2 or more minor criteria listed below are present. Localized forms of scleroderma, eosinophilic fasciitis, and the various forms of pseudoscleroderma are excluded from these criteria.

A. Major criterion

Proximal scleroderma: Symmetric thickening, tightening, and induration of the skin of the fingers and the skin proximal to the metacarpophalangeal or metatarsophalangeal joints. The changes may affect the entire extremity, face, neck, and trunk (thorax and abdomen).

B. Minor criteria

   1. *Sclerodactyly*: Above-indicated skin changes limited to the fingers

   2. *Digital pitting scars or loss of substance from the finger pad*: Depressed areas at tips of fingers or loss of digital pad tissue as a result of ischemia

   3. *Bibasilar pulmonary fibrosis*: Bilateral reticular pattern of linear or lineonodular densities most pronounced in basilar portions of the lungs on standard chest roentgenogram; may assume appearance of diffuse mottling or "honeycomb lung." These changes should not be attributable to primary lung disease.

1. Masi AT, Rodnan GP, Medsger TA Jr, Altman RD, D'Angelo WA, Fries JF, LeRoy EC, Kirsner AB, Mackenzie AH, McShane DJ , Myers AR, Sharp GC: Preliminary criteria for the classification of systemic sclerosis (scleroderma). Arthritis Rheum 23:581–590, 1980

9. Formulas of drugs used in treatment of rheumatic disease

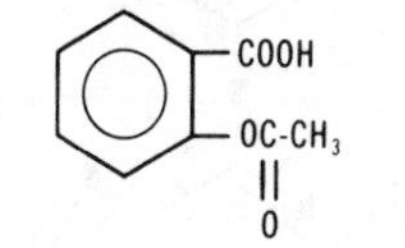

Aspirin (acetylsalicylic acid)

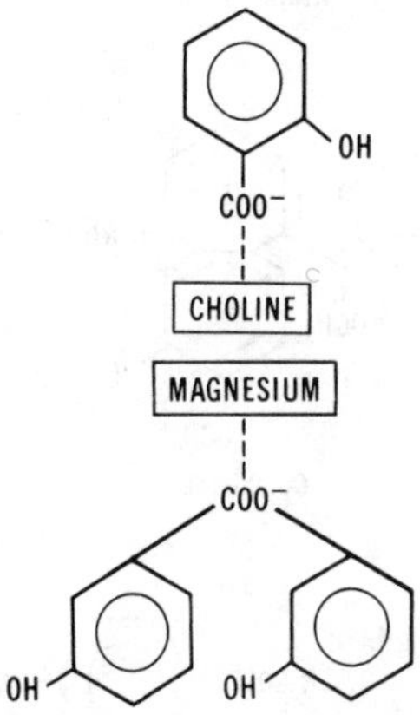

Choline magnesium trisalicylate

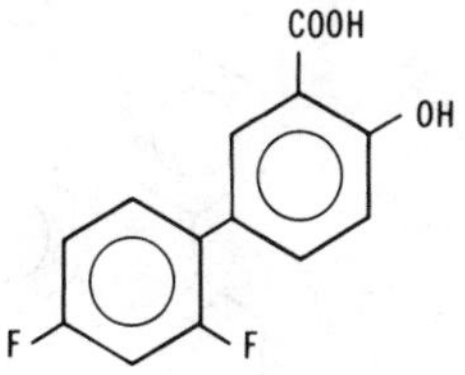

Diflunisal

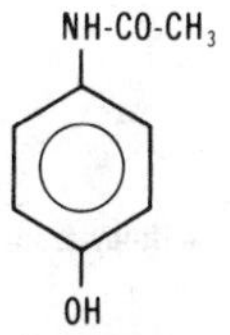

Acetaminophen

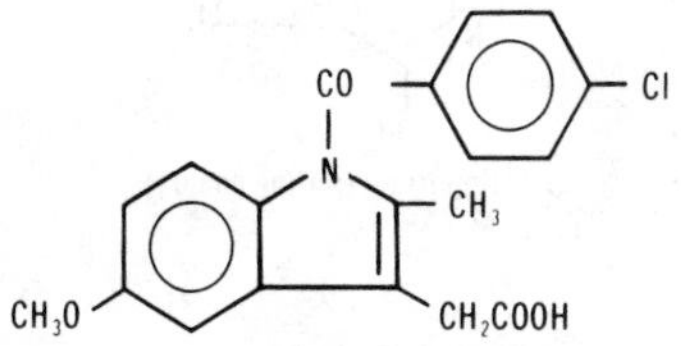

Indomethacin

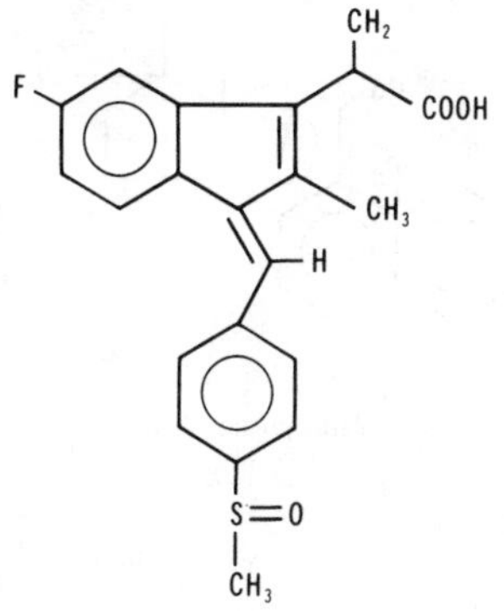

Sulindac.

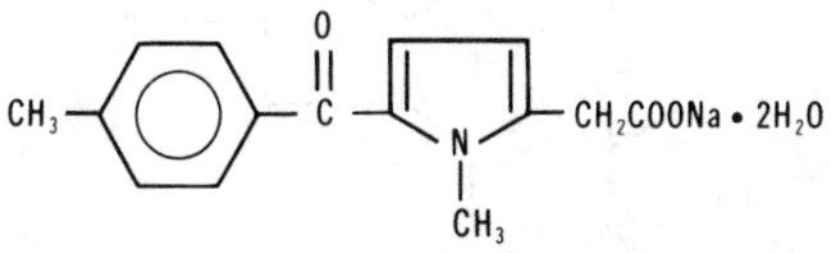

Tolmetin sodium

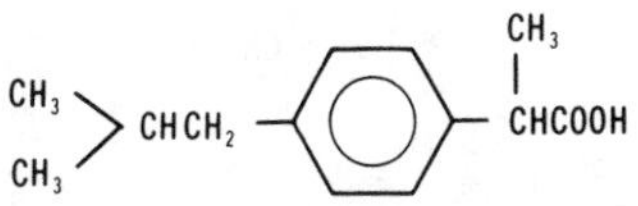

Ibuprofen

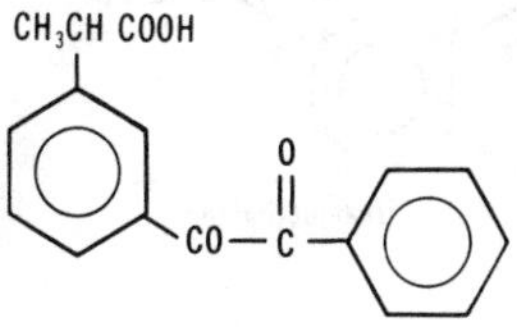

Ketoprofen

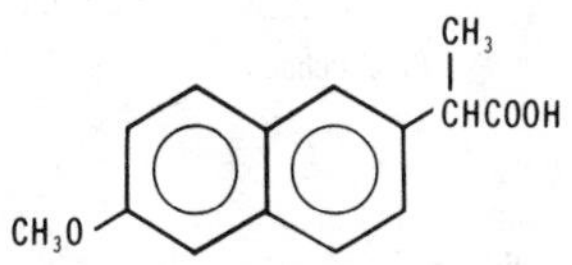

Naproxen

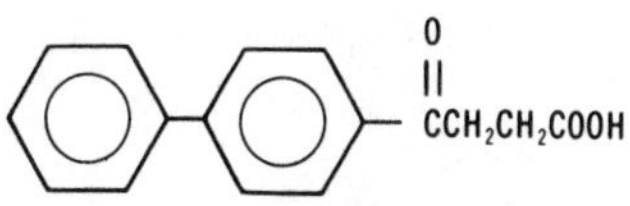

Fenbufen

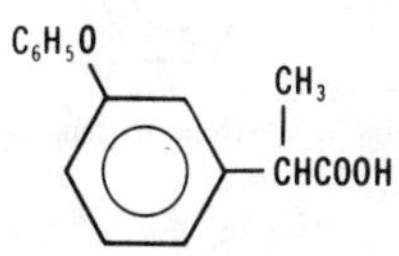

Fenoprofen

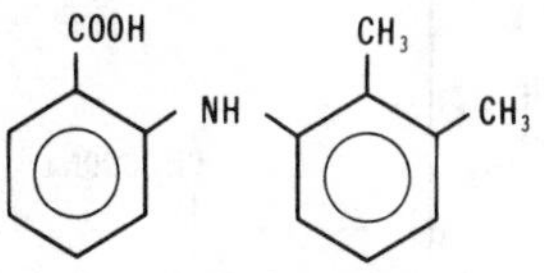

Mefenamic acid

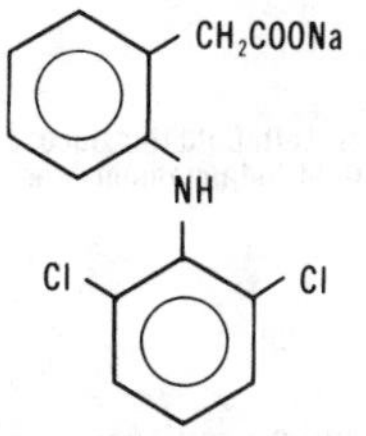

Diclofenac

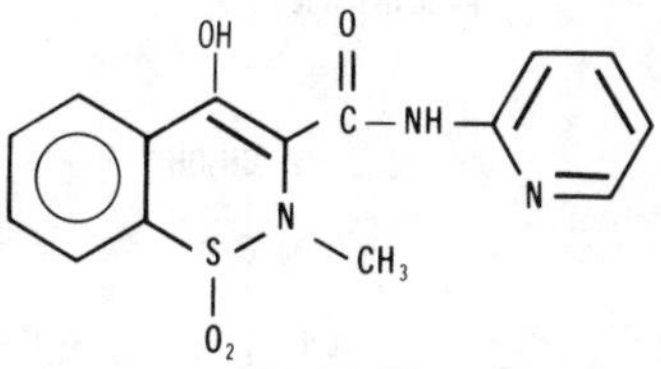

Piroxicam

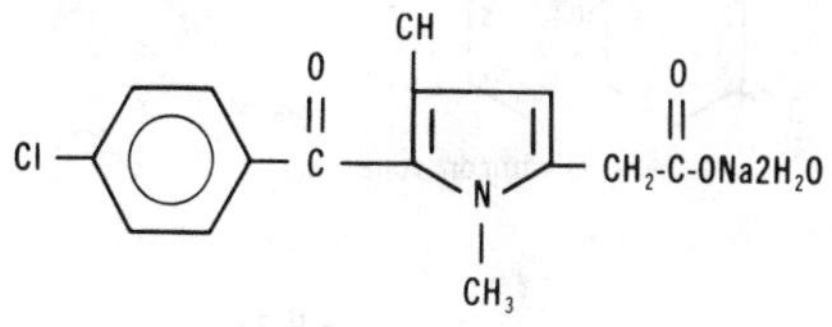

Zomepirac sodium

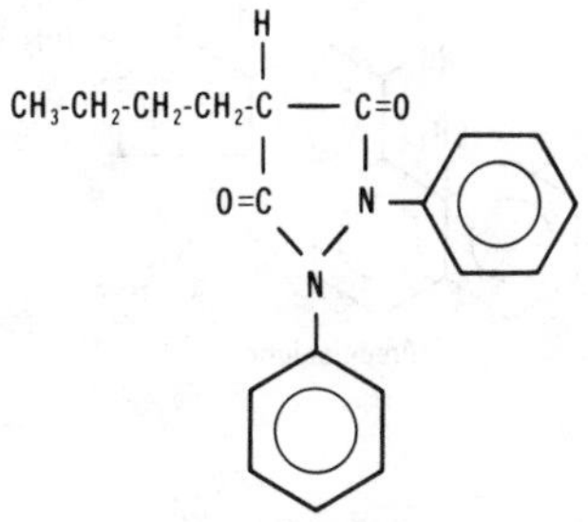

Phenylbutazone

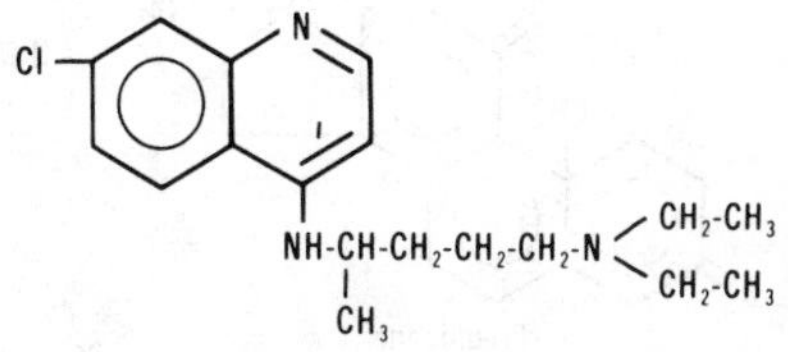

Chloroquine

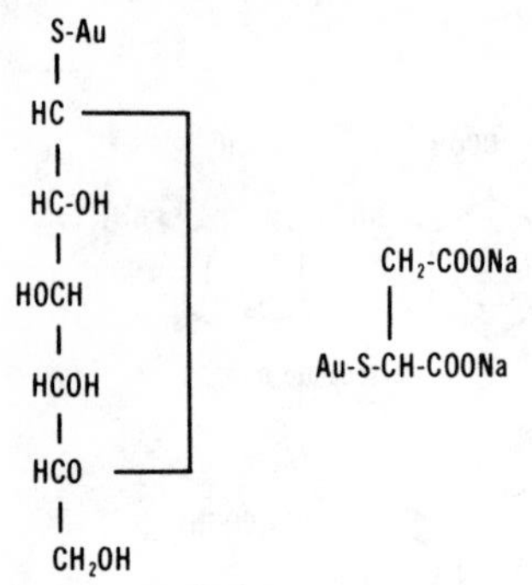

Gold salts. Left. Gold thioglucose
Right. Gold sodium thiomalate

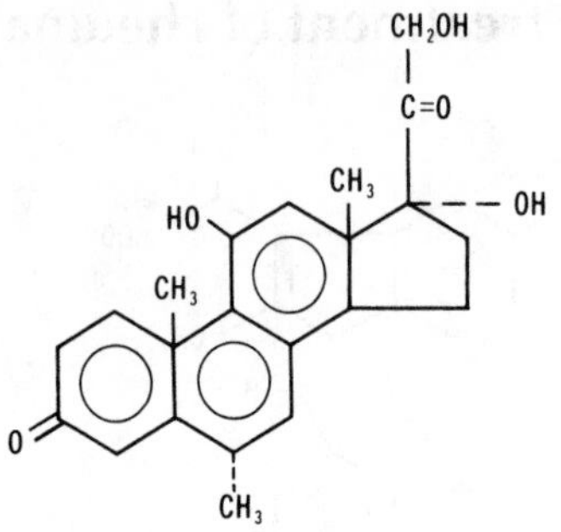

CH₂-COONa

Au-S-CH-COONa

Methylprednisolone

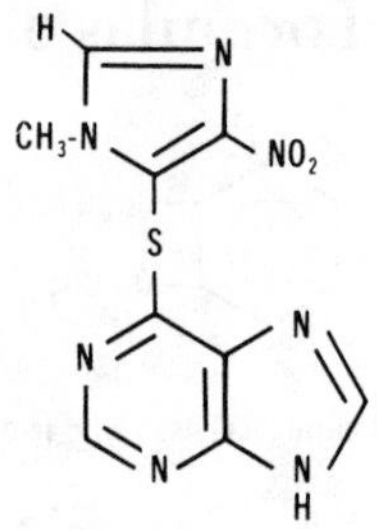

Azathioprine

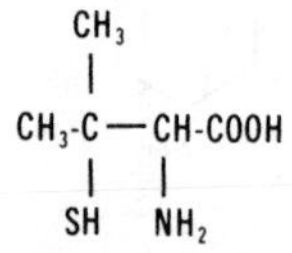

Penicillamine

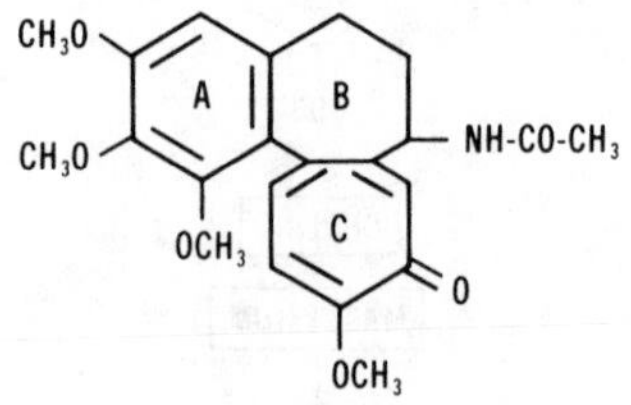

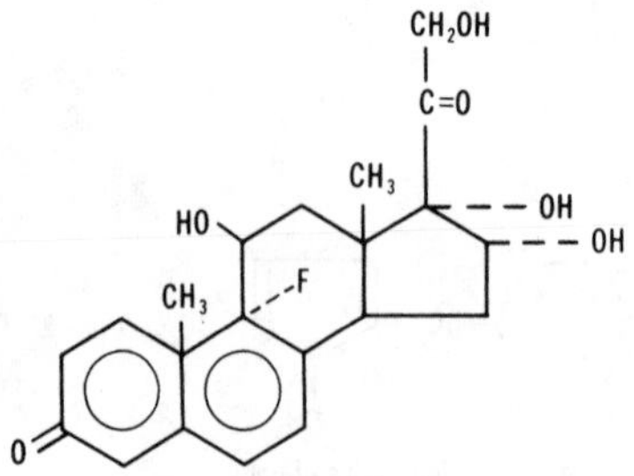

Triamcinolone

Colchicine

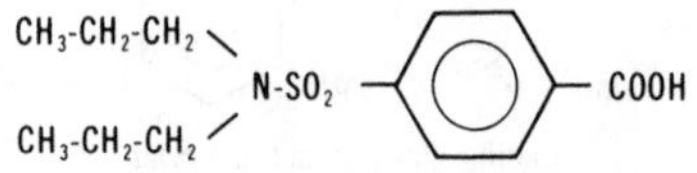

Probenecid

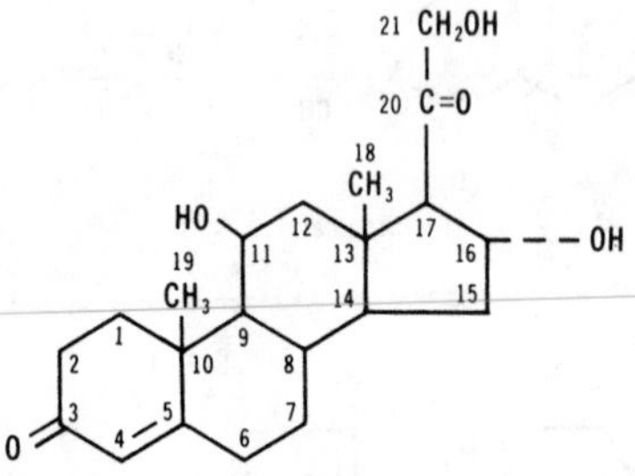

Hydrocortisone

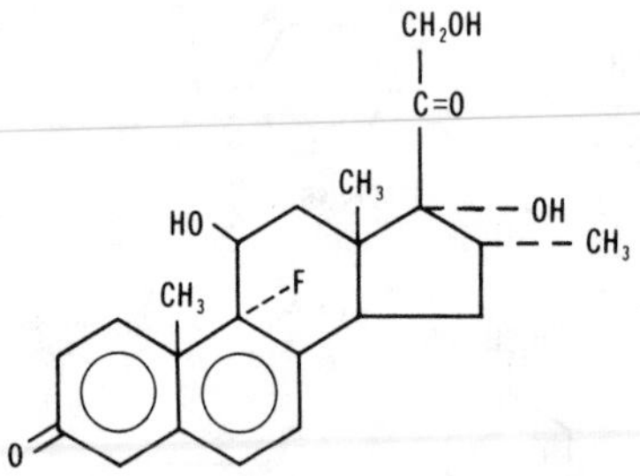

Dexamethasone

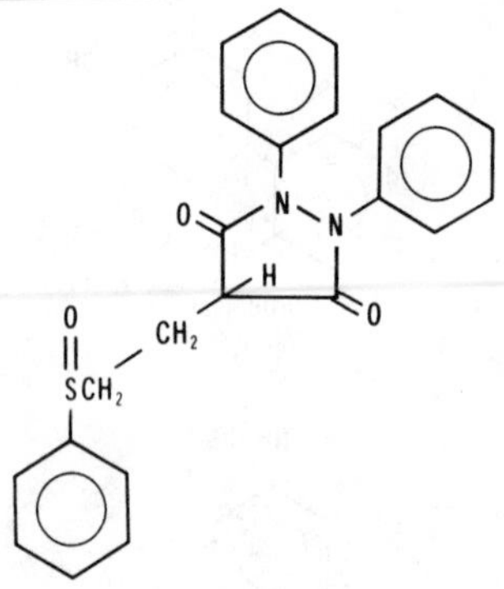

Sulfinpyrazone

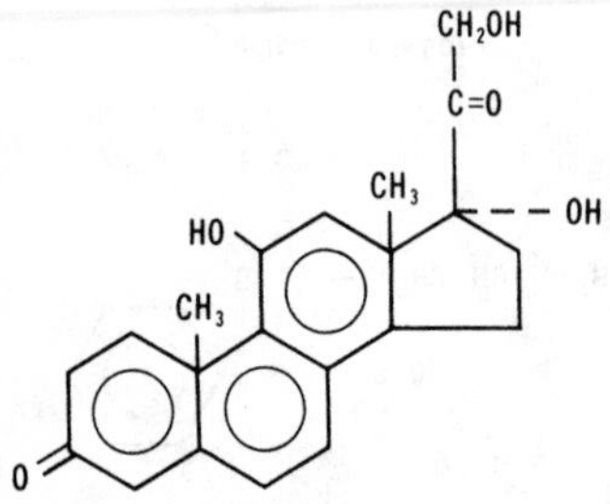

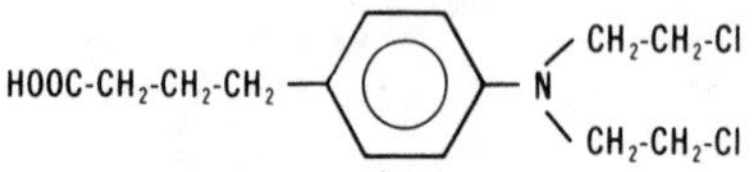

Chlorambucil

Prednisolone

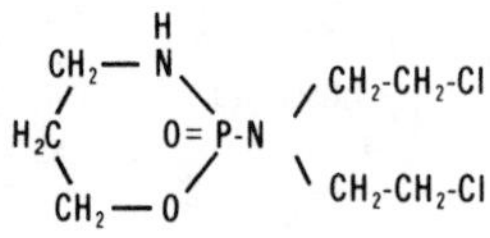

Cyclophosphamide

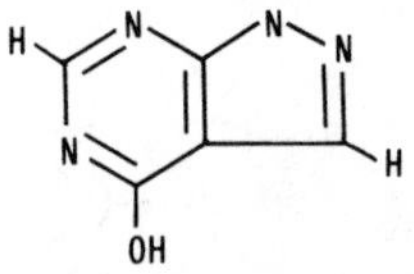

Allopurinol (purine analog)

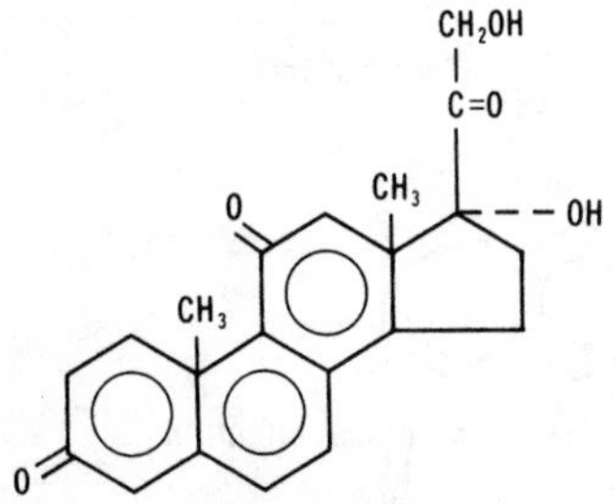

Prednisone

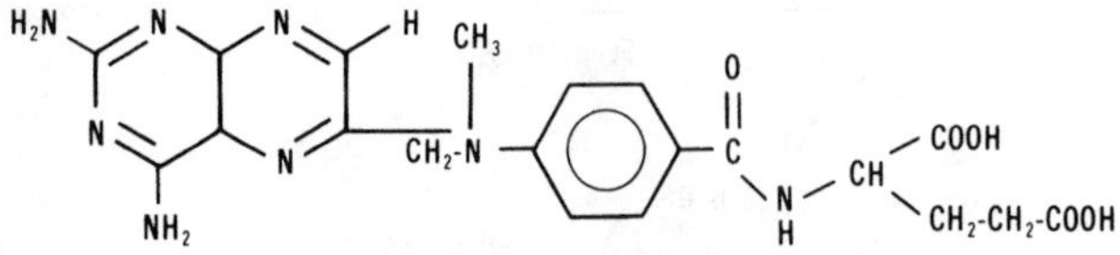

Methotrexate (folic acid analog)

10. Uniform database for the rheumatic diseases

The first edition of *A Standard Database for Rheumatic Diseases* was developed at an American Rheumatism Association (ARA) Database Workshop in September 1973 (1). The revised edition, entitled *A Uniform Database,* was published in 1976 (2) after the second Database Workshop held September 1975. At a third workshop held in Washington, DC, in September 1978 the Database was intensely reviewed and particular attention paid to reducing the number of descriptors, smoothing the terminology, interchanging the terms, and defining the descriptors (3).

An important need identified at the third workshop was the requirement for uniformly accepted definitions of many of the terms used in rheumatology. In 1980, the ARA Glossary Committee began the process of defining the elements of the Database. The first volume of this effort was published in September 1982 as the *Dictionary of the Rheumatic Diseases* (4). A sample is included at the end of this section.

The purpose of the Uniform Database for Rheumatic Disease has been to provide a common terminology to uniformly describe the varied aspects of rheumatic diseases. The resulting compendium is periodically updated and revised under the aegis of the ARA Glossary Committee to reflect information garnered from its use in the rheumatologic community.

The following is the updated Uniform Database for Rheumatic Diseases resulting from the 1978 Washington workshop and Glossary Committee revisions.

Copies of the complete Database and also sample chart formats of the database may be obtained from ARAMIS, Suite 3301, 701 Welch Road, Palo Alto, California, 94304.

1. Hess EV, Fries JF, Klinenberg, JR: A Standard Database for Rheumatic Disease. Arthritis Rheum 17:327–336, 1974
2. Hess EV, Fries JF, Klinenberg JR: A Uniform Database for Rheumatic Diseases. Arthritis Rheum 19:645–648, 1976
3. Hess EV, Fries JF, Klinenberg JR: A Uniform Database for Rheumatic Diseases. Arthritis Rheum 22:1029–1033, 1979
4. ARA Glossary Committee: Signs and Symptoms. Vol 1, Dictionary of the Rheumatic Diseases. New York, Contact Associates, 1982

SELECTED SYMPTOM REVIEW

General
- Fatigue
- Fever
- Fever type (chronic, intermittent)
- Immunizations
- Intercurrent illness
- Shaking chills
- Weight loss (due to illness)

Skin
- Alopecia (disease or drug)
- Photosensitivity
- Psoriasis
- Purpura
- Rash, malar
- Rash, other
- Raynaud's phenomenon
- Skin tightening
- Skin ulcers, digital
- Skin ulcers, non-digital
- Urticaria

Ears, eyes, nose, throat
- Conjunctivitis
- Dry eyes
- Dry mouth
- Head pain (specify location)
- Mucosal ulcers
- Nasal complaints
- Ocular inflammation, other
- Salivary gland enlargement
- Sore throat
- Tinnitus

Cardiopulmonary
- Chest pain, pleuritic
- Chest pain, other
- Cough, persistant
- Dyspnea or orthopnea
- Edema, dependent
- Edema, other
- Hemoptysis
- Wheezing

Gastrointestinal
- Abdominal pain, other
- Anorexia
- Diarrhea
- Dysphagia
- Hematemesis and/or melena
- Peptic ulcer symptoms
- Vomiting and/or nausea

Genitourinary
- Genital ulceration
- Hematuria by history
- Proteinuria by history
- Renal stone
- Significant menstrual abnormality
- Urethral discharge

Hematologic
- Anemia by history
- Leukopenia by history
- Thrombocytopenia by history

Neuromuscular–Psychiatric
- Muscle pain
- Muscle weakness
- Parenthesias
- Psychiatric (specify)
- Seizures

Other history
- Days absent from work/school
- Failure to participate in activity/school

PHYSICAL EXAMINATION

General
- Height (cm)
- Weight (kg)
- Blood pressure, systolic
- Blood pressure, diastolic
- Temperature (°C)
- Respirations (minute)
- Pulse rate (minute)

Skin
- Abnormal pigmentation
- Alopecia
- Calcinosis, dermal
- Digital, ulcers, scars
- Erythematous knuckles
- Erythema marginatum
- Erythema nodosum
- Erythema, perigungual
- Heliotrope eyelids
- Keratoderma blennorrhagica
- Nail pitting
- Psoriasis
- Purpura or ecchymosis
- Rash, discoid
- Rash, JRA
- Rash, malar
- Rash, other
- Scleroderma, acrosclerosis
- Scleroderma, facial
- Scleroderma, generalized
- Scleroderma, localized (morphea)
- Scleroderma, sclerodactyly
- Telangiectasia
- Ulcerations, other
- Urticaria

Eye
- Cataract
- Conjunctivitis
- Episcleral, scleral disease
- Fundi, abnormal
- Iritis (acute)
- Schirmer test (mm)
- Uveitis (chronic)

Head
- Lymphadenopathy
- Oral ulcers
- Salivary gland enlargement
- Thyroid, abnormal
- Xerostomia

Chest
- Pleural effusion
- Pleural rubs
- Rales
- Wheezing

Heart
- Abnormal P_2

Edema, dependent
Enlarged heart
Murmur, diastolic
Murmur, systolic
Pericardial rub

Abdomen
Hepatomegaly
Jaundice
Peritoneal signs
Splenomegaly

Genitalia
Pregnancy
Ulcerations, rashes (balanitis)
Urethral discharge

Arteries
Absent pulses (specify)
Raynaud's phenomenon (exam)
Temporal artery tenderness

Muscles
Atrophy
Tenderness
Weakness, distal
Weakness, proximal

Neurologic–Psychiatric
Neuropathy, entrapment
Neuropathy, motor
Neuropathy, sensory
Personality change
Psychosis

ARTICULAR HISTORY

Arthralgia, stiffness only (0−3+)
Course
Heel pain (0−3+)
Interval exacerbations (number)
Joint, heat/redness (0−3+)
Joint, swelling (0−3+)
Joint, pain on use/exercise (0−3+)
Joint, number of involved (0,1,2−4.>4)
Joint, number of newly involved (0,1,2-4.>4)
Low back pain (0−3+)
Morning stiffness (hours)
Myofascial pain (motion)
Myofascial pain (non-motion)
Myofascial site (general/regional)
Neck pain (0−3+)
Night pain (0−3+)
Patient estimation of arthritis severity (0−3+)
Patient estimation of pain (0−3+)
Symmetry (0,+)

ARTICULAR PHYSICAL EXAM

Upper extremity
Shoulder girdle
Sternoclavicular
Acromioclavicular
Shoulder
Elbow
Wrist
First carpometacarpal
Metacarpophalangeal
Thumb interphalangeal
Proximal interphalangeal
Distal interphalangeal

Lower extremity
Pelvic girdle
Hip
Knee
Ankle

Subtalar
Tarsal
Metatarsophalangeal
Great toe, metatarsophalangeal
Great toe, interphalangeal
Proximal interphalangeal
Distal interphalangeal

Axial skeleton
Temporomandibular
Sternomanubrial
Costochondral
Cervical spine
Thoracic spine
Lumbar spine
Sacroiliac

Articular physical findings (0,+)
Bursitis (specify)
Epicondylitis (specify)
Painful areas
Painful nodules
Radiculopathy (specify)
Subcutaneous nodules
Subungual hemorrhages
Synovial cysts (e.g., Baker's)
Tendon lesions, tenosynovitis (specify)
Tophi

FUNCTION MEASUREMENTS

ARA functional class (I, II, III, IV)

Activities of daily living (Activity Scale 0−3+)
Ability at vocation
Activity
Dressing/grooming
Eating
Functional grip
Gait/walking
Hygiene/bathing
Reach over head
Rise from straight chair
Sexual
Stairs/5 steps
Quantitative measurements of function
Chest excursion (maximum cm)
Chin-chest (cm)
Grip strength (mm/Hg total of R+L)
Interincisor (mm)
Occiput-wall
Schober test (total cm)
Time to walk 50 feet (seconds)

Other function assessments
Compliance (total, good, fair, poor)
Gait (0−4+)
Restricted range of motion
Sexual (independent, arthritis, situational)
Vocation (school, house, sedentary, active)

SOCIOECONOMIC STATUS

Discomfort
Severity
Trend

Dollars
Drugs (# or $/year)
Devices
Domestic
Employment
Hospital (days)
Lab tests (# or $/year)
Surgery
Transportation
Visits, MD (#/year)

Visits, paramedical (#/year)
X-rays

Indices
Costs, medical
Costs, out of pocket
Costs, social
Costs, total dollar
Disability index
Discomfort index
Side effects index
Status (alive, lost, dead)

LABORATORY

Chemical
Albumin
Aldolase
Alkaline phosphatase
Bilirubin, total
BUN
Calcium
Cholesterol
CPK
Creatinine
Fibrinogen
Glucose
Guaiac
LDH
Phosphorus
Salicylate level
SGOT
SGPT
Total protein
T4
Uric acid

Hematologic
Bands (%)
Basophils (%)
Eosinophils (%)
Hepatoglobin
Hematocrit
Hemoglobin (gm %)
Hemoglobin electrophoresis
Iron
Iron binding capacity/transferrin
Lymphocytes (%)
Monocytes (%)
Neutrophils (%)
Platelets
Prothrombin time
PTT
Reticulocytes (%)
Undifferentiated WBC (%)
Westergren sedimentation rate
White blood count
Wintrobe sedimentation rate

Serologic
Anti-DNA (% bound)
Anti-DNA (mg bound)
Anti-DNA (titer)
Anti-ENA
Antiglobulin
ASO titer
Australian antigen or antibody
C-reactive protein
CH50
Coombs direct
Cryoglobulins
C2
C3
C4
FANA pattern
FANA titer
FTA

HLA–B27
IgA
IgG
IgM
Immunoelectrophoresis
Latex fixation (slide)
Latex fixation titer
LE preparation
Protein electrophoresis
RNP specificity
Sm specificity
STS (VDRL)

Urine
    Casts, granular
    Casts, red cell
    Casts, white cell
    Creatinine clearance
    Glucose
    Protein
    RBC
    Urine pH
    WBC
    24-hr uric acid
    24-hr urine creatine
    24-hr urine creatinine
    24-hr urine protein

Cerebrospinal fluid
    Cells/mm^3
    Glucose (mg %)
    Polymorphs (%)
    Protein (mg %)

Joint fluid
    Crystals (urate, CPPD, apatite, steroid)
    Complement (mg %)
    Glucose (mg %)
    Mucin clot (normal, fair, poor)
    Polys (%)
    White count/mm^3

Pulmonary function
    Diffusing capacity
    One-second expiratory volume (% VC)
    Total lung capacity (ml)

Skin tests
    Candida (mm induration)
    Cocci (mm induration)

DNCB (mm induration)
Mumps (mm induration)
PPD (mm induration)
Trichophyton (mm induration)
Varidase (mm erythema)

BIOPSIES
    Kidney biopsy
    Liver biopsy
    Muscle biopsy
    Skin biopsy
    Synovial biopsy
    Temporal artery biopsy

X-RAYS
    Chest
    Chondrocalcinosis
    Degenerative changes
    Erosions
    Esophageal aperistalsis
    Periosteal new bone
    Sacroiliac

MISCELLANEOUS
    Electrocardiogram
    Fist closure, right
    Fist closure, left
    Leg length, right
    Leg length, left
    Drug reaction=1
    Drug reaction=2
    Drug reaction=3
    Side effect symptom=1
    Side effect symptom=2
    Side effect symptom=3

THERAPY

Rheumatic agents
    ACTH (units)
    Allopurinol (mg/day)
    Antimalarials (mg/day)
    Azathioprine (mg/day)
    Chlorambucil (mg/day)
    Chrysotherapy (cumulative total mg)
    Colchicine (mg/day)
    Cyclophosphamide (mg/day)
    Cytotoxics, other

Fenoprofen (mg/day)
Ibuprofen (mg/day)
Indomethacin (mg/day)
Intraarticular, other (specify joint)
Intraarticular, steroid (specify joint)
Methotrexate (mg/week)
Naproxen (mg/day)
Nonarticular, local injection (specify)
Penicillamine (mg/day)
Phenylbutazone (mg/day)
Prednisone equivalent (mg/day)
Prednisone, dosage schedule (divided, daily,
    every other day)
Probenecid (gm/day)
Salicylate (gm/day)
Salicylate type (plain, buffered, enteric-
    coated, choline, sodium)
Sulfinpyrazone (mg/day)
Sulindac (mg/day)
Tolmetin (mg/day)

Rheumatic surgery
    Synovectomy (specify joint)
    Reconstructive with prosthesis (specify joint)
    Reconstructive, without prosthesis
        (specify joint)
    Total joint replacement (specify joint)
    Other surgery

Physical and occupational therapies
    Appliances and devices
    Physical measures
    Therapeutic exercises (active, passive)

Nonrheumatic drugs
    Alpha methyl dopa
    Analgesics
    Anticonvulsants
    Antihypertensives, other
    Diuretics
    Hormones
    Hydralazine
    Isoniazid
    Oral contraceptives
    Other cardiac agents
    Penicillin
    Procainamide
    Propranolol
    Sulfa
    Tetracycline

Examples of Entries in the Dictionary

Morning stiffness

The subjective complaint of either localized or generalized lack of easy mobility of the joints upon arising. Morning stiffness is a nonspecific indication of inflammation and the duration is directly proportional to the severity of the inflammatory process. This complaint can vary from 0 hours for the patient in remission to throughout the patient's waking hours ("all day"), even though this form of persistent stiffness would not strictly be "morning stiffness."

This complaint is manifest in most types of inflammatory arthritis (e.g., rheumatoid arthritis, systemic lupus erythematosus) as well as in polymyalgia rheumatica. Patients with degenerative arthritis may also complain of morning stiffness but it tends to be brief.

Ascertainment: By history
The time elapsed between the time usual awakening (even if not in the morning) and the time the patient is as limber as she/he will be during a day involving typical activities. For those experiencing relief, the actual hours elapsed to relief should be recorded no matter how long.

Record:
The duration in hours to the nearest quarter (0.25, 0.50, 0.75) hour. For those patients with unrelenting stiffness, record 24 hours.

Raynaud's phenomenon

Sudden reversible "dead white" pallor of an acral structure (e.g., fingers, whole hand, toes, tip of nose, earlobe, or tongue), precipitated by cold exposure or emotion. This reaction is episodic, may be precipitated by even a small drop in ambient temperature or may arise without an obvious precipitating factor. The involved area may subsequently develop cyanosis and the rewarming become hyperemic. Numbness and pain may be associated.

Raynaud's phenomenon results from paroxysmal vasospasm and therefore the pallor should be uniform distal to the point of spasm. This term should not be confused with the blotchy discoloration of livedo reticularis.

Ascertainment: By history
Reversible pallor must be present to make this diagnosis.

Record:
0 = absent
1 = present

INDEX

A

Abdominal pain
  in childhood dermatomyositis, 67
  in Schönlein-Henoch purpura, 73
  in SLE, 53
Acetaminophen, 213
  for hyperuricemic gout, 126
  for osteoarthritis, 107
Acetylating enzymes, 54
Acetylcholinesterase, collagenous sequences
    in, 10
Achilles tendinitis, 163, 165
  arthrocentesis for, 199
Achilles tendon, rheumatoid nodules of, 42
Achondroplasia, 144
Acne arthralgia, 173
Acrodermatitis chronica atrophicans, 59
Acrolysis, clubbing and, 168
Acromegaly, 135
  carpal tunnel syndrome in, 160
  classification, 36
  hyperostosis of spine in, 152
  skin changes in, 59
Acromegalic arthropathy, osteoarthritis and,
    107
Acromioclavicular joint involvement in osteo-
    arthritis, 106
Acromionectomy, subtotal, 161
ACTH, 191–192
Activities of daily living, 203–204
Acupuncture, 107, 204
Acute anterior uveitis
  epidemiology of, 35
  HLA–B27 association with, 32
Acute febrile neutrophilic dermatosis, 173
Acute gouty arthritis, 122
ADCC. See Antibody-dependent cell-mediated
    cytotoxicity
Addison's disease, HLA antigens associated
    with, 78
Adenopathy in JRA, 98
Adenovirus, arthritis and, 115
Adhesive capsulitis, 37
Adolescent coxa vara, 147
Adrenocortical insufficiency, arthropathy in,
    136
Adrenocorticotrophic hormone (ACTH), 191–
    192
Adult onset Still's disease, 103–104
Adventitious bursae, 154
Agammaglobulinemia, 173
Aging, amyloidosis and, 79
Agranulocytosis
  from gold therapy, 192
  from NSAIDs, 190
Alanine in elastin, 12
Alcoholism
  Dupuytren's contracture and, 167
  gout and, 124
  osteonecrosis and, 157
Aldermanic gout, 124
Alkaptonuria, 134–135
  back pain in, 148
  classification, 36
  osteoarthritis and, 107
Allergic granulomatosis, 4
Allergic granulomatous angiitis, 71
  in children, 102
Allergic purpura, 73–74
Allergic reactions
  IgE in, 22
  mechanisms of, 25
Allergic vasculitis, 71–72
  in children, 102

Allograft rejection, cell-mediated immunity in,
    28
Allopurinol, 126, 214
Alopecia
  in childhood dermatomyositis, 101
  in MCTD, 65
  in SLE, 53
Alphamethyl dopa, SLE induced by, 54
Alternate complement pathway activation, 19
  immunoglobulins in, 22
  in Schönlein-Henoch purpura, 74
American Juvenile Arthritis Organization
    (AJAO), 5
American Rheumatism Association (ARA), 5
  criteria for diagnosis and classification,
    207–212
  disease classification of, 36
  Uniform Database, 215
Amino acids
  composition in elastic fibers, 12
  of collagen, 9
Aminosalicyclic acid
  hypersensitivity to, 81
  SLE induced by, 54
Amitriptyline for fibrositis, 142
Amphiarthrodial joints, classification, 13
Amphotericin B for fungal arthritis, 114
Amyloid, 79, 80
  in ankylosing spondylitis, 87
Amyloid neuropathy, 109
Amyloidosis, 79–81
  carpal tunnel syndrome in, 160
  classification, 36
  clinical features, 79
  immunochemical findings, 79
  in adult onset Still's disease, 104
  in familial Mediterranean fever, 118
  in myelomatosis, 137
  in Reiter's syndrome, 90
  laboratory findings in, 80
  skin changes in, 59
  treatment, 80
ANA. See Antinuclear antibodies
Analgesics, 188
Anaphylactic reactions
  cellular immunity in, 23
  leukotriene D and, 17
  mechanisms of, 25
  schematic of, 27
Anaphylactoid purpura, 73–74
  in children, 102
Anaphylatoxins in inflammation, 16
Anemia
  in giant cell arteritis, 77
  in JRA, 98
  in Kawasaki disease, 75
  in MCTD, 65
  in polyarteritis, 71
  in polymyalgia rheumatica, 77
  in PSS, 62
  in Reiter's syndrome, 91
  in relapsing polychondritis, 83
  in rheumatoid arthritis, 44
  in Schönlein-Henoch purpura, 74
  in Sjögren's syndrome, 78
  in SLE, 55
  in thrombotic thrombocytopenic purpura, 84
  in Wegener's granulomatosis, 72
Anemia, aplastic
  drug-induced, 190, 192
  in eosinophilic fasciitis, 65
Anemia, autoimmune hemolytic, 26
Anemia, hemolytic, in thrombotic thrombocy-
    topenic purpura, 84

Aneurysms
  in polyarteritis, 71
  in Takayasu's arteritis, 74
Angiokeratoma corporis diffusum universale,
    139
Angiopathy in childhood dermatomyositis, 101
Ankle and subtalar joint assessment, 186
Ankle arthrocentesis, 199
Ankle pannus, 40
Ankylosing hyperostosis, 106, 151
Ankylosing spondylitis, 85–88
  amyloidosis associated with, 79
  back pain in, 148
  classification, 36
  clinical features and diagnosis, 86
  comparison with other seronegative spondyl-
    arthropathies, 85
  epidemiologic studies of, 34–35
  etiology, 88
  first studies of, 2–3
  heel pain in, 163
  HLA antigens associated with, 35
  HLA–B27 associated with, 32, 86
  hyperostosis of the spine in, 152
  in children, 86, 100
  in women, 88
  inflammatory intestinal disease and, 92
  laboratory studies in, 87
  management, 88
  NSAIDs for, 191
  prevalence, 86
  radiologic evaluation, 87, 179–180
  surgical risks in, 200–201
  synovial fluid analysis in, 187
  total hip replacement for, 201
  Whipple's disease and, 93
Ankylosing vertebral hyperostosis, 37. See also
    Diffuse idiopathic skeletal hyperostosis
    (DISH)
Anserine bursitis, 165
Antacids, NSAIDs and, 58
Anterior uveitis in Reiter's syndrome, 89
Anti-β_2-microglobulin, 25, 26
Antibiotics
  for bacterial arthritis, 112
  for intestinal bypass arthritis, 172
  for intestinal infection in PSS, 61
  for rheumatic fever, 96
Antibodies, See also Immunoglobulins
  anti-bacterial, 21
  IgM class, 22
  in immune injury, 25
  in myasthenia gravis, 69
  in rheumatic fever, 95
  in Sjögren's syndrome, 78
  rheumatoid factors, 38
Antibody-dependent cell-mediated cytotoxicity
    (ADCC)
  in antibody-mediated reactions, 26
  IgM mediation of, 22
  macrophages in, 23
  T lymphocyte mediation of, 25
Antibody-mediated reactions, 25–27
Anticentromere antibody in PSS, 62
Anticholinesterase agents for myasthenia gra-
    vis, 69
Anticoagulant drugs, 189
  for Schönlein-Henoch purpura, 74
  hemarthrosis from, 110
  in SLE, 56
  NSAIDs interation with, 191
Anticonvulsant drugs
  for central nervous system SLE, 58
  lupus-like syndrome and, 100

Antidiabetic drugs, 189
Antigens in cell-mediated reactions, 27
Antihypertensive drugs, 58, 61, 63
Anti-idiotype antibodies in immunoregulation, 28
Antilymphocyte antibodies in antibody-mediated reactions, 26
Antimalarial drugs
  antiinflammatory action of, 18
  for rheumatoid arthritis, 47
  for SLE, 57
Antinuclear antibodies (ANA)
  first detection of, 3
  in childhood scleroderma, 102
  in childhood SLE, 100
  in chronic active liver disease, 84
  in cryoglobulinemia, 82
  in JRA, 98
  in linear scleroderma, 63
  in MCTD, 65
  in PSS, 62
  in rheumatic diseases, 56–57
  in rheumatoid arthritis, 55
  in SLE, 54, 56–57
  placental transmission of, 100
Antirheumatic drugs, clinical pharmacology of, 188–192
Anti-seizure drugs, SLE induced by, 54
Anulus fibrosus, structure, 149
Aorta, elastic fibers of, 12
Aortic arch syndrome
  in giant cell arteritis, 76
  in Takayasu's arteritis, 74
Aortic regurgitation in seronegative spondylarthropathies, 85
Aortitis syndrome, 74
Apatite crystal deposition disease, 131–132
  colchicine for, 126
Apatite crystals in osteoarthritis, 107
Aplastic anemia
  from gold therapy, 192
  from NSAIDs, 190
  in eosinophilic fasciitis, 65
Apophyseal osteoarthritis, back pain in, 148–149
Appendicitis in polyarteritis, 70
Apresoline for SLE hypertension, 58
Arachidonic acid, role in inflammation, 16
Arachnodactyly in Marfan's syndrome, 142
Arachnoid cyst, computed tomography in detection of, 184
Arboviral diseases, arthritis in, 115
Arm disorders, 164
Arterial hypertension associated with gout and hyperuricemia, 35
Arterial involvement
  in giant cell arteritis, 76
  in polyarteritis, 70
Arterial lesions, in Takayasu's arteritis, 74
Arteriosclerosis, role of elastase in, 12
Arthralgia
  in adult onset Still's disease, 103
  in Cogan's syndrome, 71
  in JRA, 98
  in Kawasaki disease, 75
  in polyarteritis, 70
  in polymyalgia rheumatica, 76
  in Schönlein-Henoch purpura, 73
  in Whipple's disease, 93
Arthritis associated with infectious agents, classification, 36
Arthritis associated with spondylitis, classification, 36
Arthritis Foundation, 5, 48
Arthritis Health Professions Association (AHPA), 5

Arthritis mutilans, 91
Arthrocentesis, 197–199
  in infectious arthritis, 111
Arthrodesis
  in neuropathic arthropathy, 109
  in rheumatic diseases, 200–202
Arthrography
  for Baker's cyst, 41
  in diagnosis of internal derangement of knee, 185
Arthrogryposis multiplex congenita, 37
Arthropan for JRA, 99
Arthropathies associated with endocrine disorders, 135–136
Arthropathies associated with hematologic diseases and storage disorders, 136–139
Arthroplasty
  for hemochromatosis, 133
  for osteoarthritis, 107
  for rheumatic disease, 200–202
Arthroscopy, 184–185
Arthus reaction, 26
Articular cartilage, biology of, 14
Aschoff, Ludwig, 1
Aschoff nodule in rheumatic fever, 95
Aseptic necrosis of bone, 157
  in SLE, 53
Asparagine, binding of glucosamine to, 7
Aspirin, 46, 57, 75, 86, 92, 96, 99, 101, 104, 107, 116, 122, 143, 156, 200, 213
  inhibition of prostaglandins, 18
  link to Reye's syndrome, 99
  pharmacokinetics, 188–189
Asthma preceding allergic granulomatous angiitis, 71
Atherosclerosis
  in gout, 35, 123
  in Takayasu's arteritis, 74
Atlantoaxial subluxation
  in ankylosing spondylitis, 180
  in JRA, 176
  in rheumatoid arthritis, 42, 175
Atrophic arthritis. See Rheumatoid arthritis
Atrophoderma Pasini-Pierini in scleroderma, 59
Atypical verrucous endocarditis associated with SLE, 3
Auranofin, 192
Auricular chondritis, 83
Aurothioglucose, 192
Aurothiomalate, 192
Auspitz, Heinrich, 3
Autoantibodies in SLE, 51
Autoimmune disease
  HLA genes and, 31
  immune deficiency associated with, 29
  mechanisms of, 28
Autoimmune exocrinopathy, 78
Autoimmune hemolytic anemia
  corticosteroids for, 196
  immunopathogenesis of, 26
  in PSS, 62
Autoimmune thyroiditis, antibody-dependent cellular cytotoxicity in, 26
Autoimmunity, 28–29
Autoreactive cells, 28
Avascular necrosis, 37
Avascular necrosis of bone, 157
  in gout, 123
Azapropazone, 189
Azathioprine, 194, 214
  for chronic active liver disease, 84
  for PM/DM, 68
  for polyarteritis, 71
  for rheumatoid arthritis, 48
  for SLE, 58
Azotemia in Wegener's granulomatosis, 72

B

B lymphocyte alloantigens, HLA disease associations and, 31
B lymphocyte antigens in Sjögren's syndrome, 78
B lymphocytes
  cell surface determinants of, 25
  differentiation of, 24
  effect of corticosteroids on, 195
  immunoglobulin classes of, 22
  in cellular immunity, 23
  in development of hypergammaglobulinemia, 51
  in proliferative states, 194
  in PSS, 63
  percentages in lymphoid organs, 25
  primary functions of, 26
Back pocket wallet syndrome, 165
Bacterial arthritis, 112
  classification, 36
  synovial fluid analysis in, 187
Bacterial endocarditis, 72
  classification, 70
  clubbing and, 168
  infectious arthritis and, 113
  rheumatoid factor in, 38
Bacterial infection, mixed cryoglobulinemia and, 82
Bacteroides fragilis, antibodies to, in intestinal bypass arthritis, 172
Baehr, George, 3
Baillie, Matthew, 1
Baillou, Guillaume, 1
Baker's cysts, 154, 165
  in rheumatoid arthritis, 41
Bamboo spine in ankylosing spondylitis, 87, 180
  radiographic appearance, 180
Bannatyne, GA, 2
Barbiturates, linked to osteomalacia, 170
Basement membrane collagens, 11
Basilar-vertebral insufficiency syndrome in osteoarthritis, 106
Basophils
  in anaphylactic reactions, 25
  in cellular immunity, 23
Bb, function, 20
Bechterew, Vladimir von, 2
Behçet's syndrome, 117–118
  classification, 36
  criteria for diagnosis, 117
  HLA associations in, 32
Benign hyperglobulinemic purpura, 70
Benzothiadiazide diuretics for SLE hypertension, 58
Bernstein, Lilli, 3
Beta thalassemia, arthropathy in, 137
Betamethasone, 191
Bezecny, Rudolf, 4
Bicipital tendinitis, 161
  classification, 37
Biliary cirrhosis
  clubbing and, 168
  in PSS, 62
Billings, Frank, 2
Biochemical abnormalities associated with rheumatic states, 36
Biofeedback, 204
Blastogenic factors, secretion by T lymphocytes, 27
Blastomycosis, infectious arthritis and, 114
Bleomycin-induced fibrosis, scleroderma and, 59
Blood dyscrasias caused by NSAIDs, 190
Blood supply to joints, 15
Blood vessels
  collagenous components of, 10

Blood vessels (cont'd)
elastic fibers of, 12
Blount's disease, 145
Bone
collagenous component of, 10
effects of prostaglandin on, 18
erosion of, 89, 175
formation, 169
proteoglycan components of, 7
resorption, 169
in PSS, 60
Bone and cartilage disorders, 37
Bone atrophy. See Osteoporosis
Bone disease, metabolic, 169–171
Bone erosion
in Reiter's syndrome, 89
in rheumatoid arthritis, 175
Bone lesions in sarcoidosis, 117
Bone marrow–derived lymphocytes. See B lymphocytes
Bone tumors, scintigraphy in diagnosis of, 184
Bony ankylosis
in ankylosing spondylitis, 180
in rheumatoid arthritis, 175
Bouchard, CJ, 3
Bouchard's nodes
in CPPD disease, 129
in osteoarthritis, 106
Bouillaud, Jean-Baptiste, 1
Boutonniere deformity in rheumatoid arthritis, 41
Bow-leg deformity, 145
Bowel disease, chronic inflammatory, associated with arthritis, 36
Bradykinin, in inflammation, 16
Brewerton, Derek, 3
Bright, Richard, 2
Brim sign in Paget's disease of bone, 156
Broch, OJ, 3
Brodie, Benjamin, 2, 4, 88
Buchman's disease, 146
Bulge sign, 186
Bunyamwera, arthritis in, 115
Bursitis, 160–161
arthrocentesis for, 197
caused by infectious agents, 36
classification, 37
in viral arthritis, 115
radiographic findings, 161
Buschke, Abraham, 3
Butterfly rash, 49, 54
in childhood SLE, 100
in PM/DM, 67
in SLE, 53
Bypass surgery for obesity, arthritis following, 172
Bywaters, Eric GL, 2

C

C1 in complement activation, 19
C1q
collagenous sequences of, 10
immunoglobulin fixation of, 22
C2 in complement activation, 19
C3
in PM/DM, 68
in Schönlein-Henoch purpura, 74
in SLE, 56
C3 deficiency in hypocomplementemic cutaneous vasculitis, 75
C3a, 20
in inflammation, 16, 18
C3b(bi), C3bBb, C3d, function, 20
C4
in complement activation, 19

C4 (cont'd)
in Schönlein-Henoch purpura, 74
in SLE, 56
C5a, C5b67, C5b6789, 20
in inflammation, 16
C-reactive protein (CRP), 79
in rheumatic fever, 96
Caisson disease, osteonecrosis, and, 157
Calcaneal periostitis, 163
in ankylosing spondylitis, 87
Calcaneal spurs in Reiter's syndrome, 89
Calcific periarthritis, apatite crystals in, 131
Calcific tendinitis of shoulder, 160–161
Calcifications in DISH, 152
Calcinosis
earliest description of, 3
in childhood dermatomyositis, 101
in PSS, 59
Calcinosis circumscripta, 60
Calcinosis universalis in PM/DM, 67
Calcitonin
for Paget's disease of bone, 156
in bone formation and resorption, 169
Calcium, in bone formation and resorption, 169
Calcium hydrogen phosphate dihydrate crystals, 132
Calcium oxalate deposition, 132
Calcium pyrophosphate dihydrate crystals in osteoarthritis, 107
Calcium pyrophosphate dihydrate (CPPD) deposition disease, 128–131. See also Chondrocalcinosis; Pseudogout
classification, 36, 130
clinical features, 128–130
myxedema and, 136
osteitis fibrosa in, 170
pathogenesis, 130
radiologic features, 130, 177
sites for, 129
synovial fluid analysis in, 187
treatment, 131
Calvé disease, 146
Cancer, first associated with dermatomyositis, 4
Candidiasis, infectious arthritis and, 114
Capillaritis in rheumatoid arthritis, 43
Capillary blood flow in PSS, 60
Caplan's syndrome, 43
Captopril for PSS hypertension, 63
Carbidopa, scleroderma and, 59
Carcinoid syndrome, skin changes in, 59
Carcinoma
dermatomyositis and, 67
hypertrophic osteoarthropathy and, 163
Cardiac involvement
in adult onset Still's disease, 103
in amyloidosis, 80
in ankylosing spondylitis, 3
in childhood scleroderma, 102
in childhood SLE, 100
in Cogan's syndrome, 71
in Ehlers-Danlos syndrome, 142
in gout, 123
in hyperlipoproteinemia, 140
in JRA, 98
in Kawasaki disease, 74
in Lyme disease, 116
in Marfan's syndrome, 142
in MCTD, 65
in Paget's disease of bone, 156
in PM/DM, 67
in polyarteritis, 70
in PSS, 4, 61
in Reiter's syndrome, 90
in relapsing polychondritis, 83
in rheumatic fever, 95

Cardiac involvement (cont'd)
in rheumatoid arthritis, 43
in Wegener's granulomatosis, 72
Cardiovascular involvement
in ankylosing spondylitis, 87
in pseudoxanthoma elasticum, 143
in SLE, 53
Carditis in rheumatic fever, 1, 95
Carpal tunnel syndrome, 159–160
arthrocentesis for, 199
classification, 37
clinical features, 159
following rubella vaccination, 115
in acromegaly, 135
in amyloidosis, 80
in eosinophilic fasciitis, 64
in gout, 123
in hypothyroidism, 136
in myelomatosis, 137
in rheumatoid arthritis, 41, 43
Carprofen, 189
Cartilage
breaking into the joint, 154
collagenous component of, 10
crystal deposition in, 128
in osteoarthritis, 104–105
proteoglycan components of, 7
proteoglycans in, 8
response to injury, 9
Cartilage destruction in relapsing polychondritis, 83
Cartilage hyperplasia in osteoarthritis, 178
Cartilaginous joints, classification, 13
Cathepsin G in inflammation, 19
Cauda equina syndrome
in ankylosing spondylitis, 87
in osteoarthritis, 106
Causalgia, 165
Cazenave, Pierre Louis Alphée, 3
Cecil, Russell L, 2
Celiac disease, HLA antigens in, 78
Cell-mediated cytotoxicity, antibody-dependent, IgM mediation of, 22
Cell-mediated immune reactions, 27–29
in PM/DM, 68
in SLE, tests for, 56
in Wegener's granulomatosis, 73
Cell surface determinants of lymphocytes, 25
Cellular hypersensitivity hypothesis in pathogenesis of rheumatoid arthritis, 39
Cellular immunity, 22–25
effect of corticosteroids on, 195
Central nervous system (CNS) involvement
in childhood SLE, 100
in SLE, 53–54
Cerebral arteritis in polyarteritis, 70
Cerebral thrombosis in MCTD, 65
Cerebral vasculitis, Sjögren's syndrome and, 78
Cerebrospinal fluid analysis in SLE, 55
Cervical collar for osteoarthritis of spine, 108
Cervical disc disease, 150
Cervical spondylitis
in JRA, 176
in rheumatoid arthritis, 175
CH50 levels in SLE, 56
Chandler's disease, 157
Charcot, Jean-Martin, 2
Charcot arthropathy, CPPD disease and, 130
Charcot joints, 108–110
classification, 37
osteoarthritis and, 107
Charcot-like steroid arthropathy, 197
Charcot-Marie-Tooth disease, 109
Chauffard, Anatole, 4
Chemically induced scleroderma-like conditions, 59

Mixed connective tissue disease (cont'd)
  systemic manifestations, 65
  treatment, 66
Mixed cryoglobulinemia, 82
  hepatitis B antigen–antibody complexes in, 27
Mixed lymphocyte culture (MLC) reaction, 31
  T lymphocyte response in, 25
MLC. *See* Mixed lymphocyte culture (MLC) reaction
Mollaret's meningitis, confusion with Behçet's syndrome, 118
Monocyte–macrophage system, 23
Monocytes, 6
  in cellular immunity, 23
Monokines in collagen synthesis, 6
Mononeuritis multiplex
  in polyarteritis, 70
  in rheumatoid arthritis, 43
  in Wegener's granulomatosis, 72
Mononuclear phagocytes in cellular immunity, 23
Mononucleosis infections
  antinuclear antibodies in, 56
  mixed cryoglobulinemia and, 82
Monophasic synovioma, 153
Monosodium urate crystals in gout, 123–124
Monosodium urate deposition, 36. *See also* Gout
Monosodium urate monohydrate crystals in gout, 122–123
Moore, DH, 3
Moore, H, 3
Moore, J. Earle, 3
Morning stiffness
  in ankylosing spondylitis, 86
  in JRA, 98
  in polymyalgia rheumatica, 76
  in rheumatoid arthritis, 40
  in SLE, 52
Morphea of scleroderma, 59, 62–63
Morquio syndrome, 143
  osteoarthritis and, 107
Morton's neuroma, 162
Mouse models of SLE, 52
MT alloantigen systems, 31
Mucin clot test, 187
  in rheumatoid arthritis, 44
Mucocutaneous lymph node syndrome, 74
  classification, 36
Mucolipidoses, 143–144
Mucopolysaccharide abnormalities, 36
Mucopolysaccharidosis, 143
Mucous membrane involvement in seronegative spondylarthropathies, 85
Multicentric reticulohistiocytosis, arthropathy in, 138–139
Multiple epiphyseal dysplasia, osteoarthritis and, 107
Multiple myeloma, amyloidosis associated with, 79
Mumps, arthritis in, 115
Muscle atrophy
  in JRA, 100
  in rheumatoid arthritis, 41
  in PSS, 61
Muscle contraction headache, cause, 163
Muscle disorders, polymyositis and dermatomyositis, 66–69
Muscle fibers, types of, 203
Muscle involvement
  in childhood dermatomyositis, 101
  in MCTD, 65
  in polymyalgia rheumatica, 76
  in sarcoidosis, 117
Muscle spasm in intervertebral disc disease, 150
Muscle tenderness in fibrositis, 141

Muscle weakness
  in carpal tunnel syndrome, 159
  in myasthenia gravis, 69
  in polyarteritis, 70
  in Takayasu's arteritis, 74
Muscular dystrophy, similarity to polymyositis, 67
Musculoskeletal examination, 185–187
Myalgia
  in adult onset Still's disease, 103
  in JRA, 98
  in polymyalgia rheumatica, 76
  in SLE, 53
Myasthenia gravis, 69
  arthropathy in, 135
  from penicillamine, 192
  HLA antigens in, 78
  immunopathogenesis of, 26
  treatment, 69
Mycobacteria arthritis, classification, 36
Mycoplasmal arthritis, 114–115
Mycoses, erythema nodosum in, 172
Myelography, for assessing disc disease, 150
Myeloma, osteopenia in, 170
Myelomatosis
  arthropathy in, 137
  back pain in, 148
Myelomeningocoele, neuropathic arthropathy and, 109
Myeloproliferative disorders, gout in, 123
Myocardial fibrosis, earliest association with PSS, 4
Myocardial infarction
  in giant cell arteritis, 76
  in polyarteritis, 70
Myocarditis
  hemochromatosis and, 133
  in JRA, 98
  in Kawasaki disease, 75
  in MCTD, 65
  in PM/DM, 67
  in Reiter's syndrome, 90
  in rheumatic fever, 95
  in rheumatoid arthritis, 43
  in SLE, 53
Myofascial neck pain, 163
Myofascial pain syndromes, classification, 37
Myoglobinemia in PM/DM, 68
Myopathy
  in MCTD, 65
  in Whipple's disease, 93
  Sjögren's syndrome and, 78
Myositis, 68
  in SLE, 53
  influenza B virus infection and, 101
  PM/DM and, 66
Myositis ossificans progressiva, classification, 37
Myxedema
  arthropathy in, 136
  carpal tunnel syndrome in, 160

N

N-acetyl neuraminic acid, occurrence in proteoglycans, 7
N-acetylglucosamine, structure and function, 7
Nail involvement
  in psoriatic arthritis, 91
  in Reiter's syndrome, 90
Nailfold changes in PSS, 60
Naproxen, 189, 213
  for gout, 126
  for JRA, 100
  for osteoarthritis, 107
Narcotics for osteoarthritis, 107
Nasal chondritis, 83
Native DNA, antibodies to, in SLE, 54, 56

Neck involvement
  in polymylagia rheumatica, 76
  in rheumatoid arthritis, 42
Neck muscle weakness in MCTD, 67
Necrotizing angiitis
  of the skin, 75
  treatment, 71
Necrotizing arteritis, 69
  in rheumatoid arthritis, 43
Necrotizing vasculitis, 69–75
  classification, 36
Neisser, Albert, 4
Neisseria gonorrhoeae, infectious arthritis from, 112–113
Neisseria infections, complement deficiency associated with, 21
Neoplasia
  from immunosuppressive therapy, 195
  PM/DM and, 67
Neoplasms
  amyloidosis associated with, 79
  back pain and, 148
  of the joints, 152–154
  rheumatic states and, 37
Neostigmine for myasthenia gravis, 69
Nephritis
  cryoglobulinemia and, 82
  in serum sickness, 27
  in SLE, 50
Nephrolithiasis preceding gout, 122
Nephrotic syndrome in Schönlein-Henoch purpura, 74
Nerve supply to joints, 15
Neurologic injury, apatite crystals in, 132
Neurologic involvement
  in Behçet's syndrome, 118
  in childhood SLE, 100
  in Dupuytren's contracture, 167
  in intervertebral disc disease, 150
  in Lyme arthritis, 116
  in MCTD, 65
  in osteoarthritis of the spine, 106
  in reflex sympathetic dystrophy syndrome, 165
  in Reiter's syndrome, 90
  in SLE, 53–54
  in thrombotic thrombocytopenic purpura, 84
  in tuberculous arthritis, 113
  in Wegener's granulomatosis, 72
Neuropathic arthropathies
  carpal tunnel syndrome, 159–160
  Charcot joints, 108–110
  chondrocalcinosis in, 177
  in MCTD, 65
  in polyarteritis, 70
  in PSS, 62
  in rheumatoid arthritis, 42, 48
  infectious arthritis in, 111
  loose bodies in, 154
  pronator syndrome, 160
  radiographic findings in, 181–182
  Sjögren's syndrome and, 78
  synovial fluid analysis in, 187
  tarsal tunnel syndrome, 163
Neuropathic disorders associated with rheumatic states, 37
Neutral proteases in inflammation, 18–19
New Zealand mouse SLE-like disease, 52
Nodular panniculitis, 171
Nomenclature and Classification Committee of the American Rheumatism Association, 36
Nonacetylated salicylates, 189
Nonarticular rheumatism, 37
Nonsteroidal antiinflammatory drugs (NSAIDs), 189–191
  antacids and, 58
  classification, 189
  drug interactions with, 191

Pannus formation (cont'd)
  in slipped capital femoral epiphysis, 147
Papular mucinosis, 59
Paraaminobenzoic acid for SLE, 58
Paraffin wax applications, 108, 204
Paramethasone, 191
Parasitic arthritis, classification, 36
Parasitic infection, mixed cryoglobulinemia and, 82
Parasternal chondrodynia, 169
Parathyroid hormone (PTH) in bone formation and resorption, 169
Parenchymatous fibrosis associated with PSS, 4
Paresthesias after intestinal bypass, 172
Parotitis in Sjögren's syndrome, 78
Pasteurella ssp, 93
Patient self-assessment in rheumatoid arthritis, 46
Pauciarticular onset JRA, 98–99
Pelvic girdle muscle weakness
  in polymyalgia rheumatica, 76
  in polymyositis, 67
Pemphigus from penicillamine, 192
"Pencil-in-cup," 92
Penicillamine, 192, 214
  antiinflammatory action of, 18
  delayed healing and, 200
  for JRA, 100
  for palindromic rheumatism, 119
  for rheumatoid arthritis, 48, 86
  for Wilson's disease, 134
  SLE induced by, 54
Penicillin
  for gonococcal arthritis, 112
  for Lyme arthritis, 116
  for rheumatic fever, 96
  hypersensitivity to, 81
  SLE induced by, 54
Pentazocine-induced fibrosis, scleroderma and, 59
Periarterial fibrosis in SLE, 49, 50
Periarteritis nodosa, 70. *See also* Polyarteritis
  early description of, 4
  immune complex damage in, 27
Pericapsulitis, 161
Pericarditis
  after intestinal bypass, 172
  cryoglobulinemia and, 82
  in adult onset Still's disease, 103
  in childhood SLE, 100
  in JRA, 2, 98
  in Kawasaki disease, 75
  in MCTD, 65
  in polyarteritis, 70
  in PSS, 61
  in Reiter's syndrome, 90
  in rheumatic fever, 95
  in rheumatoid arthritis, 43, 48
  in SLE, 53
  in Wegener's granulomatosis, 72
Pericellular collagens, 11
Periostitis
  in hypertrophic osteoarthritis, 167
  in Reiter's syndrome, 181
Peripheral nerve injury in neuropathic arthropathy, 109
Peritoneal macrophages in cellular immunity, 23
Peritonitis in familial Mediterranean fever, 118
Periungual erythema in SLE. 53
Petrone, LM, 4
Peyronie's syndrome, 167
Phagocytic cells, 22
Phagocytosis in antibody-mediated reactions, 26
Pharmacology of antirheumatic drugs, 188–192
Pharyngeal muscle weakness in polymyositis, 67

Phase-specific drugs, 193
Phenformin for erythema elevatum diutinum, 173
Phenobarbital
  for Raynaud's phenomenon, 63
  in etiology of shoulder disorders, 161
Phenotype, HLA, 31
Phenoxybenzamine for Raynaud's phenomenon, 63
Phenylacetic acid derivatives, 189
Phenylalamine metabolism, 134
Phenylalkanoic acid derivatives, 18
Phenylbutazone, 189, 213
  for ankylosing spondylitis, 86
  for bursitis, 161
  for gout, 126
  for osteoarthritis, 107
  for pseudogout, 131
  for regional rheumatic pain syndromes, 163
  for rheumatoid arthritis, 47
  for seronegative spondylarthropathies, 85
Phenylketonuria, skin changes in, 59
Phosphate in bone formation and resorption, 169
Photosensitivity
  in childhood dermatomyositis, 101
  in SLE, 53
Physical exertion liked to eosinophilic fasciitis, 65
Physical therapy, 204
  for intervertebral disc disease, 150
  for JRA, 99
  for osteoarthritis, 107
  for regional rheumatic pain syndromes, 163
  for rheumatoid arthritis, 48
Picornavirus-like structures in polymyositis, 68
Pierson's disease, 146
Pigmented villonodular synovitis, 152
  hemosiderin in, 133
  synovial fluid analysis in, 187
Piriformis syndrome, 165
Piroxicam, 189, 213
  for gout, 126
  for osteoarthritis, 107
Pirprofen, 189
Pitcairn, David, 1
Pituitary disease, clubbing and, 168
Plantar fasciitis, 163, 165
  arthrocentesis for, 199
  in ankylosing spondylitis, 87
Plantar spurs in seronegative spondylarthropathies, 85
Plantar subluxation in rheumatoid arthritis, 175
Plasma cell neoplasia, skin changes in, 59
Plasma cells
  IgE synthesis by, 25
  in cellular immunity, 23
Plasma infusion for thrombotic thrombocytopenic purpura, 84
Plasmapheresis
  for mixed cryoglobulinemia, 83
  for myasthenia gravis, 69
  for rheumatoid arthritis, 48
  for SLE, 58
Plasmin in inflammation, 16, 19
Plasminogen in inflammation, 16
Pleural macrophages in cellular immunity, 23
Pleuritis
  in rheumatoid arthritis, 43
  in Reiter's syndrome, 90
Plotz, Charles M, 2
Pneumocystis carinii infections from immunosuppressive therapy, 195
Pneumonitis
  hypersensitivity, 26
  in allergic granulomatous angiitis, 71
  in rheumatoid arthritis, 43
  in Wegener's granulomatosis, 72

Pneumonitis (cont'd)
  infectious arthritis and, 112
Pneumothorax in rheumatoid arthritis, 43
Podagra, early description of, 1
Poikiloderma, skin changes in, 59
Polyarteritis, 69, 70–71. *See also* Necrotizing vasculitis; Systemic necrotizing vasculitis; Vasculitis
Polyarteritis nodosa, 70
  classification, 36
  corticosteroids for, 191
  early description of, 4
  first description, 70
  in children, 102
  lack of epidemiologic studies of, 34
  mixed cryoglobulinemia and, 82
  overlap with PM/DM, 66
  similarity to vasculitis of rheumatoid arthritis, 43
Polyarthralgia
  cryoglobulinemia and, 82
  in MCTD, 65
  in Schönlein-Henoch purpura, 73
  in Takayasu's arteritis, 74
Polyarticular onset JRA, 98
Polycythemia, osteonecrosis and, 157
Polymorphonuclear leukocytes (PMNs), 6
  chemotaxis of, 23
  in cellular immunity, 22–23
  neutral protease production by, 18–19
Polymyalgia rheumatica, 76–77
  classification, 36
  corticosteroids for, 191
  scintigraphy in, 183
Polymyositis
  azathioprine for, 194
  complement deficiency in, 21
  corticosteroids for, 191
  early studies of, 4
  features in MCTD, 65
  from penicillamine, 192
  HLA associated with, 32
  in children, 101
  in PSS, 59
  in SLE, 53
  methotrexate for, 195
  Sjögren's syndrome and, 77
  synovial fluid analysis in, 187
Polymyositis and dermatomyositis (PM/DM), 66–69
  classification, 36, 67
  epidemiologic studies of, 34
  rheumatoid factor in, 38
Polyserositis in JRA, 98
Popliteal cyst, 165
  in rheumatoid arthritis, 42
Populations studies. *See* Epidemiology
Porphyria cutanea tarda, 59
Postdysenteric arthritis, classification, 36
Post-injection flare, 197
Postrheumatic fever arthropathy, 97
Poststreptococcal glomerulonephritis
  immune complex damage in, 27
  mixed cryoglobulinemia and, 82
Postthoracotomy syndrome, shoulder disorders in, 161
Pott's disease, 113
Poulsen, H, 1
Poynton, Frederick, J, 2
Praetorious, E, 1
Prazosin for Raynaud's phenomenon, 63
Prednisolone, 4, 18, 191, 197, 214
Prednisone, 191, 214
  for adult onset Still's disease, 104
  for Behçet's syndrome, 118
  for childhood SLE, 101
  for eosinophilic fasciitis, 65
  for giant cell arteritis, 77

Tuberculosis
  amyloidosis associated with, 79
  carpal tunnel syndrome in, 160
  erythema nodosum in, 172
  rheumatoid factor in, 38
  T$_{DH}$ cells in, 25
Tuberculous arthritis, 113–114
  osteoarthritis and, 107
  radiographic findings in, 182
  synovial fluid analysis in, 188
Tumor rejection, cell-mediated immunity in, 28
Tumoral calcinosis, 132
Type C virus, 51
Tyrosine metabolism, 134

U

Ulcerative colitis
  arthritis and, 92
  B27-associated spondylarthropathies and, 35
  clubbing and, 168
  pyoderma gangrenosum in, 174
  relapsing polychondritis and, 83
Ulcers in Behçet's syndrome, 117
Ulnar deviation in rheumatoid arthritis, 41, 175
Ultrasound for bursitis, 161
Umbilical cord, proteoglycan components of, 7
Uniform Database for the rheumatic diseases, 215–217
Unilateral arthritis in rheumatoid arthritis, 41
Unverricht, Heinrich, 4
Urate crystals, first description of, 1
Ureaplasma urealyticum in infectious arthritis, 115
Urethritis
  in gonococcal arthritis, 4
  in Reiter's syndrome, 4, 89
  in seronegative spondylarthropathies, 85
Uric acid, 1, 120
Uricosurics for hyperuricemic gout, 126
Urinary tract hemorrhage in thrombotic thrombocytopenic purpura, 84
Urticaria, 74
Uveitis
  in ankylosing spondylitis, 86
  in Behçet's syndrome, 117
  in relapsing polychondritis, 83
  in seronegative spondylarthropathies, 85

V

Vacuum phenomenon, in disc degeneration of osteoarthritis, 178
Vaginal hemorrhage in thrombotic thrombocytopenic purpura, 84
Valgus deformity
  in osteoarthritis, 106
  in rheumatoid arthritis, 41
Valine in elastin, 12
Valvulitis in rheumatic fever, 95
Van Neck's disease, 146
Varus in CPPD disease, 129
Vascular lesions
  in SLE, 53
  in thrombotic thrombocytopenic purpura, 84
Vascular pulmonary fibrosis in PSS, 4
Vasculitis
  after intestinal bypass, 172
  childhood dermatomyositis and, 67

Vasculitis (cont'd)
  complement deficiency in, 21
  foot pain in, 163
  hypersensitivity, 71–72
  immune complex damage in, 27
  in Behçet's syndrome, 117
  in children, 102
  in JRA, 98
  in mixed cryoglobulinemia, 82
  in relapsing polychondritis, 83
  in rheumatoid arthritis, 43–48
  in SLE, 49
  lack of epidemiologic studies of, 34
  Sjögren's syndrome and, 78
  systemic necrotizing, 69–75
Vasoactive amines in inflammation, 16
Vasoactive substances
  in anaphylactic reactions, 25
  in inflammation, 16
Vasomotor disorders, classification, 37
Venulitis in rheumatoid arthritis, 43
Verrucous endocarditis in SLE, 49
Vertebra plana, 146
Vestibuloauditory dysfunction in Cogan's syndrome, 71
Vidal, Emil, 4
Villonodular synovitis, 152–153
  classification, 37
Vincristine, 194
  for thrombotic thrombocytopenic purpura, 84
Vinylchloride disease, scleroderma and, 59
Viral arthritis, 115
  classification, 36
Virus
  adenovirus, 115
  arboviral group A, 115
  arthritis caused by, 115
  cytomegalic, 82, 195
  echo, 115
  Epstein-Barr, 82
  hepatitis B, 82, 115
  herpes, 115
  in adult onset Still's disease, 104
  in Behçet's syndrome, 118
  in infectious mononucleosis, 115
  in mixed cryoglobulinemia, 82
  in Paget's disease of bone, 156
  in pathogenesis of SLE, 51
  influenza B and myositis, 101
  rubella, 96, 115
  type C, 51
Virus-infected cell lysis, cell-mediated immunity in, 28
Visceral abscess, mixed cryoglobulinemia and, 82
Viscosity of synovial fluid, 15
Vision loss in giant cell arteritis, 76
Vitamin B6 deficiency, carpal tunnel syndrome from, 160
Vitamin C deficiency, associated with rheumatic states, 36
Vitamin D in bone formation and resorption, 169
Vitamin D intoxication, apatite crystals in, 132
Vitamin D resistant rickets, 144
  osteopenia in, 170
Vitamin K, osteocalcin in, 9
Vitreous humor
  collagen component of, 10
  proteoglycan components of, 7

Volar subluxation in rheumatoid arthritis, 175
von Bechterew's disease, 85
Von Gierke's glycogen storage disease, 122
Vossius, Adolf, 4

W

Waaler, E, 2
Wagner, Ernst L, 4
Waldenström's macroglobulinemia
  arthropathy in, 138
  rheumatoid factor in, 38
Weather sensitivity, 37
Weber, H, 3
Weber-Christian disease, 171
  classification, 36
Wegener, F, 4
Wegener's granulomatosis, 72–73
  aneurysms in, 71
  classification, 36
  clinical features, 72
  cyclophosphamide for, 195
  first reports of, 4
  in children, 102
  laboratory findings, 72–73
  nose deformity in, 72
  treatment, 73
Weight loss in rheumatoid arthritis, corticosteroids for, 48
Weiss, Soma, 4
Weissenbach, RJ, 3
Wells, William C, 1
Werner's syndrome, skin changes in, 59
Westphal, CF, 4
Whately, Thomas, 4
Whipple's disease, 93
  classification, 36
Wilson's disease, 134
  myasthenia gravis–like syndrome in, 69
  osteoarthritis and, 107
Wollaston, William H, 1
World Health Organization (WHO), 5
Wrist
  arthrocentesis, 199
  arthrodesis, 201
  assessment of, 186
  in rheumatoid arthritis, 41

X,Y,Z

Xanthochromia of synovial fluid, 187
Xanthomas, 153
  in hyperlipoproteinemia, 139
Xerostomia
  in Sjögren's syndrome, 77
  in SLE, 55
Xiphoid hypersensitivity, 169
Xiphoidalgia, 169
X-irradiation, 194
  osteonecrosis and, 157
Yaws, neuropathic arthropathy, 109
Yersinia enterocolitica
  erythema nodosum and, 172
  in Reiter's syndrome, 89
Yersinial arthritis, 93–94
  classification, 36
  HLA–B27 association, 32
Zomepirac, 189, 213
Zymogens in complement activation, 20

Primer on the Rheumatic Diseases

Eighth Edition

Available from the Arthritis Foundation
1314 Spring Street, NW
Atlanta, GA 30309

Price $10